Lecture Notes in Computer Science 6389

Commenced Publication in 1973
Founding and Former Series Editors:
Gerhard Goos, Juris Hartmanis, and Jan van Leeuwen

Gerhard Leitner   Martin Hitz
Andreas Holzinger (Eds.)

HCI in Work and Learning, Life and Leisure

6th Symposium of the Workgroup
Human-Computer Interaction
and Usability Engineering, USAB 2010
Klagenfurt, Austria, November 4-5, 2010
Proceedings

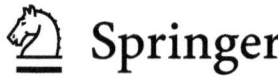 Springer

Volume Editors

Gerhard Leitner
Martin Hitz
Alpen-Adria-Universität Klagenfurt, Institute of Informatics Systems
Interactive Systems Research Group
Universitätsstraße 65-67, 9020 Klagenfurt, Austria
E-mail: gerhard.leitner@uni-klu.ac.at; martin.hitz@uni-klu.ac.at

Andreas Holzinger
Medical University of Graz (MUG)
Institute of Medical Informatics, Statistics and Documentation (IMI)
Research Unit HCI4MED
Auenbruggerplatz 2/V, 8036, Graz, Austria
E-mail: andreas.holzinger@medunigraz.at

Library of Congress Control Number: 2010936987

CR Subject Classification (1998): H.4-5, D.2, C.2, I.2, J.3, K.4.2

LNCS Sublibrary: SL 2 – Programming and Software Engineering

ISSN	0302-9743
ISBN-10	3-642-16606-7 Springer Berlin Heidelberg New York
ISBN-13	978-3-642-16606-8 Springer Berlin Heidelberg New York

springer.com

© Springer-Verlag Berlin Heidelberg 2010
Printed in Germany

Typesetting: Camera-ready by author, data conversion by Scientific Publishing Services, Chennai, India
Printed on acid-free paper   06/3180

Preface

The Human–Computer Interaction & Usability Engineering Workgroup (Arbeitskreis HCI&UE) of the Austrian Computer Society (Österreichische Computer Gesellschaft, OCG) has been serving as an international platform for interdisciplinary exchange, research and development since February 2005. While human–computer interaction (HCI) traditionally brings psychologists and computer scientists together, the inclusion of usability engineering (UE), a software engineering discipline ensuring the appropriate implementation of applications, has become indispensable. Because of the fast developments in information and communication technologies (ICT), the fields of application of HCI and UE are broader than ever. Therefore, USAB 2010 had, in comparison to past USAB conferences, quite a broad focus on all potential aspects of HCI in work environments, learning, private life and leisure activities. Each of these areas of application includes various challenges for HCI and UE, which go far beyond the classical desktop interface as well as usability norms and definitions postulated in the late twentieth century.

The contributions for USAB 2010 provide important insights on the actual research activities in the field and support the interested audience by presenting the state of the art in HCI research as well as giving valuable input on questions arising when planning or designing research projects. Because of the increasing propagation of the field of HCI research, it is not possible to address all areas within a small conference; however, this is not the goal of USAB 2010—it should be seen as a metaphorical counterpart of a wholesale, an HCI delicatessen shop providing a tasting menu with different courses (hopefully) catering to all tastes.

As a kind of appetizer, the session "Psychological Factors of HCI" puts a focus on psychological and social aspects to be considered in the development of end user applications. Based on the example of the participatory design of visual analytics, Mayr et al. illustrate the importance of human problem solving strategies. In their first paper Pommeranz et al. show how the quality of decision support systems can influence the elicitation of user preferences. Arning et al. focus their contribution on usage motives and usage barriers related to the use of mobile technologies. In their second contribution, Pommeranz et al. address the relevance of context and subjective norm on the acceptance of a mobile negotiation support system.

The session "e-Health and HCI" illustrates that although the health of the elderly is a central issue in today's discussion on demography, they are not the only group who can benefit from ICT research. Holzinger et al. sketch an alarming picture of the health status of the youth in Austria, but also show possibilities how to combine the hype of mobile devices and Web 2.0 to change health awareness within youths. Wilkowska et al. focus their contribution on the role of gender in the acceptance of medical devices and show that there are indeed

differences in specific situations. The health system of Western countries is prototypical for high public expenditure; therefore financing usability engineering
activities seems to be a difficult task. Verhoeven and Gemert-Pijnen show that
discount usability methods can even be applied to health care settings with very
low costs (which, invested in usability, exhibit a high return on investment, as
illustrated by Bias & Mayhew[1]). Another way of efficient HCI application is
the re-use of existing knowledge, e.g., on the basis of HCI patterns. Doyle et al.
present an approach to share knowledge in the health care sector by establishing
a customized pattern language structured on the needs of the area of application.

Since the group of the elderly plays an important role in today's HCI research,
it is considered also in USAB. The session "Enhancing the Quality of Life of
Elderly People" is motivated by the fact that current and future generations of
the elderly are more active than the generations of elderly in the past. To support
their activity, HCI and UE research has to focus on their needs. Schaar and Ziefle
show how e-travel services could be enhanced for this special target group. To
enhance the activity of elderly at home, Harley et al. present the possibilities
of game playing based on the Nintendo Wii console in a sheltered home. But
even when activity is already reduced, there are possibilities to support elderly
with technology, which, however, has to fulfill certain usability requirements.
Otjacques et al. present the system SAMMY, which supports the daily life of
elderly in a retirement home.

Not only the elderly, but all user groups not optimally supported by ICT are
in the focus of HCI research in order to make e-inclusion not an empty phrase.
The session "Supporting Fellow Humans with Special Needs" is therefore devoted to this heterogeneous group of users. Kranjc and his colleagues address
the possibilities to apply the user-centered design approach to enhance mobile
devices for visually impaired people, whereas Debevs et al. focus on the respective possibilities for hearing-impaired people. Finally, Curatelli and Martinengo
address motor-impaired users and present a keyboard with a specific layout based
on pseudo-syllables.

Besides e-health for different groups of people, e-learning includes various
challenges for HCI researchers. The authors' contributions to the session "Teaching and Virtual/Mobile Learning" face these challenges. Safta and Gorgan analyze the characteristics and structure of the teaching process and show how
to implement these into a system for computer-based learning. De Troyer et al.
discuss the possibilities of adaptive virtual learning environments. Gil-Rodriguez
and Rebaque-Rivas focus their contribution on online learning with mobile devices while commuting.

Another variation of HCI is presented in the session "Enhanced and New
Methods in HCI Research." Stickel et al. as well as Stork et al. focus their
contributions on visual aspects and show possible enhancements to existing approaches. Stickel et al. propose a metric which can be used for measuring the

---

[1] Bias, R. G. and Mayhew, D. J. 2005 Cost-Justifying Usability: an Update for the
Internet Age. Morgan Kaufmann Publishers Inc.

visual complexity of websites and can therefore be used as some kind of auto-mated evaluation criterion, whereas Stork et al. show how contextual cues can support the quality and efficiency of visual search. Schrammel et al. illustrate an extraordinary approach and propose body motion to be included in HCI research.

The dessert of our menu can be chosen between the special thematic sessions UXFUL[2] and WIMA[3], which put a focus on the cutting edge research topics user experience and multimedia applications, respectively. The program is rounded up by a tutorial given by Ebner et al. on the usage of iPad, iPhone & Co.

USAB 2010 received a total of 55 submissions. We followed a careful and rigorous review process, assigning each paper to a minimum of three and max-imum of five reviewers. On the basis of the reviewers' results, 10 full papers and 10 short papers were accepted in the main track of the conference. The two special thematic sessions, UXFUL and WIMA, were established with the inten-sive support of the organizing colleagues and contributed a further 13 papers to the program. Additionally, to give a selected authors the opportunity to show their work in progress, a poster presentation section was created. The scientific program, the vicinity to the melting pot of ICT research, development and ap-plication (Lakeside Science and Technology Park) and the involvement of the local industry, made USAB 2010 a platform that brought together the scientific community focused on HCI and usability with interested people from industry, business, or government as well as from other scientific disciplines. The final product can be seen as a valuable piece of the mosaic of further development of the HCI & UE community. The credit for this belongs to each and every person who contributed to making USAB 2010 a great success: the authors, reviewers, sponsors, organizations, supporters, the members of the organization team, and all the volunteers, without whose help this deli would never have been built.

November 2010

Gerhard Leitner
Martin Hitz
Andreas Holzinger

---

[2] Enabling User Experience with Future Interactive Learning Systems.
[3] Interactive Multimedia Applications.

Organization

Program Chairs

Gerhard Leitner   University of Klagenfurt, Austria
Martin Hitz   University of Klagenfurt, Austria
Andreas Holzinger   University of Technology/Meduni, Graz, Austria

Program Committee

Patricia A. Abbot	Johns Hopkins University, USA
Ray Adams	Middlesex University London, UK
Dominique Archambault	Université Pierre et Marie Curie, France
Sheikh Iqbal Ahamed	Marquette University, USA
David Ahlström	University of Klagenfurt, Austria
Henning Andersen	Risoe National Laboratory, Denmark
Keith Andrews	Graz University of Technology, Austria
Russel Beale	Birmingham University, UK
Marilyn Sue Bogner	Institute of Human Error LLC Bethesda, USA
Tiziana Catarci	University of Roma La Sapienza, Italy
Luca Chittaro	University of Udine, Italy
Andy Cockburn	University of Canterbury, New Zealand
Matjaz Debevc	University of Maribor, Slovenia
Alan Dix	Lancaster University, UK
Martin Ebner	Graz University of Technology, Austria
Judy Edworthy	University of Plymouth, UK
Jan Engelen	Katholieke Universiteit Leuven, Belgium
Pier Luigi Emiliani	National Research Council, Italy
Anton J. Fercher	University of Klagenfurt, Austria
Matjaz Gams	University of Ljubljana, Slovenia
Daryle Gardner-Bonneau	Western Michigan University, USA
Vlado Glavinic	University of Zagreb, Croatia
Sabine Graf	Athabasca University, Canada
Andrina Granic	University of Split, Croatia
Eduard Groeller	Vienna University of Technology, Austria
Sissel Guttormsen	University of Bern, Switzerland
Timo Honkela	Helsinki University of Technology, Finland
Kasper Hornbaek	University of Copenhagen, Denmark
Zahid Hussain	Quest University, Pakistan
Ebba P. Hvannberg	University of Iceland, Island
Bin Hu Birmingham	City University, UK
Bo Hu	SAP Research Belfast, UK

Homa Javahery	IBM Centers for Solution Innovation, Canada
Julie Jacko	Georgia Institute of Technology, USA
Chris Johnson	University of Glasgow, UK
Anirudha N. Joshi	Indian Institute of Technology Bombay, India
Frank Kappe	Graz University of Technology, Austria
Kinshuk	Athabasca University, USA
Georgios Kouroupetroglou	University of Athens, Greece
Christian Kruschitz	University of Klagenfurt, Austria
Effie Lai-Chong Law	University of Leicester, UK
Denise Leahy	Trinity College Dublin, Ireland
Zhengjie Liu	Dalian Maritime University, China
ZongKai Lin	Chinese Academy of Science, China
Julie Maitland	Georgia Institute of Technology, USA
Lena Mamykina	Georgia Institute of Technology, USA
Rudolf Melcher	University of Klagenfurt, Austria
Klaus Miesenberger	Johannes Kepler University Linz, Austria
Silvia Miksch	Donau University Krems, Austria
Lisa Neal	Tufts University School of Medicine Boston, USA
Alexander Nischelwitzer	University of Applied Sciences Graz, Austria
Shogo Nishida	Osaka University, Japan
Hiromu Nishitani	University of Tokushima, Japan
Nuno J Nunes	University of Madeira, Portugal
Anne-Sophie Nyssen	Universit de Licge, Belgium
Anna-Lisa Osvalder	Chalmers University of Technology, Slovenia
Erika Orrick	GE Healthcare Carrollton, USA
Philipe Palanque	Université Toulouse, France
Vimla Patel	Arizona State University, USA
Helen Petrie	University of York, UK
Margit Pohl	Vienna University of Technology, Austria
Robert W. Proctor	Purdue University, USA
Harald Reiterer	University of Konstanz, Germany
Anxo C. Roibas	University of Brighton, UK
Demetrios Sampson	University of Piraeus, Greece
Nikolai Scerbakov	Graz University of Technology, Austria
Lynne Schrum	George Mason University, USA
Anthony Savidis	ICS FORTH Heraklion, Greece
Yvonne Schikhof	Rotterdam University, The Netherlands
Albrecht Schmidt	University Duisburg-Essen, Germany
Andrew Sears	UMBC Baltimore, USA
Ahmed Seffah	EHL Lausanne, Switzerland
Klaus-Martin Simonic	Medical University Graz, Austria
Wolfgang Slany	Graz University of Technology, Austria
Cecilia Sik Lanyi	University of Pannonia, Hungary
Daniel Simons	University of Illinois at Urbana Champaign, USA
Christian Stary	Johannes Kepler University Linz, Austria

Constantine Stephanidis	ICS FORTH Heraklion, Greece
Zoran Stjepanovic	University of Maribor, Slovenia
Harold Thimbleby	University of Swansea, UK
Hironomu Takagi	Tokyo Research Laboratory, IBM Research, Japan
A Min Tjoa	Vienna University of Technology, Austria
Manfred Tscheligi	University of Salzburg, Austria
Jean Underwood	Nottingham Trend University, UK
Geoff Underwood	Nottingham University, UK
Oliver Vitouch	University of Klagenfurt, Austria
Gerhard Weber	Technische Universität Dresden, Germany
Karl-Heinz Weidmann	University of Applied Sciences Dornbirn, Austria
William Wong	Middlesex University, London, UK
Panayiotis Zaphiris	Cyprus University, Greece
Ping Zhang	Syracuse University, USA
Jiajie Zhang	University of Texas Health Science Center, USA

Organizing Committee

Christine Haas	Austrian Computer Society (OCG)
Karin Hiebler	Austrian Computer Society (OCG)
Andreas Holzinger	Austrian Computer Society (OCG)
Eugen Mühlvenzl	Austrian Computer Society (OCG)

Local Hosts

Martin Hitz	University of Klagenfurt, Austria
Christian Kruschitz	University of Klagenfurt, Austria
Gerhard Leitner	University of Klagenfurt, Austria
Kerstin Smounig	University of Klagenfurt, Austria

Members of the WG HCI and UE of the Austrian Computer Society

(as of August 2010)

Ackerl, Siegfried	Bärnthaler, Markus
Ahlström, David	Baumann, Konrad
Aigner, Wolfgang	Bechinie, Michael
Albert, Dietrich	Behringer, Reinhold
Andrews, Keith	Bernert, Christa
Auer, Michael	Biffl, Stefan
Auinger, Andreas	Binder, Georg
Baillie, Lynne	Bloice, Marcus

Breiteneder, Christian
Brugger, Martin
Burgsteiner, Harald
Christian, Johannes
Debevc, Matjaz
Derndorfer, Christoph
Dirnbauer, Kurt
Dorfinger, Johannes
Dorner, Stefan
Ebner, Martin
Eckhard, Benedikt
Edelmann, Noelle
Ehrenstrasser, Lisa
Erharter, Dorothea
Errath, Maximilian
Fasswald, Markus
Ferro, Bernhard
Figl, Kathrin
Flieder, Karl
Freund, Rudi
Frühwirth, Christian
Fricht, Reinhard
Geierhofer, Regina
Geven, Ajan
Glavinic, Vlado
Goldmann, Thomas
Gorz, Karl
Graf, Sabine
Graf, Sylvia
Granic, Andrina
Grechenig, Thomas
Grill, Thomas
Groeller, Edi
Gross, Anne
Haas, Christine
Haas, Rainer
Haberfellner, Tom
Hable, Franz
Hacker, Maria
Hackl, Erich Patrick
Hailing, Mario
Haug, Bernd
Hauser, Helwig
Heimgärtner, Rüdiger
Hellberg, Philip von

Herget, Martin
Hitz, Martin
Hoeller, Martin
Holzinger, Andreas
Hruska, Andreas
Huber, Leonhard
Hussain, Zahid
Hyna, Irene
Jaquemar, Stefan
Jarz, Thorsten
Kainz, Regina
Keki, Susanne
Kempter, Guido
Kingsbury, Paul
Kittl, Christian
Kleinberger, Thomas
Kment, Thomas
Kohler, Kirstin
Koller, Andreas
Koeltringer, Thomas
Kotsis, Gabriele
Kreuzthaler, Markus
Krieger, Horst
Kriegshaber, Ursula
Kriglstein, Simone
Kroop, Sylvana
Krümmling, Sabine
Kuenz, Andreas
Lanyi, Cecilia
Leeb, Christian
Leitner, Gerhard
Leitner, Hubert
Lenhardt, Stephan
Linder, Jörg
Loidl, Susanne
Lugmayer, Artur
Luneski, Andrej
Maier, Edith
Maitland, Julie
Makolm, Josef
Mangold, Pascal
Manhartsberger, Martina
Mayr, Stefan
Meisenberger, Matthias
Melcher, Rudolf

Messner, Peter
Miesenberger, Klaus
Miksch, Silvia
Mittenecker, Georg
Motschnig-Pitrik, Renate
Müller, Regine
Musil, Sabine
Mutz, Uwe
Nedbal, Dietmar
Nemecek, Sascha
Nischelwitzer, Alexander
Nowak, Greta
Oppitz, Marcus
Osterbauer, Christian
Otjacques, Benoît
Parvu, Andrej
Peischl, Bernd
Pellegrini, Tassilo
Pesendorfer, Florian
Pohl, Margit
Purgathofer, Peter
Ramkinson, Arun
Rauhala, Marjo
Reichl, Peter
Richter, Elisabeth
Richter, Helene
Riener, Andreas
Robier, Hannes
Safran, Christian
Sahanek, Christian
Schaupp, Klaus
Scheugl, Max
Schloegl, Martin
Schreier, Gnther
Schwaberger, Klaus
Schwantzer, Gerold
Searle, Gig W.
Sefelin, Reinhard
Seibert-Giller, Verena

Seyff, Norbert
Simonic, Klaus-Martin
Slany, Wolfgang
Sorantin, Erich
Sorantin, Felix
Spangl, Jürgen
Sproger, Bernd
Stanglmayer, Klaus
Stary, Christian
Stenitzer, Michael
Stickel, Christian
Stiebellehner, Johann
Stjepanovic, Zoran
Thümer, Herbert
Thurnher, Bettina
Tjoa, A Min
Tscheligi, Manfred
Urlesberger, Berndt
Vecsei, Thomas
Vogler, Robert
Waclick, Olivia
Wagner, Christian
Wagner, Claudia
Wahlmueller, Christine
Wally, Bernhard
Wassertheurer, Sigi
Weidmann, Karl-Heinz
Weippl, Edgar
Werthner, Hannes
Wimmer, Erhard
Windlinger, Lukas
Wöber, Willi
Wohlkinger, Bernd
Wolkersdorfer, Peter
Wotawa, Franz
Zagler, Wolfgang
Zellhofer, Norbert
Ziefle, Martina
Zorn-Pauli, Gabriele

Sponsors

We are grateful to the companies, institutions and organizations for their support in our aims to bridge Science and Industry. Their logos are displayed on **http://usab2010.uni-klu.ac.at/**

Published with the support of the Research Council (Forschungsrat) of the University of Klagenfurt out of the sponsorship of the City of Klagenfurt.

Table of Contents

Supporting Fellow Humans with Special Needs

Teaching and Virtual/Mobile Learning

Enhanced and New Methods in HCI Research

Enabling User Experience with Future Interactive Learning Systems (UXFUL 2010)

Interactive Multimedia Applications (WIMA)

Tutorial

Posters

e-Health and HCI

Mapping the Users' Problem Solving Strategies in the Participatory Design of Visual Analytics Methods

Eva Mayr[1], Michael Smuc[1], Hanna Risku[1], Wolfgang Aigner[2], Alessio Bertone[2],
Tim Lammarsch[2], and Silvia Miksch[2]

[1] Research Center KnowComm, Danube University Krems,
Dr. Karl Dorrek Str. 30, 3500 Krems, Austria
{Eva.Mayr,Michael.Smuc,Hanna.Risku}@donau-uni.ac.at
[2] Department of Information and Knowledge Engineering (ike), Danube University Krems,
Dr. Karl Dorrek Str. 30, 3500 Krems, Austria
{Wolfgang.Aigner,Alessio.Bertone,Tim.Lammarsch,
Silvia.Miksch}@donau-uni.ac.at

Abstract. Especially in ill-defined problem spaces, more than one exploration way leads to a solution. But often visual analytics methods do not support the variety of problem solving strategies users might apply. Our study illustrates how knowledge on users' problem solving strategies can be used in the participatory design process to make a visual analytics method more flexible for different user strategies. In order to provide the users a method which functions as a real scaffold it should allow them to choose their own problem solving strategy. Therefore, an important aim for evaluation should be to test the method's flexibility.

Keywords: Problem solving strategies, information visualization, visual analytics, evaluation.

1 Introduction

"The goal of visual analytics is to create software systems that will support the analytical reasoning process" [19]. Following this rationale, we are currently engaged in a research project which aims to support the daily work processes of business consultants by means of novel visual analytics methods. To ensure that the methods successfully support data exploration, prototypes are iteratively evaluated in real-world settings with real users and refined based on evaluation results.

A successful visual analytics method allows users to generate insights and supports exploratory data analysis. Therefore, evaluation techniques building on task completion time and number of errors were criticized as restricted in the past [2]. In more recent evaluations researchers code and count the insights gained [13][17]. Though insights are an outcome of cognitive processes during exploratory data analysis, they are not directly linked to the task at hand. To understand the users' cognitive processes while they are completing a task (or failing to do so) we proposed to analyze the problem solving processes [10]. Problems are the users' subjective representations of

G. Leitner, M. Hitz, and A. Holzinger (Eds.): USAB 2010, LNCS 6389, pp. 1–13, 2010.

an objectively given task [11]. Therefore, analyzing problem solving strategies can help us to understand how individual users approach the tasks in evaluation studies.

To gain meaningful results from evaluations, it was proposed that users have to solve ecologically valid tasks during the evaluation procedure [12]. Therefore, we asked experts to provide not only real-world data sets, but also real-world tasks of different complexity for the evaluation in our research project DisCō. During earlier stages in the participatory design process of two visual analytics methods, we observed that users apply many different strategies to solve these tasks. There was not one single problem solving strategy that led to a correct solution – as many ways lead to Rome, users reached a solution via different paths. Still, some of the strategies that were applied did not yield a sufficient solution. Interestingly, the question of how problem solving strategies interact with characteristics of the method/visualization and task completion was not addressed in prior research.

In this paper we argue that though some users may have taken a wrong path, for others the method probably impeded a successful strategy. In our view a successful information visualization allows for a variety of different problem solving strategies. By analyzing users' problem solving strategies we can understand how a visual analytics method supports or impedes the problem solving processes – better than by coding and counting insights alone. In addition, we can generate ideas how the method should be improved to allow for frequently used problem solving strategies. By looking more deeply into the problem solving processes, the evaluation produces results beyond task completion, number of insights, time, and errors.

To prove our point, we first give some background information on problem solving and discuss how an information visualization or visual analytics method can act as a scaffold. To show how the flexibility of a method can be evaluated and improved we present results from our experimental study.

2 Problem Solving

"Research in situated and everyday problem solving (e.g., Lave, 1988) makes clear distinctions between convergent problem-solving thinking and the thinking required to solve everyday problems" [7]. Therefore, it is important to distinguish between different types of problems and identify which problem solving strategies are applied to solve them.

2.1 Problem Types

In cognitive psychology, two major types of problems are distinguished [7]: Well-defined problems have one correct solution and provide all information needed to solve them. Typical locating- (e.g., finding a date) or identifying-tasks (e.g., finding the maximum) [20] can be associated with such kind of problems. In contrast, ill-defined problems have more than one solution and often include only fragmentary information. Exploratory data analysis only seldom converges in one single correct solution; therefore, it can be classified as ill-defined.

2.2 Problem Solving Strategies

These two types of problems not only differ in the number of correct, respectively plausible solutions, but also in the processes needed to get to a solution. A problem solving strategy is "a technique that may not guarantee solution, but serves as a guide in the problem solving process" [5].

Ill-defined, everyday problems can be solved in different ways, probably leading to different solutions. This is a very creative process [7]. Therefore, it is difficult to predict either solutions or strategies applied for such problems.

People who are able to successfully solve well-defined problems cannot necessarily solve ill-defined problems, too [14]. To solve well-defined problems, one has to know rules and strategies and know when to apply which. For ill-defined problems one has to generate different solutions and evaluate them based on one's own knowledge and opinions.

This could be explained by different kinds of problem solving strategies applied to well-defined and ill-defined problems: In well-defined problems, users are more likely to have a schema (including knowledge on procedures, relevant information, and goals) which can be applied to solve the problem. In contrast to these schema-based problem solving strategies [5], ill-defined problems might require a search-based problem solving strategy [5] to reach a solution. Users have to search for relevant information, decompose the problem into sub-problems (which can again be more well- or ill-defined), and identify goals. Which strategy is applied, depends to a great extent on the expertise of the user (does he have a schema available?) and the problem at hand.

2.3 Scaffolding Problem Solving

The aim of visual analytics is to support the problem solving process [19]. From the view of situated cognition, the visual representations serve as scaffolds [3] for the problem solving process. By visualizing and pre-processing the information, these methods reduce the need to process and store data in memory.

Experts are more suited to solve problems, as they can faster and better identify the type of problem at hand and have a bigger repertoire of problem solving strategies [7]. To serve as real scaffold, the visual analytics method should consequently allow for multiple problem solving strategies to support the creative process of solving ill-defined problems at work.

Let us exemplify our point with an example from everyday life: You want to tighten a screw, but do not have a screwdriver at hand. With good skills and strength, you might be able to tighten it with a simple coin, a key, or a pocket knife. But if you are provided a Swiss army knife, you will solve this problem more easily.

To ensure that a visual analytics method is such a flexible scaffold, we evaluated how many different problem solving strategies our method supports and which strategies it impedes.

3 Identifying Problem Solving Strategies in Participatory Design

In a study within the research project DisCō we compared two different prototypes, GROOVE [9] and a variant of the Multiscale visualization [16]. Whereas GROOVE allows users to interactively fold and unfold time scales, the Multiscale visualization shows all temporal granularities one below the other.

3.1 The Aims of and Visualizations Used in the Project DisCö

The project DisCö[1] aims at designing novel interactive Visual Analytics methods that support users to discover temporal patterns and their relationships. In doing so, a large number of time-related aspects need to be considered [1]. One aspect that is especially worth exploring is the calendar aspect. The structures of time strongly determine phenomena which can be found in time-oriented data. For instance, the patterns of monthly sales vary strongly due to differences in the arrangement of workdays, weekends, and holidays.

Our target users handle application scenarios of data analysis in different industrial or service sectors (e.g., transportation, call centers, retail, health care) and in the public sector. Users reported that they are often confronted with ill-defined problems [18]. To solve such problems, temporal analysts have to identify temporal patterns of different time granularities in the data. Consequently, our users have to (1) gain an overview of the data set, (2) identify relevant and define specific time granularities (e.g., one business day can last from 6am to 6pm, from midnight to midnight), and (3) find anomalies and relevant patterns, trends, and relations within this data set. To provide visualizations that suit these requirements, we researched various advancements on the basis of pixel-based visualizations.

Pixel-based visualizations [8] use position in two dimensions and color to encode data. For time-oriented data, the position within a two-dimensional grid can be determined by the timestamp of a data element. In such visualizations, it is necessary to find a way to encode the value of single data points, as both axes are used for time granularities. One way is using different colors for different values.

The tripartite Multiscale visualization [16] (see figure 1) is a further development of pixel-based visualizations. It uses a parallel overview of average values as a guidance and information source as well. The daily scale data area shows squares for each month. Each square contains a small pixel-based visualization in itself, arranging the data using week of month and day of week as coordinates. The monthly scale data area shows the same squares filled with a single color based on the monthly average. The yearly scale data area shows only one square per year, with the color based on the yearly average. However, the overview is not optimal as guidance, as it is spatially apart from the details. The eye of the beholder constantly has to jump between the two parts, which is rather a long distance, comprising the danger of mistakes and straining working memory.

We have developed a visualization called GROOVE that contains several advancements compared to the Multiscale visualization [16] [9]. The central advancements are overlay techniques that provide an overview which is integrated with the details more closely and interactive methods for changing the view. For the study described in this paper, we excluded the overlay possibilities in order to get a clear comparison between parallel views and interactive change of detail level. The interactive visualization (see figure 2) we compared to the Multiscale visualization works as follows: Users are shown an overview with large areas coloured based on average

---

[1] http://www.donau-uni.ac.at/disco (accessed on May 4, 2010).

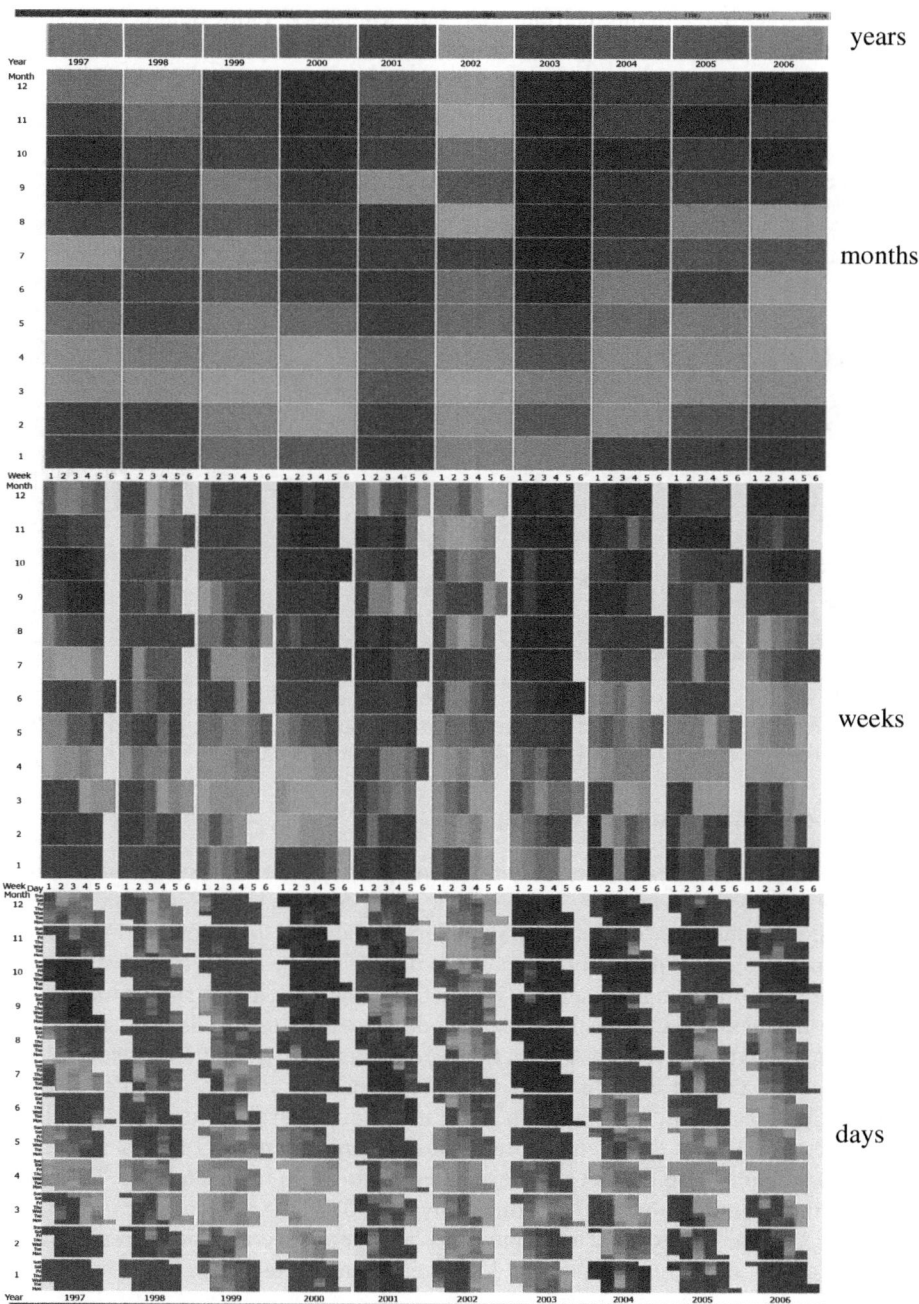

Fig. 1. Multiscale visualization of meteorological data set with yearly, monthly, weekly and daily views

values. By clicking left on such an area, they can show more details consisting of smaller pixels. By clicking right inside an area, the detail level is reduced. It is also possible to align the detail level for the whole visualization using a double-click.

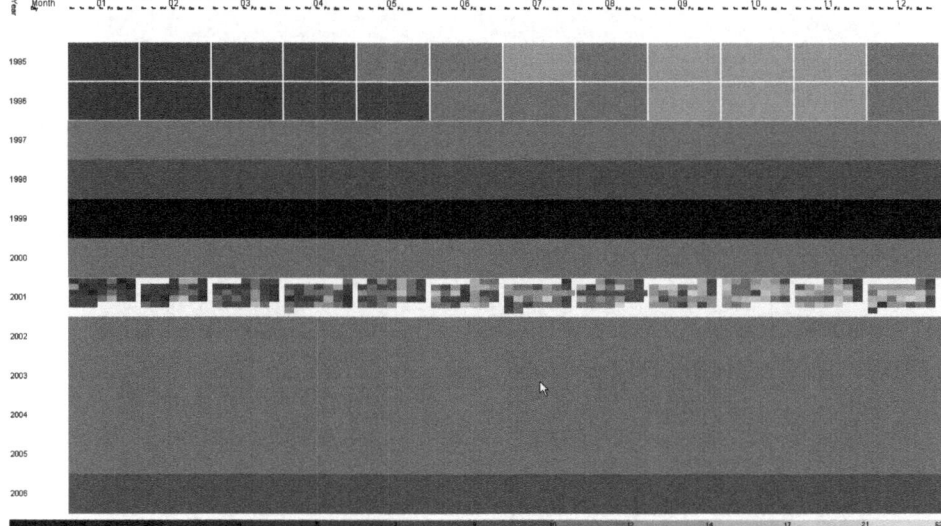

Fig. 2. Our interactive test environment of the traffic dataset: For most of the years, only an average value is shown. For the first two years 1995 and 1996, a more detailed view for the months has been opened. For 2001, average daily values are displayed.

3.2 Experimental Setting: Material

We used five different datasets of similar complexity from different domains in our study: meteorology, economy, traffic, education, and finance. The data values are presented in quantiles, with temporal granularities ranging from hours up to decades.

The meteorology dataset shows gauging data from the Traisen, a river in Lower Austria for the time-range of several years. The economy dataset shows turnover data from the business area of gastronomy for one year. The traffic dataset shows traffic accidents of novice drivers in Austria between the ages of 18 and 30 for several years. The education dataset contains total access statistics for infovis-wiki.net, a wiki for Information Visualization which is heavily used for e-learning purposes. Finally, the finance dataset shows the exchange rates of the Euro and the US Dollar over the last two decades. For these datasets, our users had to solve up to seven tasks, for example "What's the quantile value on Christmas Day in 2007?", "Are there clues for errors in the data?", "When looking at separate days, are there several typical trends over the hours of day?", or "Which global and local trend can you identify?".

3.3 Experimental Setting: Participants

Twelve people who are experienced in the exploration and analysis of time-oriented business data participated in our study. They had to solve the above mentioned well- and ill-defined problems with five temporal data sets (one for familiarisation, two using GROOVE, two using Multiscale visualizations, compare table 1). Participants were randomly assigned to versions A and B. For each data set, users solved two general tasks and a set of three to five domain-specific tasks.

Table 1. Research design

Data Set	meterology	economy	traffic	education	finance
Method Version A	GROOVE	GROOVE	GROOVE	Multiscale	Multiscale
Method Version B	Multiscale	Multiscale	Multiscale	GROOVE	GROOVE

A problem solving process includes different cognitive [7] and perceptual [6] processes. Therefore, we used multiple process measures to study the participants' problem solving strategies. We logged participants' interaction with the method, tracked their eye movements, observed their behaviour, and asked them to think aloud during the experiment [17]. We integrated these data sources, segmented them according to the tasks, and documented the users' strategies and success levels.

In the context of data visualizations and visual analytics methods, three levels of graph comprehension can be differentiated [4]: (1) reading the data (i.e. extracting data, locating), (2) reading between the data (i.e. finding relationships, integrating), and (3) reading beyond the data (i.e. extrapolating from the data, generating). Well-defined problems require level 1 and sometimes level 2, whereas ill-defined problems require all three levels to be solved successfully. In the following we will present two exemplary problems – one from level 1, reading the data, and one from level 3, reading beyond the data.

3.4   Well Defined Problem: Extracting a Concrete Value

For each data set and method, our users had the same task to solve: to name the data value on Christmas day in a concrete year (the other tasks compare Section 3.2). This is a rather narrow and well-defined task, as it has a single correct solution. But despite this fact, we observed a variety of different strategies that were applied.

Two excerpts from one participant shall illustrate the variance of strategies:

Economy data set (Groove):
"Christmas Day 2007, okay. [...] now I'll try to find Christmas. Oh, there are weeks, not month. I have to calculate back. It has to be 51 or 52. [...] Oh, when Monday ends earlier on this day, it has to be Christmas. [...] And I assume that this orange is somewhere in the range of 365."
Finance data set (Multiscale visualization):
"Christmas Day 2007. There is 2007. Mostly it's the end of the year. Okay I assume this is the 31st of December. Actually it does not matter, somewhere here. Everything is the same colour, and it's the darkest. [...] about 1.36, okay."

Problem Solving Strategies. To solve this problem, users had to identify the location of this date and to associate a value to the data point. We analyzed the different process measures described above and observed seven problem solving strategies which were applied either individually or in combination with each other: (1) count days from the beginning of December or (2) from the end of December; (3) map specific

data characteristics (e.g., shop closes earlier on 1 day, less activity) onto the characteristics of Christmas day (see the economy excerpt above for an example); (4) use external scaffold (e.g., calendar on mobile phone) to determine the associated day of
week; (5) remember the correct day of week from a prior dataset; (6) approximate the
location by searching for week 51; (7) estimate roughly (see the finance excerpt above
for an example).

The strategies applied differed highly between participants, but also within participants. No one used one single problem solving strategy consistently. A more detailed
look at the variations showed that participants applied problem solving strategies
differently in dependence of the method and the data set at hand (see figure 3).

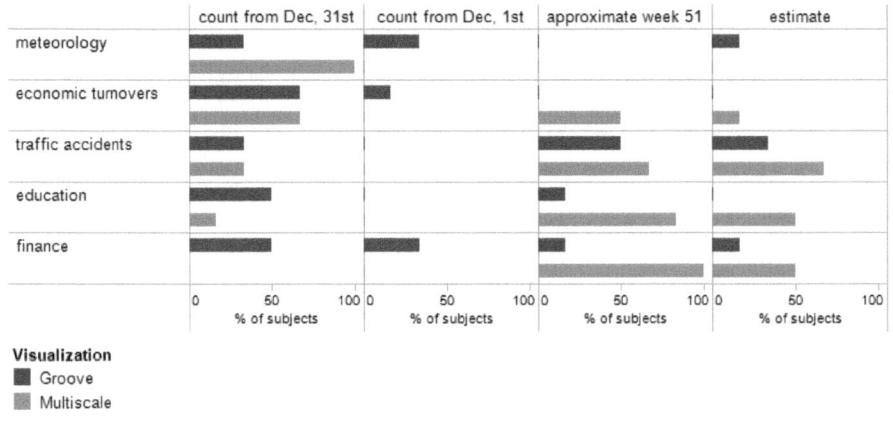

Fig. 3. Percentage of users applying different problem solving strategies for 5 data sets

Obviously some data sets suggest specific strategies. For example, the financial
data set had only little variance within weeks. Therefore, approximating the location
and roughly estimating the correct value was a highly efficient strategy, leading to
correct solutions in 82 % of all cases. The economic turnover data set, on the other
hand, was only solved correctly by 17 % of the participants. It has high variance
within the data and is visualized on a weekly rather than on a monthly basis. Therefore, only participants who counted from the end of the year solved this problem.
Every fourth participant was not able to generate any solution at all.

A clear difference exists also between the two methods, GROOVE and Multiscale
visualization, in the problem solving strategies applied. This can be seen clearly in the
traffic accidents data set, where all Multiscale visualization users counted from the
end of the year, whereas the GROOVE users applied a variety of problem solving
strategies. This difference also results in different solution probabilities: When participants used the GROOVE, they solved the task in 50 % of the time; whereas when
they used the Multiscale visualization, only 27 % solved the task. With the Multiscale
visualization, they often experienced problems to find the data point (33 %), but also
for the second step in solving the problem: to differentiate between colours (10 %)
and to associate the colour to the scale (10 %).

Design Implications. To improve the two methods, participants made some remarks which can be turned into suggestions for improvements directly:

- Labelling the figure on both sides
- Showing date and value on mouse over
- Ease making the association of data points with the legend

Besides, many users experienced problems to locate the Christmas day. Therefore, the methods should be improved, for example, by providing a tooltip or a search function for specific dates (e.g., with a calendar overlay).

With the Multiscale visualization, users experienced many problems in identifying a specific data point and in differentiating between the colours used. This problem could be solved by providing an optical zoom function and (a user-customized) colour scale to increase the contrast for specific scale segments.

3.5   Ill Defined Problem: Drawing an Inference from the Data

For the economy data set, participants were asked from which gastronomic business these data are from (e.g., snack restaurant, bakery, or coffee house). This is a clearly ill-defined problem as it allows for different plausible answers (even though the data stem from one concrete business) and as a wide range of information sources is relevant. To make this conclusion, users had to build on the different features of the visualization and draw inferences from their insights. They had to identify patterns and compare them to patterns from their own prior knowledge, raise hypotheses and test them against the patterns found.

An excerpt from one participant (female, Multiscale visualization, implausible solution) shall illustrate the nature of this task. She does identify the daily and weekly sales patterns, but ignores the opening hours, the annual sales pattern, and the amount of turnover.

> *"They sell a lot in the afternoon, mostly. Which kind of business? Nonsense, it's not afternoon, but rather evening. I would say: after-work. But also in the morning. I would say a café. No it's too late for a café. They are already eating. But also earlier, about 10 am or 9 there is a lot. That's strange, it does not fit. Evening restaurant. Especially on Saturday there is nearly anyone there. Yes, it's a café-restaurant."*

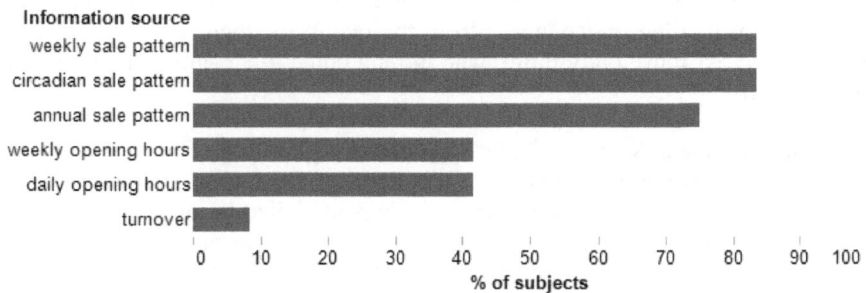

Fig. 4. Percentage of participants who used a specific information source

Problem Solving Strategies. For this very open task, users relied on six different information sources to infer the problem solution (see figure 4): Whereas the sale patterns (circadian, weekly, and annual) were used by most participants, only some also took the opening hours (weekly and daily) into account. Only one participant considered the amount of the turnover as a relevant information source.

No difference existed between the two methods, GROOVE and Multiscale visualization, in the information sources used and the quality of the solution gained. Overall, 17 % of the users were not able to generate any solution for this task. Half of the remaining participants generated a plausible, near-to-correct solution (42 %), the other half no plausible solution (42 %).

We compared the problem solving strategies used by these three groups and found that the quality of the solution correlated with the number of information sources participants took into account (see figure 5): If they considered only two or three different kinds of information they were likely to generate a wrong solution. If they considered three to four information sources, they did not generate any information ("I give up. I've no idea what this could be."). Only if they considered a higher number of more than four different information sources, were they likely to generate a plausible, correct solution.

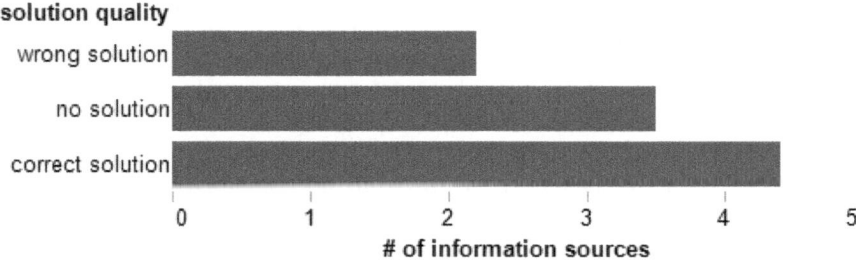

Fig. 5. Number of information sources used in dependence of the solution quality

When we look at these kinds of information more qualitatively, we see a tendency that those participants who considered the weekly and daily opening hours were more likely to come to a correct solution. A frequent wrong solution neglected the information that the business closed before 8 pm and, therefore, could not be a dinner restaurant.

The difference cannot be explained by a motivational deficit as participants took a similar amount of time, independent from the quality of their solution (correct: 3.1 min, incorrect: 2.1 min). Only those, who did not come to a solution at all, took more time (8.3 min).

Design Implications. A crucial factor to generate a plausible solution for this task is to take into account not only the temporal patterns of the data set, but also the temporal boundaries of the visualization. Many participants failed because they did not take the daily and weekly opening hours into account. To make the daily opening hours more salient, one could highlight the closing hours by showing not only labels for those hours of the day where data exist, but also for those where no data exist. Another possibility would be to increase the size of the labels.

Another question (that remains to be solved) is how participants can be encouraged to test their hypotheses against more information sources and thereby become more likely to discover wrong assumptions.

A possibility within the GROOVE would be to lead users through all granularities step by step and thereby make it easier to check possible solutions against all temporal granularities. A disadvantage of such a solution is that the user looses freedom of action.

4 Conclusions

In this paper we presented two examples of how users' problem solving strategies can be analyzed and how this knowledge be used to improve a visual analytics method during the participatory design process. For the well-defined problem (finding a date and naming the associated value) users applied various strategies. We observed that for different data sets different problem solving strategies led to a correct solution. Similarly the two visual analytics methods afforded different strategies – and different success rates. But there was no single strategy, nor a combination of strategies that always led to a correct solution.

For the ill-defined problem we identified a concrete information source as necessary prerequisite to generate a plausible solution. In ill-defined problem solving, it seems to be important that users do not abort the search-based problem solving process too early, but engage in multiple rounds of generating and testing hypotheses against the data at hand.

Our results confirm that the best problem solving strategy varies from data set to data set and from visual analytics method to method. Especially expert users are more likely to select the most appropriate strategies for the situation at hand [15]. Because experts are more likely to adjust their strategies and use them more flexibly, a visual analytics method should enable the application of a variety of problem solving strategies. Even within the short time frame of the experiment (1 to 1.5 hours) we observed that some users adjusted their problem solving strategies to the possibilities provided by the visual analytics method. Such adaptive behaviour is even more likely when the visual analytics method is used over a longer time period (even though method-specific schemata for problem solving are likely to be built up over time as well). Despite the possibility to open new ways to solve a problem, the method should not impede established and successful problem solving strategies. Therefore, we propose to let users cut their own path and provide them with the visual analytics methods required to find *their own* way to the problem's solution.

In the field of information visualization and visual analytics, different assumptions exist concerning the effectiveness of a visualization [1][12][13][19]. We argue that an effective information visualization or visual analytics method allows for multiple ways to solve a problem. Our results confirm that different problem solving strategies are applied in dependence of the user's expertise, the task, the data set, and the method at hand. To develop a successful visual analytics method, users should be allowed to choose between different ways to the problem's solution. In the participatory design process of novel visual analytics (but also other) methods, we can enhance a method by analyzing the users' problem solving strategies and by mapping them closely in the next design phase.

Acknowledgements

This research was conducted within the DisCō research project, supported by the program "FIT-IT Visual Computing" of the Federal Ministry of Transport, Innovation and Technology, Austria (Project number: 813388).

References

1. Aigner, W., Miksch, S., Müller, W., Schumann, H., Tominski, C.: Visual Methods for Analyzing Time-Oriented Data. IEEE T. Vis. Comput. Gr. 14, 47–60 (2008)
2. Bertini, E., Perer, A., Plaisant, C., Santucci, G.: BELIV 2008: Beyond time and errors – novel evaluation methods for information visualization. In: Proceedings of BELIV 2008, pp. 3913–3916. ACM Press, New York (2008)
3. Clark, A.: Being There. Putting Brain, Body, and World Together Again. The MIT Press, Cambridge (1997)
4. Friel, S.N., Curcio, F.R., Bright, G.W.: Making sense of graphs: Critical factors influencing comprehension and instructional implications. J. Res. Math. Educ. 32, 124–158 (2001)
5. Gick, M.L.: Problem-solving strategies. Educ. Psychol. 21, 99–120 (1986)
6. Grant, E.R., Spivey, M.J.: Eye movements and problem solving: Guiding attention guides thought. Psychol. Sci. 14, 462–466 (2003)
7. Jonassen, D.H.: Instructional design models for well-structured and ill-structured problem solving learning. Educ. Tech. Res. 45, 65–94 (1997)
8. Keim, D., Kriegel, H.-P., Ankerst, M.: Recursive Pattern: A Technique for Visualizing Very Large Amounts of Data. In: Proceedings of IEEE Visualization (Vis 1995), pp. 279–286 (1995)
9. Lammarsch, T., Aigner, W., Bertone, A., Gärtner, J., Mayr, E., Miksch, S., Smuc, M.: Hierarchical Temporal Patterns and Interactive Aggregated Views for Pixel-based Visualizations. In: Proceedings of IV 2009, pp. 44–49. IEEE Computer Society Press, Los Alamitos (2009)
10. Mayr, E., Smuc, M., Risku, H.: Many Roads Lead to Rome. Mapping Users' Problem Solving Strategies. In: Proceedings of BELIV 2010. ACM Press, New York (2010)
11. Newell, A., Shaw, J.C., Simon, H.A.: Elements of a theory of human problem solving. Psychol. Rev. 65, 151–166 (1958)
12. Robertson, G.: Beyond time and errors – position statement. In: BELIV 2008 (2008), http://www.dis.uniroma1.it/~beliv08/pospap/robertson.pdf
13. Sarayaia, P.B., North, C., Duca, K.: An insight-based methodology for evaluating bioinformatics visualizations. IEEE Trans. Vis. Comput. Graph 11, 443–456 (2005)
14. Schraw, G., Dunkle, M.E., Bendixen, L.D.: Cognitive processes in well-defined and ill-defined problem solving. Appl. Cognitive Psych. 9, 523–538 (1995)
15. Schunn, C.D., McGregor, M.U., Saner, L.D.: Expertise in ill-defined problem solving domains as effective strategy use. Mem. Cognition 33, 1377–1387 (2005)
16. Shimabukuro, M., Flores, E.F., de Oliveira, M.C.F., Levkowitz, H.: Coordinated views to assist exploration of spatio-temporal data: A case study. In: Proceedings of the 2nd International Conference on Coordinated and Multiple Views in Exploratory Visualization (CMV 2004), pp. 107–117. IEEE CS Press, Los Alamitos (2004)
17. Smuc, M., Mayr, E., Lammarsch, T., Aigner, W., Miksch, S., Gärtner, J.: To score or not to score? Tripling insights for participatory design. IEEE Comput. Graph. 29(3), 29–38 (2009)

18. Smuc, M., Mayr, E., Lammarsch, T., Bertone, A., Aigner, W., Risku, H., Miksch, S.: Visualizations at first sight. Do insights require training? In: Holzinger, A. (ed.) HCI and Usability for Education and Work, pp. 261–280. Springer, Berlin (2008)
19. Thomas, J.J., Cook, K.A.: Illuminating the Path: The Research and Development Agenda for Visual Analytics. IEEE Computer Society Press, Los Alamitos (2005)
20. Valiati, E.R.A., Pimenta, M.S., Freitas, C.M.D.S.: A taxonomy of tasks for guiding the evaluation of multidimensional visualizations. In: Proceedings of BELIV 2006, pp. 1–6. ACM Press, New York (2006),
    http://doi.acm.org/10.1145/1168149.1168169

User-Centered Design of Preference Elicitation Interfaces for Decision Support

Alina Pommeranz, Pascal Wiggers, and Catholijn M. Jonker

Section Man-Machine Interaction, Delft University of Technology,
Mekelweg 4, 2628 CD Delft, The Netherlands
a.pommeranz@tudelt.nl

Abstract. A crucial aspect for the success of systems that provide decision or negotiation support is a good model of their user's preferences. Psychology research
has shown that people often do not have well-defined preferences. Instead they
construct them during the elicitation process. This implies that the interaction between the system and a user can greatly influence the quality of the preference
information and the user's acceptance of the results provided by the system. In
this paper we describe a user-centered approach to design preference elicitation
interfaces. First, we extracted a number of criteria for successful design of preferences elicitation interfaces from literature and current systems designs. Second
we constructed four new intermediate designs that are compositional with respect to different criteria and, furthermore correspond to different thinking styles
of the user. Last, we offer first insights from an initial formative evaluation of our
designs.

Keywords: Preference Elicitation, Prototypes, User-Centered Design,
Evaluation.

1 Introduction

Knowing what a user likes and dislikes, i.e., his preferences, is important for intelligent systems in many domains. A user's preferences are part of an accurate user model,
which is needed to create system responses that are adapted to the user, e.g. his learning
style in an eLearning system, and for the creation of personalized content. We focus our
work on preference elicitation for decision or negotiation support systems. These systems are similiar to Recommender Systems which support people to find right products
and services online. Decision support systems, however, focus more on the decision
process itself. This includes helping the user to discover and enter their preferences,
understand the link between preferences and decision outcomes and analyzing the steps
taken in the process. Particularly in negotiation support, the quality of the outcome depends to a large extent on the quality of the preparation of the negotiators and their interaction. Both preparation and interaction should focus on discovering the preferences
of both parties [15]. Often decision support systems are used in difficult and important
decision situations, that have serious consequences, e.g. in health care [18].

Existing interfaces aiming at eliciting preferences from users range from systems that
explicitly ask their users to fill in a long list of values for all the attributes of a certain

G. Leitner, M. Hitz, and A. Holzinger (Eds.): USAB 2010, LNCS 6389, pp. 14–33, 2010.

product to systems that implicitly learn preferences from the user's ratings and comparison to other users of the system [28]. Both extremes are not likely to be successful if we want the user to stay engaged with the system and trust the system's advice. First of all it is not sensible to ask a large number of elicitation questions that are cognitively demanding to the user. Using implicit techniques to get a preference model on the other hand bears the danger that the elicited model is not accurate [5]. This might lead to the problem that the users cannot comprehend the advice from the system.

Recently, researchers in the AI [5] and HCI [27] communities have already pointed towards the constructive nature of human preferences and the implications for intelligent systems. Preference models based on economists' views of stable and known preferences might not always be accurate since people do not possess stable preferences that reside in their heads. Often they construct their preferences during the elicitation process. Therefore, it is important to design that process carefully, so that the user is able to construct an accurate model. We believe that a major factor in the process is the interaction between the system and its user via a preference elicitation interface. Therefore, in order to create more successful systems that can elicit accurate preferences we have to focus on the design of the user interface. Even the best underlying algorithms and reasoning frameworks do not give successful results if the user has problems interpreting information presented by the system and entering his preferences [25].

Our goal is to design interfaces that help users build their own preference profile in a way that is intuitive and comprehensible to them. To achieve that goal we set up a list of criteria for the design of such interfaces extracted from social sciences, psychology and HCI literature on human preferences. Next, we created a number of interface elements addressing the different criteria and combined them into four first prototypes. They also take into account people's different styles of perceiving and processing information. Last, we evaluated the different interface elements with people using the prototypes and held a creative session where the same participants combined the elements to new interfaces. The data collected in the evaluations informed our further design process.

2 Related Work

People's preferences have been the interest of researchers in many fields including psychology, behavioral science, consumer research, e-commerce, intelligent (interactive) systems, as well as decision support. We do not aim to give a complete overview of the work in all these fields, but focus on topics relevant for designing user interfaces for preference elicitation for intelligent systems. Many algorithms and interaction techniques have been proposed in current systems to elicit and model the users' preferences. Before giving an overview of the state-of-the art systems, we would like to give the reader insights into how people construct their preferences, since this is the process we want to support the user in with adequate interfaces. Last, we will give a short introduction into Participatory Design, since it is relevant for our evaluations and creative design sessions described later on.

2.1   Constructive View on Preferences

Carenini and Poole [5] describe a conceptual shift for classical decision theory towards constructive preferences [24] and the implications for AI research. Opposing the prevailing economist view of rational and stable preferences, see e.g. [10], psychology studies have confirmed that preferences are not stable but constructive. This means that people do not have well-defined preferences in most situations but rather construct them when necessary, i.e., in the decision making context. This allows people to re-construct their preferences whenever they get new information that is important for the decision. There are different views on how people construct their preferences.

Simon and colleagues [32], for instance, found in their experiments that while people processed the decision task, their preferences of attributes in the option that was chosen increased whereas those for attributes of rejected options decreased. Similar effects have been found in negotiation settings reported by [8]. This is in line with one of the meta-goals named by Bettman and Luce [1], i.e. trying to maximize the ease of justifying a decision. Another aspect of constructing preferences has been brought forward by Fischer et al. [14] focusing on the goals of the decision task in relation to a so-called prominence effect. This effect occurs when people prefer an alternative that is superior only on the most important attribute. They confirmed in three studies that the prominent attribute will be more heavily weighted when the goal was making a choice between alternatives than when the goal was to arrive at a matching value. Johnson and colleagues [18] found anchoring effects and effects that occur when complicated information is presented in the choice task. They conclude that different ways to measure preferences can lead to different results, which is not the intention of eliciting preferences. To help people to construct their preferences in health care scenarios, the authors suggest presenting defaults choices that have led to the best outcome for most patients and presenting information in a way that helps the patient to understand the outcomes of each choice. Another view is the so-called PAM (preferences-as-memory) framework [36], which assumes that "decisions (or valuation judgments) are made by retrieving relevant knowledge (attitudes, attributes, previous preferences, episodes, or events) from memory in order to determine the best (or a good) action."

Consumer research looked at the interplay between affect and cognition on decision making [31]. They investigated the influence of available processing resources when confronted with a decision task. In cases where people have only few resources available affective reactions tend to have a greater impact on choice, whereas with high availability of resources cognitions related to the consequences of the choice are more dominant. This finding can be influenced by personality and by the representation of the choice alternatives.

In conclusion, we can record that there are many factors influencing preference construction and elicitation. To avoid unwanted effects we have to think carefully about the way we pose a preference elicitation task to the users.

2.2   Preference Elicitation - Current Systems

Chen and Pu [7] provide an overview of existing systems that elicit user preferences. They mention techniques commonly used, e.g. knowledge-based find-me techniques

[2], example critiquing and tweaking [11,29], active decisions and clustering or collaborative filtering [28]. Collaborative filtering and clustering techniques are used mainly to create profiles for new users of recommender systems based on clusters of existing users and similarity. For an overview see [28]. There are also hybrid systems combining different approaches [3]. In knowledge-based systems, preferences are elicited by example-similarity; the user rates a given item and requests similar items. Tweaking can be used to limit the similar items to only those satisfying the tweak. In example-critiquing approaches [29] the user is presented with a set of candidates (e.g. products) that can be critiqued. The user can either choose one of them or critique some of their attributes. An interesting example-critiquing interface is the Apt Decision Agent [29]. In this system people initially provide a small number of criteria for an apartment. Based on those they get a number of sample apartments. They can react to any attributes of any apartment. Interesting here is that the preference feedback by the user gets more and more detailed during the interaction. At the same time the user is not forced to go into more detail, but is free to give only the feedback the user wants to give.

Not all techniques mentioned are relevant for decision support systems due to a lack of user-involvement. The user will be less likely to trust the advice by the system, if the system has created a user profile implicitly. A majority of the literature presenting these systems focuses on technical implementations rather than the user. Therefore, it is not always clear how the interface designs support the constructive nature of human preferences. Lately, some researchers have acknowledged this gap and made attempts to set up guidelines for user-involved preferences [23,27].

2.3 Participatory Design

Participatory design (PD) is a design approach where the user is involved not only as an experimental subject or someone to be consulted but as an active member of the design team [9]. PD can be seen as a form of user-centered design (UCD). For a more detailed description of the relation between PD and UCD see Caroll [6]. PD originated in Scandinavia, in the 1980s and has since then been growing rapidly in terms of numbers of practices, extent of theoretical development, numbers of practitioners etc. [21]. To give practitioners guidance in which techniques are best applicable in which circumstances Muller and colleagues provide taxonomy of PD practices. It is based on the dimensions of point of time in the design cycle and who is participating with whom (designers in user's world or vice versa). In addition, they give an indication of optimal group size for every PD technique. Techniques range from ethnographic methods and contextual inquiry [17] to various forms of cooperative prototyping, e.g. paper prototyping [22] and evaluation. One interesting PD technique, that inspired our approach, is PICTIVE [20], which makes use of low-tech objects of system functionality (plastic icons, post-its, colored pens etc.) which are used in a brainstorming session to express the participant's ideas.

3 Design Criteria for Preference Elicitation

From the related literature presented above the following design criteria are derived, which appear to be influential to the success of a preference elicitation interface.

(1) Support of human process of constructing preferences

A major outcome from the studies presented in the related work section is that people do not possess stable preferences, but construct their preferences when confronted with a decision task. This construction process is highly influenced by the decision context and the way the preference questions are posed. The work of [27] provides a number of more detailed guidelines addressing this criterion:

> *(1.1) show decision context, that also allows people to see the consequences of their decisions.*
> *(1.2) provide examples that can be critiqued by the users to refine their preferences.*
> *(1.3) give immediate visual feedback.*

(2) Affective feedback

The role of affect in preference construction was explored in consumer research. As described above, there is an interplay between cognition in affect when people construct their preferences. Therefore, combining cognitive (e.g. choosing from a list of values) and affective (e.g. emoticons) elements in an interface might lead to more insights into the user's preferences.

(3) Value-Focused Preferences

In opposition to the traditional approach of alternative-focused thinking, Keeney proposed [19] value-focused thinking. In this approach the decision-maker should focus on fundamental values that are relevant for a decision before identifying possible decision alternatives and assessing their desirability. Generally, values are seen as more stable than preferences over attributes [30]. This idea has been used in a small number of preference elicitation interfaces, e.g. Personal Choice Point, a financial aid system showing consequences of a decision in terms of lifestyles [12] and Teaching Salesman [34], a product recommender focusing on needs and features.

(4) Transparency

A major aspect influencing the success of decision support systems is the user's trust in the system [26]. System transparency is one aspect that can enhance the user's trust [33]. Take a recommender system that implicitly learns your preferences and then recommends a product to you. Often you wonder 'why this product'? You do not understand the relation between the product and your preferences since you do not know the preference profile the system created. Furthermore, you did not get the chance to construct your preferences in the first place. If the recommendation was a movie, you might watch it anyway. However, if the system gave you advice on buying a house you might be more reluctant. To avoid this situation it is important that the system is transparent for the user, i.e. the user knows what the system is doing, why it asks certain elicitation questions and how the current profile looks.

(5) User-System Interaction/Collaboration

For a long time already designing user interfaces is not only about graphical designs but much more about designing the interaction between the system and the user. For decision support it is important that the user and the system collaborate in establishing a good user profile. We define three criteria for the interaction:

(5.1) Natural Interaction

Natural interaction refers to the usual way in which the users act in the physical world [35] applied to computer systems. People use gestures, expressions, speech and movement to communicate.

(5.2) Real World Metaphors

Part of designing the interaction with a system as natural as possible is using real-world metaphors. Users know them and can relate to them easily, e.g. the trashcan on the windows desktop. In the physical world preferences of people show by what people say, their emotional reaction to something or the way they order things or actions.

(5.3) Mixed-Initiative

An aspect often studied with regard to user-system interaction is the level of initiative. For collaborative problem solving (e.g. constructing a preference profile) between user and system mixed-initiative is a popular approach [13].

4   User-Centered Prototype Design

As part of our design of a novel negotiation support system we are in the process of designing prototypes for the preference elicitation interface. Our domain is job contract negotiations. Given the set of design criteria in the previous section we selected appropriate existing interface elements (e.g. ValueCharts [4], a virtual job agent) and created new ones (e.g. job offer clusters, post-it notes with preference information). Next, we combined these elements into four interfaces. There are, of course, many combinations of elements possible, which would lead to an exponential number of prototypes. Instead of creating this high number of prototypes we combined the elements in a way that each prototype differs in the way the system interacts with the user. Each way of interaction supports a different thinking style based on the theory by Gregorc [16]. By this we can create meaningful combinations, each supporting a different user group. In the evaluations we did not try to find the best prototype to choose and develop further, but rather evaluate the different design elements used. In the following creative session we then gave the participants the chance to combine them in different ways that they preferred and found more usable. We implemented the designs as hi-fi prototypes because this was the best way to ensure that the users get a feeling for the interaction with the system. In the following we describe the four prototypical interfaces highlighting the interface elements used (*italic font*).

4.1 Conversation: Abstract-Random Style

This prototype (Figure 1) focuses mainly on design criterion 5 and in particular the natural interaction (5.1) between the user and the system employing mixed-initiative (5.3). A natural way of building a preference model is being questioned by an expert, who can understand what you want by asking the right questions. In real life this could be a job agent. Since this is a known and intuitive way for people to express their preferences we designed a very simple interface based on a conversation with a *virtual agent*. Another design criterion used in this prototype is criterion 4. We tried to reach transparency of the system by two means: the affective state of the agent and the "thoughts" of the agent regarding the user's preferences. In the first simple version there are three states of the agent implemented, speaking with positive expression, thinking and confused. The second feature is a *thought bubble* above the agent's head. In the beginning of the conversation it is empty. It gets filled with tags (forming a *tag cloud*) whenever the agent could retrieve an interest or issue from the chat that seems to be important to the user. To ensure natural interaction during the evaluation sessions the prototype was implemented as a client-server application for a Wizard-of-Oz testing, i.e. the role of the agent was taken by a real person.

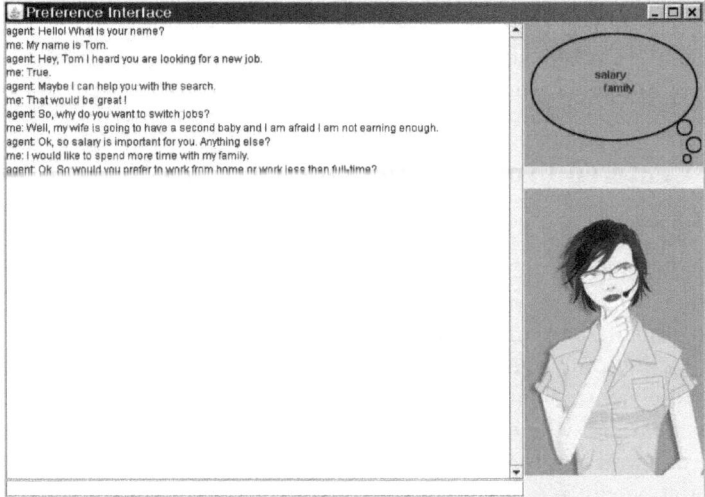

Fig. 1. User interface for conversation with intelligent agent

4.2 Post-its: Concrete-Random Style

This prototype uses different design elements based on criteria 1, in particular 1.1 and 1.3, and 5.2. The focus lies on supporting the constructive nature of human preferences (1). Two things inspired the interface shown in Figure 2. First, preferences are rather unstructured to begin with. They are not necessarily linked to each other. Second, preferences change dependent on the context.

We used *post-it notes* as a real-world metaphor (5.2). The interface allows dragging as many post-it notes onto the so-called preference view as the users want. They can then write the important issues on the notes, add a value and specify whether they like, want, dislike or do not want these issues. At any time they can remove, add or drag around the post-its to structure their profile. More important issues can be dragged further up and less important ones down.

At the same time we provide the users with the needed context (1.1) to make their choices of how to structure the notes. The context is a number of job offers in the *outcome view* that get arranged into *clusters* according to good fit to the current preference profile. This could be done in real-time while the user is interacting with the notes to give immediate visual feedback (1.3). For simplicity reasons the arrangement takes place after pressing the "update offers" button. In the evaluation we discussed both options.

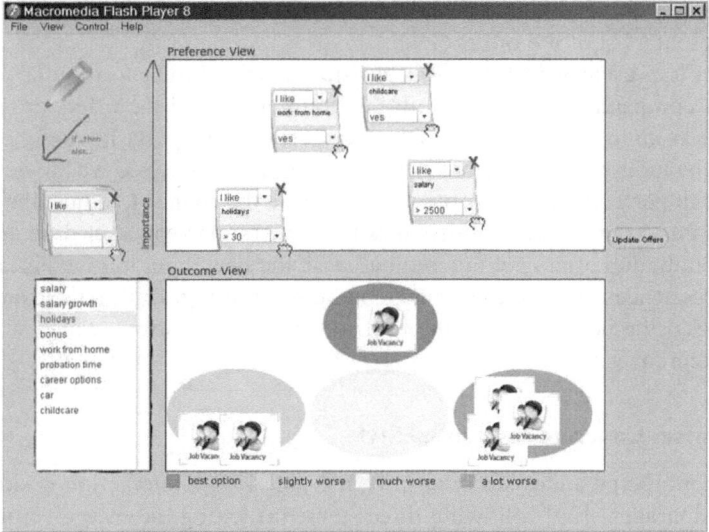

Fig. 2. Visual construction of preference profile

4.3 Comparison: Abstract-Sequential Style

This prototype (Figure 3) employs criteria 1.1 and 1.3 as well as 3. Based on the value-focused thinking approach (3) the user chooses from a list of *interest profiles*: family-oriented, money-oriented, career-oriented, or self-fulfillment. We chose these profiles because they represent life goals that are linked closely to jobs. In a real system this needs to be scientifically proven. In order to help people choose a profile we added a visual stimulus to each profile. We chose a moodboard-like collection of images as often used in advertising to convey a certain feeling or style. Each moodboard consists of a collection of images that represent the particular profile at a glance. The selection of images aimed at giving a diverse view of the profile (e.g. career profile: doctor, model, business man etc.) in order to avoid that users focus too much on a particular image. In

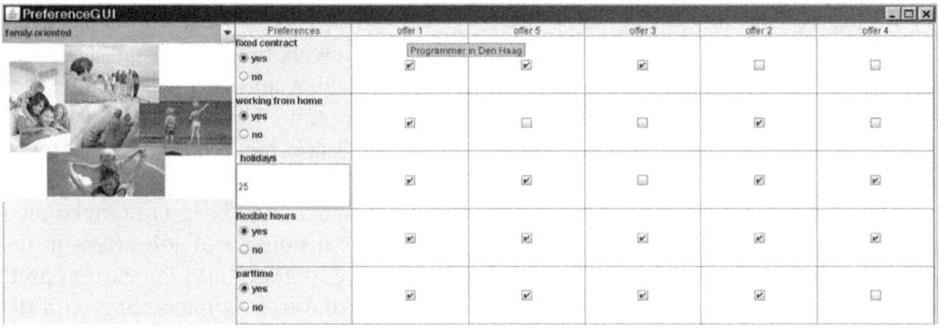

Fig. 3. Choosing and adjusting a default profile

the second step, the user received a filled-in list of preferences that fit the chosen profile. To give the user context to understand their preferences and refine the preselected ones we also present a list of job offers (1.1).

The data is presented in form of a *decision matrix* similar to the ones often used on product comparison websites. Both the preferences and the offers are ordered by importance, from top to bottom and left to right respectively. By hovering over the job offer with the mouse the user gets a description of the jobs. Since we are not expecting that people fit perfectly into a profile the users have the chance to adjust the preference values as well as the ordering. As soon as they enter a new value or drag and drop the rows around the job offers get ordered based on the new input to give visual feedback of the consequences (1.3). We use a lexicographic ordering. During the evaluations we also discussed the possibility for the user to drag the job offers, which will result in adapted preferences.

4.4   Stepwise: Concrete-Sequential Style

Our fourth prototype addresses criteria 1, 2, 3 and 4. The interaction is similar to the APT Decision agent [29] following three steps: (a) letting the user give only a small number of preferences, (b) then receiving a list of offers to compare and (c) giving feedback to attributes that appear in the offers. We adapted this approach and ask the users in the first stage about their three most important interests (e.g. work-life balance or professional development) instead of negotiable issues. By that we follow the value-focused thinking approach [19] (3). After choosing the interests the user enters the interface depicted in Figure 4. The interface aims at helping the user explore several job offers (1.1) with regard to the user's interests and by that construct his preference profile. To compare the offers we used *ValueCharts*, developed by Carenini and Loyd [4]. The user can adjust the (initially equal) importance of the interests. He receives immediate visual feedback (1.3) on how well the job offers match his interests, while adjusting the importance by growing or shrinking of the job offer bars. By double clicking on an interest the job offers get ordered according to good fit. The interface also offers the possibility to critique any attribute of a job offer (1.2). Once the user chooses to look at a job offer in more detail the table on the right gets filled with all values for existing attributes in the job offer. The users are free to give *affective feedback* (2) on any

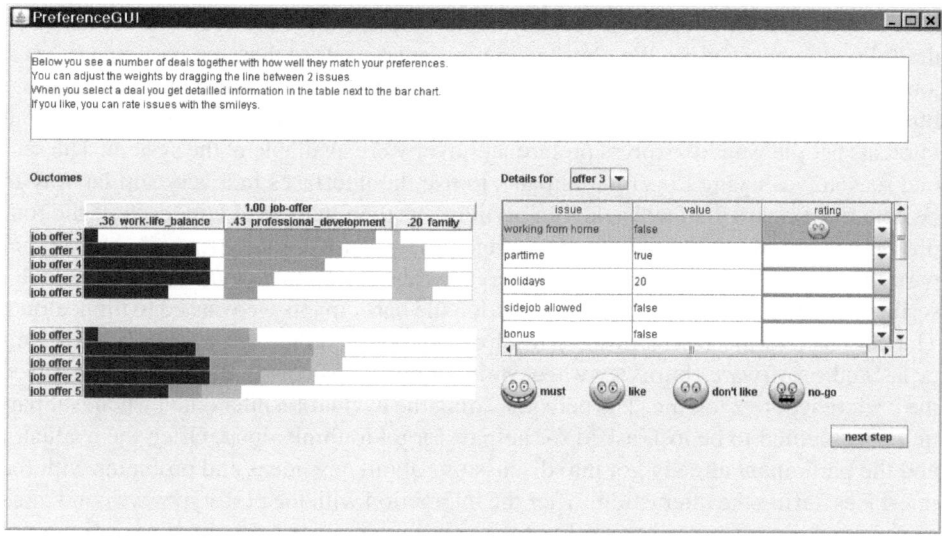

Fig. 4. Preference elicitation using ValueCharts and affective feedback

issue-value pair they want, but are not forced to rate all of them. We included "musts" and "no-goes" as hard constraints in the system, i.e. a job that does not comply with either will not be an option to the users. When the user is done exploring his options, the interface reveals an overview over elicited preference profile, which supports the transparency of the system (4).

5 Formative Evaluation

As a first step in our iterative cycle of designing new preference elicitation interfaces we conducted eight evaluation sessions with one participant at a time and one creative session with all eight participants. In the individual sessions the participants had the chance to interact with all four prototypes and give verbal feedback.

5.1 Individual Sessions

Participants. We included 5 male and 3 female participants. The participants were people with different backgrounds, i.e. computer science, artificial intelligence, agent technology, affective computing, design, linguistic and visual perception. We intended to have a mixture of people with diverse backgrounds in order to get different views on the interfaces.

Procedure. The sessions were carried out in a lab setting. The participants were first briefed about the background of the evaluation and the intention. We emphasized that we would like to receive constructive feedback on the different elements of the prototypes that we can feed back into the design process rather than focusing on usability issues. After the briefing we provided the participants with the scenario described in the following subsection. We chose using a scenario rather than the participants' real job preferences for two reasons. The first is of practical nature: Since our interfaces are limited regarding their domain knowledge, we wanted to make sure that the issues and interests people want to express preferences over were available in the system. The second reason was trying to get participants to use the interfaces in a very similar way to be able to compare the feedback. The participants then interacted with each of the four prototypes for about 10 minutes on average. The order of prototypes was changed per participant. Their task was to fill in preferences about jobs that would fit the person described in the scenario. During the interaction the participants were asked to think aloud. The actions and the voices of the participants were recorded by the help of the Camtasia Studio software (http://www.techsmith.com/camtasia.asp). Each prototype saved the preferences to a log file. The person leading the evaluation intervened whenever participants seemed to be lost, asked for help or forgot to think aloud. Often the evaluator and the participant already got into discussions about new ideas and problems with the interfaces during the interaction. After the interaction with the prototypes we conducted an informal interview to get a grasp of the user's experiences, constructive critique and new ideas. We used printed screenshots of each interface to remind the participant what they looked like. Together with the evaluator new ideas were developed and discussed and drawn onto the printed screenshots.

Scenario. "Bob, a 35 year old programmer with some experience in consulting and project management, is searching for a new job. He and his wife recently moved into a new house because they are going to have a baby soon. It will be their second child- their daughter is 5 years old. Bob likes to spend time with his family. He enjoys playing with his daughter and is excited about the new baby. Generally, he is a very social person, involved in many activities besides his work that he values highly. Having luxury is not one of his concerns. However, in the current situation regarding the new house and baby, it is important for him to earn a decent salary and to have a secure job. In his current job he earns about 2850 EUR (before taxes) monthly. He thinks it is okay for a programmer, but since the working hours are long and overtime is unpaid he wants to change jobs."

Wizard of Oz set-up. The prototype based on a conversational approach was implemented for a Wizard of Oz testing. Instead of implementing an intelligent agent that could interact with the user we developed a client-server chat application. The participants in our evaluation used a Java client which included a chat window, a virtual agent and a thought bubble above the agent's head (Figure 1). The wizard was sitting in a different room and was thus not visible to the participant. He received an SMS from the evaluator about 3 minutes before the chat started in order to get ready. The connection between the server and client applications was made before the evaluation session started. Within the server application used by the wizard, he could reply in text form, change the agent's state between talking, confused or thinking, and put in tags that appeared in the thought bubble on the user side. The participant initiated the conversation by talking to the agent. The wizard followed a script while talking to the participant.

The script included greeting and ending of the conversation as well as a number of questions that he could pose fitting the scenario. He also had a number of tags that he could use. However, since the user input could be arbitrary the wizard was free to adapt to the conversation.

5.2   Collaboration Session

After the individual sessions we held a creative session with all eight participants. Goal of this session was to create new ideas for preference elicitation interfaces. The session consisted of two parts, a group discussion and participatory design session aimed at creating new paper prototypes.

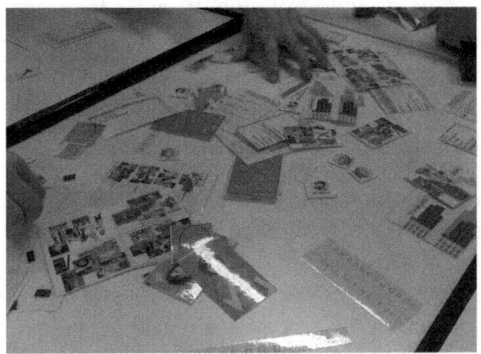

Fig. 5. Interface Elements for Creative Session

Material. We created paper versions of all interface elements we had used in the four hi-fi prototypes (Figure 5), e.g. the virtual agent, the post-its, the value charts or the tag cloud, as well as standard interface elements such as text fields, check boxes, sliders, comboboxes, etc. Additionally, we had a number of blank papers, pens and scissors to give the participants the chance to create their own interface elements. These materials were used by the participants in the second part of the session to design their own preference elicitation interfaces.

Procedure. After a short introduction to the meeting including a reminder of all four interfaces and the agenda, we started a general discussion about the interface elements. The discussion took part with the whole group and took about 20 minutes. After that we split all participants into two groups of four participants each. Each group was provided with the same set of materials described above and instructed to use the material to create their own version of a preference elicitation interface. They were encouraged not only to combine the elements existing in the four presented prototypes but also create new ones. This part of the creative session was planned for about 30 minutes. However, since both groups were not done within that timeframe, the session went longer (ca. 1 hour). The creative session was concluded with a presentation of the two groups' results to each other. During the presentation new discussions arose about design decisions.

6   Informing the Design Process

We gained detailed feedback on the four prototypes as well as new ideas, including tips and new combinations of the prototypes' elements. We will use this data to inspire our further design process. Therefore, the analysis was focused on extracting ideas instead of drawing general conclusions about the four different prototypes. In order to extract ideas we annotated the recordings from the individual sessions using NVivo (www.qsrinternational.com). Based on the annotations we created a table with feedback on each prototype per participant. In addition, we made a list of observations of how users used the prototypes and a list of new ideas that were discussed in the individual and the collaborative session. In the following we will give a detailed account of the feedback we got per prototype element. We will combine data coming from the individual sessions and the group discussion, because the same issues were discussed in both settings. Finally, we will describe the new designs that came out of the creative session.

6.1   Feedback from Individual and Collaborative Sessions

Virtual agent (Conversation prototype). From observation we can say that the conversational prototype with the virtual agent was engaging and straight forward. The opinions of whether it is a useful interface for eliciting preferences, however, were rather diverse. Whereas some participants doubted mostly the feasibility, others thought of it as a natural way to enter preferences. Main critique points were that it was generally too slow in getting to a complete preference profile, it is rather vague, the profile that is saved by the system is not clear and it does not offer any comparison of job offers. Positive points mentioned were the ease of use, the fact that it is open, that the user does not need to work within the programs constraints and that it is easier than giving each issue a number. A few times the idea was mentioned that this could be a nice interface for eliciting underlying interests from the participants. Another point mentioned often was that the success of this kind of interface depends on how good the agent is and how much the user can trust her.

Tag Cloud/ Thought bubble (Conversation prototype). Most participants, regardless of positive or negative attitude towards the complete interface, liked the tag cloud because it gave them a hint of what the system was "thinking".

Post-it notes (Post-its prototype). The post-it notes were discussed both in the individual and collaborative sessions. The majority of participants had a positive attitude towards them. Only one participant thought it was too difficult to operate and another said there were too many hidden things. From the other participants we got a lot of feedback regarding improvements of this prototype. Besides smaller usability issues like the way you drag the post-it notes on the preference view or that the "best"-cluster should not be red, we received feedback about the visualizations and ideas for combinations with other interfaces. Most participants agreed that the process of dragging the post-it notes and filling them takes quite long. Therefore they suggested that this interface could be combined with a profile selection, either with pictures or a short chat. In the next step the relevant preferences for the chosen profile could already be in place. The user just needs to 'fine-tune' them. One idea for fine-tuning was using scenarios, i.e., job offers that people have to decide between. This is similar to the example critique approach mentioned in the related work section. An easier way to represent the post-its would be on a horizontal line, where the more important preferences would be further right. The line could be colored with a gradient from red to green, indicating the importance from low to high. The colors would help people to judge the importance better than in the current version. Equally important preferences could be stacked onto each other. The outcome view could be enhanced, e.g., by aligning the offers in a diagonal line from bottom left to top right, whereas the best option would be on the top right.

Outcome view/ clusters of offers (Post-its prototype). Participants generally liked seeing and exploring the offers in the outcome view. One participant in the individual sessions mentioned the importance of the "tie between what you are doing (preferences) and the consequences (job offers)". This was also an aspect that most participants agreed on in the group discussion. Many ideas arose to improve the interaction. One participant had the idea that when you mark one preference it should be highlighted in the outcome view how well the offers fit regarding just that preference. Generally, participants agreed that the offers should be dragable and trigger an update in the issue preferences. Several participants mentioned that when the user wants to drag a worse offer to a better cluster the user needs to give a reason to the system why he likes this offer. In turn the user should also have the possibility to ask the system why a particular job offer scores badly with the current preferences. One participant suggested the possibility to zoom into the cluster view and see more details the further you zoom in. Furthermore, the offers themselves could be colored according to how well they match the preferences.

Interest Profiling (Comparison prototype). In general, participants liked the idea of choosing a profile. However, most had trouble deciding on one profile that fits them best. Different ideas were mentioned to overcome the problem, e.g., allowing combinations of profiles, using a chat to understand which profile the user fits in or already showing the default preferences of each profile. In addition, after choosing a profile the user should still have the chance to remove and add issues from the pool of all issues. This was also an element discussed a lot with the whole group of participants. It was discussed to give people the choice of choosing a default or starting with an empty profile. In order to choose a profile different ways were mentioned, e.g. using a set of questions or pictures. An idea that appealed to a number of participants was the combined use of pictures and sliders for each profile. The users can select with the slider how important each profile is to them. This solves the problem of fitting into exactly one profile.

Decision matrix (Comparison prototype). One participant liked the matrix with preferences and job offers, because it reminded her of the product comparison websites online. The other participants had a negative attitude towards the matrix. One main critique point of the interface was the visualization. Most participants had trouble understanding that issues and jobs were ordered and that it was possible to drag them around to adjust the preferences. One user said that the table gives a static impression. Instead we could show the rows as free-floating bars or the selected row could be overlaying the other ones to make it clear that they are not fixed. Another option would be to use arrows behind each row indicating that it can be moved up or down. Another point mentioned was that most of the interface is occupied by the checkmarks and not by the preferences, although the latter are what it is all about. One participant mentioned that the user should maybe have the chance to select a couple of offers and compare them in detail instead of all five offers.

ValueChart (Stepwise prototype). The ValueChart got a lot of positive feedback and was also a major discussion point in the group session. People needed a first period of understanding how to operate it. Most participants found it appealing since it gives an overview of how the job offers fit the profile but without losing the detailed information of how well each interest/issue scores in an offer. This is something that is, e.g. not visible in the clustering (outcome view in constructive prototype). Participants particularly liked the immediate visual feedback while interacting with them. One participant had the idea to use the chart for profile selection. Another idea was to attach ValueCharts to the job offers in the constructive prototype to enhance the visual feedback of how good a job is. A major critique point of the whole interface was that there is no link between the ValueChart on the left and the table with issue ratings on the right side. Almost all participants were expecting that when you rate the issues it will have an effect on the bars in the ValueChart. One participant mentioned that if there is no connection there should be a clearer distinction, e.g., between your life goals (ValueChart) and your current job preference (table).

Affective feedback (Stepwise prototype). A problem that occurred with the affective feedback was that the must-have smiley was not interpreted as a hard constraint but rather for something that is liked a lot but not a must. One participant suggested using smileys with a continuous scale with clear extremes instead of static ones. This could help avoiding misunderstandings of the static smileys.

Summary (Stepwise prototype). Another element that was liked was the summary of preferences in the last step. However, it was also mentioned that this summary should already appear while you are adjusting your preferences and that it needs more interactivity (dragging issues into different categories, adding new ones, etc.). This element could, generally, be combined with any other prototype to give the users a clear picture of their preferences.

6.2   Overall Feedback

From the individual evaluations we could discover a tendency towards the post-it notes interface but combined with other approaches, e.g. having pre-set default profiles. Other ideas that came up besides the ones mentioned above were: including standards in the interface, e.g. the typical number of holidays based on the user's age or typical salary for a certain position; and giving people the option to choose only a few job offers that they want to compare (instead of a fixed number). In general, it seemed that the participants were exploring the options and the link between their preferences and job offers a lot. In the group discussion most participants generally agreed, that the visual and real time feedback is important for to get an understanding of their preference adjustments and the consequences. They played around to figure out how the job offers' order changed when they adjusted their preferences. Some even emphasized that they wanted to be in control of the process. One participant aptly formulated that "it is better when you feel involved in the process. If it is your own creation you feel more attracted than when the computer says: 'this is your profile'".

6.3 New Interfaces

After the discussion we split the participants into two groups of four people to each design their version of a preference elicitation interface. The results are depicted in figure 6. Group 1 designed an interface consisting of three parts (views). In the upper left is a profile selection. Each of the four profiles is presented with an image. The user can give both an affective rating with a smiley as well as an importance rating with a slider for each profile. The lower left part of the interfaces shows based on the profile input a small number of filled-in preferences in form of an ordered list. The user can add new ones (presented by the post-it in figure 6) or manipulate the existing ones. At the same time the user gets an outcome view on the right side of the interface which shows a number of offers including a full description of all issues. To each job offer a ValueChart is attached consisting of two rows. The first shows the fit of the different profiles for the offer and the second one the fit of a number of issues that can be selected by the user in the preference view. In turn the user can also directly drag an interesting issue from a job offer to the preference list on the left. The idea of the group was that all three views are connected and manipulation of one affects the other two. In addition, each view can be minimized or maximized (lines in the upper right corners of each view in figure 6). Some users might prefer not to see all views at the same time and should be able to choose.

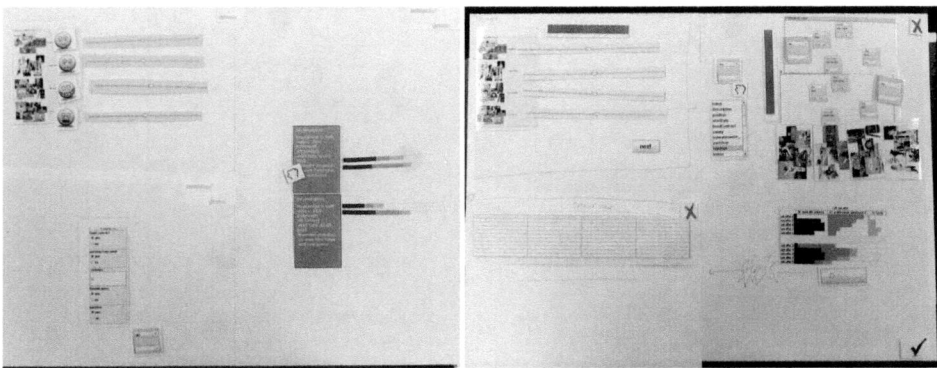

Fig. 6. Design proposal group 2 (left) and group 1 (right)

Group 2 decided to start the process with a so-called profiles wizard, a separate
screen where the user decides on a profile that fits him. Pictures help to visualize the
four profiles and the importance of each profile to the user is put in by positioning a
slider. A colored bar from red to green helps the user, red indicated low importance,
green high. Once the user clicks a 'next' button the screen is closed and the user gets
to a new screen. This one is split into two parts similar to the constructive prototype.
In the top half the user already gets a number of post-it notes with preferences. These
are arranged in a 2D space according to importance on the y-axis and the four profiles
on the x-axis. The user can still adjust the preferences by changing the values, adding
or removing issues. The bottom part of the interface contains a visualization of how
good five job offers score according to the current preferences using a ValueChart. The
job offers are only described in short summary here. By selecting one and clicking the
'detail' button the user can get a table (pop-up) that shows all issues and values of the
selected offer. The users can interact with the preferences and job offers, as they wish,
and the respectively other view gets adjusted automatically.

6.4   Design Implications Leading to Current Work

This first formative evaluation provided us with insights into how people would like to
enter their preferences, what they find important and which elements support the process. Regardless of the interface elements used, an important aspect for people was to
understand and explore the link between the preference input and the order or fit of job
offers. An element that the participants found highly useful for this exploration were the
ValueCharts, because they give immediate visual feedback while keeping details about
the selected interests/issues. Another well-liked element supporting the construction of
preferences was the post-it note. Furthermore, using default profiles was anticipated

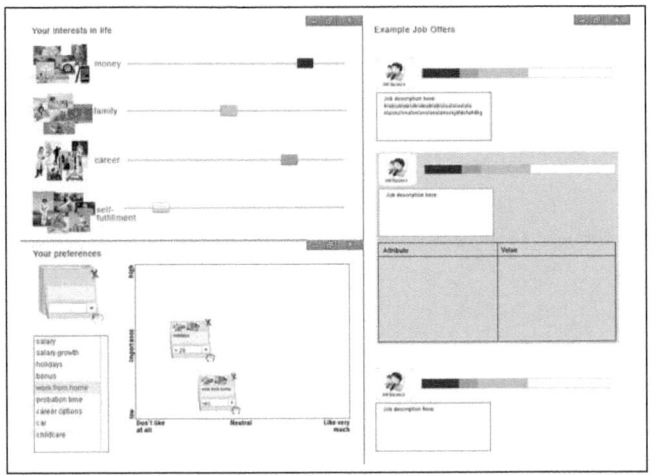

Fig. 7. Design for Preference Elicitation Interface for NSS Prototype

since it gets the elicitation process started more easily. Based on a given profile a number of common preferences can already be displayed. Carefulness needs to applied with designing the interface in this case. Most people had trouble fitting themselves into one of the four given profiles.

Based on these findings and the created interface proposals (Figure 6) we designed a preference elicitation interface for our first prototype of a novel NSS (Figure 7). We picked up the idea of having three panels: (1) one where people can specify their interests, (2) one for entering preferences using the post-it notes and (3) one for showing job offers with ValueCharts indicating how they fit the interests. Each panel can be minimized if not needed. We are currently in the process of defining the concrete interaction between the three views, i.e. how changes in one view affect the other two. As a follow up we will test the interface in the context of our NSS prototype with real users in a preparation for a negotiation.

7 Conclusion and Future Work

We presented the first stages of our approach to designing new preference elicitation interfaces for decision/negotiation support systems. Unlike many existing systems we put the focus on how to involve the user in the process of constructing his preference profile. Our scientific contribution is a number of design criteria based on the literature about human preferences and a number of design elements combined to four new interfaces. Our user-centered design process involving users actively in designing new interfaces provided insights into how people perceive the interface elements and envision complete interfaces. We noticed that participants in the creative session focused only on existing elements although we encouraged them to create their own new ones. Therefore, having separate creative sessions with other potential users that have not seen the prototypes could help more to facilitate creation and inclusion of new elements for preference elicitation.

Our work on evaluating, combining and improving the interfaces in an iterative way is still in progress. Therefore, we cannot give any generalizations on which interface would work the best. Certainly this is also dependent on the characteristics (e.g. thinking styles) of the user and the goal of the system. However, we believe, the work we have done so far, offers a new view on designing preference elicitation interfaces focusing more on the users and their cognitive abilities. We hope to be able to motivate researchers from diverse fields dealing with preferences to put more focus on the constructive nature of human preferences and acknowledge the importance of well-designed interfaces supporting the users in that process. Our work can be seen as a starting point for further research in the following directions: (a) the influence of initiative between the user and the system, (b) how to achieve system transparency (e.g. by the system's explanation based on reasoning with the preferences), (c) intelligent interaction between the user and a virtual agent eliciting preferences, or (d) the influence of different thinking styles of people on the accuracy of the elicited preference profile.

Acknowledgments

We thank the project team and all participants of the evaluation. This research is supported by the Dutch Technology Foundation STW, applied science division of NWO and the Technology Program of the Ministry of Economic Affairs. It is part of the Pocket Negotiator project with grant number VICI-project 08075.

References

1. Bettman, J.R., Luce, M.F., Payne, J.W.: Constructive consumer choice processes. Journal of Consumer Research 25(3), 187–217 (1998)
2. Burke, R.: Knowledge-based recommender systems. In: Kent, A. (ed.) Encyclopedia of Library and Information Systems, vol. 69. Marcel Dekker, New York (2000)
3. Burke, R.: Hybrid recommender systems: Survey and experiments. User Modeling and User-Adapted Interaction 12(4), 331–370 (2002)
4. Carenini, G., Loyd, J.: Valuecharts: analyzing linear models expressing preferences and evaluations. In: Proceedings of the Working Conference on Advanced Visual Interfaces, AVI 2004, pp. 150–157. ACM Press, New York (2004)
5. Carenini, G., Poole, D.: Constructed preferences and value-focused thinking: Implications for ai research on preference elicitation. Tech. rep. (2002)
6. Carroll, J.: Encountering others: Reciprocal openings in participatory design and user-centered design. Human-Computer Interaction 11(3), 285–290 (2009)
7. Chen, L., Pu, P.: Survey of preference elicitation methods. Tech. rep., Swiss Federal Institute of Technolog. In: Lausanne, EPFL (2004)
8. Curhan, J.R., Neale, M.A., Ross, L.: Dynamic valuation: Preference changes in the context of face-to-face negotiation. Journal of Experimental Social Psychology 40(2), 142–151 (2004)
9. Dix, A., Finlay, J., Abowd, G.D., Beale, R.: Human-Computer Interaction. Prentice-Hall, Englewood Cliffs (2004)
10. Doyle, J.: Prospects for preferences. Computational Intelligence 20(2) (2004)
11. Faltings, B., Pu, P., Torrens, M., Viappiani, P.: Designing example-critiquing interaction. In: Proceedings of the 9th International Conference on Intelligent User Interfaces, IUI 2004, pp. 22–29. ACM Press, New York (2004)
12. Fano, A., Kurth, S.W.: Personal choice point: helping users visualize what it means to buy a bmw. In: Proceedings of the 8th International Conference on Intelligent User Interfaces, IUI 2003, pp. 46–52. ACM Press, New York (2003)
13. Ferguson, G., Allen, J.: Mixed-initiative systems for collaborative problem solving. AI Magazine 28(2) (2006)
14. Fischer, G.W., Carmon, Z., Ariely, D., Zauberman, G.: Goal-based construction of preferences: Task goals and the prominence effect. Management Science 45(8), 1057–1075 (1999)
15. Fisher, R., Ury, W.L., Patton, B.: Getting to Yes: Negotiating Agreement Without Giving In. Penguin, Non-Classics (1983)
16. Gregorc, A.: The Mind Styles Model: Theory, Principles, and Practice. AFG (2006)
17. Holtzblatt, K., Jones, S.: Participatory design: Principles and practices. In: Associates, C./.L.E. (ed.) Contextual Inquiry: A Participatory Technique for System Design, pp. 177–210 (1993)
18. Johnson, E., Steffel, M., Goldstein, D.: Making better decisions: from measuring to constructing preferences. Health Psychology 24(8), 17–22 (2005)
19. Keeney, R.: Value-Focused Thinking: A Path to Creative Decision Making. Harvard University Press, Cambridge (1992)

20. Muller, M.J.: Pictive - an exploration in participatory design. In: CHI 1991, pp. 225–231. ACM Press, New York (1991)
21. Muller, M.J., Wildman, D.M., White, E.A.: Taxonomy of pd practices: A brief practitioner's guide. Communications of the ACM 36(4), 24–28 (1993)
22. Osman, A., Baharin, H., Ismail, M., Jusoff, K.: Paper prototyping as a rapid participatory design technique. Computer and Information Science 2(3) (2009)
23. Payne, J.W., Bettman, J.R., Schkade, D.A.: Measuring constructed preferences: Towards a building code. Journal of Risk and Uncertainty 19(1-3), 243–270 (1999)
24. Payne, J., Bettman, J., Johnson, E.: The Adaptive Decision Maker. Cambridge University Press, Cambridge (1999)
25. Peintner, B., Paolo Viappiani, N.S.: Preferences in interactive systems: Technical challenges and case studies. AI Magazine 29(4) (2008)
26. Pu, P., Chen, L.: Trust-inspiring explanation interfaces for recommender systems. Knowledge-Based Systems 20(6), 542–556 (2007)
27. Pu, P., Faltings, B., Torrens, M.: User-involved preference elicitation. In: Workshop Notes of the Workshop on Configuration, the Eighteenth International Joint Conference on Artificial Intelligence (IJCAI 2003), pp. 56–63 (August 2003)
28. Rashid, A.M., Albert, I., Cosley, D., Lam, S.K., McNee, S.M., Konstan, J.A., Riedl, J.: Getting to know you: learning new user preferences in recommender systems. In: Proceedings of the 7th International Conference on Intelligent User Interfaces, IUI 2002, pp. 127–134. ACM Press, New York (2002)
29. Shearin, S., Lieberman, H.: Intelligent profiling by example. In: Proceedings of the 6th international Conference on Intelligent User Interfaces, IUI 2001, pp. 145–151. ACM Press, New York (2001)
30. Shiell, A., Hawe, P., Seymor, J.: Values and preferences are not necessarily the same. Health Economics 6(5), 515–518 (1997)
31. Shiv, B., Fedorikhin, A.: Heart and mind in conflict: the interplay of affect and cognition in consumer decision making. Journal of Consumer Research 26(3), 278–292 (1999)
32. Simon, D., Krawczyk, D.C., Holyoak, K.J.: Construction of preferences by constraint satisfaction. Psychological Science 15(5), 331–336 (2004)
33. Sinha, R., Swearingen, K.: The role of transparency in recommender systems. In: Extended Abstracts on Human Factors in Computing Systems, CHI 2002, pp. 830–831. ACM Press, New York (2002)
34. Stolze, M., Ströbel, M.: Dealing with learning in ecommerce product navigation and decision support: the teaching salesman problem. In: Proceedings of the Second Interdisciplinary World Congress on Mass Customization and Personalization (2003)
35. Valli, A.: The design of natural interaction. Multimedia Tools Appl. 38(3), 295–305 (2008)
36. Weber, E.U., Johnson, E.J.: Constructing Preferences from Memory. Cambridge University Press, Cambridge (2006)

"Same Same but Different"
How Service Contexts of Mobile Technologies
Shape Usage Motives and Barriers

Katrin Arning, Sylvia Gaul, and Martina Ziefle

RWTH Aachen University
Communication Science, Human Technology Centre (HumTec),
Theaterplatz 14, 52056 Aachen, Germany
{Arning,Gaul,Ziefle}@humtec.rwth-aachen.de

Abstract. As wireless technologies evolve, mobile technologies and services will increasingly affect our lives, accompanied by positive and negative effects. This development requires a high acceptance of users to the presence of mobile services in various usage contexts. In an exploratory focus-group-interview approach (n = 63), this research investigates usage motives as well as barriers, which are perceived by users of wireless mobile technologies. In order to understand the impact of specific usage contexts, in which mobile services are applied, an ICT context was contrasted to a medical service context. Outcomes show that acceptance factors are neither static nor independent from the specific usage or service context in which a technology is applied. Rather, acceptance reveals to be a product of individual usage motivations, situation-specific evaluations, and individual user profiles.

Keywords: Usage motives, usage barriers, acceptance, ICT, medical technologies, system design.

1 Introduction

The distribution of mobile devices represents one of the fastest growing technological fields ever. Mobile information and communication technologies (ICT) have interpenetrated all professional and private fields in last decades. According to recent statistics, 4 billions of GSM connections exist worldwide [1]. Mobile information is delivered by different device types (mobile or smart phones, navigation or medical devices), which provide increasing functionalities. Also, continuously diverse service options are available [2], ranging from control services for technical processes (e.g., programming TV), mobile computing, social networks, entertaining and gaming, Internet access up to administrating personal concerns (e.g., managing accounts). It is predicted that by 2013, over 445 million people will be regularly using their mobile phone to purchase goods and electronic services [3]. Beyond their ubiquity, these technologies have fundamentally changed the nature of social, economic and communicative pathways in modern societies and they will bring essential changes to our lives [e.g., 4, 5, 6, 7]. Communication and information are present everywhere and at

G. Leitner, M. Hitz, and A. Holzinger (Eds.): USAB 2010, LNCS 6389, pp. 34–54, 2010.
© Springer-Verlag Berlin Heidelberg 2010

any time and they overcome physical as well as mental borders [e.g., 8]. Mobile technology is increasingly incorporated in smart homes, (walls, furniture or clothes, [9,10]) and might overstep personal intimacy limits, raising concerns about privacy, data security and loss of control [11, 12]. Sensitive and detailed information regarding various topics is available everywhere and anytime. Decision makers in education, politics, and business may use this information in real time. This may implicate both positive effects (productivity, mobility and growth) but also negative effects (violations of privacy, security concerns [6], infrastructure constraints and user distrust in mobile applications). Current developments require a high acceptance and impose high responsibility to all persons and organizations involved: users, decision makers, technical designers, but also industry, economics and legislation.

Over the last years, a lot of research activities were carried out and a solid body of knowledge is prevalent regarding the design of mobile systems as well as technical, socioeconomic and usability issues [e.g., 13, 14, 15]. Though originating from different disciplinary backgrounds and perspectives, all research approaches pursue the same goal: to develop a successful product, which is adopted and accepted by the user. Technical disciplines focus on technical feasibility and safety, as well as the planning, deployment and implementation of wireless technologies [e.g., 16, 17]. Marketing research focuses on the economic potential of new market segments, services, customer profiles, as well as adoption determinants [e.g., 18, 19, 20, 7]. Cognitive ergonomists and human-computer-interaction experts examine usability issues [e.g., 21, 21, 23] and interface designs that are easy to use and learn. Also, the impact of user diversity [e.g., 24, 21, 25] on the interaction and communication with technology receives broad attention as well as the determinants of technology acceptance [e.g., 26, 24, 27].

Technology acceptance has become a key concept for the successful rollout of technical devices [e.g., 26, 27]. On the long run technical products are only successful if users perceive them as useful, and easy to use [e.g., 11, 27, 28]. Both criteria, ease of use and usefulness, are the key determinants of technology acceptance, a concept originating from the 1980s [27], in which personal computers entered offices area-wide. Though research has made significant efforts in explaining and predicting technology acceptance of ICT, the knowledge about factors, determinants and situational aspects affecting acceptance is still limited. Due to the increasing diversity of users, technical systems (visible vs. invisible, local vs. distributed) and usage contexts (fun and entertainment, medical, office, mobility), more aspects are relevant in understanding users' acceptance – beyond the ease of using a system and the perceived usefulness. In addition, studies dealing with technology acceptance mostly considered ICT within the work context [e.g., 29], and it is highly disputable if outcomes are transferable to other technologies and using contexts. Furthermore, most studies are limited to technology acceptance of young, experienced and technology-prone persons, thus a user group, whose acceptance towards technology might not be prototypical for the broad variety of users nowadays confronted with technology [e.g., 30].

Yet, comparably few studies concentrated on the diversity of users and their acceptance patterns [e.g., 31, 11, 32, 15, 33], even though it is obvious that people may have different adoption behaviours due to individual characteristics (etc. age, gender, abilities, beliefs). In addition, only limited knowledge is available regarding the acceptance of mobile services and service-enabling technologies [e.g., 5, 21, 34]. Still more important, there is a considerable knowledge gap [e.g., 21], in which respect and to which extent the specific *usage context*, in which a specific technology is used, affects acceptance patterns. If we want to learn about the impact of technology adoption as well as its consequences for people's social lives, a deeper understanding of technology acceptance is needed, in combination with a more differential approach.

Our assumption is, that mobile technology acceptance is neither static, nor independent from the specific usage context. Rather, we assume mobile technology acceptance to be a product of individual usage motivation (using motives as well as perceived barriers) and situation-specific evaluations, driven by individual needs and demands. A mobile device once used as a communication device in the ICT context (e.g. communication with others) should evoke different perceived benefits and costs or barriers than the same device (and technology) in a medical context (e.g. monitoring of vital parameters, [e.g., 28]). The acceptance pattern for the same device in two different usage contexts could also be different, if persons evaluate the usefulness of the device for themselves, or for others [e.g., 11]. Thus, a motivation "cartography" is needed, in which acceptance and technology adoption of mobile services are considered in relation to the underlying motivational structure, and usage contexts.

2 Methodology

In the following, the methodological approach of this study is detailed.

2.1 Research Aims

Following an exploratory approach, the studies' goals were: (1) an identification of peoples' utilization motives and perceived utilization barriers for and against using mobile technology in two differing service contexts. One service scenario was an ICT-scenario, i.e. the usage of mobile technologies such as mobile phones, handhelds, smart phones, or netbooks for information exchange and communication purposes. The other service scenario was taken from the medical technology context (MedTec), where mobile communication networks are used for transferring patient data to and from, e.g. medical caring centers or physicians. Examples of these kinds of medical technologies are monitoring devices like a cardio messenger (a device that monitors heart activity in risk patients) or devices for controlling vital parameters like blood pressure levels. (2) The second aim was to contrast usage motives and barriers in both contexts in order to gain deeper insights into the specificity of acceptance patterns regarding ICT and MedTec service contexts. (3) As third aim, we strived for an investigation of the impact of user characteristics such as age, gender or technical experience on acceptance patterns.

2.2 Variables

In order to learn more about usage motives and barriers of mobile technologies in an ICT and MedTec service context, *two independent variables* were investigated by conducting semi-structured interview sessions. The first independent variable was "service context", which consisted of the two levels "ICT" and "MedTec". As second variable the within-factor "target person" with the two levels "oneself" and "others" was under study (Table 1).

Table 1. Independent variables "service context" and "target group"

Service context	Target group	
	oneself	others
ICT		
MedTec		

As *dependent variables*, Likert-scale ratings of an introductory screening part of the interview guideline were analyzed. In order to analyze participants' motive structure, their undirected and spontaneous statements regarding (1) usage motives for oneself and others (in the following referred to as "pro's"), (2) usage barriers (in the following referred to as "con's") as well as (3) "no-go's", (indicating a barrier which hinders persons to use the technology at all) for oneself and others were qualitatively analyzed and numerically recoded into a category system. The category system will be presented in the results' section.

2.3 Materials and Procedure

Focus group interviews were run in order to identify usage motives and barriers. Interview sessions were conducted in form of single or group interviews, depending on the availability of participants. Interviewers (n=5) were professionals from social sciences (psychologists, sociologists) and received an interview training in order to guarantee a standardized interviewing procedure. An interview workbook was developed and given to participants, in which they could write down their statements. The workbooks were collected after they were filled in and were used for data documentation.

In the beginning of the interview session, participants were informed about the general goals of our study and about the procedure of the interview. Also, the interview guideline was presented and participants were asked to answer the screening questions. In a next step, the interviewer presented the ICT- respectively the MedTec service scenario. Participants had to write down personal statements regarding usage motives and barriers on small cards (green cards for usage motives, red cards for usage barriers). In case of group interviews, participants were allowed to discuss their statements after writing them down. Questions to the interviewer were also answered in order to ensure a full understanding of the ICT or MedTec service scenarios. The interview sessions lasted between 30-60 minutes, depending on the responsiveness to discussion.

2.4 The Interview Guideline

The first part of the semi-structured interview guideline (1 – 3) was assessed for screening purposes (demographics, previous technical experience, literacy regarding mobile technologies as well as individual proneness to health concerns due to mobile technologies); the second part (4 – 5) was assessed in order to get insights into participants' motive structure regarding the usage of mobile technologies. The interview guideline (Figure 1) was structured as follows: (1) demographic questions (age, gender, education, profession, family status, children); (2) technical experience with ICT or MedTec (duration of mobile phone or medical device usage, usage frequency and intensity), interest, level of information and knowledge about mobile technologies in the ICT or MedTec context, respectively; (3) perceived threat by mobile technologies and risk perception [35]; (4) utilization motives ("pro's"); (5) utilization barriers ("con's") and absolute "no-go's" for oneself and others.

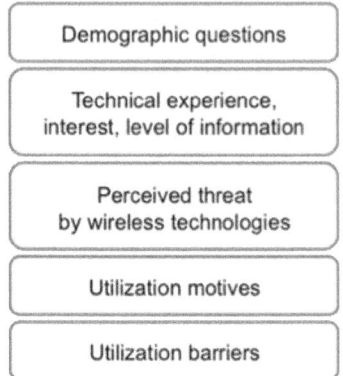

Fig. 1. Interview guideline structure

    The interview guideline contained a mixture of open and closed questions. Questions in the screening part (demography, technical experience and interest, level of information, knowledge and risk perception) had to be answered on six-point Likert scales. For the ratings of perceived threat by mobile technologies a visual analog scale was used, where participants had to mark the degree of perceived threat with a cross on a line between the end poles "very low and very high" [35]. Questions in part 4 and 5 (utilization motives and barriers) were open questions, where the brainwriting-method was applied. Participants were asked to think about pro's and con's of ICT or MedTec utilization for oneself and for others and had to write them down. The number of possible statements regarding usage motives and barriers was not limited.

2.5 The Sample

Participants in the current study were recruited by announcements in newspapers and open places in which they were invited to take part in a structured interview about the perception of mobile technologies either in an ICT- or in a medical context.

    A total of 63 participants took part in the study with an age range from 21 to 75 years. Participants were randomly assigned to either the medical context, or to the ICT context (independent study design). The sample allocated to the medical scenario consisted of 32 users (M = 42 years, 72% women), the ICT scenario sample consisted of 31 people (M = 39 years, 42 % women).

    In order to assess expertise with mobile technologies, participants were asked whether they own a mobile phone respectively a medical device, how long they own it and how frequently they use it. Table 2 gives an overview of participants' expertise with mobile technology (ICT and MedTec).

Table 2. Expertise with ICT and MedTec devices and services

	ICT (100% owner)			MedTec (21.9% owner)		
	Total N	Mean	SD	Total N	Mean	SD
Years	31	9.2	2.6	6	11.2	10.3
Usage frequency*	31	3.2	1.05	6	1.8	1.3

*scale ranging from 0 = "rare" to 4 = "several times a day".

3   Results

In the following section, the results concerning the two different service contexts (ICT vs. MedTec) as well as the impact of user factors on perceived utilization motives and barriers are presented. Data was non-parametrically analyzed. In order to determine differences within and across the two different service contexts, nonparametric testing was complemented by parametric testing procedures (ANOVAs). Bivariate correlations were also calculated. The level of significance was set at 5%; results reaching a level of 10% are referred to as marginally significant.

3.1   Effects of Service Context (ICT vs. MedTec) on Usage Motives and Barriers

Quantitative Analysis of Usage Motives and Barriers. First, perceived utilization motives and barriers for the two service contexts (ICT and MedTec) were contrasted quantitatively. Summarized over the number of all statements (pro's and con's) participants made 32% more statements in the ICT service context than participants in the MedTec service context ($F(1,61) = 12.6$; $p < 0.001$; ICT: in total 377 statements, 12.1 statements per person, SD = 4.5; MedTec: in total 257 statements, 8.0 statements per person, SD = 4.7). In a further step, the different statements (number of con's, no-go's and pro's) were analyzed according to differences within service contexts (ICT vs. MedTec) or target group (oneself vs. others). Overall, participants made significantly more statements about usage motives for (pro's: $F(1,61) = 11.3$, $p < 0.001$) and against (con's: $F(1,61) = 4.9$, $p < 0.05$) mobile device usage within the ICT service context compared to the MedTec service context (Table 3). Moreover, participants made more pro-statements for themselves than for the usage of mobile technology for others in both service contexts ($F(1,61) = 20.7$, $p < 0.001$). An interaction between service context and target groups for pro-statements did not exist. For no-go-statements, no effects of service context or target group were found.

Qualitative Analysis of Usage Motives and Barriers. Detailing participants' motive structure regarding mobile technologies, two independent experts qualitatively analyzed motive and barrier statements. A category system for usage motives and barriers regarding the usage of mobile technologies in the ICT and MedTec service context was developed and applied, i.e. participants' statements were numerically recoded. The category system for both service contexts was identical in most parts. Due to context-specificity, some categories were added either in the ICT- or MedTec-Scenario, or categories received a context-specific phrasing.

Table 3. Mean number of pro, con and no-go statements for service contexts and target groups (n = 63)

	ICT	MedTec	p
Pro's oneself	3.0	2.3	$p < 0.001$
Pro's other	2.3	1.0	$p < 0.001$
Con's	3.5	2.6	$p < 0.05$
No-go oneself	1.7	1.3	n.s.
No-go other	1.7	0.9	n.s.

Overview over Usage Motives and Barriers. The first research question of this study was directed towards an identification of utilization motives ("pro's") and barriers ("con's") for respectively against using mobile technologies in two differing service contexts (ICT vs. MedTec). In the following, the extracted categories for usage motives and barriers, which were reported by participants, are described (in alphabetical order). The categories, which are marked with an asterisk, where only reported as potential motives or barriers for others, not for participants themselves.

Usage motive categories ("pro's")

Availability	to be able to reach someone anytime at any place and, in turn, be reachable by others
Communication	information exchange with other persons
Documentation	precise and "seamless" documentation of (health) parameters
Economic reasons	cost reduction in health care budgets (e.g. the decrease of doctor's appointments due to MedTec usage)
Facilitation of daily life	organization, reduced frequency of doctor appointments, relief for medical practices
Flexibility	to act flexibly
Functions	specific functionality, and applications provided by mobile devices (such as SMS, MP3 player)
Improved medical care	better and quick diagnosis, higher quality of medical care
Information	to get information everywhere quickly, to get information about one's own health status (MedTec)
Mobility	to be independent of place
Surveillance	monitoring gives certainty about someone's health status and well-being (MedTec), or localization (e.g. knowing where your child is)
Other	statements, which could not be allocated to a specific category
Safety	feeling more safely by using the technology
Social aspects	facilitation of social networking, staying in touch with friends, family, etc.
Status symbol*	design, brand or price of a specific device to indicate someone's status
Warning	emergency calls or alarm signals in case of critical health parameters (MedTec) (in contrast to the "feeling of safety" the motive "warning" refers to an action or function)

Usage barrier categories ("con's and no-go's")

(Data) Privacy	concerns about violations of data protection and privacy, protection of personal rights and loss of privacy
Annoyance	noise "pollution" or disturbance due to loud ringtones or phone talks
Availability	feeling uncomfortable due to permanent reachability
Costs	hidden or unnoticed costs while using ICT (roaming costs)
Dependency of technology	the feeling of being dependent from technology (e.g. the usage of ICT devices is indispensable for someone, or the belief the usage is vital (MedTec))
Health damage	fears of physical threat, cancer, heart diseases, brain damages and tumors were subsumed
Manipulation	fear of data manipulation, criminal misuse of personal data and of active manipulation through someone else
Others	statements, which could not be allocated to a specific category
Radiation	fear of radiation emitted by mobile technologies
Social aspects	loss of personal communication and contacts, loss of personal care (MedTec), lower extent of commitment
Surveillance	localization of someone's' position (ICT context), the feeling of being constantly controlled and observed
Technical alternative*	especially mentioned for No Go's – "I never would use this technology if I would have alternatives"
Unaesthetic cell phone towers	refers to the visual appearance or design of cell phone towers
Usability*	problems while interacting with a technical device due to a lack of competence on the user side and the "non-user-friendly" design of a device and its interface on the device side

After introducing the category system, the results regarding the total distribution of usage motives and barriers, which perceived participants for themselves, are presented. As the number of possible statements regarding usage motives and barriers was not limited, i.e. multiple responses were allowed; participants' statements were aggregated in a "multiple response set procedure". The following figures (Figure 2 and Figure 3) and results provide an overview over the total proportion of usage motives and barriers (for themselves), which where stated by participants, combined over the two service contexts.

The most important *usage motive* for mobile technologies, which perceived participants for themselves, was the facilitation of daily life activities, followed by an improved availability of oneself and others (Figure 2). The third-important usage motive was functions or applications provided by mobile technologies such as SMS, MP3 player, camera function, etc. Improved mobility and flexibility were further perceived advantages of mobile technologies, followed by a facilitation of information, i.e. sending and retrieving data. An improved medical care, i.e. diagnosis, therapy and long-term care was a frequently mentioned usage motive, as well as warning functions such as emergency calls or alarm in case of critical health conditions, and safety aspects. Further, but less frequently mentioned usage motives, were communication, documentation, i.e. the seamless recording of data, surveillance, i.e. knowing the location of one's child, social aspects and economic reasons.

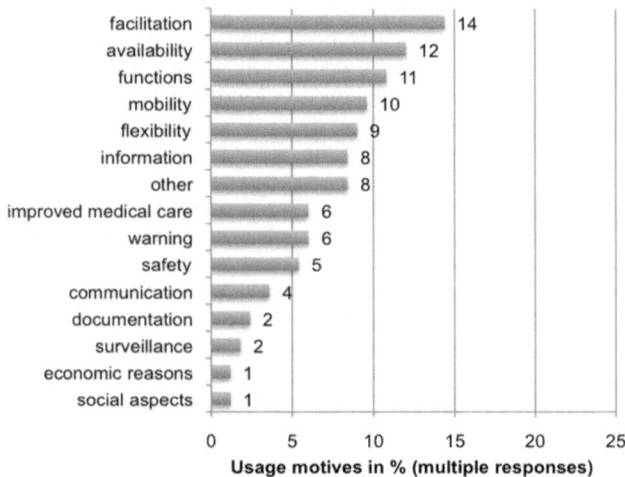

Fig. 2. Usage motives for participants themselves in % (multiple responses)

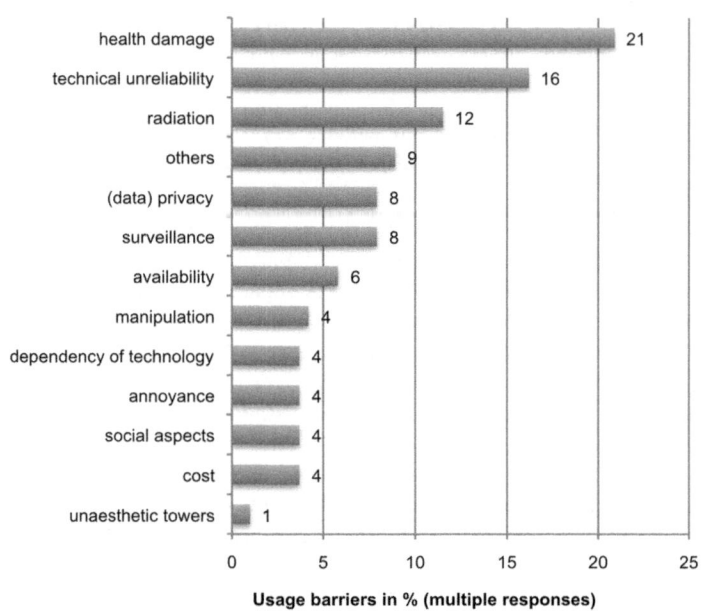

Fig. 3. Usage barriers in % (multiple responses)

The most prominent *usage barrier* of mobile technologies for participants them-selves (Figure 3) refers to health damage, i.e. the fear of damages caused to some-one's health. Some examples for negative health consequences are cancer, infertility or reduction of cognitive abilities such as concentration. The second most important usage barrier was technical unreliability such as faulty connections with the conse-quence of data loss. The fear of radiation was also a frequently made statement, which has a strong association to the aspect of negative health consequences. Further usage barriers of mobile technologies were surveillance, i.e. the positioning of a persons' location or the tapping of telephone conversations; data privacy, i.e. the fear that the access to personal data is uncontrolled and unprotected; availability, manipulation of data and costs. Less frequently named usage barriers were social aspects, i.e. negative effects on social relationships due to the usage of mobile technologies; annoyance by acoustic "noise", (ringtones or telephone conversations of others); dependency of technology and unaesthetic visual appearance of cell phone towers.

Service Context-Specific Differences in Usage Motives and Barriers. The second aim of the study was to learn more about the service' context-specificity of users' acceptance patterns of mobile technologies. Therefore, usage motives ("pro's") and barriers ("con's" and "no-go's") for the ICT and MedTec service context were contrasted. As dependent variable the number of statements per single usage motive or barrier was calculated and used for statistical analyses (ANOVAs).

Table 4. Average no. of statements per person for a specific usage motive in the ICT and MedTec service context

Usage motive	ICT	MedTec	p
flexibility	0.4	0.1	p < 0.05
communication	0.2	0.0	p < 0.01
availability	0.6	0.0	p < 0.05
functions	0.6	0.0	p < 0.001
warning	0.3	0.0	p < 0.05
documentation	0.0	0.1	p < 0.05
facilitation of daily life	0.1	0.7	p < 0.01
improved medical care	0.0	0.3	p < 0.01

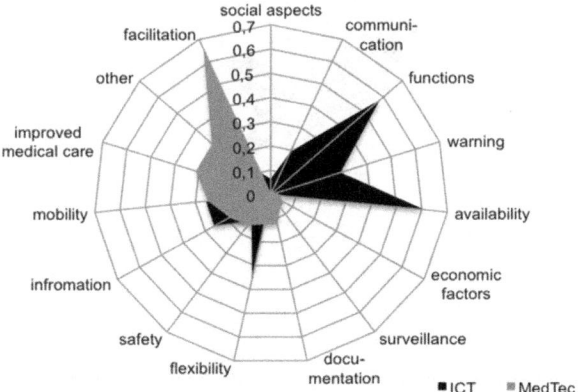

Fig. 4. Pattern of usage motives in the ICT- and MedTec service context

Regarding *usage motives* ("pro's") significant differences between the ICT and the MedTec service context were found, indicating that users perceive *different* patterns of motives and barriers in a specific service context. In the ICT service context (black area in Figure 4) participants significantly more strongly pronounced the following motives: flexibility, communication, availability, functions and warning function (Table 4). In the MedTec service context (grey area in Figure 4), the usage motives documentation, facilitation of daily life, and improved medical care were significantly named more frequently. For other motives no differences between the two service contexts were found.

The contrast of service contexts (ICT vs. MedTec) for *usage barriers* ("con's") also revealed highly significant differences (Figure 5). The usage barriers of surveillance, cost and availability were more frequently stated in the ICT service context (black area in Figure 5). In contrary, the fear of technical unreliability and of data manipulation was more strongly present in the MedTec service context (grey area in Figure 5).

Table 5. Average no. of statements per person for a specific usage barrier in the ICT and MedTec service context

Usage barrier	ICT	MedTec	p
surveillance	0.4	0.1	$p < 0.05$
costs	0.3	0.0	$p < 0.05$
availability	0.4	0.0	$p < 0.05$
technical unreliability	0.2	0.8	$p < 0.01$
manipulation	0.0	0.3	$p < 0.05$

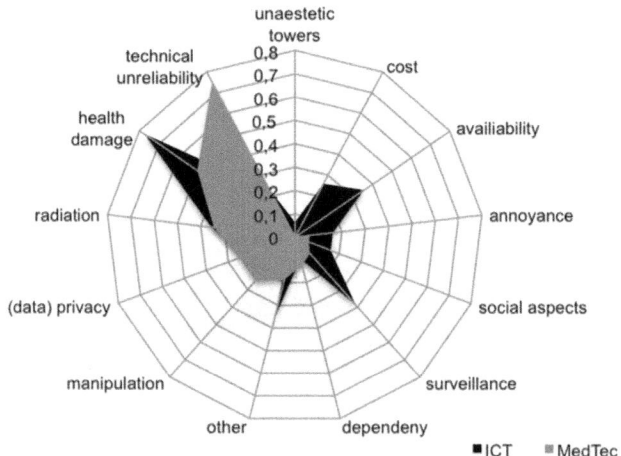

Fig. 5. Pattern of usage barriers for the ICT- and MedTec service context

For the *no-go*-statements ("I would never use the technology, if..."), service-specific differences were also prevalent. Interestingly, they only referred to a limited number of usage barriers. In the ICT service context (black area in Figure 6) participants more often mentioned the fear of damage to someone's health and overcharged costs (Table 6). The no-go "technical unreliability" was more dominant in the Med-Tec context (grey area in Figure 6).

Table 6. Average no. of statements per person for no-go statements in the ICT and MedTec service context

No-go	ICT	MedTec	p
health damage	0.8	0.3	$p < 0.01$
costs	0.3	0.0	$p < 0.05$
technical unreliability	0.0	0.4	$p < 0.01$

Summarizing the findings so far, we can conclude that the same technological base of devices and services, i.e. mobile technologies, rises different advantages and concerns in potential users.

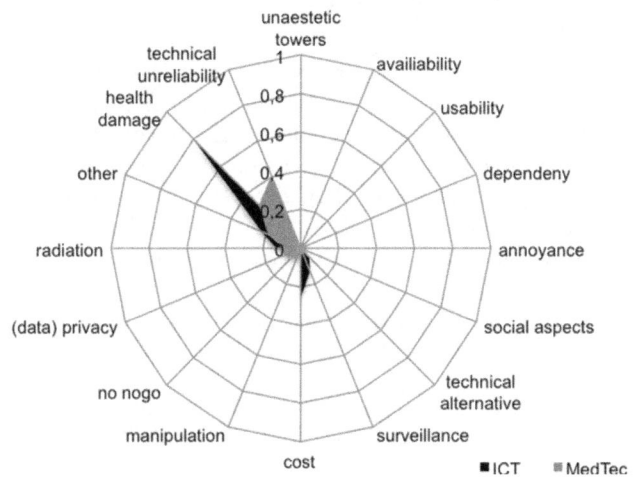

Fig. 6. Pattern of no-go statements in the ICT and MedTec service context

3.2 Effects of User Factors on Usage Motives and Barriers

In a further step the impact of certain user factors on specific using motives and barriers was analyzed. Besides prevalent factors like age and gender, knowledge of and interest in technology, using frequency, average years of using the device and the perceived threat (caused by a specific technology) as well as risk perception were also considered as user factors.

In order to analyze age effects, participants were divided in three age groups (Table 7). Participants were also assigned to three different risk perception groups: those who tended to be *unconcerned* about possible risks, those who were *undecided* whether or not risks exist and those who tended to be *concerned* about possible risks of mobile technologies. Two participants in the ICT condition and four in the MedTec condition could not be assigned to any group because of missing responses.

By differentiating participants according to the perceived threat extent, three groups were formed according to their score on the 10-point scale: high threat (>4.6), medium threat (2.6 - 4.5) and low threat (<2.5).

Overview of the Total Sums of Con's and Pro's. First, it was analyzed whether user groups differ in their number of statements. While there were no significant differences for age, gender and risk perception, the extent of perceived threat affected the number of usage barriers in the MedTec service context. People with a high degree of perceived threat reported significantly more usage barriers ($F(2,29) = 4.33$; $p < 0.05$; 3.7 statements per person; $SD = 0.82$) than people with a medium (1.9 statements per person; $SD = 1.6$) and a low degree of perceived threat (2.3 statements per person; $SD = 1.7$). The second user factor that revealed a significant difference was the using frequency in the ICT service context. Participants, which use their devices more than once a day reported more usage motives for others ($F(1,29) = 4.62$; $p < 0.05$; 2.9 statements per person; $SD = 1.85$) than people who use their device less frequently (1.7 statements per person, $SD = 1.1$).

Impact of Age and Risk Perception. In a second step the impact of user factors on the total distribution of usage motives and barriers in both contexts was analyzed. As shown in table 7, only for the ICT service context significant age effects were found.

Within the usage motives, the enhanced feeling of *safety* and the simple fact to *communicate* with people was more often reported by the youngest group (< 30 years). In contrast to that, it was the oldest group (50+) that stated much more the usage barrier *annoyance* as reason against using an ICT device.

Table 7. Mean number of motive and barrier statements for service contexts and age groups

ICT	age			p
	0-30 (N = 11)	31-50 (N=10)	51+ (N=10)	
safety	0.6	0.2	0	p < 0.05
communication	0.73	0.1	0.2	p < 0.05
annoyance	0	0.1	0.7	p < 0.05

Moreover, effects of risk perception on motive patterns were found (Table 8). Within the ICT service context, the usage motive *flexibility* was mostly named by *concerned* persons. Within the usage barriers, *cost* was more often named by *unconcerned* people, and not at all by *concerned* persons. For the *undecided* group it is the usage barrier of *permanent availability*, that distinguishes this group from the other two, because they named this kind of argument more frequently. Within the MedTec context, *radiation* as usage barrier is significantly more often reported by *concerned* users than by *undecided* and *less concerned* user groups. The usage barrier *technical unreliability* is mostly reported by *undecided* people but also by the *concerned* group.

Table 8. Mean number of statements for service contexts and 'risk groups'

	'risk groups'			
ICT	No concern (N = 17)	Undecided (N = 9)	concerned (N = 3)	p
flexibility	0.2	0.4	1.6	p < 0.05
costs	1.0	0.3	0	p < 0.05
availability (barrier)	0.4	1.2	0.7	p < 0.05
MedTec	**N = 18**	**N = 7**	**N = 3**	
radiation	0.3	0.3	1.7	p < 0.01
technical unreliability	0.6	2.9	1.0	p < 0.05

Impact of "Technical Expert" Factors and Perceived Threat. Finally, the scores on the perceived threat scale, as well as all technical experience factors (knowledge, interest, using frequency, mean years of device use) were correlated with the number of statements in each category, separated by service context and separated by target group (usage for themselves or others). For a better understanding of the correlation results: Higher values indicate a higher level or frequency of the variable (e.g. high values in interest ratings express a high level of interest).

Figure 7 shows a correlation model for the ICT service context. At first sight, it becomes evident that more usage barrier statements show significant correlations to user factors than positive usage motive statements. Among all user characteristics considered, the degree of *perceived threat* as well as the *using frequency* showed the strongest associations to motives and especially usage barriers -meaning they are correlated to a greater amount of arguments.

Correlation patterns show, that the higher the degree of a perceived threat by technology, the higher the fear of possible health risks. On the other hand, people who do not report to perceive any threat have greater fears of high (and also unknown) costs and fear of (data) privacy loss. People with a low degree of perceived threat also state, that they would only refrain from using their mobile device if costs will be too high (no-go).

Experience-related using factors (domain knowledge, interest and using frequency) were found to be predominately related to positive usage motives, indicating that the active handling of technology leads to a more positive perception of technology. Though, participants, who use their device very often (more than once a day), also complained about *technical unreliability* (usage barrier), apparently recurring to frequent experience with this problem. The barrier *social aspects* – loss of personal contact due to technology usage – is negatively correlated to the level of domain knowledge, technical interest and years of using the device. Thus, frequent device users and technically experienced persons deny fearing that mobile technology usage leads to a decrease in social contact.

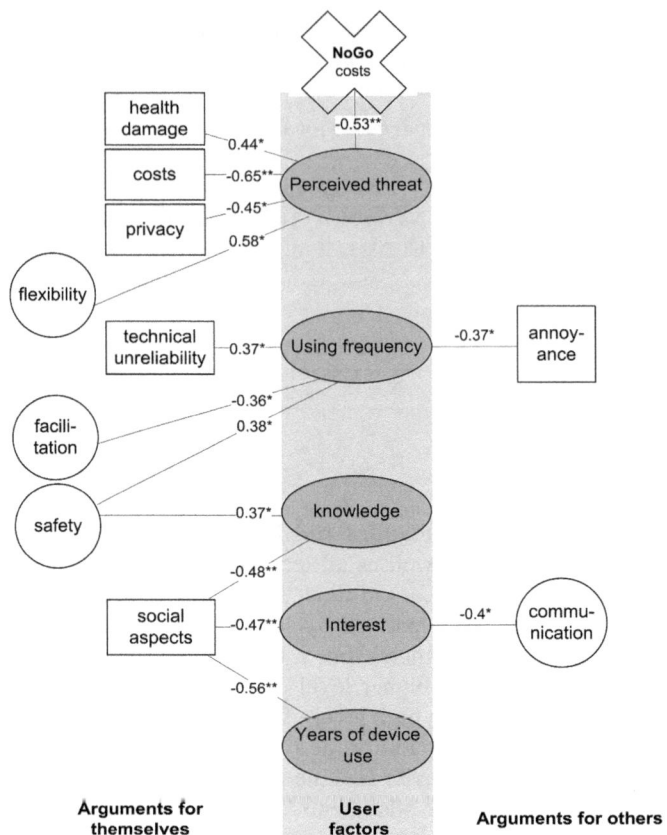

Fig. 7. ICT service context: Correlation of arguments and user factors differentiated by arguments for themselves and for others ("barriers" in squared boxes, "motives" in circles; *p<0.05; **p<0.01)

Concerning arguments, which militate in favor for usage of the respective technology for others, there were two prominent factors among assessed user characteristics, which show significant correlations. The usage motive *communication* was negatively correlated to the level of interest and the usage barrier *annoyance* was negatively related to using frequency. We conclude, that especially older people, who use their device less frequently, react very sensitive to "noise pollution" (annoyance) by mobile devices (e.g., ringtones).

In Figure 8 (previous page), the correlation pattern for the MedTec service context is depicted. As can be seen, about the same number of statements were given as positive usage motives for oneself and for others. Within the MedTec context, additional and different motives and barriers were associated to user factors in comparison to the ICT service context. In the MedTec context, the level of domain knowledge was the most relevant user factor, which showed associations with usage motives and barriers. Moreover, the usage barriers *radiation, fear of data manipulation* and *fear of being controlled* (surveillance) were positively correlated with perceived threat in the

MedTec service context. In contrast to the ICT service context, there were much more correlations of arguments in the MedTec service context, which militate in favor of usage the technology for others. Finally, it is noteworthy, that in both service contexts expertise-related factors were more strongly correlated to positive usage motives, meanwhile usage barriers were more strongly related to the degree of perceived threat.

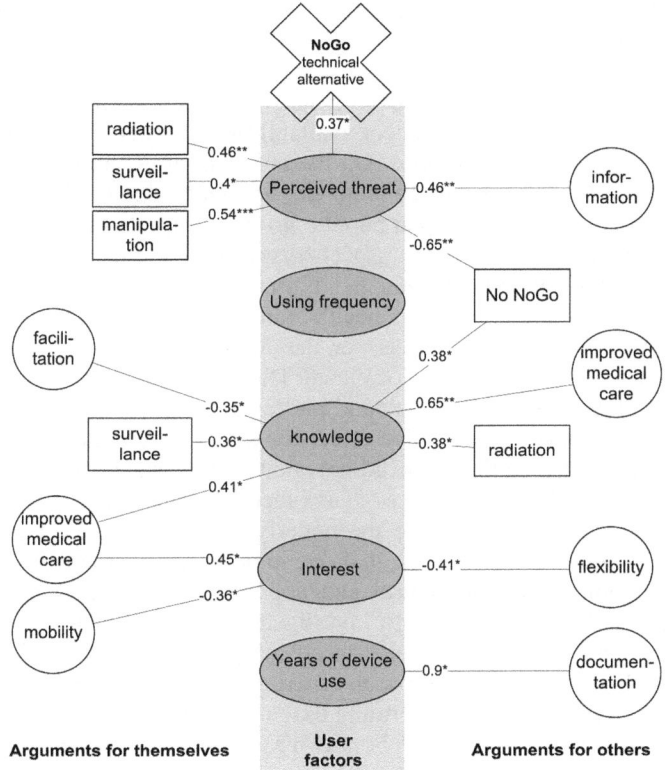

Fig. 8. MedTec service context: Correlations between usage arguments and user factors, differentiated by arguments for themselves and for others ("Con's" are given in squared boxes, "pro's" in circles). *p<0.05; **p<0.01

4 Discussion

In the following sections the findings and implications of our study are discussed.

4.1 Identification of Usage Motives and Barriers

The analysis of user statements regarding pro's and con's of ICT and MedTec device usage revealed an comprehensive image of usage motives and barriers – which is especially valuable for the development and marketing of technical service systems.

These motives and barriers are involved or cognitively activated when users think about using or adapting to a specific technical service. We identified different types of factors, which affect the adoption of specific technologies or services: a) usage motives, which can be seen as "benefits" or "promoters" of technology usage, b) usage barriers, which reduce the probability of a product's success on the market, and c) no-go's, which should be seriously considered in system design, because they can "kill" the acceptance of a product in the market.

Interestingly, some categories regarding motives or barriers had a high similarity or even congruence with regard to their content. An example for a category, which was present "on both sides" (pro's and con's), was *availability*, which was either perceived positively (in terms of improved reachability of oneself and others) *or* negatively (in terms of annoying permanent availability). Another "Janus-faced" category was *social networks or relationships*. On the one hand users appreciated the facilitation of staying in touch with family members or friends due to ICT services, but on the other hand they also complained about a growing superficiality and low commitment in social relationships. For the aspect *surveillance* we also uncovered diverging "Janus-faced" statements: One the one hand, users made positive statements about the improved certainty about someone's health status (MedTec), well-being or localization (e.g. knowing where your child is); on the other hand users disliked the feeling of being of constantly controlled or localized. The aspect *health awareness* was also mentioned ambiguously: on the one hand participants appreciated - especially in the medical service context – the positive effects on someone's health awareness, but, on the other hand, they stated that they did not want to be permanently reminded of their health status. After identifying these "Janus-faced" usage motives and barriers, one central question emerges: What are the underlying factors or mechanisms of these "double-sided" motives? We assume that one important moderator is "perceived control", i.e. behavioral situation control and not "affective" control of a technology. However, future studies will have to investigate the effects of potential moderators such as control on these specific "Janus-faced" usage motives and barriers.

The overall high number of motive and barrier statements suggests, that users seem to integrate several motives when forming usage decisions and to balance benefits and risks against each other. This corroborates previous findings and approaches [10], where the acceptance and intention to use technologies is explained in terms of a cost-benefit analysis. It is assumed that users weigh individually expected benefits and costs (e.g. investment of money and energy, personal efforts and frustration while learning to use the system) before adopting a new technology. Future studies will have to provide a deeper insight in the genesis of acceptance decisions. To this end, a research approach is necessary, which allows the analysis of the interaction between different usage motives and barriers, i.e. the determinations of their relative importance by using conjoint analyses. The findings of the present study will provide a sound basis for conjoint analyses and the identification of critical and potent decision criteria.

4.2 Is There a Service-Specificity in Motive Patterns?

The contrast of usage motives and barriers in the ICT- and MedTec service context convincingly confirmed our assumption of the presence of service-specificity in motive patterns. Motive patterns in the two service contexts revealed to be quantitatively and qualitatively different.

Referring to quantitative differences, participants made over one third fewer statements for the MedTec service context. We assume, that due to the smaller diffusion rate of MedTec in comparison to ICT, participants had not yet enough concrete experience with the MedTec service context to produce a comparable number of usage motives and barriers. Therefore, in following studies a bigger group of actual MedTec users should be recruited. Another interesting finding was that potential users made more statements about usage motives and barriers for themselves than they claimed for others. Especially in the MedTec service context, we expected more statements directed to the usage of medical technology for others. This expectation was based on the effect of "comparative optimism" [36], according to which (health) risks for others are perceived to be higher than for one self. Hence, we assumed that "others" would be perceived as the main target group of MedTec services rather than oneself. On the other hand we cannot exclude, that the (cognitive) change of perspective was difficult to realize, which is necessary to find usage motives and barriers for others. With regard to user factors, this might also explain the contradictory finding of a larger number of correlations between user factors and arguments for others in MedTec service context than in the ICT service context. We assume that participants' lower personal experience with medical technology might have activated more unspecific public opinions, rather than arguments based on own experience, which in turn results in a more uniform picture of correlations in MedTec service contexts.

Regarding qualitative differences it was revealed, that potential users in fact perceive *different* patterns of motives and barriers in a specific service context. For example in the ICT service context the motives of flexibility, communication, availability, functions, and warning function were more dominant, whereas aspects of documentation, facilitation of daily life, and improved medical care were more important in the MedTec context. One finding is especially noteworthy in this context. Although both service types are based on the same (mobile) technology, the fear of health damage as a consequence of electromagnetic radiation is considerably more prominent in the ICT service context than in the MedTec service context. The critical question is, why potential users of MedTec services do not think about potential negative effects on their health. We assume that users make a "trade-off" between costs (usage barriers) and benefits (usage motives) in their decision process and that specific usage motives in the MedTec service context have a higher relevance (i.e. improved medical care, facilitation of daily life) in this decision process. Hence, further research is necessary in order to find out, why the very same usage barrier is evaluated differently in two differing contexts.

4.3 The Role of User Factors

This study pointed out, that in the context of mobile (wireless) technologies the 'expert' factors and perceived risk respectively perceived threat are appropriate factors to differentiate between user groups. The most important user factors with regard to acceptance patterns in both technical service contexts were "perceived threat" and "risk" as well as 'technical expertise' factors (e.g. domain knowledge, using frequency or interest). For example, people who use their mobile device not that frequently, who are not that interested in the topic or report to have less technical knowledge, stated more usage barriers, especially regarding social aspects. Interestingly, positive usage motives were correlated with 'expert' factors; perceived threat was more strongly correlated with usage barriers. It is not sufficient to consider just one sort of user factor for classifying but to take both factors into account in order to get an understanding of both sides of acceptance - this is especially important with regard to the identified "Janus-faced" usage motives. Gender had no effect on motive patterns, in contrast to age, which revealed some significant effects. However, we assume, that age effects were moderated by expertise effects. Therefore, in future studies age should always be considered in combination with other user factors such as expertise.

4.4 Limitations of the Present Study and Future Research

As the present study had a strong exploratory character, a number of research questions were uncovered. Future studies will therefore have to address more aspects in acceptance-relevant motives as well as further mobile service contexts, e.g. social software services, such as Facebook, or telemedical assistants in the MedTec context. Also, future work should integrate broader user groups (i.e. older users and frail persons) and more actual users of MedTec devices (i.e. patients, which already use mobile medical devices) in order to supplement the investigation of "anticipated usage scenarios" by "actual usage experience". Apart from the assessment of motives and barriers of users in structured interview situations, one research focus should be laid on the analysis of user's behavior in real usage situations. Future research activities should finally investigate the interaction of acceptance-relevant usage motives and barriers in more complex decision situations, where several motives and barriers have to be integrated at the same time by the user. Accordingly we will apply conjoint analyses in a next research step.

Acknowledgments. We thank Johanna Kluge, Christina Vedar, Oliver Sack, and Jenny Figueroa Diaz for research support. Thanks also to Anne-Kathrin Schaar for constructive discussions during paper preparation.

This research was funded by the Excellence Initiative of the German state and federal government.

References

1. Tech Crunchies – Internet Statistics and Numbers, http://techcrunchies.com/distribution-of-gsm-connections-worldwide/2009
2. Rao, B., Minakakis, L.: Evolution of Mobile Location-based Services. Communications of the ACM 46, 61–65 (2003)
3. Informa Telecoms and Media's global media forecasts (2008), http://www.intomobile.com/2008/
4. Hargittai, E.: Second Level digital divide: Differences in peoples online skills. First Monday 7, 1–18 (2002)
5. Iacucci, G., Kuutti, K., Ranta, M.: On the move with a magic thing: role playing in concept design of mobile services and devices. In: Proceedings of the 3rd Conference on Design Interactive Systems, Practise, Methods and Techniques, pp. 193–202. ACM, New York (2000)

6. Lalou, S.: Identity, Social Satus, privacy and face-keepting in the digital society. Social Science Information 47, 299–330 (2008)
7. Pagani, M.: Determinants of adoption of third generation mobile multimedia services. Journal of Interactive Marketing 18, 46–59 (2004)
8. Korupp, S.: No Man is an Island: The influence of Knowledge, Household Settings, and Social Context on Private Computer Use. International Journal of Internet Science 1, 45–57 (2006)
9. Meyer, S., Mollenkopf, H.: Home technology, smart homes, and the Aging user. In: Schaie, K.W., et al. (eds.) Aging Independently: Living Arrangements and Mobility, pp. 148–161. Springer, Berlin (2002)
10. Mynatt, E.D., Melenhorst, A.-S., Fisk, A., Rogers, W.: Aware Technologies for Aging in Place: Understanding user needs and attitudes, pp. 36–41. IEEE CS, Los Alamitos (2004)
11. Gaul, S., Ziefle, M.: Home Technologies: Insights into Generation-Specific Acceptance Motives. In: Holzinger, A., Miesenberger, K. (eds.) USAB 2009. LNCS, vol. 5889, pp. 312–332. Springer, Heidelberg (2009)
12. Grabner-Kräuter, S.D., Kaluscha, E.A.: Empirical research in on-line trust: a review and critical assessment. International Journal of Human-Computer Studies 58, 783–812 (2003)
13. Schröder, S., Ziefle, M.: Icon design on small screens: Effects of miniaturization on speed and accuracy in visual search. In: Proceedings of the 50th Conference on Human Factors and Ergonomics Society, Santa Monika, pp. 544–549 (2006)
14. Schröder, S., Ziefle, M.: Making a completely icon-based menu in mobile devices to become true: A Methodology for its development. In: ter Hofte, H., Mulder, I., de Ruyter, B. (eds.) Proceedings of the 10th International Conference on Human-Computer Interaction with Mobile Devices and Services, pp. 137–146. ACM, New York (2008)
15. Ziefle, M., Bay, S.: Mental models of Cellular Phones Menu. Comparing older and younger novice users. In: Brewster, S., Dunlop, M.D. (eds.) Mobile HCI 2004. LNCS, vol. 3160, pp. 25–37. Springer, Heidelberg (2004)
16. Hanly, S., Mathar, R.: On the optimal base station density for CDMA cellular networks. IEEE Transactions on Communications 50, 1274–1281 (2002)
17. Imhof, L., Mathar, R.: The geometry of the capacity region for CDMA systems with general power con'straints. IEEE Transactions on Wireless Communications 4, 2040–2044 (2005)
18. Daghfous, N., Petrof, J.V., Pons, F.: Values and Adoption of Innovations: A Cross-Cultural Study. Journal of Con'sumer Marketing 16, 314–331 (1999)
19. Bonfadelli, H.: The Internet and Knowledge Gaps: A theoretical and empirical Investigation. European Journal of Communication 17, 65–84 (2002)
20. Tarasewich, P.: Mobile commerce opportunities and challenges: Designing mobile commerce applications. Communications of the ACM 46 (2003)
21. Arning, K., Ziefle, M.: Effects of cognitive and personal factors on PDA menu navigation performance. Behaviour and Information Technology 28, 251–268 (2009)
22. Ryan, C., Gonsalves, A.: The effect of context and application type on Mobile usability: An empirical study. In: 28th Australasian Computer Science Conference, pp. 115–125. Australian Computer Science, Newcastle (2005)
23. Tuomainen, K., Haapanen, S.: Needs of the active elderly for mobile phones. In: Stephanidis, C. (ed.) Universal Access in HCI, pp. 494–498. Laurence Erlbaum Associates, Mahwah (2003)
24. Agarwal, R., Prasad, J.: Are Individual Differences Germane to the Acceptance of New Information Technologies? Decision Sciences 30, 361–391 (1999)

25. Arning, K., Ziefle, M.: What older adults expect from mobile services: An empirical survey. In: Pikaar, R.N., Konigsveld, E.A., Settels, P.J. (eds.) Proceedings IEA 2006. Meeting Diversity in Ergonomics. Elsevier, Amsterdam (2006)
26. Agarwal, R., Prasad, J.: A Conceptual and Operational Definition of Personal Innovativeness in the Domain of Information Technology. Information Systems Research 9, 204–215 (1998)
27. Davis, F.D.: Perceived Usefulness, Perceived Ease of Use, and User Acceptance of Information Technology. MIS Quarterly 13, 319–340 (1989)
28. Arning, K., Ziefle, M.: Different Perspectives on Technology Acceptance: The Role of Technology Type and Age. In: Holzinger, A., Miesenberger, K. (eds.) USAB 2009. LNCS, vol. 5889, pp. 20–41. Springer, Heidelberg (2009)
29. Agarwal, R., Prasad, J.: The Role of Innovation Characteristics and Perceived Voluntariness in the Acceptance of Information Technologies. Decision Sciences 28, 557–581 (1997)
30. Wilkowska, W., Ziefle, M.: Which factors form older adults' acceptance of mobile information and communication technologies? In: Holzinger, A., Miesenberger, K. (eds.) USAB 2009. LNCS, vol. 5889, pp. 81–101. Springer, Heidelberg (2009)
31. Arning, K., Ziefle, M.: Understanding differences in PDA acceptance and performance. Computers in Human Behaviour 23, 2904–2927 (2007)
32. Melenhorst, A.S., Rogers, W.A., Caylor, E.C.: The use of communication technologies by older adults: exploring the benefits from the user's perspective. In: Proc. of the Human Factors and Ergonomics Society 45th Annual Meeting, Human Factors and Ergonomics Society, Santa Monica, CA, USA (2001)
33. Ziefle, M., Michel, T., Strenk, J., Schroeder, U.: How young and older users master the use of hyperlinks in small screen devices. In: Proceedings of the SIGCHI Conference on Human Factors in Computing Systems 2007, pp. 307–316. ACM, New York (2007)
34. Venkatesh, V.: Mobile commerce opportunities and challenges: Understanding usability in mobile commerce. Communications of the ACM 46 (2003)
35. Wiedemann, P., Schütz, H.: Mobile fears? – Risk perceptions regarding RFEMF. In: Proceedings JRC/EIS-EMF Workshop, Ispra, Italy (2004)
36. Sheppard, J.A., Carroll, P., Grace, J., Terry, M.: Exploring the causes of comparative optimism. Psychologica Belgica 42, 65–98 (2002)

Social Acceptance of Negotiation Support Systems

Alina Pommeranz, Pascal Wiggers, Willem-Paul Brinkman, and Catholijn M. Jonker

Section Man-Machine Interaction, Delft University of Technology,
Mekelweg 4, 2628 CD Delft, The Netherlands
a.pommeranz@tudelt.nl

Abstract. We investigate people's attitudes towards the possible use of mobile negotiation support systems (NSS) in different social contexts and the consequences for their design. For that purpose we developed an online survey based on existing models of technology acceptance. In the questionnaire we showed five filmed scenarios of NSS use contexts. The data collected from 120 respondents, showed (a) that subjective norm is an important factor influencing the intention to use the system and (b) that the acceptance of NSS depends on the use context. Therefore, we argue that NSS should be designed not merely as tools being used in the actual negotiation but as social devices harnessing social networks to provide support in all negotiation phases.

Keywords: Negotiation Support Systems, Social Settings, Technology Acceptance, User Study.

1 Introduction

A skillful negotiator has to carefully balance the issues at stake, have a good understanding of his own and the opponent's needs and since negotiation is a social activity, manage relationships and handle emotions [22]. Often negotiating involves overlooking a vast amount of options, deciding on strategies and evaluating bids with multiple attributes. Computational power can facilitate these processes. Within different research areas, e.g. management science, e-commerce and artificial intelligence [11,18,19,23], researchers have been dealing with supporting people electronically in negotiations. Existing negotiation support systems (NSS) can significantly improve the human performance in negotiations and increase the number of win-win outcomes if the negotiation space is well-understood [7,10].

Most existing NSS have been developed either as stand-alone applications [11] or Web-based applications [10] and are currently used for training and research rather than in real-life negotiations. The advance of mobile technology, however, opens up a whole new range of possibilities for NSS. Since negotiation is an activity that can take place in almost any setting instead of being tied to, e.g., an office, mobile technology enables people to have their NSS at hand at any time they are involved in a negotiation. Current mobile devices such as mobile phones, PDAs, handheld computers etc., offer among other things the opportunities to store and compute large amounts of data, access online sources and show graphical data on color screens. In addition, the number of people using portable Internet devices is rapidly growing [8]. We would like to take advantage

G. Leitner, M. Hitz, and A. Holzinger (Eds.): USAB 2010, LNCS 6389, pp. 55–70, 2010.

of these trends and develop a new kind of NSS for mobile use, a so-called Pocket Negotiator (PN) as described by [7]. Our vision is to develop a mobile system that is able to collaborate with its users in order to reach win-win outcomes in negotiations. The PN will enhance the negotiation skills and performance of the user by increasing the user's capacity for exploration of the negotiation space, i.e. possible bids and deals, reducing cognitive task load and preventing mental errors. The functionality of the device will be focused on handling computational complexity issues and providing bidding- and interaction advice. Our idea is to cover all negotiation phases (preparation, joint exploration, bidding and closure) [22] with the support from the system.

The mobile nature of the system will allow users to refer to this support not only when they prepare themselves at home, but also when they are on the move or even during the face-to-face situation with the other negotiation partner. This entails several advantages. The users can, e.g., collect relevant information for the negotiation and enter it immediately into the NSS or update information about their preferences in case they change due to new information. They can practice the different negotiation steps and review tips and strategies at any time. In a face-to-face situation it might also be useful to enter information, e.g., revealed by the opponent (i.e. spoken words or information about the opponent's behavior, emotions etc.). Based on this input the NSS will be able to give context-relevant advice or it could just serve as a reminder for information entered by the user during earlier preparation. Also the possibility of connecting to a wireless network enriches the functionality of the NSS, e.g. by providing online market information. With this new freedom mobile NSS offer, new questions and problems occur. Besides technical restrictions like the small screen size or short battery times the question of social implications arises. When putting NSS into the social setting of a face-to-face negotiation or using it in public spaces, we have to consider appropriateness and acceptance regarding the user, the opponent or bystanders. Entering information or consulting the NSS during a negotiation might interrupt the flow of the communication or bother the opponent for other reasons. Furthermore, the user might be concerned about his or her image when using a mobile NSS in public. These are issues worthwhile investigating.

Therefore, we conducted an online survey (a) to find out in which situations people consider a mobile NSS socially acceptable, (b) to find the factors and relationships that influence this acceptance in the different situations and social contexts and (c) to investigate the consequences of people's attitudes towards NSS for their design.

We would like to stress at this point that the system has not been implemented yet. Before designing the concrete functionality of a Pocket Negotiator and implementing it we would like to investigate the social acceptance of mobile NSS in different situations. This will enable us on the one hand to inform the further design process and on the other hand find answers to why current NSS are not used in real negotiations.

2   Related Work

The majority of existing NSS has been used for training and research purposes, but has not been applied to real life negotiations [9]. A recent study on user acceptance of Web-based NSS [23] predicts that 80 percent of the users would use the system to prepare and train for negotiations but only 61 percent would use it in the negotiation. Why is the acceptance for real cases so low? One possible answer is that NSS development is too focused on the technical aspects and disregards human concerns. Bui [3] points out that research on NSS concentrates on technological solutions, while the social problems they intend to solve are secondary or completely neglected. Swaab and colleagues [21] argue for a careful analysis of social and psychological processes in order to design good NSS and claim that the success of an NSS depends on the understanding of the activity that the system will support.

Negotiation is inherently a social activity, since it involves communication between at least two parties and is influenced by the social setting in which it takes place. Literature on business science [6] has, e.g., emphasized the influence of relationships on negotiation processes. Moreover, based on results from expert focus groups [17] we know that people's attitudes towards NSS differ widely and that social contexts might play a role when choosing to use a system or not. Therefore, we believe that in order to design NSS that will be successfully used we first need to investigate whether people are willing to accept the use of NSS in different social settings.

Researchers focusing on the adoption of mobile technology in general have recently included social context into their models. Social impacts of mobile technology have been widely studied [12,13,14,15], especially the pervasive nature of mobile phones in public places. Most of the literature in this area focuses on the distraction of bystanders by people talking loudly on the phone or by the mix-up of geographic spaces (current physical space the mobile phone user is in and the space created by a phone conversation) [12,13,20]. In the case of using a mobile NSS, distraction is, of course, especially an issue when the NSS user is in an active, ongoing communication with the other negotiation party (face-to-face or on the phone). The interaction with the device might disrupt this communication and therefore be less socially acceptable. Furthermore, the other party might not accept the interaction with the NSS because it allows the user to have an advantage and other party might feel excluded. In other situations where the NSS is used for preparation, social acceptance might be less of an issue.

3   Research Questions

We looked at several detailed research questions. **RQ 1**: Is there a relationship between the user characteristics and (perceived) usefulness, attitude towards negotiation, behavioral control and social acceptance? The user characteristics include demographic data and experience in computer usage and with negotiations. We expect that age and possibly gender influence the acceptance of a mobile NSS in different situations. In focus groups with negotiation experts we conducted [17] it was anticipated that younger people are more open to technology use in public places and social situations than older people because younger generations grow up with technology around them. This is reflected in **RQ 1a**: Is there a negative impact of the user's age on the acceptance of a NSS in a face-to-face situation?

Based on the results of focus groups we did with end-users (5 groups with 3 high school students each, aged 15 to 18 ($M = 16.73$, $SD = 0.88$), 6 groups with 6 highly-educated women each, aged between 31 and 70 ($M = 49.86$, $SD = 9.16$)), we expect that people with low negotiation skills and a negative attitude towards negotiation are more likely to use an NSS. Due to their own lack of knowledge about negotiations or insecurity they might find an NSS more useful than people, who enjoy negotiating and consider themselves good at it. This leads to the questions: **RQ 2**: Is there a negative relation between a person's attitude towards negotiations and the attitude towards NSS? **RQ 2a**: Is there a relationship between on the one side negotiation skills and experience and on the other side the attitude towards negotiations?

We believe that the acceptance of a NSS in a social context has an impact on the intention to use it. The social acceptance is measured by two variables, one describing how acceptable people find it to use an NSS in a situation (SN1) and the other describing in how far they believe that the opponent would find it acceptable (SN2). Whereas in a face-to-face situation it might play a big role what the opponent thinks, it might become less influential in a phone scenario. Therefore, our last research questions are: **RQ 3**: Is there a relationship between the social acceptance of an NSS and the intention to use it? **RQ 3b**: Does the negotiation situation determine the social acceptance?

4   The Model

The relations between usefulness, attitude towards a system and intention to use as well as the influence of subjective norm and behavioral control that we are interested in are well-studied for information systems within the scope of the Technology Acceptance Model (TAM) [5] and the Theory of Planned Behavior (TPB) [1]. Both models are extensions to the Theory of Reasoned Action introduced by Martin Fishbein and Icek Ajzen [2].

Based on our research questions we created a model to explain possible factors influencing the social acceptance and use intention of an NSS in different situations that combines both models and extends them with a number of factors that we think are influential specifically for mobile NSS.

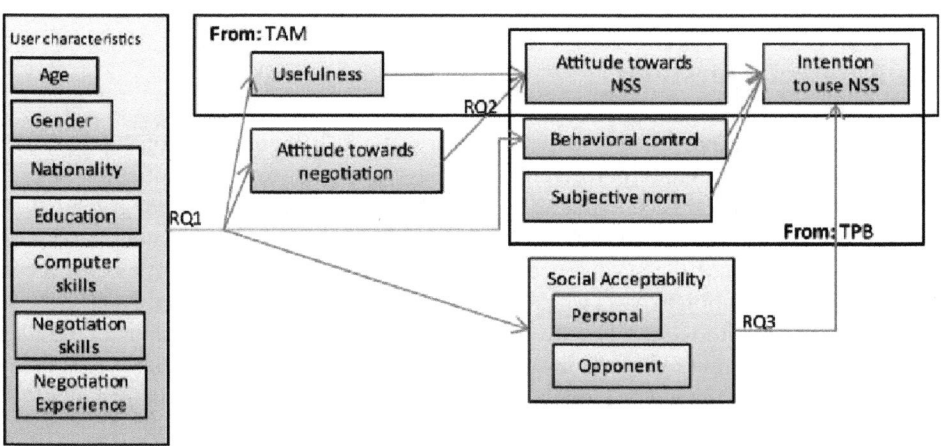

Fig. 1. NSS Social Acceptance Model

4.1 TPB and TAM Model

The TPB is a well known model in social psychology to explain the link between attitudes and behavior. It identifies the attitude towards a behavior, subjective norm (an individual's perception of others' beliefs whether he or she should perform the behavior) and perceived behavioral control (an individual's perceived ease or difficulty of performing the particular behavior) as indicators for the intention to use. The perceived behavioral control and the intention to use determine together the actual behavior regarding the use of a system.

The TAM has been widely used to explain people's attitude towards the use of technological systems. It identifies perceived usefulness and perceived ease of use as two independent factors that influence the intention to use a system and its actual use.

Since our study takes place before the implementation of the system, we are not able to measure the actual use of a system or the ease of use. To be able to measure usefulness and behavioral control we showed either videos or storyboards of NSS use cases. We kept the attitude towards NSS influencing the intention to use, but added the general attitude towards negotiations as an influential factor of attitude towards NSS. As mentioned earlier the use of such systems might depend on different situations and how socially acceptable it is to use a system in that situation. Therefore, we added social acceptance as an extra factor influencing the intention to use. Last, we added a number of user characteristics including: age, gender, nationality, education, computer and negotiation skills and experience.

5   The Survey

To give respondents an idea about the contexts and type of functionality that an NSS could perform we identified, together with a negotiation coach, five distinct situations for NSS use: face-to-face with the boss with concealed use of the NSS, face-to-face with open use at a car dealer, distant negotiation on the phone, collaborative preparation of a couple and short preparation being mobile on a train (Figure 2). For each situation we wrote and filmed a scenario (see e.g. http://mmi.tudelft.nl/video/scenario1/, Dutch voiceover, for other scenarios change the 1 to a number between 1 and 5) to be shown in the questionnaire.

5.1   Scenarios

Scenarios are useful in the design process since they capture the consequences and trade-offs of designs [4]. The narrative nature of scenarios enables users to imagine the use situations and contexts of new or existing technology. For each of the five use contexts we wrote a scenario presented in the following in summary. Italic text is taken from the original texts of the scenarios. In the project we currently focus on two example domains for NSS use: job contract and real estate negotiations. We chose to write two scenarios illustrating a job negotiation, two with real estate content and one about buying a car. All scenarios were checked by a professional negotiation coach to make sure that they were sufficiently realistic. Each scenario is briefly discussed below.

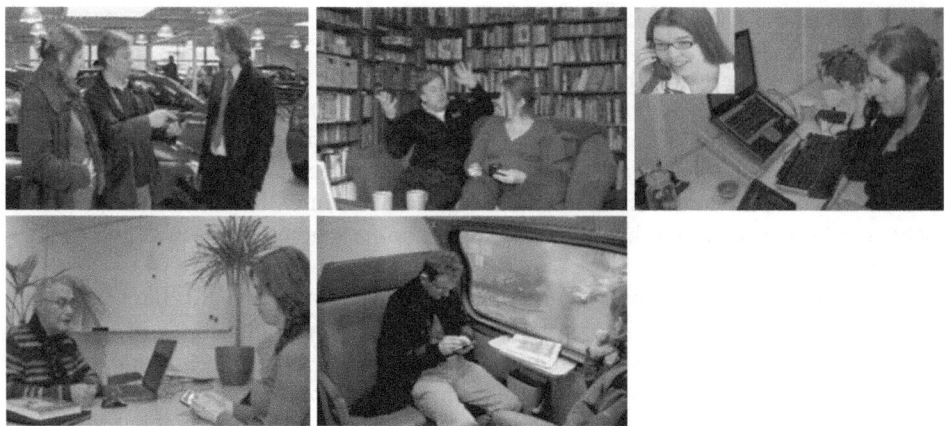

Fig. 2. Scenarios (Screenshots from videos) from left to right, top row: open use at car dealer, collaborative preparation before buying a house, on the phone with real estate agent, ; bottom row: evaluation talk with boss, preparation for job interview on the train

Mobile Preparation with Time Constraints (train). Preparation is one of the negotiation phases stressed in the literature, e.g. [6]. In this scenario we describe a preparation situation with special constraints. The job applicant Martin is already on his way to the interview. Therefore, he has limited time to prepare himself. In addition, the mobile setting constitutes another constraint, namely limited resources. Both constraints require special regard when it comes to the functionality of the device. Just before getting on the train Martin has received a mobile NSS from a friend. He uses the device's speed preparation function to prepare himself in the short time he has left. Among other functions the device allows him to receive knowledge about the job negotiation domain.

He wonders how much money he could ask for. He chooses 'expert opinion' on the interface and types in 'salary'. The PN suggests a website that has a forum where you can discuss current average salaries for IT consultants with an expert in the field. After reading through the forum Martin has a quite good idea what he can ask for with his kind of educational background and experience. With that knowledge he feels more secure and relieved.

Later in the scenario Martin makes use of the training module of the NSS which enables him to go through a simulated interview with a virtual agent. He receives on-the-fly advice about his and the opponent's actions. The scenario ends with Martin being more relaxed, knowing what to expect in the upcoming negotiation.

Face-to-Face Negotiation, Secret Use (F-2-F). The situation described in this scenario is a negotiation between an employee, Bianca, and her boss. Bianca is using a mobile NSS. The emphasis in this scenario is the concealed use of the NSS. Bianca is hiding the fact that she has support from an NSS by telling her boss she is using her device only to take notes.

Bianca has been working for a big telecommunication company in The Hague for 2 years now. Today her annual evaluation with her boss is due. Bianca wants to take this meeting as an opportunity to re-negotiate some parts of her contract. Since her husband

got a new job in another city, they decided to move further away. Therefore, she wants to discuss opportunities with her boss to handle the new situation. She knows that she worked hard and well in the last year and should get what she wants, but she does not consider herself a good negotiator. Therefore, she recently got the PN *and prepared herself for this negotiation with the device.*

Throughout the negotiation described in the scenario Bianca receives help from the device. Several functions are described in this scenario including, e.g., the management of emotions, generating new options, and receiving advice from the system. The scenario ends with a deal in which both parties gain something and are satisfied with.

Collaborative Preparation (Coll. Preparation). Negotiation involves a lot of emotions on both sides of the bargaining table, but also within one party, e.g., between two partners buying a house together. In this case the first step is to merge the demands and preferences of both partners before starting a negotiation with the opponent side. Our scenario describes a couple that is planning to buy a house together and uses the NSS during the preparation to sort out their preferences and to download domain knowledge about real estate.

The 'collaborative preparation' module starts up. After a short introduction the PN *asks each of them to put in their preferences for a house separately. Since they also have the* PN *software installed on their laptop they put in their preferences in parallel. From both preference profiles the* PN *creates a matching profile and shows the clashes of their preferences. It advices the couple discussing the clashes and trying to find trade-offs between them that suit both.*

During this process of compromising the couple gets into a quarrel in which both insist on their own wishes without even communicating the underlying reasons in detail. In this case our device takes on a proactive role and interrupts the couple to give advice on how to handle the conflict.

The PN *senses the noise and the angry voices in the room and assumes an argument. The* PN *suggests calming down [and] prompts them to put in an emotional value on a scale from 'I don't care at all' to 'I would die for this' for each variable they have different preferences on.*

After having sorted out all their preferences they start looking for houses. In the last scene of the scenario the couple visits a house and takes advantage of the PN's feature of taking pictures and storing them together with other information about the house in a database.

Negotiation on the phone (Phone). A negotiation in which both parties are not situated in a face-to-face setting, but are distant from each other offers different design challenges for a NSS. First of all one party does not see the other party and therefore the use of a NSS can take place without each others' notice. Especially in real estate situations, e.g. when buying a house another aspect to consider is that the negotiation is split into a number of phone calls. This gives the user time in between the calls to use the system in each step of the negotiation. Our scenario describes a couple negotiating for a house. Before the interaction with the opponent they prepare themselves with the help of the NSS.

Furthermore, the PN *has downloaded housing domain knowledge, such as contracts and legal issues and the prices of similar houses in the neighborhood to take into account. Before Mary came to work this morning she had decided with Piet to set a first bid around 450.000 Euro.*

At work Mary calls the agent and starts negotiating. Before and during the phone calls she uses the NSS on her laptop to receive advice about different steps in the negotiation, e.g. the PN advises her to not start the negotiation with offering a price, but instead talk about other issues and options.

The bidding goes on for a while and the PN *shows a visualization of the bids in the outcome space based on the preferences of Piet and Mary and the estimated preferences of the agent. After a while the* PN *detects that the bidding is not reaching a win-win situation.*

After finding new variables to include in the negotiation to reach an agreement that suits both parties they finally close a deal.

Face-to-Face Negotiation, Open Use (Car Dealer). We decided to include another scenario that has a face-to-face setting, but showing an open use of the NSS meaning that the other party is aware of the use. This scenario is about a couple buying a car. Our belief is that the car dealer's setting enables people to use the NSS more openly. When buying a car it is usually not necessary to stick to one specific car dealer. No long-term relationship needs to be considered. Therefore, the couple in the scenario openly states that they will be using the NSS and explain what they can do with it.

The focus of the scenario lies in the advice of time-outs at strategic points during the negotiation. During the process of looking at cars and refining their preferences for the new car, they enter information about the state of the negotiation into the NSS. They receive strategic advice on how to proceed and when to take the time to recapitulate.

He [the car dealer] *shows them a range of more sporty looking family cars and the couple chooses their favorite. They enter that into the* PN. *The* PN *advices them to take a time-out and check whether they have considered all their preferences and whether all the information they need has been disclosed.*

After they have found an interesting car the bidding starts in the car salesman's office. The NSS assists the couple by comparing prices with similar cars online. They disclose to the salesman that the market price is lower than his offer. The salesman drops his price. They negotiate about a few extras and finally leave with a new car and a deal they are satisfied with.

5.2   The Questionnaire Structure

The questionnaire is based on the model shown in Figure 1. For details about the constructs and questions, see Appendix A. After a short introduction we collected the user characteristics. The factors intention to use (IU), subjective norm (SN) and social acceptability (SA) were measured after each scenario presented to the respondent. At the end of the survey we collected more general information about the attitude towards NSS (PNA), including behavioral control (BC) and usefulness (USE). For the majority of questions we asked the respondents to rate their agreement with a number of statements on a 7-point Likert scale and for an explanation for the ratings after each scenario to explore why people might accept the system in one scenario but not in another.

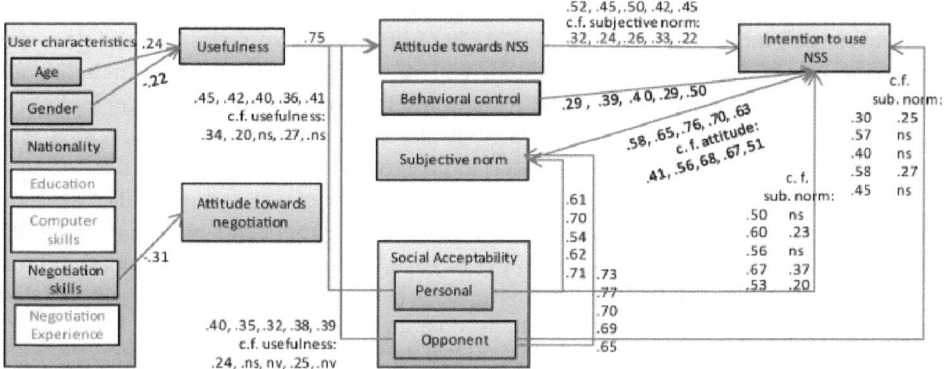

Fig. 3. Model with (partial) correlations, 5 numbers: per scenario, cf = controlled for, ns = not significant, nv = no value

5.3 Versions

We setup a Dutch version with short videos (3 min) and a Dutch and English version each with screenshots from the videos and text explaining the situation. The version with videos took about 45 minutes to fill in and the picture versions 10-15 minutes. To avoid order effects we shuffled the order of scenarios and statements.

5.4 Survey Distribution and Response

With NetQuestionnaires (www.netquestionnaires.com) we administered and distributed the survey online. We used an opportunity sample strategy to select participants for the study. We took advantage of personal networks and online forums to invite people to participate. We also asked each invited participant to motivate other friends and colleagues to participate. The questionnaire was approached by 365 people, and 178 started filling it in. In the following statistical analysis we included 120 (74 male, 46 female) from 18 countries, who completed the questionnaire. From these 120 participants 72 completed the English, 31 the Dutch version with videos and 17 the Dutch version with pictures. The most represented countries were the Netherlands (48), Sweden (19), Germany (15) and Greece (10). The age span ranged from 20 to 68 ($M = 32.28$, $SD = 10.36$). Participants are mostly familiar with computer usage, with the average number of hours spent at the computer being 44.86 ($SD = 20.14$) and highly educated (102 with university degrees). The negotiation experience of the sample is rather low. Only about a fourth of the participants are regularly engaged in negotiations in their jobs (31 participants). On average participants have bought 0.65 ($SD = 0.97$) and sold 0.47 houses ($SD = 2.43$) and have had less than seven job interviews ($M = 6.65$, $SD = 10.33$).

6   Results

6.1   Measurements of Contructs

For an overview of all constructs used in the questionnaire see Appendix A. We used Cronbach's alpha to test the reliability of the constructs usefulness (USE) (.95), and behavioral control (BC) (.72) and calculated aggregated measures for both including all original items. The Cronbach's alpha for attitude towards negotiation (NAT) including all four original items is very low (.04), but increases to .69, if the items NAT 1 and NAT 4 are deleted. Therefore, we decided to keep only the items NAT 2 and NAT 3 and combined them to an aggregated measure. For the construct negotiation skills (NSK) we keep the three items NSK 1, NSK 4, NSK 5 reaching a Cronbach's alpha of .71, while removing NSK 2 and NSK 3. The reliability of social acceptance (SA) was measured per scenario (Cronbach's alpha between .81 and .94). We did not calculate an aggregated measure for the acceptance, but kept them separate in the further analysis.

Table 1. Results of regression analysis for each scenario

Scenario	R	R^2	Adj. R^2	SE	df_{reg}	df_{res}	F	p
Train	.684	.467	.453	1.341	3	116	33.90	<.001
F-2-F	.762	.580	.569	1.143	3	116	53.39	<.001
Coll. Preparation	.674	.455	.439	1.434	2	69	28.78	<.001
Phone	.764	.584	.577	1.151	2	117	82.15	<.001
Car Dealer	.577	.333	.327	1.521	1	118	58.83	<.001

6.2   Data Analysis

We used correlation analysis to check our hypotheses. Significant correlation coefficients can be found in Figure 3.

User's background. We found a positive correlation between age and usefulness and a negative one between gender and usefulness. Computer skills and negotiation experience were not correlated with usefulness, attitude towards negotiation or behavioral control. We removed the item education from the model, since our data was not heterogeneous enough to draw any conclusions on the effects of education level. We also removed nationality because the data was not equally distributed. Interestingly, we found that negotiation skills are negatively correlated with the attitude towards negotiation opposing our initial hypothesis. However, negotiation skills were rated subjectively by the respondents themselves, which might not correspond to their actual negotiation skills. This issue needs further research.

Usefulness, Subjective Norm and Social Acceptance. We found a positive correlation between usefulness and the attitude towards NSS, which confirms the relationship predicted by TAM. We found that social acceptance, (personal (SA 1) and opponent

Table 2. Estimated coefficients of regression models for each scenario

Scenario	B	SE	β	t	p	VIF
Train						
Constant	-.77	.644		-1.19	.24	
SN	.46	.111	.394	4.10	<.001	2.01
BC	.38	.126	.237	3.04	.003	1.33
SA	.22	.105	.188	2.11	.04	1.73
F-2-F						
Constant	-1.25	.523		-2.39	.02	
SN	.52	.097	.441	5.33	<.001	1.89
SA	.36	.088	.339	4.08	<.001	1.91
BC	.24	.095	.157	2.56	.01	1.04
Coll. Preparation						
Constant	-.41	.794		-.51	.61	
SN	.67	.102	.595	6.53	<.001	1.05
BC	.34	.144	.215	2.36	.02	1.05
Phone						
Constant	-.37			-.71	.48	
SN	.82	.076	.704	10.88	<.001	1.18
BC	.21	.102	.131	2.03	.05	1.18
Car Dealer						
Constant	1.01	.383		2.63	.01	
SN	.70	.092	.577	7.67	<.001	1.00

(SA 2) view), is correlated with the attitude towards NSS and the intention to use for all scenarios. However, when controlled for usefulness in the first case and subjective norm in the second, the correlations are either weaker or not significant. This suggests that the attitude towards an NSS is mainly influenced by how useful people consider it. The intention to use the system depends mainly on the subjective norm, i.e. whether others relevant to the respondent believe he or she should use it.

The dominance of subjective norm was further analyzed by regression analysis (Table 1) for each individual scenario. We used a stepwise method with the dependent variable intention to use NSS in a particular scenario and the following independent variables: attitude towards negotiation (NAT), behavioral control (BC), subjective norm (SN) and social acceptance (SA). Table 2 gives an overview of the regression models with included variables and coefficients. We can see that subjective norm has the major influence in predicting intention to use in all scenarios. In the car dealer scenario it is even the only variable included in the model (β= .58, t(118) = 7.67, p < .001). In the collaborative preparation and the phone scenarios behavioral control were also included in the model. In the face-to-face and the train scenario behavioral control as well as social acceptance was included in the model. Whereas face-to-face the social acceptance is the second strongest indicator before behavioral control, in the train scenario it is the other way around. This is not surprising since in the situation with the boss social rules are much more important and can have stronger consequences than when sitting on a train. People using mobile devices on a train are a common sight and therefore social acceptance has less influence. More interesting is that in the other three scenarios social acceptance is not included in the model. In the phone and collaborative preparation scenario this might be due to the lack of a public setting.

Looking at the comments respondents gave voluntarily, we get deeper insight into how people see social acceptance considering the opponent's view in the different scenarios. People tend not to care whether the opponent accepts the NSS if they are not in eye contact ("This [on the phone] seems like the best application of the NSS, because it is invisible to the 'opponent'.") In the face-to-face scenarios people value the opponent's opinion highly. In the car dealer scenario some respondents doubt the acceptance of the NSS by the opponent. However, usefulness, the competitive situation ("I think the opponent will accept it because otherwise people would go to the competitor.") or the ability to put pressure on the opponent ("I like the secret weapon!") cause people to care less about the opponent. In the job scenario between an employee and her boss, most respondents are worried about the opponent's opinion on the use of an NSS. The comments show different views considering not being honest ("I think it is not acceptable because she lies about using an NSS."), impolite ("Its very impolite to use an electronic device during a face-to-face negotiation."), embarrassed ("I would be embarrassed to use an NSS in this situation."), nervous ("Stealth mode would make me extremely nervous.") or appearing weak ("In a face-to- face negotiation this would make you look like you cannot think for yourself."). A dominant opinion was that the interaction with the device will interrupt the communication flow ("The boss could get angry for not paying attention, the communication would be disturbed").

As shown in Figure 4, the social acceptance generally depends on the situation in which the NSS is used. Whereas most scenarios have an average rating above the scale's mean (4), the face-to-face situation with the boss got a low rating (3.06) lying significantly below the average ($t(119) = -6.25$, $p < .001$). This means, in the latter scenario people do not accept the use of an NSS. The situations which are most favorable for NSS use are negotiations on the phone and preparation on the train. At the car dealer or during the collaborative preparation NSS are accepted, but the average rating is closer to the neutral value.

7   Design Implications

Bringing the results of the data analysis into perspective of NSS design, we learned that not only functionality and usefulness play a role, but also social aspects like the subjective norm and social acceptance. An NSS is not only a tool people use to fulfill a certain task but it is a social device depending on the use context. Therefore, the designer has to determine in which context the device should be used and fit the design to the context and its social norms. Furthermore, our survey has shown that the respondents value the opinions of close friends or family highly, both for deciding whether to use an NSS and when taking decisions during the negotiation. Some respondents mention explicitly that they consult others before an important negotiation. ("I would take others' opinions into consideration as well, [. . .]", "In buying something like a car [. . .] I get advice for prices online, from friends.") This behavior made us contemplate about the idea to create NSS that are connected to social networks. Friends using the same type of NSS could be connected to each other, and whenever one needs to take a decision they could provide help or generally comment on each others' actions.

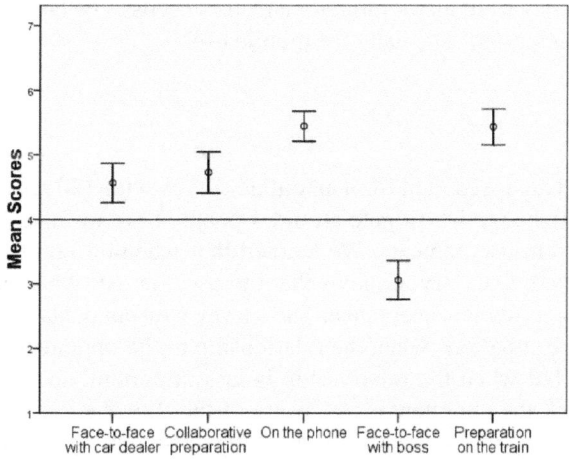

Fig. 4. Mean social Acceptance ratings (1=low to 7=high)

Another idea is storing negotiations within this network in a database that every NSS can access. This will enable users to see what strategies friends used in similar negotiations. These ideas fit social computing trends [16] by bringing mobile information spaces to the user and using social networks to enhance the system's functionality. Also, if people like to ask friends for advice when negotiating, a good NSS should be designed to behave in a similar manner. Surely, there are more ways designers can think of to make NSS more social devices.

8 Limitations

The study presented in this paper has a few limitations. First of all, the participants were not offered the chance to interact with an implemented system. Since we are at the beginning of the development of a novel NSS there is no implementation at hand yet. Furthermore, this study intended to inform the design process of this new NSS, instead of evaluating an existing design. On purpose we tried to focus rather on the use situations than the functionality the NSS could offer. We believe that by showing scenarios of use contexts in the questionnaire we found a good way to give participants a vision of what the system could be able to do, but on such a level that it does not distract from the focus on the situation. We think that people could get a feeling for the usefulness of the system and judge whether they would be able and willing to use it. Since the TAM model is based on constructs which can be perceived by the user when interacting with a real system, we excluded variables from the model that could not be perceived by only watching videos or seeing pictures, e.g. perceived ease of use.

Further limitations concern the number of participants in the study and the opportunistic sample. Unfortunately, these aspects did not allow us to make any general claims about the acceptance of NSS with regard to cultural or educational backgrounds or differences depending on age groups. Despite this, we believe that we offer interesting results that put NSS into a different light. The fact that both subjective norm and situation dependency were major influential factors needs to be taken into consideration when designing new NSS, especially for mobile use.

9   Conclusion

We presented and analyzed data from an online survey with 120 respondents with little negotiation experience to investigate attitudes people have towards an envisioned mobile NSS in different use contexts. We learned that when designing NSS social issues cannot be neglected. Our survey shows that the use context of an NSS is an important factor influencing its social acceptance. The survey's respondents would not accept the use in face-to-face situations when the relationship to the opponent was important, i.e. with one's boss, but when the relationship is less important, i.e. with a car dealer. In situations in which the opponent is not aware of the NSS, e.g. on the phone, it is most accepted. Surprisingly, the subjective norm is the most dominant factor influencing the intention to use a mobile NSS. People value opinions of their close ones high when deciding whether to use an NSS and they also ask them for advice when negotiating.

We were able to obtain these results by giving people a vision of how a new kind of mobile NSS could be used by the help of filmed scenarios. This enables us to inform the design process of our envisioned system in an early stage. After implementing first prototypes in the near future we will be able to investigate more factors, which can only be perceived during the interaction with a prototype, e.g. ease of use. Other aspects to be considered for future research are the influences of educational and cultural background of the user on attitudes towards negotiation and NSS.

Overall, when designing novel, mobile NSS we should aim for creating NSS not merely as tools but as social devices considering the use context and social networks.

Acknowledgments

We thank the project team and all participants of this study. This research is supported by the Dutch Technology Foundation STW, applied science division of NWO and the Technology Program of the Ministry of Economic Affairs. It is part of the Pocket Negotiator project with grant number VICI-project 08075.

References

1. Ajzen, I.: The theory of planned behavior. Organzational Behavior and Human Decision Processes 50, 179–211 (1991)
2. Ajzen, I., Fishbein, M.: Understanding Attitudes and predicting Social Behavior. Prentice-Hall, Englewood Cliffs (1980)
3. Bui, T.: Evaluating negotiation support systems: A conceptualization. In: HICSS 1994. IEEE Computer Society Press, Los Alamitos (1994)
4. Carroll, J.M.: Making Use: Secenrio-based Design of Human-Computer Interactions. MIT Press, Cambridge (2000)
5. Davis, F.: Perceived usefulness, perceived ease of use, and user acceptance of information technology. MIS Quarterly 13(3), 319–339 (1989)

6. Essentials, H.B.S.: Negotiation. Harvard Business School Publishing Corporation, Boston (2003)
7. Hindriks, K., Jonker, C.: Creating human-machine synergy in negotiation support systems: Towards the pocket negotiator. In: HuCom 2008. ACM Press, New York (2008)
8. ITU: Itu internet reports: The portable internet, Tech. rep., ITU (2004), `http://www.itu.int/portableinternet`
9. Kersten, G.: Negotiation support systems and negotiating agents. In: Modles et Systmes Multi-Agents pour la Gestion de lEnvironement et des Territoire (1999)
10. Kersten, G., Lo, G.: Aspire: an integrated negotiation support system and software agents for ebusiness negotiation. International Journal of Internet and Enterprise Management 1(2), 293–315 (2003)
11. Kersten, G.E., Lai, H.: Negotiation support and e-negotiation systems: An overview. Group Decision and Negotiation 16, 553–586 (2007)
12. Ling, R.: "One can talk about common manners!": the use of mobile telephones in inappropriate situations. in themes in mobile telephony. Tech. rep., COST 248 Home and Work group (1997)
13. Love, S., Perry, M.: Dealing with mobile conversations in public places: Some implications for the design of socially intrusive technologies. In: CHI 2004, pp. 1195–1198. ACM Press, New York (2004)
14. Mallat, N., Rossi, M., Tuunainen, V., Rni, A.: The impact of use context on mobile services acceptance: The case of mobile ticketing. Information Management 46, 190–195 (2009)
15. Palen, L., Salzman, M., Youngs, E.: Discovery and integration of mobile communications in everyday life. Personal Ubiquitous Computing 5(2), 109–122 (2001)
16. Parameswaran, M., Whinston, A.: Social computing: An overview. Communications of the Association for Information Systems 19, 762–780 (2007)
17. Pommeranz, A., Brinkman, W., Wiggers, P., Broekens, J., Jonker, C.: Towards design guidelines for negotiation support systems: An expert perspective using scenarios. In: ECCE 2009 (2009)
18. Rangaswamy, A., Shell, G.: Using computers to realize joint gains in negotiations: Towards an electronic bargaining table. Management Science 43(8), 1147–1163 (1997)
19. Schoop, M., Jertila, A., List, T.: Negoisst: a negotiation support system for electronic business-to-business negotiations in e-commerce. Data and Knowledge Engineering 47(3), 371–401 (2001)
20. Srivastava, L.: Mobile phones and the evolution of social behavior. Behaviour and Information Technology 24(2), 111–129 (2005)
21. Swaab, R., Postmes, T., Neijiens, P.: Negotiation support systems: Communication and information as antecedents of negotiation settlement. International Negotiation 9, 59–78 (2004)
22. Thomson, L.: The Heart and Mind of the Negotiator. Pearson, Prentice Hall (2005)
23. Vetschera, R., Kersten, G., Koeszegi, S.: User assessment of internet-based negotiation support systems: An exploratory study. Journal of Oganizational Computing and E-Commerce 16(2), 123–132 (2006)

A   Questionnaire - English Version

(Unless otherwise specified in the footnotes the answers were measured by a 7-point Likert scale)

Item/Construct	Question	Item included
	Before all scenarios	
GEN	What is your gender? (male/female)	
COU	What is your nationality? (open)	
EDU	What is your level of education?	
	(No degree, vocational training, university degree)	
AGE	How old are you? (open)	
CSK	How many hours do you spend using computers per week? (open)	
(NEX)		
NEX 1	How many houses have you sold? (open)	
NEX 2	How many houses have you bought? (open)	
NEX 3	How many job interviews have you had? (open)	
NEX 4	Is negotiation an important part of your job? (yes/no))	
(NAT)		
NAT 1	Negotiation is a game.	
NAT 2	I try to avoid negotiations.	*
NAT 3	I enjoy negotiations.	*
NAT 4	Negotiations are a necessary must.	
(NSK)		
NSK 1	I am a good negotiator.	*
NSK 2	I would rather negotiate myself if the negotiation task is simple.	
NSK 3	I would let someone else negotiate for me if the negotiation task is simple.	
NSK 4	I would rather negotiate myself if the object of the negotiation is important for me.	*
NSK 5	I would let someone else negotiate for me if the object of the negotiation is important for me.	*
	After each scenario	
IU	I would use the Pocket Negotiator (PN) in the situation shown in the video/picture.	
SN	Most people who are important to me would think a Pocket Negotiator is useful in this situation.	
(SA)		
SA 1	I think it is socially acceptable to use a PN in this situation.	*
SA 2	I think the opponent would think it is socially acceptable to use a PN in this situation.	*
Specific		
train	I expect a PN to prepare me in a short (1-2 hours) time before a negotiation.	
f-2-f	A PN would be useful to propose new options for the negotiation.	
coll.prep.	I expect a PN to help me organizing data (e.g. information from the Internet).	
phone	I expect from a PN to give me a clear overview of the negotiation process.	
car dealer	I believe the advice that the PN gives is useful for the negotiation.	
Comment		
COM	Could you please explain what you based your ratings on? (open)	
	After all scenarios	
PNA	My attitude towards using a PN is positive.	
BC		
BC 1	I would probably feel comfortable using a PN on my own.	*
BC 2	Learning to operate a PN would probably be easy for me.	*
BC 3	I would probably understand how to use a PN.	*
USE		
USE 1	A PN would help me to reach a better outcome in a negotiation.	*
USE 2	I would feel more confident in the negotiation while using a PN.	*
USE 3	I will learn how to negotiate better through using the PN.	*
USE 4	Using a PN would increase my productivity.	*
USE 5	Using a PN would increase my negotiation performance.	*
USE 6	Using a PN would enhance my effectiveness in negotiations.	*
USE 7	Using a PN would make negotiations easier for me.	*
USE 8	Overall, I find the PN useful for house/job negotiations.	*
OCM	Please feel free to enter comments here: (open)	

Chances of Increasing Youth Health Awareness through Mobile Wellness Applications

Andreas Holzinger[1,2], Stefan Dorner[1,2], Manuela Födinger[3],
André Calero Valdez[4], and Martina Ziefle[4]

[1] Medical University Graz, A-8036 Graz, Austria
Institute for Medical Informatics (IMI), Research Unit HCI4MED
[2] Graz University of Technology, A-8010 Graz, Austria
Institute for Information Systems and Computer Media (IICM)
andreas.holzinger@medunigraz.at,
sdorner@student.tugraz.at
[3] Kaiser Franz Josef Spital, A-1100 Wien, Institut für Labordiagnostik
manuela.foedinger@wienkav.at
[4] RWTH Aachen University, D-52056 Aachen, Human Technology Centre (Humtec)
{ziefle,calero-valdez}@humtec.rwth-aachen.de

Abstract. The poor general state of health of the Austrian youth – which is possibly representative for the western industrial world – will have dramatic effects on our health care system in years to come. Health risks among adolescents, including smoking, alcohol, obesity, lack of physical activity and an unhealthy diet, will lead to an increase in chronic diseases. A preventive measure against such a development could be to reinforce health awareness through the use of web and mobile applications supporting self observation and behavior change. In this paper, we present an overview of the latest developments in the area of mobile wellness and take a look at the features of applications that constitutes the current state of the art, as well as their shortcomings and ways of overcoming these. Finally, we discuss the possibilities offered by new technological developments in the area of mobile devices and by incorporating the characteristics that make up the Web 2.0.

Keywords: Wellness, Health, mobile computing, self-observation, behavior change, Web 2.0, prevention.

1 Introduction and Motivation for Research

The poor general state of health of Austrian youths will have dramatic effects on our health care system in the future. According to Chini & Dorner from the Austrian Medical Association [1] we will have to face additional costs of 1.6 billion Euros in 2030, increasing to 3.7 billion Euros in 2050.

This will be mainly due to smoking, alcohol, obesity, lack of physical activity and insufficient consumption of fruit, leading to common diseases such as diabetes, hypertension, myocardial infarction, stroke, renal insufficiency, osteoporosis and chronic back. *"Today's unhealthily living youths will be tomorrow's chronically ill"*, as

G. Leitner, M. Hitz, and A. Holzinger (Eds.): USAB 2010, LNCS 6389, pp. 71–81, 2010.

Dr. Walter Dorner, president of the Austrian Medical Association pointed out. This trend will not only lead to increased costs in health care, but it will also result in a lack of available manpower in the job market. As suggested by Chini, these costs should better be reallocated to preventive costs. Through successful prevention, health care costs arising from people older than 65 can be reduced significantly.

A preventive measure against such a development can be by enforcing a permanent change in the lifestyle and health-awareness of adolescents by the use of wellness management and self-observation. Such measures fit well into the description of the health continuum by Saranummi [2], who emphasizes the advantage of proactive management of health and illness compared to reactive action. Saranummi also states that the provision of knowledge and tools for self-management is another important part of the health continuum. This can be achieved through the use of wellness applications that offer their end users assistance in performing self-observation and motivate them to improve their lifestyle over a long-term period. Mobile applications offer some important advantages for this task such as pervasive and permanent availability. In this paper we take a look at the current state of the art in the area of mobile wellness supporting applications.

We describe some features of current applications, the technologies used, as well as the shortcomings these applications may hold and ways of overcoming these. We also take a look at new technological developments in the area of mobile devices and the possibilities they provide, combined with the characteristics that make up the Web 2.0, they offer in the invention of new wellness supporting applications.

2 Related Work: Applications Supporting Health Awareness

During the last years several web and mobile applications have been developed with the aim of supporting self-care. Most of these applications were intended to be used by chronic disease patients, but the main goal of motivating their users to a healthier lifestyle can also be applied to young, healthy individuals. The technologies used for these applications ranged from web services and web applications using RIA (rich internet application) methods to client side technologies such as the Java2 Micro Edition (J2ME) and native client device applications.

2.1 Personal Health Applications

Personal Health Applications (PHAs) allow users to store and manage their personal health information, thereby supporting patient empowerment and facilitating the flow of information between patients and health care providers.

Along with the users' personal data the application can store a variety of health related data like laboratory medical conditions, test results, medications and allergies. Amongst the most prominent of these applications are Google Health, Microsoft HealthVault or LifeSensor. Microsoft's solution puts special effort on the possibility to connect to external health devices including blood pressure monitors, pedometers, glucometers. The main strengths of Google Health are it its ability to connect to external health providers such as hospitals in order to integrate their data as well as the possibility for external applications to access Google Health functions through the Health Data API.

Andry et al (2008), [3] created LifeSensor Diabetes, a web application which is built atop the LifeSensor Personal Health Record (PHR) and the ICW eHealth Framework. Users can start using the application by filling in basic profile information (gender, age, height, weight). They can also specify personal targets for specific diabetes markers. Data that already exist in the user's PHR on LifeSensor can be imported, new data are entered regularly. Since the ICW eHealth Framework supports device integration, the project is working on implementing automatic data gathering from glucometers. The application aims to motivate its users to access their application regularly, so much effort is put into high interactivity und good usability features. To achieve this, modern web technologies including AJAX and FLEX were used for implementing the client application [4], [5]. Another motivating feature is the possibility for users to define action plans that provide them the possibility to plan and track their progress towards achieving defined personal goals.

Analyzing the granularity of the visualized observations showed, that data differed in both the frequency of measurement and the types of values [6]. Some data has to be measured several times a day, while other data will be measured on a yearly basis. The different types of values were assigned to two different types of graphs: health targets (e.g. blood glucose or cholesterol) can be represented using 2D line charts and candle-like charts, activities (e.g. exercise, diet or medication) were assigned ordinal values (poor, fair, good, very good) and displayed using histograms. The visualization itself is handled by a generic graph container which can display one or two modules out of eight currently implemented modules (exercise, diet, medication, blood glucose, weight, cholesterol, HbA1c, blood pressure / heart rate). By displaying two modules inside the same container and synchronizing their time axis, data correlations can be discovered visually.

2.2 Mobile Applications Supporting Wellness

The rapid improvement of mobile devices regarding their usability and their technological abilities as well as their high pervasiveness and availability makes them a popular platform for wellness supporting applications. The Wellness Diary as described by [7], [8] is a mobile application that can be used for recording and managing personal health data. The system is able to monitor weight, exercise, diet, alcohol usage, sleep, smoking, stress and step data per default, but it is also customizable, so users are able to adapt the data model to their needs and preferences. The mobile application is no web application but a standalone application storing the data, which is manually entered by the user, on the mobile device itself.

The developers also created a web service counterpart to the mobile application that allows for data synchronization between the mobile device and a central server.

iBody [9] is a commercial iPhone application and makes use of the GPS functionality provided by the iPhone. The application allows to monitor various sportive activities including running or cycling. GPS is used in order to track the covered route and distance. The measured distance combined with information about the type of activity and the user's weight can then be used to calculate the calorie consumption. It is also possible to view the route covered in Google Maps. Similar to other wellness supporting applications, one can enter health related data, e.g. body weight, adipose, blood pressure, pulse or blood-test results and offers graphical reports of these.

2.3 Mobile Applications for People with Chronic Diseases

The majority of mobile health supporting applications found, are not aimed at supporting healthy people in their daily wellness related activities but rather in supporting people with chronic diseases and people recovering from certain illnesses. Despite the different target groups, their goals, namely patient empowerment and motivation, are largely the same.

Walters et al. (2010) [10] developed a mobile application, based on Wellness Diary used for home-based care of cardiac rehabilitation patients. The application is able to monitor blood pressure through an external device and to estimate physical activity through a step counter provided by the mobile phone. Additionally to these automatically measured data the patients can manually enter other parameters like weight, body fat percentage, additional exercise information, stress, sleep times and tiredness as well as nutritional, smoking and alcohol consumption information. Weekly consultations with their mentor who is able to access all entered data helps in setting reasonable goals and discuss the progress toward recent goals. The project also makes use of motivational and multimedia messages provided by the mentor through the mobile phone. The mentored phase lasts for 6 weeks but the patients are encouraged to keep using the application for self management.

The Confidant system by [11] is another mobile application used for chronic disease management. Similar to the cardiac rehabilitation application by [10] it combines collected (blood glucose, blood pressure, weight) and manually entered (count, customized questions) data with the informative messages provided on a daily basis. The application consists of two communicating modules, a native client-side program and a server application running on a web server.

A rich internet application (RIA) developed by [12] and usable on handheld devices aims to bring modern RIA technology into the fields of telemedicine and mobile health. Their web based application enables a communication path between handheld devices and hospital information systems.

Some of their main aims for this system were to enable access to medical data, to tele-consultation as well as to educational means.

By creating a web based application suited to be used by mobile devices, no installation on the client side was required and the application was independent of platform and hardware. Due to the outsourcing of application logic to the mobile client less network traffic was needed and the server side application gained higher scalability. The main technologies used were a content management system (CMS) using Adobe Flex and a mobile application using the Flash Lite platform.

The Diabetes Living Assistant by Calero-Valdez et al. [13], [14] is a diabetes management program developed with Java2ME for mobile devices.

It includes a diabetes diary, health parameter-tracking, BE-calculator and a reminder tool for medical intake. It also includes graphical analyses for key health factors. The diabetes diary goes beyond simple tracking and logging of glucose readings and food intake by suggesting adjusted insulin dosages in regard to current glucose measurement, activity level and planned eating, thus simplifying the patients tedious calculations for everyday insulin administration (see Fig. 1).

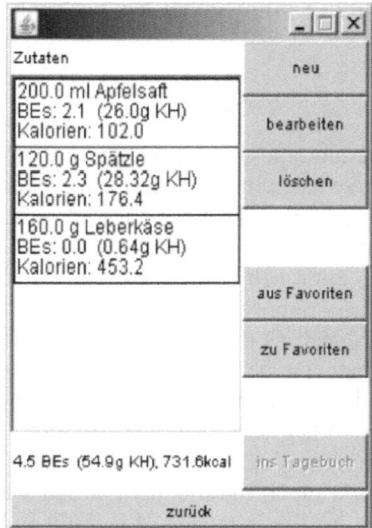 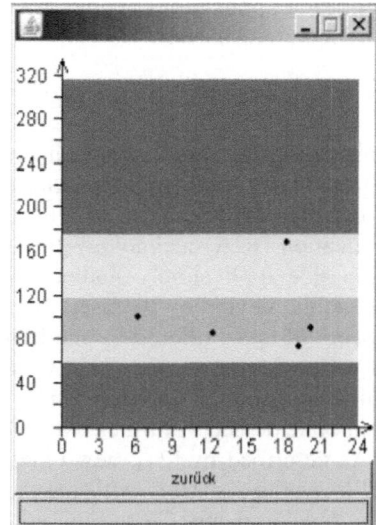

Fig. 1. Screenshots of the Diabetes management program showing the "Favorite Dishes" (left) and "Graphical Analysis" (right) function of the device

BE-calculations are also simplified by allowing users to store and retrieve favorite dishes and use them in the diary. In order to ease switching from paper-based tracking to a mobile device, user interface layouts are based on the commonly used paper-based diabetes diaries. Acceptance testing of a prototype of the Diabetes Living Assistant yielded good acceptance rates [15].

3 Potential for Improvement

3.1 Results from User Studies on Wellness Applications

A number of user experience studies on Wellness Diary [16], [17], [18] and [19] have been performed and [20] present concepts to improve the application based on the received feedback. One of their main improvement aims was to increase the long-term motivation of their users. Furthermore, many users did not use the application regularly due to forgetfulness or during their holidays. According to the authors, long-lasting motivation could be achieved by making the application generally more enjoyable to use. Another flaw of current wellness applications was the users' effort of entering wellness data that was by far too high as compared to the results obtained from the application. Features that could increase the motivation of the users might be alarms, rewards and detailed analysis of the user data. A high level of interactivity is also regarded as a good means of motivating users to continue using the wellness application.

Regarding user support by mentors, the study done by [17] showed two different user positions. While some users preferred to use the application privately, others would welcome professional feedback on their data. Considering this result, wellness supporting applications should allow the possibility of professional feedback but not force it onto its users.

3.2 Impact of New Technologies

Considering the rapid advancement in mobile technologies, using a web application instead of an application running on the client device will increase the number of applicable mobile devices to all offering a supported browser. By using rich internet application (RIA) technology the application can offer the look and feel of a pure client side application. Another advantage of this approach is that no installation on the mobile device by the user will be necessary. As opposed to this approach is the concept of apps, offered by modern smart phones such as the iPhone or phones running Google's Android – native applications that can be easily acquired through online app stores. Developing such native apps allows the application to better utilize the mobile device's abilities but makes porting it to other devices more difficult.

As described by [21], new emerging interface technologies including multi-touch and low priced sensors will make user interaction a much more enjoyable feature of new developments. Gesture-based devices including the Nintendo Wii, built-in pedometers and GPS enabled mobile devices offer new possibilities of integrating physical activity into future wellness applications. Similar to the utilization of a step counter by the application developed by [10], new tools may use GPS to track the user's running activity, including speed and distance. The W3C Geolocation API [22] provides support for retrieving and working with location information inside web pages using JavaScript and is already supported by the major browsers.

This location information can not only be retrieved from IP addresses but can also utilize GPS data as provided by many mobile devices. Employing these new ways of gathering activity data can significantly decrease the effort of entering wellness relevant data into a mobile device.

In March 2010 Nintendo released two games (Pokémon HeartGold and Pokémon SoulSilver) for their mobile gaming platform Nintendo DS that require the usage of a pedometer for game success and is aimed at the younger audience (ESRB-Rating: E). The player takes out one of his virtual pets on a walk in order to train the pet to become stronger inside the game and to earn virtual currency within the game. Players can also engage in competition with each other comparing the strength of their virtual pets. Bayer also released a Nintendo DS game, which in conjunction with a special glucosemeter, teaches children with diabetes good glucose testing habits. Regular testing is rewarded with in-game bonus points that can be redeemed both inside the game and on a social networking site for kids with diabetes. Effectiveness of educational gaming has been studied with stationary gaming consoles for teaching health related topics in general [23] and for diabetes in particular [24] leading to positive changes in behavior, self-efficacy and communication with parents.

Web 2.0, often also called the "social web", is described by several characteristics [25] including collaborative activity, greater levels of participation and high interactivity as well as high applicability in educational settings [26]. These attributes can be seen in applications including wikis, blogs, podcasts, social bookmarking, collaborative tagging, social networking and online social gaming. These applications can play a significant role in providing more motivational features in wellness supporting applications.

While wikis, blogs, podcasts or social bookmarking can be employed in order to give the user access to information about all aspects of their personal wellness, social networking allows them to share their experience and efforts with other same minded users. Several studies suggest, that peer groups can have a significant effect on the weight of adolescents, especially of females [27], [28]. Social networks could utilize this effect in order to support a healthier lifestyle. Online social gaming can increase the fun effect of their activities while offering a good opportunity to include a system of goals and rewards, thereby offering strong incentives for a long-term use of the application. A social game with a competitive character about the accomplishment of goals can offer very high motivation to its users.

The combination of the possibilities of modern mobile devices including GPS, cameras or step counters with aspects of Web 2.0 like social networking or social gaming offers very interesting possibilities for future wellness supporting applications. [21] describes Geocaching, an outdoor sport similar to a paper chase game which combines GPS with social gaming in order to create a game encouraging physical activity together with like-minded people.

3.3 Abilities, Motivation and Cognitive Mindsets for Health Awareness

So far, this paper discuss new mobile applications, and devices, which had been developed to support health-related behaviors. The availability of mobile technical solutions is definitely an important way to increase the general health awareness.

However, there is also another component, which should be considered and adequately addressed when designing and developing new health applications and interfaces. However, from a psychological point of view, we should be aware that the usage of (mobile) technology, their success and sustainability, strongly depends on the extent to which human properties -cognitive, affective and motivational aspects- are taken into account. Even though mobile technology and mobile applications are one of the fastest growing industrial sectors ever, considerable friction losses with respect to usability concerns are to be noticed [29], [30], [31]. Users often get stuck and overwhelmed when using technical devices and need to be supported to come to terms with sophisticated technology [32]. The still-present gap between technological genius and usability demands might represent a serious obstacle for the acceptance of technology by a broad user group if not adequately addressed by designers and manufacturers [33]. Devices must meet the demands and cognitive abilities of a broad user group and respond to users' diversity likewise. As long as mobile interface and information designs are not easy to use, technical innovations will not have sustained success. One may argue that the usability problem will vanish whenever the old technically inexperienced generation died off, relying on the idea that children and teens, which have a different technical upbringing and used to technology from early on might less affected by a low interface usability. Even though technical experience is definitely advantageous for device handling, see e.g. [34] it could be shown that especially children and teenagers are highly sensitive for suboptimal user interface design [35], [36]. Facing an increase in the usability of functions announced by manufacturers, this is of central interest. Independently of which and how many functions will be implemented in future devices, Coopers' (1999), [37] warning will have to be exigently followed: 'You can predict which features in any new technology will get used and which not. The usage of features is inversely proportional to the amount of interaction needed to control it' (Cooper, 1999, p. 33).

In addition to the ease of using aspect, mobile health applications should be developed in a way that users want to use it. This seems of specific impact in the context of disease management and health behaviours. Within public perception, the prevalent image of medical technology still is stigmatizing, intrusive, and difficult to use. Also, using medical technology is seen as a necessary evil, and only tolerated when patients do not have any alternatives. In this sense, medical technology is functional, but associated with disease and health deficits [38]. Especially, the implementation of mobile wellness applications requires a broadening of the classical focus and should include emotional or affective designs. In this perspective, the quality of "good interfaces" relies on more than the orientation on mere functional aspects, but the inclusion of hedonic aspects emphasizing individuals' well-being, pleasure and fun [39]. Accordingly, studies show that users desire more than the mere functioning of technology, but prefer interfaces with a high social or hedonic value. Hedonic functions are providing stimulation, identity, and valuable memories [40], [41], [42].

A medical application or device, which is joyful to use, which is elegant and "cool", would definitely increase the motivation for using it and the compliance behaviors regarding health and disease management.

By combining positive characteristics and human desires with medical engineering, the medical application would be redefined from being a marker of shortcomings and deficits to a driver of individual quality of life decisions [38].

A vivid and very convincing example for such an approach can be seen is the piano staircase (http://www.thefuntheory.com/piano-staircase). The grounding question of this showcase was whether we can we get more people to choose the stairs over the escalator by making it fun to do. The on-site scene is at a Swedish underground stop over, at which the stairs were transformed to huge piano keys. Each step on these keys resulted in a tone. The question whether hedonic interfaces would motivate people to behave „healthy" by choosing the stairs over the escalator can be clearly answered. 66% more people chose the stairs, and the video clips taken from there show that the enthusiasm about choosing the stairs was high, independently of the age and culture of the pedestrians.

4   Conclusion

Supporting adolescents in leading a healthier lifestyle is an essential preventive measure against the development of chronic diseases. This proactive way of health management can be an important factor in the reduction of future health care costs. One way of providing this support can be through the use of a mobile application. Mobile devices offer the advantage of high pervasiveness, especially in our target group of adolescents. There are already a number of applications for personal health support like Personal Health Applications, mobile applications for persons with chronic diseases and also some mobile wellness supporting applications. A very important factor for the success of such applications is their ability to motivate people to use them constantly and over a long time. The combination of aspects of Web 2.0 like social networking or social gaming with technological features of mobile devices like GPS, cameras or step counters offers very interesting possibilities for making wellness supporting applications motivating and even fun to use for young people.

References

1. Chini, L. W., Dorner, W.: Kranke Kinder, was tun? Bessere Prävention macht auch Volkswirtschaft gesünder, Pressetext 2010-03-23, `http://www.aerztekammer.at` (last access: 2010-08-19)
2. Saranummi, N.: IT applications for pervasive, personal, and personalized health. IEEE Transactions on Information Technology in Biomedicine 12(1), 1–4 (2008)
3. Andry, F., Freeman, L., Gillson, J., Kienitz, J., Lee, M., Naval, G., Nicholson, D.: Highly-Interactive and User-Friendly Web Application for People with Diabetes. In: IEEE International Conference on Communication Systems, HEALTHCOM 2008, pp. 118–120 (2008)
4. Holzinger, A., Hoeller, M., Bloice, M., Urlesberger, B.: Typical Problems with developing mobile applications for health care: Some lessons learned from developing user-centered mobile applications in a hospital environment. In: Filipe, J., Marca, D.A., Shishkov, B., Sinderen, M.v. (eds.) International Conference on E-Business (ICEB 2008), pp. 235–240. IEEE, Los Alamitos (2008)
5. Holzinger, A., Mayr, S., Slany, W., Debevc, M.: The influence of AJAX on Web Usability ICEB, pp. 124–127. IEEE, Los Alamitos (2010)
6. Mandryk, R.L., Atkins, M.S.: A fuzzy physiological approach for continuously modeling emotion during interaction with play technologies. International Journal of Human-Computer Studies 65(4), 329–347 (2007)
7. Koskinen, E., Sahninen, J.: A customizable mobile tool for supporting health behavior interventions. In: 2007 Annual International Conference of the IEEE Engineering in Medicine and Biology Society, vol. 1-16, pp. 5908–5911. IEEE, Los Alamitos (2007)
8. Yang, Y.: The design and implementation of a Web mobile-based behavior change application system. In: 5th International Conference on Information Technology and Applications in Biomedicine (ITAB 2008) in Conjunction with 2nd International Symposium & Summer School on Biomedical and Health Engineering (IS3BHE 2008), pp. 491–494. IEEE, Los Alamitos (2008)
9. Welsch, H., Müller, K.: iBody, `http://www.ihanwel.com/?page_id=269` (last access: 2010-08-19)
10. Walters, D.L., Sarela, A., Fairfull, A., Neighbour, K., Cowen, C., Stephens, B., Sellwood, T., Sellwood, B., Steer, M., Aust, M., Francis, R., Lee, C.K., Hoffman, S., Brealey, G., Karunanithi, M.: A mobile phone-based care model for outpatient cardiac rehabilitation: the care assessment platform (CAP). BMC Cardiovascular Disorders 10 (2010)
11. Katz, D.L., Nordwall, B.: Novel interactive cell-phone technology for health enhancement. Journal of Diabetes Science and Technology 2(1), 147–153 (2008)
12. Constantinescu, L., Pradana, R., Kim, J., Gong, P., Fulham, M., Feng, D.: Rich internet application system for patient-centric healthcare data management using handheld devices EMBC. In: 2009 IEEE Engineering in Medicine and Biology Society, pp. 5167–5170 (2009)
13. Calero-Valdez, A., Ziefle, M., Alagöz, F., Holzinger, A.: Mental Models of Menu Structures in Diabetes Assistants. In: Miesenberger, K., Klaus, J., Zagler, W., Karshmer, A. (eds.) ICCHP 2010. LNCS, vol. 6180, pp. 584–591. Springer, Heidelberg (2010)
14. Calero Valdez, A., Ziefle, M., Horstmann, A., Herding, D., Schroeder, U.: Effects of Aging and Domain Knowledge on Usability in Small Screen Devices for Diabetes Patients. In: Holzinger, A., Miesenberger, K. (eds.) USAB 2009. LNCS, vol. 5889, pp. 366–386. Springer, Heidelberg (2009)

15. Calero-Valdez, A., Ziefle, M., Schroeder, U., Horstmann, A., Herding, D.: Task perform-
    ance in mobile and ambient interfaces. In: IEEE International Conference of the I-Society,
    Does size matter for usability of electronic diabetes assistants? Full paper at the, IEEE
    (2010) (in press)
16. Mattila, E., Korhonen, I., Lappalainen, R., Ahtinen, A., Hopsu, L., Leino, T.: IEEE, Nuadu
    Concept for Personal Management of Lifestyle Related Health Risks. In: 2008 30th An-
    nual International Conference of the IEEE Engineering in Medicine and Biology Society,
    vol. 1-8, pp. 5846–5850. IEEE, Los Alamitos (2008)
17. Mattila, E., Parkka, J., Hermersdorf, M., Kaasinen, J., Vainio, J., Samposalo, K., Merilahti,
    J., Kolari, J., Kulju, M., Lappalainen, R., Korhonen, K.: Mobile diary for wellness man-
    agement - Results on usage and usability in two user studies. IEEE Transactions on Infor-
    mation Technology in Biomedicine 12(4), 501–512 (2008)
18. Ahtinen, A., Ramiah, S., Blom, J., Isomursu, M.: Design of mobile wellness applications:
    identifying cross-cultural factors. In: Proceedings of the 20th Australasian Conference on
    Computer-Human Interaction: Designing for Habitus and Habitat, pp. 164–171 (2008)
19. Ahtinen, A., Mattila, E., Vaatanen, A., Hynninen, L., Salminen, J., Koskinen, E., Laine,
    K.: User experiences of mobile wellness applications in health promotion: User study of
    Wellness Diary, Mobile Coach and SelfRelax Pervasive Computing Technologies for
    Healthcare. In: 3rd International Conference on Pervasive Health 2009, pp. 1–8 (2009)
20. Mattila, E., Korhonen, I., Salminen, J.H., Ahtinen, A., Koskinen, E., Sarela, A., Parkka, J.,
    Lappalainen, R.: Empowering Citizens for Well-being and Chronic Disease Management
    With Wellness Diary. IEEE Transactions on Information Technology in Biomedi-
    cine 14(2), 456–463 (2010)
21. Falchuk, B.: Visual and interaction design themes in mobile healthcare. In: 2009 6th An-
    nual International Mobile and Ubiquitous Systems: Networking & Services, MobiQuitous
    2009, pp. 1–10. IEEE, Los Alamitos (2009)
22. Popescu, A.: Geolocation API Specification,
    http://www.w3.org/TR/geolocation-API/ (last access: 2010-08-19)
23. Lieberman, D.A.: Interactive video games for health promotion: Effects on knowledge,
    self-efficacy, social support, and health. In: Street, R.L., Gold, W.R., Manning, T. (eds.)
    Health Promotion and Interactive Technology: Theoretical Applications and Future Direc-
    tions. Lawrence Erlbaum, Mahwah (1997)
24. Brown, S.J., Lieberman, D.A., Gemeny, B.A., Fan, Y.C., Wilson, D.M., Pasta, D.J.: Edu-
    cational video game for juvenile diabetes: Results of a controlled trial. Medical Informat-
    ics 22(1), 77–89 (1997)
25. Ward, R., Moule, P., Lockyer, L.: Adoption of Web 2.0 Technologies in Education for
    Health Professionals in the UK: Where are we and why? Academic Conferences Ltd.,
    Reading (2008)
26. Holzinger, A., Kickmeier-Rust, M.D., Ebner, M.: Interactive Technology for Enhancing
    Distributed Learning: A Study on Weblogs. In: HCI 2009 The 23nd British HCI Group
    Annual Conference, pp. 309–312 (2009)
27. Trogdon, J.G., Nonnemaker, J., Pais, J.: Peer effects in adolescent overweight. Journal of
    Health Economics 27(5), 1388–1399 (2008)
28. Renna, F., Grafova, I.B., Thakur, N.: The effect of friends on adolescent body weight.
    Economics & Human Biology 6(3), 377–387 (2008)
29. Ziefle, M., Bay, S.: How older adults meet complexity: aging effects on the usability of
    different mobile phones. Behaviour & Information Technology 24(5), 375–389 (2005)
30. Ziefle, M., Bay, S.: How to overcome disorientation in mobile phone menus: A compari-
    son of two different types of navigation aids. Human Computer Interaction 21(4), 393–432
    (2006)

31. Holzinger, A., Searle, G., Kleinberger, T., Seffah, A., Javahery, H.: Investigating Usability Metrics for the Design and Development of Applications for the Elderly. In: Miesenberger, K. (ed.) ICCHP 2008. LNCS, vol. 5105, pp. 98–105. Springer, Heidelberg (2008)
32. Ziefle, M., Bay, S.: Transgenerational Designs in Mobile Technology. In: Lumsden, J. (ed.) Handbook of Research on User Interface Design and Evaluation for Mobile Technology, pp. 122–140. IGI Global (2008)
33. Arning, K., Ziefle, M.: Barriers of information access in small screen device applications: The relevance of user characteristics for a transgenerational design. In: Stephanidis, C., Pieper, M. (eds.) ERCIM Ws UI4ALL 2006. LNCS, vol. 4397, pp. 117–136. Springer, Heidelberg (2007)
34. Ziefle, M.: The influence of user expertise and phone complexity on performance, ease of use and learnability of different mobile phones. Behaviour & Information Technology 21(5), 303–311 (2002)
35. Bay, S., Ziefle, M.: Children Using Cellular Phones. The Effects of shortcomings in user Interface Design. Human Factors 47(1), 158–168 (2005)
36. Bay, S., Ziefle, M.: Landmarks or surveys? The impact of different instructions on children's performance in hierarchical menu structures. Computers in Human Behavior 24(3), 1246–1274 (2008)
37. Cooper, A.: The Inmates are Running the Asylum: Why High-Tech Products Drive Us Crazy and How to Restore the Sanity. Sams, Indianapolis (IN) (1999)
38. Borchers, J., Jakobs, E.-M., Ziefle, M., Russell, P., Schmitz-Rode, T.: Health@Home. Technology supporting personal quality of life decisions. White Paper at RWTH Aachen University, Germany (2010)
39. Ziefle, M., Jakobs, E.-M.: New challenges in Human Computer Interaction: Strategic Directions and Interdisciplinary Trends. In: 4th International Conference on Competitive Manufacturing Technologies, pp. 389–398 (2010)
40. Hassenzahl, M.: The effect of perceived hedonic quality on product appealingness. International Journal of Human-Computer Interaction 13(4), 481–499 (2001)
41. Hassenzahl, M.: The Thing and I: Understanding the relationship between user and product. In: Blyhte, M.A., Overbeeke, K., Monk, A.F., Wright, P.C. (eds.) Funology. From Usability to Enjoyment, pp. 31–42. Kluwer, Dordrecht (2004)
42. Wright, P., Mc Carthy, J., Meekinson, L.: Making sense of experience. In: Blyhte, M.A., Overbeeke, K., Monk, A.F., Wright, P.C. (eds.) Funology. From Usability to Enjoyment, pp. 43–53. Kluwer, Dordrecht (2005)

A Small but Significant Difference – The Role of Gender on Acceptance of Medical Assistive Technologies

Wiktoria Wilkowska, Sylvia Gaul, and Martina Ziefle

RWTH Aachen University
Communication Science, Human Technology Centre (HumTec),
Theaterplatz 14, 52056 Aachen, Germany
{Wilkowska,Gaul,Ziefle}@humtec.rwth-aachen.de

Abstract. The current research aimed to study user diversity with a focus on gender differences in adoption of medical assistive technologies in general, and in particular. In order to understand the gender impact, we conducted two consecutive studies and considered gender as a key moderator of acceptance aspects in the medical context. The first study focused on general aspects of medical technology acceptability: users' willingness to use it, the importance of privacy and trust as well as the general attitude across gender and specified age groups. For a deeper insight into this topic the second study was conducted in order to analyze gendered acceptance on specific health-related device. As results showed people's general attitude towards medical technology and their willingness to use such medical assisting devices is throughout positive. However, gender differences emerge at the time when it comes to an assessment of a concrete medical tool (here smart textiles).

Keywords: Gender, smart home technology, privacy, trust, control, perceived usefulness, TAM, medical technology, smart textiles.

1 Introduction

Adoption of medical assistive devices is an important topic when facing the profound demographic changes in many countries of the world and the considerable bottlenecks arising from the fact that increasingly fewer people are present which may take over the nursing and decreasing supply shortfalls of societal health insurance funds [1]. As several studies in the last years have shown, technology acceptance is a crucial factor for a successful rollout of medical technologies, like for instance electronic health systems (ehealth), smart health, ambient assisted living (AAL), or personal health care systems [2], [3], [4], [5], [6]. Although in the past decades there is growing academic research and societal interest in understanding factors that determine acceptance in this sensitive context of medical assistive devices for elderly people, there is still a great demand for further researches and deeper insights.

In this paper two studies are presented focusing on two points that have not been really considered in the recent literature on acceptance of medical assistive technology yet – especially in their combination – namely age and gender. Before presenting

G. Leitner, M. Hitz, and A. Holzinger (Eds.): USAB 2010, LNCS 6389, pp. 82–100, 2010.

those, the underlying principles and theories of technology acceptance as well as the specifics regarding medical context of it are described. And also, the role of gender in acceptance research will be illustrated.

1.1 Technology Acceptance

The technology acceptance model (TAM) [7] and its refinement UTAUT [8], [9] build the theoretical framework in this research. TAM states that the perceived ease of using a system and the perceived usefulness are the key components of technology acceptance. However, with increasing diversity of users as well as diversity of technical systems (visible vs. invisible, local vs. distributed) and using contexts (fun and entertainment, medical, office, mobility) the end-users are confronted with, more aspects might be relevant for understanding their acceptance patterns – beyond the ease of using a system and the perceived usefulness. For this purpose, user characteristics (economic status, culture, gender, age, experience, and the voluntariness of system usage) had been added to the original model and considered in the comprehensive UTAUT-model [9].

With regard to technology acceptance within the medical context several studies were concerned with acceptance of medical and ehealth technologies from the human perspective [10], [11], [12], [13], [14]. Outcomes showed that it is highly questionable that acceptance for medical technologies can be fully understood on the base of the prevailing knowledge of technology acceptance drivers so far. Rather, the acceptance for medical technology sector seems to be more complex than it is for other technical systems, out of different reasons.

A first argument in this context is that ehealth technologies predominately address seniors, who are increasingly prone to diseases with increasing age. Ageing, dependency and illness are – still – negatively connoted in our societies and thus, they carry a stigmatizing potential, which could impact the acceptance of medical technology. Therefore, apart from ageing as a biological factor there is a great need for identification of the supposed stigmatizing factors that prevail in societal culture and cognitive models, in order to counteract these and adequately consider in development and design of medical supporting devices. Last but not least there is a prominent need for an age-sensitive communication concept, which provides reliable and updated information about technical developments in the medical sector and their benefits as well as drawbacks.

A second reason for the higher complexity of technology acceptance in medical context refers to the fact that many technologies incorporated in smart homes (walls, furniture or clothes) might overstep personal intimacy limits and result in justifiable worries about privacy, intimacy and loss of control. Until recently, the most privacy-related aspects in the research concern individual data protection needs in terms of security requirements (e.g., [15]). However, user's perception of privacy needs in terms of intimacy and unobservability with respect to medical technology usage has not been appropriately considered yet. The intension to optimize acceptance in this regard makes it therefore indispensable to take users' subjective perceived importance of privacy and their preference to be or not to be seen by others while using medical device into account.

Furthermore, it should be considered that the status of health and resulting feelings of independency or dependency on technology could additionally impact the general attitude towards and, by this, the willingness to accept and to use ehealth applications. For similar reasons, the question of trust in medical technology arises. Trusting a technology means to believe that a tool, machine or equipment will not fail [16], [17]. It can be assumed for certain that nobody would accept and rely on technology, which is not satisfactorily reliable and/or appropriately certified by accredited test institute, especially when it is the matter of one's own health. Thus, understanding trust in relation to other aspects of the health care systems is important for the assessment and design and provides insights into how medical technologies may be used.

Finally, and this is of specific interest in the present study, the acceptance of medical technology might be also influenced by age and gender.

1.2 The Gender Impact on Use of Technology

The impact of gender on the acceptance of medical technologies is, until now, not widely examined. A few studies focused on gender differences in attitudes towards ageing concepts and related medical care respectively life-prolonging technologies. Studies revealed that women in general were less likely to want treatments to prolong life [18], [19]. Further, women voiced "other oriented" reasons for their opposition, particularly not wanting to be a burden for others [20].

Another aspect concerning usage of medical technology that is widely examined is the gender difference in the (social) ageing process. Elderly men reveal to have more problems organizing their daily life when living alone, due to the fact that most of the required activities were in the traditional role allocation the wife's part. This is also the reason why women in older age have fewer problems to maintain social contacts although they are living alone [21]. Regarding coping strategies, there are also significant gender differences, since women tend to search for help in their social environment more often than men do [22].

Gender differences concerning the use of technology and the attitude towards technology is another broad research field. Whereas gender is widely researched in the context of information technologies, it has not been subject studies on acceptance of medical technologies, yet.

Several studies revealed that men have a greater interest and a more positive attitude regarding computer usage, due to a higher self-esteem and greater experience with information technologies [23], [24]. In the context of technology adoption in workplace studies showed that there are different aspects that influence the decision to adopt new computer technologies of men and women. For men it is mainly their attitude towards using a new technology whereas women are more influenced by subjective norm and behavioral control [25], [26].

With regard to technology acceptance within the medical context it seems to be necessary to not just notify, whether gender differences regarding the willingness to adopt these technologies exist, but to get a deeper understanding of the underlying principles of why they exist.

Assuming that women and men may draw on different aspects of their identities, life-experiences and knowledge base when considering the complexity associated with acceptance of medical technologies, it seems to be reasonable to examine gender in combination with age.

1.3 Questions Addressed

For the evaluation of acceptance regarding ehealth technologies, especially age and gender are assumed to play a prominent part. However, different age groups may consider medical assistive technology from different perspectives of perception. In the same way it could be assumed that men and women differ in their perception of medical devices due to their social roles and (technical) experiences. Furthermore, gender roles may vary between age groups, as well as perception and assessment of medical technologies that goes in hand with it.

For young and technology-experienced adults (about 20-30 years of age), which are not personally affected by the necessity of usage medical devices in the near future, the medical technology could represent highly useful and appropriate technological solutions for societal health-related problems. The middle-aged adults (about 45-60 years of age) could adopt another attitude: as they have the duty to care for their older parents, medical technologies could support the well-being of their parents by monitoring critical bodily functions, reminding of medication, etc. In addition, modern medical technologies could help save them costs (e.g. for nursing homes) and could spare them family caring duties. Finally, from the perspective of the older adults (70+ years olds) still different and controversial aspects could impact the degree of medical technology acceptance. On the one hand, medical technologies could allow them to feel safe in the privacy of one's home and to stay independently from the help of others. On the other hand, feelings of being permanently controlled in combination with low trust in technology could provoke ambivalent feelings towards medical technologies.

From these considerations arises the question of "how much impact has user diversity with particular attention to gender divergence on acceptance and usage behavior of medical technologies?" These factors should be examined in the following two studies.

2 Study 1

In the first study we attend to examine the general attitude towards usage of assistive medical technologies (e.g. blood pressure meter) with regard to user diversity (gender, age). Firstly, effects of age and gender on the attitude towards and the willingness to use this kind of technical devices are assessed. Later on, effects of the same users' characteristics are verified with respect to acceptability aspects like importance of privacy, trust in system's reliability and the perceived necessity of control of own health status.

2.1 Method

Questionnaire. As the method to collect the data we chose a questionnaire. The questionnaire was developed as a result of previously conducted focus groups, whereby specific details and information about peoples' perception and opinions about medical technologies were collected.

The questionnaire was formulated in German – the native language of all participants. It contained closed questions about attitudes toward technology, in general, and about the (intended) usage of assistive medical devices, in particular. Regarding medical technology usage, questions were designed to measure the attitude towards, and the willingness to use medical technology. Respondents had to express their degree of approval or rejection on a 5-point Likert-scale (from 'I fully agree' to 'I do not agree at all') rating statements like for instance: "Medical assistance devices enable older or diseased persons to improve their life quality by keeping them longer independent from health care facilities", "I would rather use/learn to use medical assistance technology than become burden to my family or friends".

In addition, the questionnaire explored the role of aspects, which are potentially highly associated with usability and a successful rollout of medical devices. These are the importance of privacy (= not being seen as diseased using medical device), the question of trust (= degree of confidence about device's reliability) and the perceived control (= periodical health check on selected vital functions). The items were designed in terms of usage motives and were to be rated on a 5-point Likert-scale like above. Here are some examples:

- -"I would not / I do not use medical devices because I do not wish other people to see that I am ill or diseased" (privacy),
- -"I (would) use medical devices because it gives me the feeling of a better control over my critical vital bodily functions" (control),
- -"I (would) use a medical device only when it is trustworthy certificated and satisfactory attested"(trust).

In order to assure that all participants respond to the asked questions about usage motives, a previous scenario introduced them to empathize with a chronically ill person, who's health status requires regular collection and storing of vital parameters data (blood pressure meter, pulse, body temperature and weight). In this way each respondent felt involved and the results brought a broad range of comprehensive opinions with regard to (anticipated) medical technology usage behavior.

Before distributing, the questionnaire was revised by an usability expert with respect to issues of comprehensibility and wording of items, and it was test-run by a sample of different aged adults (n = 12). The fill in took 20-30 minutes.

Variables. In the first instance we refer to the *independent variables*. As the topic of the current paper is to identify – when existent – gender differences in usage or intention to use medical devices, the parameter gender is considered as an independent variable in all statistical analyses. Moreover, aspiring high diversity of the respondents and, consequently, a wide spectrum of differently founded perspectives, different aged persons were addressed in the survey, and age itself was analyzed as independent variable too. Thereby, four age groups with varying technical backgrounds and technical affinity were built: (1) the group of the youngest respondents, (2) the younger middle-aged group, (3) the older middle-aged group, and (4) the oldest age group. A detailed description of these age groups is given in the following section.

As *dependent variables* firstly the general attitude towards medical technology usage was assessed (built as the sum of items with respect to usefulness, necessity, perceived advantages and benefits; Cronbach's α = .93). Secondly, influence of age and gender on the willingness to use medical assistance was analyzed (differently poled items regarding, amongst others, the readiness for monitoring of vital functions, preference for medical attendance: nursing vs. medical devices; Cronbach's α = .77). And thirdly, the impact of independent variables on aspects of privacy, control and trust in context of medical technology usage – as exemplarily showed above – was examined.

Participants. In the first place it is noteworthy that – according to the comments of people asked to participate in this survey – participants showed an extraordinary high interest for the topic and a high motivation to join this research. This motivation reflects an evident public awareness of societal needs for medical technology, but also a controversy of attitudes within this topic.

The sample consisted of 126 participants, aged between 20 and 80 years with the overall proportion of 46% female and 54% male respondents. For the purpose of statistical analyses in order to find relevant effects with respect to the diversity of (potential) users of healthcare related devices or applications, the sample was split in four age groups, whereby the division corresponds approximately to the current demographical proportion of younger in comparison to older people. The first and *the youngest* age group contains $n = 25$ persons aged between 20 and 30 years ($M = 26.3$, $SD = 2.7$; 40% female). The second age group – *the younger middle-aged* – consists of $n = 41$ of 31-45 year-olds ($M = 37.3$, $SD = 4.9$; 49% female). The third age group ($n = 36$) – we call them *the older middle-aged* – is composed of males (55%) and females (45%) at the age between 46 and 60 years ($M = 53.8$, $SD = 4.4$). And finally *the oldest* age group is made up of $n = 24$ respondents within the age range between 61 and 80 years including 50% women and 50% men ($M = 68.9$, $SD = 5.3$).

Participants were reached on different ways using advertisement in local newspapers (Aachen, Germany), authors' existing network as well as social contacts of respondents, which were asked to pass the information of recruitment by interest on to their family members and friends. There was not other gratification than a "thank-you-very-much" for the participation.

The sample covered a broad range of professions (from teachers, engineers, physicians, notaries, university lecturers trough office administrators, nurses, police officers to hairdressers, farmers and housekeepers) and according to this a broad range of different educational levels as well as economic backgrounds (see figure 1).

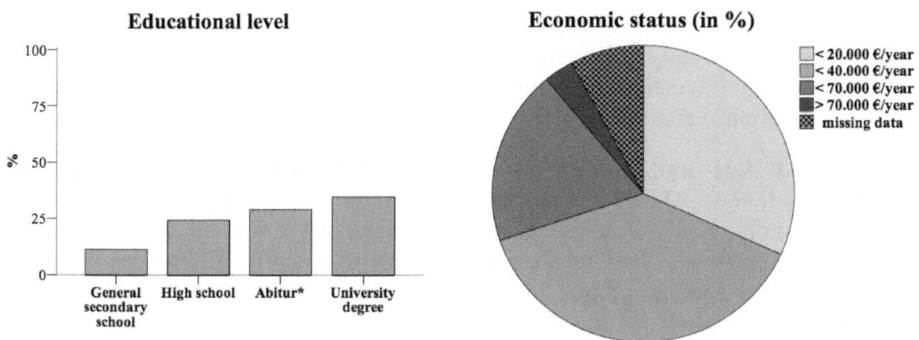

*General qualification for university entrance in Germany

Fig. 1. Educational level ($n = 123$; left) and economic background ($n = 116$; right) in the sample

It was intended to survey different aged people picked randomly out of the population in order to explore their current attitude towards medical technology and their usage behavior of general accessible assistive healthcare devices at home (e.g., blood pressure meter, blood sugar meter). Thereby, as it was assumed that frequent usage of common information and communication technologies (ICT), like for instance personal computer or mobile phone, would be associated with easier access to and navigation of medical devices, respondents were also asked about the usage frequency and perceived fun in private and job-related context. Looking at the whole sample participants referred to use technical devices quite frequently in both aspects of life (private: $M = 5$, $SD = 1.2$; work: $M = 4.7$, $SD = 1.7$ out of maximum 6 points). When regarding both gender groups separately significant differences in private using context and in having fun using technical devices appear. Men show considerably more frequent private usage ($M = 5.3$, $SD = 1$) and declare to have more fun ($M = 4.5$, $SD = 1.2$ out of maximum 6 points) in comparison to women when interacting with ICT (private usage: $M = 4.5$, $SD = 1.3$; having fun: $M = 3.8$, $SD = 1.4$). The differences in job-related interaction with technology is similar oriented but nonessential. These initial findings go along with the results of many previous studies and confirm the popular image of male-dominated preference in technical matters.

2.2 Results

The results of the first study were analyzed by bivariate correlations, multivariate and univariate analyses of variance with a level of significance set at 5%. Outcomes within less restrictive significance level of 10% are referred as marginally significant or significant by trend. The significance of omnibus F-Tests in ANOVA-analyses was taken from Pillai values. Mean value differences were analyzed with T-test.

The impact of age and gender was examined in all analyses, which in the result section of Study 1 are presented as follows: at first, the impact of independent variables on respondents' attitude towards medical technology and their willingness to use it is tested; with the next step correlative relationships of the presented variables are evaluated; and finally effects of user diversity on aspects assumed to be associated with usability and acceptance of medical assistance devices, i.e. privacy, trust and control, are variance analyzed.

Influence of Age and Gender on the General Attitude Towards and the Willingness to Use Medical Technology. Regarding the general attitude towards medical technology as well as peoples' willingness to use it, neither age nor gender effects could be found. This result evidences the absence of differences within the examined gender and age groups with respect to those parameters. Considering them separately, it was observed that the general opinions about medical technology are thoroughly positive and high pronounced reaching average values from about 42 to 44 out of maximum 55 points. More precisely it means that men and women independent of their age have a similar positive attitude towards usage of medical assistance devices.

Also, the willingness to monitor one's critical bodily functions by dint of medical technology is much more preferred than a permanent sick nursing of external caregivers or even family members (mean values ranging from 28 to about 31 out of maximum 35 points). Interestingly, a marginally significant interacting effect of age and gender was encountered in this regard (F (3,118) = 2.5, $p < 0.1$), identifying in particular younger women and younger middle-aged men to be the most willing to use medical technology in comparison to the dependency of caregivers' support (see figure 2). What is more, the willingness to use medical assistance is decreasing in women over the years, while the referred opinions of male respondents deviate in different age groups. However, considering the eldest, and at the same time those with the highest probability of chronic diseases – and consequently highest requirement to use medical assistance –, men more than women are motivated to use it. This result is the opposite way around to the opinions in the youngest age group.

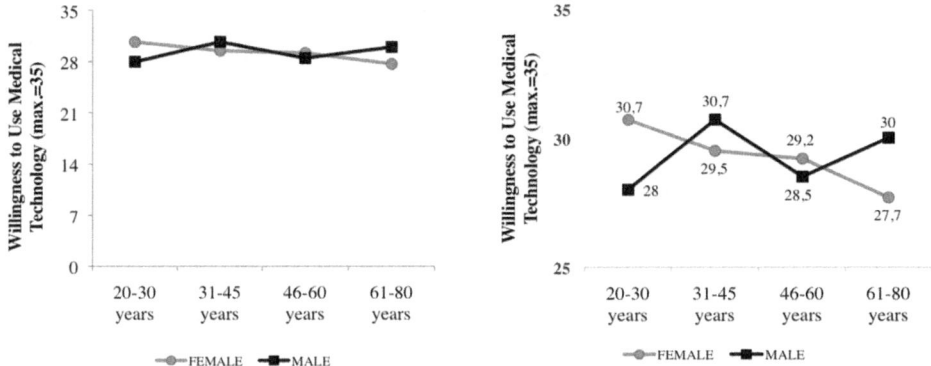

Fig. 2. Interacting effect of age and gender on the willingness to use medical technology ($N = 126$); on the right side a zoomed copy of the resulting mean values

Impact of User Diversity on Aspects of Acceptability (Privacy, Control, Trust). Tending to ascertain, which factors may additionally shape the acceptability and usage behavior of medical assistance technologies, in the present study we examined participants' assessments regarding perceived importance of privacy, of control and of trust towards assistive health technologies.

Considering the interrelation among these acceptability aspects it is firstly to observe that importance of privacy is rather weakly related to the perceived necessity of regular control of own health status ($r = 0.2$, $p < 0.05$). This indicates that some of the respondents do not wish to be disturbed from third parties by their private health measures. Secondly, a strong connection of trust and control regarding medical technology was found ($r = 0.6$, $p \leq 0.001$). Apparently the intention of periodical health check is strongly encouraged by the feeling of greater confidence and trust in its reliability. However, while the latter results are still evident in both gender groups (females: $r = 0.58$, $p \leq 0.001$; males: $r = 0.6$, $p \leq 0.001$), a significant connectivity of privacy and control disappear when men and women are considered separately.

Using multiple analyses of variance we investigated the effects of age and gender on the mentioned acceptability aspects. The MANOVA revealed an omnibus effect of age (F (9,354) = 2.4, $p < 0.05$) and an interacting effect of age and gender on importance of privacy, perceived control and trust (F (9,354) = 2.5, $p < 0.05$). Gender alone does not significantly influence these factors according to our findings.

As showed in figure 3 (on the left) the referred importance of privacy is most present in the younger middle-aged group of respondents (31-45 years) and the means for the judgments drop down with increasing age. Interestingly, the resulting average values of the youngest and the oldest participants are equally valued, meaning that both population groups would make the fewest effort, not to be seen outward as diseased because of using a medical device. One possible explanation for this fact could be the distance to the illness itself: while very young people do not feel the real nearness to it yet, the older aged adults are so close to it, that the question of privacy in this case has rather the lowest priority.

The same age groups of the questioned sample – the youngest and the oldest – show lower confidence in medical devices' reliability in comparison to the middle-aged groups (figure 3 on the right). The opinions of the latest resulted slightly higher. However, in all age groups the observed trust judgments are highly pronounced proving a high belief in devices' reliable functionality, in general.

Regarding respondents' perception of control about their own health by means of assistive medical devices (figure 3 in the middle), the 31 to 45 year olds show the highest confidence in medical technology. Surprisingly – as it is often assumed that this group is the most technically affine – the youngest participants' results are the lowest ($M = 7.7$, $SD = 1.3$ out of maximum 10 points) amongst the investigated age groups, which is probably arising from the absent closeness to or realistic imagination of (chronically) illness and the surplus value of using medical assistance technology. However, the overall resulting high means of all respondents with respect to this aspect prove a quiet positive perception and reliance on the possibility to regular check of (critical) vital bodily functions by means of medical devices at home.

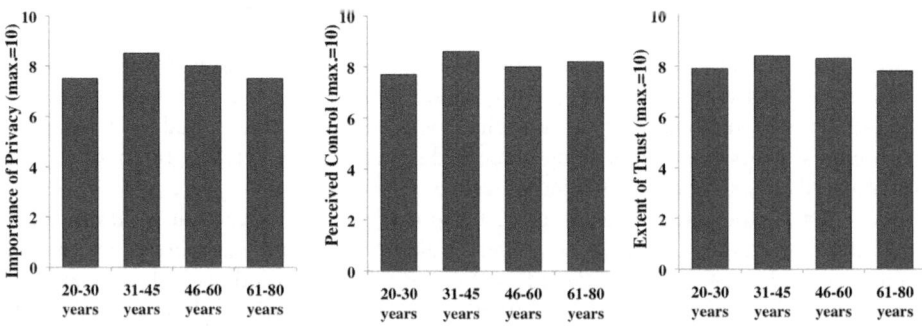

Fig. 3. Main effect of age on privacy, control and trust towards medical technology usage ($N = 126$)

Furthermore, in figure 4 the interaction of age and gender in the acceptability aspects discussed here is presented.

With regard to privacy (figure 4 left) the interaction effect becomes especially apparent in older middle-aged and oldest participants. The oldest women in comparison to those younger ones report significantly lower importance of using medical technology exclusively in private or even hiding it from the outside world. This finding is the opposite to opinions of the men in the same age group who reach distinctly higher mean values for privacy aspect of using medical technology in home environment. Apparently, the ambition of being seen as healthy and full of vigor is prevailing a male domain in the age beyond 60'ies. Looking at the whole sample, the oldest men and the middle-aged women seem to emphasize privacy in context of medical technology at the most.

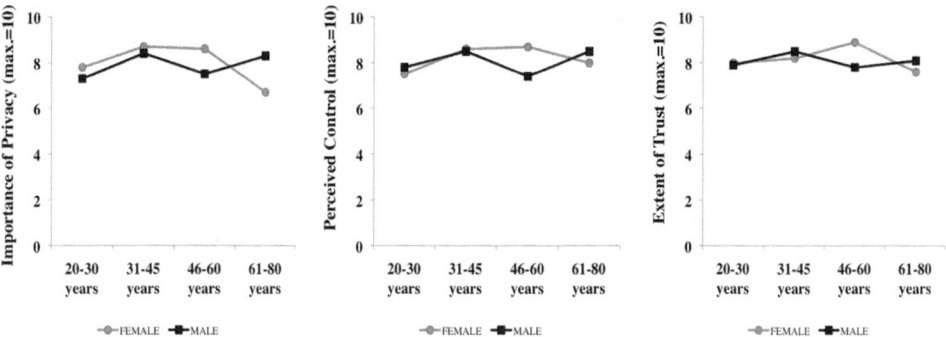

Fig. 4. Interacting effect of age and gender on privacy, control and trust towards medical technology usage ($N = 126$)

Moreover, regarding perceived control and extent of trust using accessible medical devices the major gender differences result in participants aged between 46 and 60 years (figure 4 middle and right). In this age group women attach more importance than men to the regular control of their health parameters considering a higher confidence in medical devices' reliability at the same time. Unlike, in the group of the oldest respondents it is the men who report higher trust in medical technology and a higher necessity to periodical control of their vital bodily functions. In the younger age groups, however, the perception of health control and trust in devices' reliability is comparable. Female and male respondents reach in both aspects very similar relatively high-pronounced mean values ranged in the top third of the scale.

3   Study 2

The second study aims to determine whether gender differences exist concerning the acceptance of a specific medical device – a smart textile [27]. A smart textile was introduced as a part of a mobile system, whose major function is the monitoring of the nutritional and water balance of human bodies.

3.1   Method

In order to examine a large number of participants the questionnaire-method in combination with a scenario technique was chosen as empirical approach.

Participants. A total of $N = 280$ respondents participated, with an age range between 14 and 92 years of age ($M = 46.7$), including 149 women (54%). Participants were recruited through the social network of authors and came from a broad range of professions. All participants volunteered to take part and showed a very high and personal interest in the topic, what can be taken from – for questionnaire studies – high response rates of about 80%. Participants were not gratified for their efforts. There were participants of all ages, which indicated to suffer from a chronic disease (26.4% women, 25.4% men) and which reported to use medical technical devices (18% women, 19% men), respectively. Additionally to the demographical data people were asked to specify the sector in which they are actually working in, in order to control for prior experience effects. As pointed out in figure 5, participants were almost equally distributed in four different profession areas.

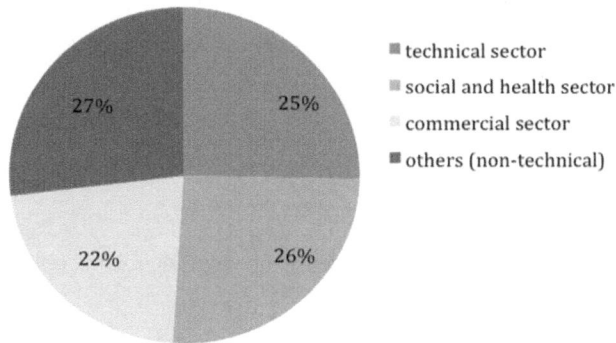

Fig. 5. Working area of participants ($n = 246$) in the sample in %

Questionnaire. At the beginning of the questionnaire participants were introduced into a medical scenario:

"Imagine that in the year 2025 a vast majority of people in our societies are 65 years and older. Many of these people will be frail and therefore reliant on medical care. Due to shortcomings in the caring sector (economic bottlenecks and a decreasing number of nursing staff) it is a basic question how older people can live independently at home, and have access to medical services. Yet, there are already mature technical developments, which enable continuous medical care at home. One example for these developments is a so-called smart textile. Smart textiles are able to monitor the nutritional and water balance of human bodies. This is especially important in cases of weak health as well as for older people who often forget to drink enough. For the attending doctors it is quite difficult to diagnose such dehydration because the symptoms are not very clear. As a consequence, the hospitalization is extended and the mortality increases dramatically. To avoid such serious effects and to improve the quality of life for all persons concerned, it is important to control the nutritional status and water balance of the body. The smart textiles enable the continuous mobile measurement of nutritional parameters, 24 hours a day, 7 days a week."

In order to ensure respondents' understanding of the scenario and its consequences, the described scenario was tested in a sub-sample before the main data collection began.

After the introduction, socio-demographic variables were assessed, followed by the items to individual aging concepts. After that participants should evaluate their intention to use the specified device, as well as the usage motives and utilization barriers. In the end they were asked about their technical experience, their attitudes towards technologies in general and medical technologies in particular.

In the following, dimensions and items are described in detail.

Variables. In order to assure a high measuring quality, reliability of the (latent construct) scales was analyzed prior to testing.

Independent variables: Independent variable is the biological gender of participants. As there are several important variables that could potentially confound gender differences in acceptance of medical assistive devices, we assessed mediating factors like technical expertise, individual health status, usage of medical devices, and attitude towards technologies.

Technical Expertise (TE)
Cronbach's Alpha amounts .80 for TE, suggesting high reliability.

Table 1. Items for Technical Expertise (1 = totally disagree to 4 = totally agree)

Which of the following actions apply to you?
I can assemble a prefabricated object (e.g., furniture) from pieces by myself
I can hang up a picture on the wall by myself
If something breaks I usually seek to repair it by myself
I easily handle a mobile phone and use it regularly
I easily handle a computer and use it regularly

Attitude towards Technologies in general (AT)
Items presented in table 2 assessed attitude towards technologies and technical progress. Reliability analysis for the latent construct AT revealed a Cronbach's Alpha of .69, which is acceptable.

Table 2. Items for Attitude towards Technologies (1 = totally disagree to 4 = totally agree)

Which of the following attitudes apply to you?
Technical progress bodes well for people
Technology allows people to live comfortably
Technology is more a threat than a benefit for people
Technology limits people in their personal liberty
Technical devices are often opaque and difficult to control
I like trying out new technical equipment

Dependent Variables: Dependent variables were the perceived usefulness of the smart textiles and the intention to use them if necessary. Items were formulated from the perspective of participants (first person), in order to enhance comprehensibility. Items had to be confirmed or denied on a four-point Likert-scale from 1 (totally disagree) to 4 (totally agree).

Intention to Use (IU)
Participants were given the in table 3 following answers regarding their intention to use technology, if necessary. Cronbach's Alpha values for IU reached satisfactory .93.

Table 3. Items for the Intention to Use (1 = totally disagree to 4 = totally agree)

Using the medical device… (smart textiles)
…would increase my contentment and satisfaction
…allows a sensible medical care
I can imagine using the device to…
… longer live independently at home
…facilitate your living conditions

Usefulness
Usefulness was assessed by usage motives (UM) and usage barriers (UB) as described in the following:

Table 4. Items for Usage Motives and Barriers (1 = totally disagree to 4 = totally agree). "Under which conditions would you use the smart textiles?".

I would use the smart textiles… ($\alpha = .79$)
…in order to save caring costs
…in order to escape from the indignity of being cared for
…in order to keep independency
…because I can take them off
No, I would be reluctant to use the smart textiles… ($\alpha = .79$)
…because I fear that they are not reliable
…because others would come to know about my health status
…because I do not want to be dependent on a technical device
…because I fear high costs for acquisition or maintenance

3.2 Results

Results were analysed by ANOVA - procedures (differences between gender groups) and bivariate correlation analyses (Spearman) to assess the interrelation between factors and variables. In a further step we used regression analyses to examine in particular the role of gender.

Gender Differences. The descriptive statistics (means and standard deviations), categorized by gender as well as intercorrelations of the constructs and age are given in table 5.

Table 5. Descriptive statistics and intercorrelations of research variables (N = 280; gender coding: men = 0, women = 1)

	Women		Men		Gender	Age	AT	TE	UM	UB	IU
	M	SD	M	SD							
AT	2.80	0.41	2.96	0.41	-.18**	-.25**		.34**	.35**	-.33**	.23**
TE	3.10	0.72	3.56	0.54	-.37**	-.42**	.34**		.19**	-.15*	.16**
UM	2.87	0.73	2.88	0.70	-.02	-.13*	.35**	.19**		-.36**	.62**
UB	2.49	0.69	2.28	0.64	.18**	.06	-.33**	-.15*	-.36**		-.39**
IU	2.54	0.76	2.67	0.82	-.08	-.16**	.23**	.16**	.62**	-.39**	

*$p < 0.05$; **$p < 0.01$.

With the exception of usage motives (UM) and intention to use (IU) the mean values between men and women were statistically different ($p < 0.05$). Age revealed a significant correlation with all constructs except for usage barriers (UB).

The Influence of Gender on the Intention to Use (IU). Multiple linear regressions were used to analyze the hypothetical relationships. We introduced gender as a dummy variable to test the moderation of the different relationships by gender. Results indicated that the relationship between UB and IU were moderated by gender, as well as the relationship between AT and UB.

By further analyzing the data for women and men separately, it appears that women's intention to use smart textiles is influenced by using motives (UM), using barriers (UB), and attitude towards technology in general (AT) while men's intention is predicted only by usage motives (UM). This result can be also confirmed in a gender-separated correlation analysis. In men there is exclusively a significant association between usage motives and intention to use smart textiles ($r = 0.7$, $p \leq 0.001$). In contrast to that, women's intention to use such a medical assistance device is statistically relevant related to several variables: usage motives ($r = 0.7$, $p \leq 0.001$) as well as to a lower extent usage barriers ($r = -0.3$, $p \leq 0.001$) and the attitude towards technology ($r = 0.3$, $p \leq 0.001$).

As presented in table 6 factors explained about 50% of variance in the intention to use smart textiles within both groups. Although age was included into the analyses, it had no significant effect on the other variables.

Table 6. Regression models for men's and women's intentions to use smart textiles

	Women		Men	
Predictor	**Adj. R^2**	**β**	**Adj. R^2**	**β**
	.50		.51	
TE		.09		.08
UM		.64**		.65**
UB		-.22**		-.09
AT		-.18*		.05
Age		-.08		.03

*$p < 0.05$; **$p < 0.01$.

4 Discussion

The major goal of this paper was to lighten the role of gender and user diversity when analyzing acceptance of medical assistive devices. For this purpose two studies were conducted. In the first study the general attitude towards and willingness to use medical technology in general were examined with regard to the effects of gender and age. The second study focused on gender influences when analyzing acceptance of specific health assistive technology using smart textiles as example.

Summing up the results of study 1, we can now state that the general attitude towards medical technology and the willingness to use it do not differ in the specified age and gender groups but the reported opinions about both aspects are overall highly pronounced. Considering the absence of age and gender differences, and the high acceptance values in this regard it is thus to conclude that there is in general a positive tendency towards and a high readiness to use medical devices, which confirms findings of the recent research [28], [29], [30].

In opposition to the rather male-dominated positive attitude towards popular information and communication technologies, the findings of our survey prove that regarding health-related technologies there is an essential difference in thinking about it. It is not longer divided in male and/or female specific domains, and it is not fun driven any more. Facing the own health status it is rather much more important how reliable the system works and how it is going to deal with the sensitive data. In this context questions about the importance of privacy and trust arise. As could be shown, those aspects in turn split the opinions of the (potential) users. The oldest and the youngest respondents report the lowest priority of privacy in comparison to middle-aged persons, and on the other side the lowest trust in reliability of medical devices amongst other age groups.

However, the general confidence about their functionality is, on average, highly pronounced. It is likely that the findings regarding privacy matters represent two poles of the same phenomenon, namely the distance to the necessity of medical technology usage. While the oldest respondents – due to their rather frail health condition and the higher probability to use medical technology in the near future – disregard or give privacy only the secondary importance, the youngest persons feel possibly not close enough to the necessity to use it [28], [29]. In contrast to that middle-aged persons attach more importance to the unobservability, unobtrusiveness, and invisibility by third parties when using medical devices. Here, social prestige, professional esteem, and societal status might play a significant role, which possibly make potential users to maintain a specific person image that might be not compatible to using and needing medical technology.

Regarding gender as separate variable, no explicit differences could be identified in the general attitudes towards medical technology matters. However, gender interacting with age revealed certain diverseness in attitude patterns. Women's reported opinions about the willingness to use ehealth applications, their privacy importance and trust in this regard show similar patterns, decreasing with increasing age. At the same time the judgments of male respondents vary much more among the different age groups. Opinions of the latter with respect to the examined variables move up and down depending on the stage of their life.

In contrast to the general attitudes towards acceptability of medical solutions a somewhat different picture emerges when analyzing more concrete ehealth technologies. The results of the second study revealed that gender plays an important role by forming underlying structures of acceptance. Although we could not detect differences between men and women regarding their reported intention to use smart textiles – both gender groups showed, alike to study 1, a relatively high willingness – significant differences appeared in analysis of usage barriers as well as in technical experience and attitudes towards medical technologies. Women tend to experience greater barriers when facing the usage of the medical device and have in general less positive attitude than men. These findings and even the higher technical experience of men are in line with prior research in the context of information technologies [23].

Furthermore, regression analysis revealed different structures of factors for predicting the intention to use the smart textiles of men and women. Whereas for men just one variable – usage motives – explains 51% of variance in the intention to use, for women three factors (attitude, usage barriers, and usage motives) are needed to explain about 50% of variance in their intention to use the smart textiles. These results suggest two conclusions: first, the intention to use smart textiles in the female part of the population is more complex to communicate, whereas for male users only the perceived usefulness of a device is decisive for their usage intention. Second, and most important, these results show that formation of acceptance patterns is gendered when focusing on a concrete device.

Taking results of both studies into account, it becomes clear that – besides age – gender plays an important role and needs to be considered when looking at technology acceptance in medical context [31]. Although both studies showed that there are no significant gender differences for the acceptance of medical technology in general, especially results of study 2 pointed out that taking a deeper look into the role of gender putting medical support in concrete terms (i.e. smart textiles) reveals very well differences for males and females – similar to the results of comparable studies (e.g., [32], [33]).

Understanding the different structures in acceptance motives of both gender groups is particularly important in the development of assistive medical devices considered for diseases that, due to their prevalence, affect either men or women more frequent. With an increasing comprehension of factors forming the usage acceptance of medical technologies in men and women, developers, designers as well as marketing experts can profit in creating user adjusted technology and advertisements.

Moreover, the knowledge about gender-specific acceptance of medical assistive devices may contribute – especially in old age – to the maintaining personal independency and mobility in everyday life, and by this, users' stay away from long-term care facilities. Thinking even further ahead, implementing gender-suited medical technologies in home environments could advantage several aspects of life quality like for instance an enhanced patient-physician communication (e.g., VoIP), better control of health status (monitoring of bodily functions), maintenance or improvement of memory performance (brain jogging), etc.

Last but not least, developing well-adapted medical support devices would probably launch new services and break into new markets. It is even conceivable, that adjusted medical systems in private homes would induce not only cost reduction but also relief in currently considerable overburdened medical healthcare sector.

5   Limitations and Suggestions for Future Research

Though results are insightful, a cautionary note has to be considered regarding methodological specificity, and the basic vulnerability to artifacts. The results described and discussed here are based on a questionnaire method, in which participants envision to use the respective technology, which they are not familiar with. On this base they evaluate the pros and the cons of the envisioned usage of these technologies.

However, we cannot finally exclude that this method provokes artificial findings. It is reasonably to assume that any envisioning of being ill and needing a specific technology might lead to an unrealistic assessment, and possibly to an overstressing of negative feelings due to the unfamiliarity with the interaction, and the basic fear to foreign matters and circumstances. And also, it is just possible that persons, who are not chronically ill, actually underestimate the worries and threats of needing to use medical technology. This, on the other hand, could be gendered as female users are known to be rather cautiously regarding the usage of technology and tend to underestimate their self-competence when using technical devices [34], [35], [36]. Therefore, future studies will have to validate the findings by using other empirical methods, including a real interaction with medical technologies.

Acknowledgments. Authors would like to thank all participants, who took part in these studies, to patiently fill in the questionnaires and to allow us to gain insights into a sensible topic. Many thanks also to Carola Caesar, Oliver Sack, and Simon Himmel for their research assistance.

This research was supported by the excellence initiative of the German federal and state governments.

References

1. Wittenberg, R., Comas-Herrera, A., Pickard, L., Hancock, R.: Future Demand for Long-Term Care in England. PSSRU Research Summary (2006)
2. Leonhardt, S.: Personal Healthcare Devices. In: Mukherjee, S., et al. (eds.) Malware: Hardware Technology Drivers of Ambient Intelligence, pp. 349–370. Springer, Dordrecht (2006)
3. Gaul, S., Ziefle, M., Arning, K., Wilkowska, W., Kasugai, K., Röcker, C., Jakobs, E.-M.: Technology Acceptance as an Integrative Component of Product Developments in the Medical Technology Sector. In: Proceedings of the Third Ambient Assisted Living Conference (AAL 2010), January 26 - 27. VDE Verlag, Berlin (2010), CD-ROM
4. Gaul, S., Ziefle, M.: Smart Home Technologies: Insights into Generation-Specific Acceptance Motives. In: Holzinger, A., Miesenberger, K. (eds.) USAB 2009. LNCS, vol. 5889, pp. 312–332. Springer, Heidelberg (2009)
5. Röcker, C.: Living and Working in Automated Environments - Evaluating the Concerns of End-Users in Technology-Enhanced Spaces. In: Mahadevan, V., Jianhong, Z. (eds.) Proceedings of the Second International IEEE Conference on Computer and Automation Engineering, Singapore, February 26 - 28, pp. 513–517 (2010)
6. Jähn, K., Nagel, E.: E-Health. Springer, Berlin (2004)
7. Davis, F.D.: Perceived Usefulness, Perceived Ease of Use, and User Acceptance of Information Technology. MIS Quarterly 13, 319–337 (1989)

8. Venkatesh, V., Davis, F.D.: A Theoretical Extension of the Technology Acceptance Model: Four Longitudinal Field Studies. Management Science 46, 186–204 (2000)
9. Venkatesh, V., Morris, M.G., Davis, G.B., Davis, F.D.: User acceptance of information technology: Toward a unified view. MIS Quarterly 27, 425–478 (2003)
10. Arning, K., Ziefle, M.: Different Perspectives on Technology Acceptance: The Role of Technology Type and Age. In: Holzinger, A., Miesenberger, K. (eds.) USAB 2009. LNCS, vol. 5889, pp. 20–41. Springer, Heidelberg (2009)
11. Ziefle, M.: Age perspectives on the usefulness on e-health applications. International Conference on Health Care Systems, Ergonomics, and Patient Safety (HEPS), Straßbourg, France (2008)
12. Meyer, S., Mollenkopf, H.: Home technology, smart homes, and the aging user. In: Schaie, K.W., Wahl, H.-W., Mollenkopf, H., Oswald, F. (eds.) Aging Independently: Living Arrangements and Mobility, pp. 148–161. Springer, Heidelberg (2003)
13. Demiris, G., Hensel, B.K., Skubic, M., Rantz, M.: Senior residents' perceived need of and preferences for "smart home" sensor technologies. International Journal of Technology Assessment in Health Care 24(1), 120–124 (2008)
14. Stronge, A.J., Rogers, W.A., Fisk, A.D.J.: Human factors considerations in implementing telemedicine systems to accommodate older adults. Telemed Telecare 13, 1–3 (2007)
15. Kalloniatis, C., Kavakli, E., Gritzalis, S.: Using Privacy Process Patterns for Incorporating Privacy Requirements into the System Design Process. In: 2nd International Conference on Availability, Reliability and Security, pp. 1009–1017. IEEE, Los Alamitos (2007)
16. Sheridan, T.B.: Humans and Automation, vol. 3. John Wiley & Sons, Santa Monica (2002)
17. Montague, E., Kleiner, B.M., Winchester, W.W.: Empirically Understanding Trust in Medical Technology. International Journal of Industrial Ergonomics 39(4), 628–634 (2009)
18. Carmel, S.: The will to live: Gender differences among elderly patients. Social Sciences and Medicine 49, 1401–1408 (2001)
19. Ditto, P.H., Smucker, W.D., Danks, J.H., Jacobson, J.A., Houts, R.M., Fagerlin, A., Coppola, K.M., Gready, R.M.: Stability of older adults' preferences for life-sustaining medical treatment. Health Psychology 22, 606–615 (2003)
20. Arber, S., Vandrevala, T., Daly, T., Hampson, S.: Understanding gender differences in older people's attitudes towards life-prolonging medical technologies. Journal of Aging Studies 22, 366–375 (2008)
21. Peplau, L.A., Bikson, T.K., Rook, K.S., Goodchilds, J.D.: Being old and living alone. In: Peplau, L.A., Perlman, D. (eds.) Loneliness: A Sourcebook of Current Theory, Research and Therapy, pp. 327–347. Wiley, New York (1982)
22. Lehr, U.: Psychologie des Alterns, 9th edn. Quelle & Meyer, Wiebelsheim (2000)
23. Schumacher, P., Morahan-Martin, J.: Gender, internet and computer attitudes and experiences. Computers in Human Behavior 17, 95–110 (2001)
24. Meelissen, M.R.M., Drent, M.: Gender differences in computer attitudes: Does the school matter? Computers in Human Behavior 24(3), 969–985 (2008)
25. Venkatesh, V., Morris, M.G., Ackerman, P.L.: A Longitudinal Field Investigation of Gender Differences in Individual Technology Adoption Decision Making Processes. Organizational Behavior and Human Decision Processes 83(1), 33–60 (2000)
26. Morris, M.G., Venkatesh, V., Ackerman, P.L.: Gender and age differences in employee decisions about new technology: an extension to the theory of planned behavior. IEEE Transactions on Engineering Management 52(1), 69–84 (2005)
27. Beckmann, L., Kim, S., Jungbecker, N., Ingerl, G., Leonhardt, S.: Entwicklung intelligenter Textilien für die Überwachung des Ernährungs- und Wasserhaushalts. In: Deutscher AAL Kongress 2009, Berlin, vol. 2 (January 27-28, 2009)

28. Wilkowska, W., Ziefle, M.: User diversity as a challenge for the integration of medical technology into future home environments. In: Ziefle, M., Röcker, C. (eds.) Human-Centred Design of eHealth Technologies. Concepts, Methods and Applications. Hershey, P.A. IGI Global (in press)
29. Ziefle, M., Wilkowska, W.: Technology acceptability for medical assistance. In: 4th Conference on Pervasive Computing Technologies for Healthcare 2010, ICST 2010, Munic, Germany (2010)
30. Ziefle, M., Röcker, C.: Acceptance of Pervasive Healthcare Systems: A comparison of different implementation concepts. In: 4th ICST Conference on Pervasive Computing Technologies for Healthcare 2010, User-Centred-Design of Pervasive Health Applications (UCD-PH 2010) (2010)
31. Gaul, S., Wilkowska, W., Ziefle, M.: Accounting for user diversity in the acceptance of medical assistive technologies. In: Proceedings of the 3rd International ICST Conference on Electronic Healthcare for the 21st Century, eHealth 2010 (2010, in press)
32. Ziefle, M., Schaar, A.K.: Gender differences in attitudes towards invasive medical technology. Electronic Journal of Health Informatics (2010, in press)
33. Ziefle, M., Schaar, A.K.: Technical Expertise and its Influence on the Acceptance of Future Medical Technologies. What is influencing what to which extent? In: Leitner, G., Hitz, M., Holzinger, A. (eds.) HCI in Work & Learning, Life & Leisure, 6th Symposium of the WG HCI&UE of the Austrian Computer Society, USAB 2010, pp. 138–155 (2010)
34. Baltes, M.M., Freund, A.M., Horgas, A.L.: Men and women in the Berlin aging study. In: Baltes, P.B., Mayer, K.U. (eds.) The Berlin Aging Study. Aging from 70 to 100, pp. 259–281. Academic Press, Oxford (1999)
35. Busch, T.: Gender differences in self-efficacy and attitudes toward computers. Journal of Educational Computing Research 12, 147–158 (1995)
36. Brosnan, M.J.: The impact of computer anxiety and self-efficacy upon performance. Journal of Computer Assisted Learning 14, 223–234 (1998)

Discount User-Centered e-Health Design: A Quick-but-not-Dirty Method

Fenne Verhoeven and Julia van Gemert-Pijnen

University of Twente, Department of Psychology and Communication of Health and Risk,
Building Citadel H400, P.O. Box 217, 7500 AE Enschede, The Netherlands
{f.verhoeven,j.e.w.c.vangemert-pijnen}@utwente.nl

Abstract. The philosophy of discount usability engineering perfectly fits the health care setting, where cost-cutting is ubiquitously present. We adapted Nielsen's discount usability approach for the health care setting by combining traditional thinking aloud (n=18) and Card Sorting (n=18) with online prototyping (n=5) and simplified thinking aloud (n=5). We used the approach to design an efficient and effective website with infection control guidelines for nursing home staff leading to high levels of satisfaction within a time frame of three months for the total cost of €7195. Based on our experiences, we would advocate using this discount user-centered approach for the design of e-health applications. Future research should concentrate on integrating the principles of creative co-design methods and online research into the discount usability approach.

Keywords: Discount usability engineering; user-centered design; usability testing; health care; infectious diseases; thinking aloud; Card Sorting; prototyping.

1 Introduction

1.1 Web-Based Infection Control Guidelines

Health care-associated infections cause thousands of preventable deaths each year in several types of care settings, including nursing homes [1]. Therefore, it is crucial that nursing home staff adhere to infection control guidelines. Although most nursing home staff are aware of the rationale for infection control practices, adherence is generally poor [2].

In addition to contextual reasons such as negative management values and a high workload, the insufficient tailoring of infection control guidelines as a communication means to nursing home staff needs might account for low adherence rates. Previous research has demonstrated that health care workers repeatedly encounter problem with the usability of the guidelines, which could be detrimental to their uptake in clinical practice [3-5]. The problem with infection control guidelines as a communication means is that they are rather expert-driven. Expert-driven guideline communication can be characterized by a strong focus on scientific validation, regulation, and legislation [6]. In the design process, higher priority is given to a consensus on content-related issues among experts than to nursing home workers' practical information needs. This can make the document difficult for individual nursing home workers to use as a resource and to identify procedures for daily work practice [7].

G. Leitner, M. Hitz, and A. Holzinger (Eds.): USAB 2010, LNCS 6389, pp. 101–123, 2010.
© Springer-Verlag Berlin Heidelberg 2010

A possible solution to enhance the usability of the expert-driven guideline format is to communicate the traditional, paper-based guidelines in a format that better fits the practical information needs of the nursing home staff. Presenting guidelines on a website facilitates the inclusion of hyperlinks to additional resources and multimodal functionalities, such as instructional videos. Consequently, in-depth information can be available without affecting the guidelines' readability [8].

1.2   User Involvement in the Design Process

The development of a website allows the direct involvement of nursing home staff, which can lead to a higher level of usability. In a user-centered design process, nursing home workers can be invited to make their tacit knowledge concerning infection control explicit, stimulated to make their own decisions about directions and strategies for improvement, and are led in those actions [4, 7]. Considering usability prior to development of a first prototype of a website may prevent uncovering pitfalls in the system after its implementation, which can be costly and avoid reluctance among intended users [9].

Various research methods are available to develop communication means with a high level of usability. These methods can be divided into usability testing and usability inspection [10-12]. In usability testing, representative users work on typical tasks using the system (or the prototype) and the evaluators use the results to see how the user interface supports the users to do their tasks. The most common employed methods are thinking aloud, field observation, and questionnaires [10]. In usability inspection, usability specialists and sometimes software developers or other professionals, examine usability-related aspects of a product or system. Various inspection methods are available, such as heuristic evaluation, cognitive walkthroughs, and action analysis.

Since it is often thought that experts are not able to identify real user problems [13], and problems with the quality of guideline communication are particularly caused by their expert-driven character, it is better to perform usability testing rather than usability inspection when improving the format of infection control guidelines. With this in mind, design of web-based guideline communication should incorporate the tools and methods applied in user-centered design: requirements gathering, analysis, design, implementation, testing, and deployment [14]. Previous studies have shown the benefits of involving users via usability testing in the design process of e-health applications [3-5]: First, user input can be taken into account before the application's release so the application's content, structure, and lay-out are completely tailored to the user needs. This leads to a high level of satisfaction among users. Second, early analysis and modeling of the mental processes involved in users' activity helps prevent failures and future costs [14, 15]. Third, it may be that user's involvement in the design process creates ownership, fosters applicability of the application, and leads to a willingness to integrate the application into daily routine [7].

Approaches based on usability engineering recently have been introduced into medical informatics [16, 17]. However, usability testing that follows a stringent approach is expensive, even if what a "modest" usability lab is constructed and staffed. The cost of using these techniques might be one important reason for the fact that usability testing is not used as a standard in medical informatics [18]. Or rather, the reason is the *perceived* cost of using these techniques, as it has been shown that many usability techniques can be deployed quite cheaply [19].

1.3   Discount Usability Engineering as a Premise

A method that is increasingly becoming popular to overcome the aforementioned problems related to time- and cost investments is "discount usability engineering". Discount usability engineering is a phrase popularized by Jakob Nielsen [19], a long-time proponent of smaller, cheaper usability studies for projects with small budgets for usability. Discount usability engineering is originally based on the use of the following three techniques: prototypes, simplified thinking aloud, and heuristic evaluation. The premise for this approach is that it is simple and has more a chance of being employed in practical situations [14]. The approach utilizes a small number of users who are tested and statistical analysis cannot be applied [20]. Usability testing is not intended to be a research experiment from which we induce a generalizable conclusion. According to Dumas and Redish, a research study seeks to know "whether or not some phenomenon exists", while a usability test aims "to uncover problems" and thereby improve an application's design [21]. Rather, the findings are qualitative in nature [22]. The methods are quick, and if one is not developing an aircraft cockpit interface with lives at stake, the risk of not finding every last usability problem is not serious [20].

Formal usability engineering can be costly to any project budget but by employing discount usability engineering, a cost effective method which provides clear identification of problems is applied. It is simple in design, and in the real world, stands a better chance of being applied and reaping the rewards towards an improved product 19]. Multiple variations of the discount usability engineering approach could be identified in the literature, with costs ranging from 62000 dollar [19] to almost nothing [16], and time spans varying between a year [19] to one day [23] or even 30 minutes [24]. The philosophy of discount usability engineering perfectly fits the health care setting, in which budgets are restrained and cost-cutting is ubiquitously present.

1.4   Discount Usability Engineering for the Design of New (e-Health) Applications

Although usability testing and inspection are steadily gaining ground in the health care setting [16], only few papers could be identified that focused on discount usability engineering in a context of medical informatics. Beuscart-Zéphir et al [15] adapted discount usability engineering to support the choice between several prototypes of a clinical information system. Discount usability engineering was used by Kaplan and colleagues [16] to evaluate a prototype of a computer-based clinical case intended for educational purposes. Yao and Gorman applied the method for the redesign of a web-based clinical library [14]. In all these studies, discount usability engineering was employed for the evaluation of existing systems or system prototypes. In here, the question rises whether the discount approach also holds for the design of new applications, as in our case a website with infection control guidelines for the nursing home setting. In other words: Are the available, existing discount usability methods suitable for the design and development of new technological applications, or do other research methods have to be incorporated? This paper is focused around this question.

1.5 Objectives

With this study, we aim to identify a discount approach for user-centered design of a completely new e-health application (without a prototype being available). We tried to achieve this by employing efficient and effective methods for both planning, administering, and analyzing the study within a time frame of three months, for cost lower than 7500€, including the design, implementation, and evaluation of the application.

We intend to demonstrate that although our method is quick, it definitely is not dirty, since our methodology is based on scientific design principles and still enables data analysis at an academic level. The user-centered design process of a website with infection control guidelines in a nursing home setting served as a casus.

2 Methods

2.1 Research Context

The "Health care Foundation Marga Klompé" is a coordinating organization that facilitates both domiciliary care as well as nursing home care. The organization comprises 23 nursing homes, scattered over six cities in the East of the Netherlands, and employs approximately 1750 people. The organization together hosts 1100 intramural clients, 110 transmural clients, and yearly offers 80000 hours of domiciliary care (extramural). The organization hires an infection control nurse from the hospital for 16 hours weekly. One of the core tasks of the infection control nurse is to write and implement the infection control guidelines [25]. The purpose of infection control guidelines is to educate HCWs about the direction on the prevention and control of infectious diseases and uphold standards of safe work practice.

In the last few years, Marga Klompé's infection control nurse observed low adherence rates to the guidelines and wondered whether the quality of the documentation contributed to this. She therefore intended to replace the paper-based guidelines with a website in order to overcome the usability problems experienced with the paper-based guidelines. In order to do so, she called in the help of a behavioral scientist (FV). Considering the restricted budget in time and money, the infection control nurse and the behavioral scientist agreed to apply the principles of discount usability engineering.

The research project concerns the development, implementation, and evaluation of a website with infection control guidelines. The users concerned by the project are all physicians, nurses, and assistant-nurses within the organization.

2.2 Methods

"Discount usability engineering" is a method based on the use of the following three techniques [19]:

1. Prototypes (referred to by Nielsen as scenarios): Prototypes are essentially a simple version of a system, such as paper mock-ups. This technique saves costs on system development by delaying development until the majority of testing is complete.

2. Simplified thinking aloud: Test users think aloud as they attempt to complete tasks while observer takes notes. The method provides insight into users' thoughts as they use an interface. Also, this method saves costs on equipment since it does not require videotaping or even a lab and does not require recruiting or accommodating large numbers of people.
3. Heuristic evaluation: A method of inspecting a system's usability that supplements user testing. A small number of evaluator examine the interface and assess whether it complies with usability principles or heuristics, such as "consistency and standards", "aesthetic and minimalistic design", and "recognition rather than recall".

We did not choose however to blindly copy Nielsen's usability engineering method. We assume there is not one "golden standard" to conduct user-centered e-health design, for two reasons.

First, the specific context of each case requires a careful consideration of the available research methods, time and time again. Particularly in the health care setting, the context in which the system is used is inherently tied to the application [26]. In our case, we believed that solely employing simplified usability methods would not serve the purpose of developing a website with infection control guidelines for nursing homes. Since no prototype was available, we preferred to start with a more traditional, ethnographic thinking aloud method in order to identify problems encountered with the current, paper-based infection control guidelines. The results were used as input to build the mock-up prototypes, and from there on, standard discount methods could be applied: prototypes and simplified thinking aloud.

Second, although heuristic evaluation is one of Nielsen's discount usability methods, we did not apply this method of usability inspection. Since it is often thought that experts are not able to identify real user problems [13], and problems with the quality of guideline communication are particularly caused by their expert-driven character, we perceived it better to perform usability testing rather than usability inspection when improving the format of infection control guidelines. Besides, while usability heuristics are useful, they are not applied by rote, and they can require interpretation. Heuristics are not uniformly interpretable, and this causes competing forces [27].

In short, for the case of this study, we adapted Nielsen's discount usability approach because (1) it is less appropriate for the design of *new* applications and (2) heuristic expert evaluation will not play its full right given the fact that in our case, the expert-driven character of the existing guidelines is the major cause of usability problems. Therefore, we complemented Nielsen's method with traditional thinking aloud to make it suitable for *new* applications, and replaced the heuristic evaluation with a more user-centered method: Card Sorting. Together, the methods generated the optimal content, structure, and lay-out of the website. Each of our selected methods will be elaborated on below.

Traditional thinking aloud (content). Of all usability testing methods, thinking aloud has been most often used in the health care domain [29]. Thinking aloud involves having an end user continuously verbalizing thoughts while using a system, which provide insight into the underlying causes for usability problems and requirements for improvement [10, 12]. At the beginning of a design process, traditional thinking aloud methods work better than simplified thinking aloud, since traditional thinking aloud aims to uncover and articulate existing work practices [26]. In the beginning of our research, no single user need was known to the researcher and in order to gain a broad a possible vision of the nursing home staff's needs and problems they encountered with using existing control guidelines, no restrictions on administration and analysis of the thinking aloud data were imposed. Therefore, we started our research with 18 traditional thinking aloud sessions to identify the usability problems that occurred with the paper-based guidelines, so input for the website could be generated.

Card Sorting (structure). Card Sorting is often applied as a user-centered method for designing the information structure of a website [29]. The process involves respondents sorting a series of cards, each labeled with a piece of content or functionality, into groups that make sense to respondents. Card Sorting can provide insight into users' mental models, illuminating the way that they often tacitly group, sort and label tasks and content within their own heads. Those patterns are often referred to as the users' mental model. By understanding the users' mental model, we can increase findability, which in turn makes the product easier to use. We applied the principle of Open Card Sorting since this is useful as input to information structures in new or existing sites and products [30]. Respondents were given cards showing site content with no pre-established groupings. They were asked to sort cards into groups that they felt are appropriate and then describe each group.

Prototyping (lay-out). A prototype is a draft version of a website. Prototypes allow the exploration of ideas among users before investing time and money into development. It is much cheaper to change a product early in the development process than to make changes after the application has been developed. A prototype can be anything from paper drawings (low-fidelity), click-through of a few images or pages, or a fully functioning website (high-fidelity). There is an on-going debate in the literature about using low- versus high-fidelity prototyping [31]. Opinions vary a great deal about how much a prototype should resemble the final version of the design. In theory, low-fidelity sketches are quicker to create. An advantage is that using rough sketches users may have an easier time suggesting changes. High-fidelity prototypes take the users as close as possible to a true representation of the user interface. We tried to stroke the golden mean by opting for "medium-fidelity" prototypes: two different homepage mock-ups were created and sent by e-mail to intended users, who provided their comments via e-mail.

Simplified thinking aloud (synergizing content, structure, and lay-out). Once the content, structure, and lay-out are fixed, the first functional prototype could be built. We used Nielsen's simplified thinking aloud technique used to as a formative evaluation of the website before it was launched online, with the purpose of "test running" various aspects of the website and to verify whether the design team did not miss any errors [32]. With this approach users were prompted to speak out loud their thoughts about what they are doing and expecting as they are evaluate a piece of software. Users are in a unique position to provide early, authentic feedback. They know what they need and want and can respond to the design. All relevant topics that were raised during the simplified thinking aloud were solved before the website was officially launched online.

2.3 Subjects

A limited number of subjects is one of the showpieces of discount usability engineering. In terms of feasibility, discount engineering requires only three to six users to identify prominent problems. Nielsen and Landauer demonstrated that the benefits from user testing are much larger than the costs, no matter how many subjects are used [33]. Based on mathematical modeling, they showed that the maximum benefit-cost ratio is achieved when using between three and five subjects. With this number of test users, approximately 75% of a system's or website's usability problems for a target user group can be detected.

A random sample involving nursing home staff from different types of wards and with varying occupations (physicians, nurses, assistant-nurses) was selected by the infection control nurse. Respondents were recruited on a voluntary basis. Eligible nursing home staff were at least 18 years old and Dutch-speaking. All respondents were staff at one of the nursing homes of the Marga Klompé Institution in the East Netherlands. They did not need to have prior knowledge or experience with the use of either paper- or web-based infection control guidelines. The numbers of respondents included in each research phase are presented in Table 1. We used different users in each study to avoid any learning effects.

For the traditional thinking aloud, we maintained the mathematical of Nielsen and Landauer to determine the number of respondents. Since our goal was to detect as many usability problems experienced with the use of the existing, paper-based guidelines, we included 18 respondents in order to find 99% of problems [33]. For the prototyping and the simplified thinking aloud, we included five users, as suggested by Nielsen and Landauer.

Table 1. Numbers and types of respondents for each of the research methods

Method	Number per occupational group	Total
Traditional thinking aloud	4 nursing assistants 8 nurses 4 physicians 2 infection control nurses	18
Card Sorting	4 nursing assistants 8 nurses 4 physicians 2 infection control nurses	18
Prototyping	1 nursing assistant 2 nurses 1 physician 1 infection control nurse	5
Simplified thinking aloud	1 nursing assistant 2 nurses 1 physician 1 infection control nurse	5

2.4 Procedure and Materials

The complete design process, including conducting and processing the study and creating and implementing the website, took place between May and July 2009.

Traditional thinking aloud and Card Sorting were combined in one session. This implied the 18 respondents were confronted with the two methods subsequently. Respondents were advised to allow 1.5 hour per test session. The tests were conducted in a quiet room somewhere in the nursing home in which the respondent was employed, under the control of a researcher that was equipped with the paper-based infection control guidelines, the interview scheme, and the materials for the Card Sorting method (cards, paper clips, Post-Its, pencil, envelope). Upon arrival for the test sessions, respondents were greeted and thanked for their participation. The respondents were then given an overview of the tasks and expectations during the session. Thinking aloud instructions were provided. The tasks consisted of what if-tasks. A total of 19 different tasks were formulated, each representing on one the chapters in the paper-based guideline document. An example is: *"You read a patient's temperature and wonder what to do with the thermometer. Using the guidelines, can you say aloud which preventive measures you must take?"* The tasks were created in consultation with an infection control nurse who ensured that the tasks represented questions from daily clinical practice. The simulated tasks were adapted for the three categories of respondents: nursing assistants, nurses, and physicians (geriatrists). During the sessions of 45 minutes, respondents described what they were doing and explained it while doing it, sometimes volunteering information and sometimes in response to questions the evaluator asked. No time limit was imposed on the respondents to work on a task, implying that respondents performed as much tasks as they could during 45 minutes. Key literature on usability evaluation suggests that spending roughly 45 minutes per test subject is sufficient to gain an overall idea about the usability [34, 35]. The researcher used a Philips digital voicetracer 660 to record the respondents' verbalizations.

After 45 minutes of thinking aloud, the Card Sorting started. The infection control nurse selected 59 major themes that represented the comprehensive content of the existing guidelines. Each theme, for instance: *"The risks of using chlorine solution for surface disinfection"*, was written on a separate card. The cards were uniquely numbered on the back. Before handing the cards to the respondent, we shuffled the cards and placed them in a pile on a large empty table in front of the respondent. We then asked the respondent to sort the cards into piles according to similarity. We encouraged them not to produce piles that were too small or too large as they perceived it, but we asked that they not aim for a specific number of cards in each pile. After a user had sorted the cards into piles, we asked the respondent to invent a name for each group. They wrote this name of a Post-It note and place it on the group of cards. The respondents typically finished the Card Sorting in about 30 minutes. When finishing the Card Sorting, respondents were given the opportunity to provide additional comments regarding the website and after 90 minutes, respondents were thanked again for their participation. No problems occurred during each of the 18 sessions.

Prototyping: In the next phase, five respondents were approached by e-mail and were required to answer several questions regarding the grading of two mock-up prototypes (see Figures 1 and 2) that the designer developed based on the results from the traditional thinking aloud and Card Sorting. The two mock-ups of the website's homepage were attached to the e-mail. In the e-mail itself, respondents were kindly requested to look at the mock-ups attentively and answer a set of identical questions for each of the prototypes. Questions concerned their first impression of each prototype, their opinion according to prototype's structure, use of color, depiction of images and text, font, etc., three positive and three negative aspects of the prototype, and suggestions for improvement. The survey ended by asking respondents to indicate their preference for prototype 1 or 2. Respondents mentioned that it took them no longer than 15 minutes to complete the survey. Many developers and designers use good old pen and paper to conduct prototyping, but we decided to conduct this part of the study online since this saved time and it obliged respondents to formulate clear and concise answers. A qualitative analysis of the answers was conducted to help decide between prototype 1 and 2.

Simplified thinking aloud: In order to "test run" the first functional prototype of the website, we employed direct user testing where we observed five respondents during a 30 minute test. In the test, users were asked to complete a series of the same tasks as were used in the traditional thinking aloud sessions. The procedure was identical to the traditional thinking aloud, with the only difference that respondents this time used the website to complete tasks and the verbalizations were not recorded with a voice recorder, since data analysis could be done based on the researcher's notes instead of by data transcription. We verified whether the problems that occurred with the paper-based guidelines were prevented with the web-based guidelines.

2.5   Analysis

A major difference between traditional user-centered design methods and discount engineering concerns data analysis: Data analysis can for instance be done based on the researcher's notes instead of by data transcription [23]. Because we wanted the website to prevent as much usability problems as possible, we recorded and transcribed data of the traditional thinking aloud data. Once the functional prototype was developed, data transcription was not necessary for the mock-up prototyping and the simplified thinking aloud, since the aim was no longer perfection, but to find recommendations for improvement [19].

Thinking aloud: Data collected included time it took for users to complete the task, whether they completed the task successfully or not, and comments voiced during and after task completion. Data were analyzed using deductive analysis, implying that the coding categories were derived from a conceptual framework developed earlier for the identification of usability problems with infection control guidelines [4].

Card Sorting: Hand sorted card data were entered into WebSortTM tool, and analyzed with IBM's EZ sort application [36], which visualizes the differences and similarities between items in a tree-diagram based on cluster analysis, providing the website's optimal navigation structure. Besides, a qualitative analysis of the labels and the interviews was conducted to assign names to the categories. Cluster analysis provides a level of rigor to the approach, which removes unconscious biases by providing an objective tool for analysis, brings order to what is potentially an unwieldy process, and lends credibility to the results and thus fosters acceptance of them [30].

Mock up prototyping: Comments provided through e-mail by the respondents were categorized into usability issues by the researcher. The comments were reduced to a series of comments that indicated: like or dislike for aspects of the website, suggestions for site improvements and confusion about the site. The researcher grouped comments into these categories and compared the issues among prototype 1 and 2.

The prototype with the fewest comments was selected. The constructive feedback given by the respondents was processed into the functional prototype of the website.

Simplified thinking aloud: Nielsen describes the main difference between simplified and traditional thinking aloud as follows: In simplified thinking aloud, analysis is based on the observer's notes instead of on transcribed verbalized data [12]. The researcher used standard approaches for qualitative data. She took detailed notes during the sessions. Notes included navigational choices each respondent made as he or she worked through the tasks, his or her comments while thinking aloud, responses to the questions the researcher asked, times when actions occurred, and remarks made during debriefing sessions. The notes were translated into practical design recommendations that the designer processed before the website's final launch.

2.6 Time and Cost Investments

Table 2 shows the time span, man-hours and cost in Euros for both the research and design process. From Table 2 can be derived that both the usability testing and the website engineering were realized within a time frame of three months for the total cost of €7195.

Table 2. Time, effort, and cost of various phases of the user-centered e-health design process

Activity	Time span (2010)	Hours	Cost in Euros
• Development of research instruments (traditional thinking aloud, Card Sorting, prototyping, simplified thinking aloud)	May 1st- May 10th	10 [1]	175
• Conducting traditional thinking aloud and Card Sorting	May 10th- May 20th	27 [1]	472.50
• Transcribing thinking aloud data	May 20th- May 30th	54 [1]	945
• Coding of thinking aloud data	June 1st- June 7th	40 [1]	700
• Processing hand-sorted Card Sorting data into WebSort™ software and cluster analysis	June 1st- June 7th	5 [1]	87.50
• Translating thinking aloud data into design recommendations for website lay-out	June 8th	5 [1]	87.50
• Creation of two mock-up prototypes	June 8th- June 10th	10 [2]	600
• Conducting prototyping by e-mail	June 10h- June 15th	1 [1]	17.50
• Analyzing prototyping results	June 16th	3 [1]	52.5
• Creating first functional prototype of website, including content management system	June 16th - July 15th	55 [2]	3300
• Conducting simplified thinking aloud (n=5)	July 16th- July 18th	5 [1]	87.50
• Translating thinking aloud data into recommendations for website optimization	July 19th	4 [1]	70
• Processing thinking aloud recommendations into final version before website launch	July 20th- July 30th	10 [2]	600
Total	3 months	229 [3]	7195

Remark. The hours and cost do not include the man-hours (40 hours) spent by the infection control nurse to improve the content of the paper-based guidelines and make it suitable for web-based communication.

[1] Conducted by a student-assistant with an hourly rate of €17.50, including social security premiums.

[2] Conducted by an engineer with an hourly rate of €60.00, including social security premiums.

[3] Of these 229 hours, 154 refer to usability testing and 75 to website development.

3   Results

3.1   Traditional Thinking Aloud (Content)

Together, the 18 respondents worked on 192 tasks (10.7 tasks per respondent in 45 minutes, on average). Almost one third of the performed scenarios was not completed successfully (32.8%). Furthermore, it took the respondents an average of 199 seconds (3.3 minutes) to finish a task. Given that in reality, health care workers abandon a search after about two minutes, the effectiveness and efficiency of the paper-based guidelines can be rated as low [37]. The observations and the think-aloud verbaliza-tions made clear what the main usability problems were. Table 3 shows the relation between the number of verbalizations and the type of usability problems.

Table 3. Overview of usability problems encountered when using paper-based guidelines (N=18)

Problem type	Frequency of problem	Percentage
Mismatch between nursing home staff's and expert vocabulary	167	42%
Incomprehensible information	100	25%
Incomplete information	69	18%
Inadequate information structure	54	14%
Inaccurate information	3	1%
Total	393	100

Table 2 shows that the tasks could not be completed successfully due to the follow-ing causes:

1. Mismatch problems (42% of problems): Respondents could not retrieve relevant information because of the volume of the guidelines (80 pages) and a mismatch between the search terms used by nursing home staff (e.g., "treatment") and the vocabulary applied in the guidelines (e.g., "decontamination procedure");
2. Incomprehensible information (25% of problems): Based on the information in the guidelines, respondents got even more confused about what to do in clinical practice, or did not comprehend the jargon used in the guidelines, e.g., the word "alkaline";
3. Incomplete information (18% of problems): For instance, the guidelines did make clear which protective clothing should be worn when entering an isolation room, but did not elucidate in which order the clothing should be taken on and off. Re-spondents indicated that the information was too concise to enable them to make a safe decision for clinical practice;
4. Inadequate information structure (14% of problems): For instance, nursing home staff expected to find the required information in a particular section of the paper document or by employing a specific search strategy, but the opposite appeared to be true, as the following citation illustrates: *"Now I have to read the complete index. An alphabetically ordered-index would make it more practical, so I can*

immediately and more quickly find what I need." Other examples of information structure problems that were encountered with the paper-based guidelines were:

- Difficulties with finding specific pages;
- Lack of list-wise presented information;
- Lack of decision trees;
- Lack of tables;
- Little space between the lines;

5. Inaccurate information (1% of problems): Outdated information, and a discrepancy between the guideline's rules and the possibilities of performing them in practice. E.g., the guideline requires each (suspicious) patient carrying a multiresistant micro-organism to be treated in preventive isolation, while on particular wards no isolation facilities are available.

We intended to prevent these problems by tailoring the website's functional requirements to the identified problems:

1. Mismatch problems and incomprehensible information: In order to communicate the guidelines' content to dovetail with nursing home staff's vocabulary, we used words on the website such as "get rid of bacteria" instead of "eradication therapy", "take swabs" instead of "perform screening cultures", "outbreak" rather than "epidemic situation", etc. A dedicated content management system enabled the infection control nurse to add and delete keywords to the search engine's database that aid in matching system with nursing home staff's vocabulary. Furthermore, mouse-overs were raised when the user moves or "hovers" the cursor over a word that they perceived as "difficult";
2. Incomplete information: Multiple key questions relating to everyday work practice were found for which the guidelines did not provide an adequate answer. Because we strived to provide nursing home staff with complete, comprehensible, and accurate guidelines that enable them to deliver safe health care, we included links, literature sources, pictures, videos, and other relevant multimedia examples to complement the guidelines;
3. Inaccurate information: Revision dates and the latest news were included in order to keep information accurate;
4. Inadequate information structure: Each guideline theme was presented according to a standardized format based on usability guidelines [38], with important items placed consistently at the top center. For each guideline, the standardized structure was: Title, target, indication, when to use, location, definitions, responsibilities, materials needed, correct procedure, comments, references. In order to make the search process more efficient, the system should allow the user to rapidly switch from one search strategy to another and enables users to keep track of their location within the system. Therefore, guidelines were retrievable through a search engine, a menu structure with categories, and frequently asked questions. The incorporation of three search options enabled nursing home staff to find the relevant information more rapidly with less effort (i.e., more efficient).

3.2 Card Sorting (Structure)

The Card Sort Study resulted in ten categories according to which the 59 themes derived from the guidelines content could be structured. The categories, each with an example to illustrate the practical approach of the website, are presented in Table 4. Compared to the general tables of content of infection control guidelines, it is remarkable that the search structure based on the Card Sort Study included a category on "To work or not to work", and a separate category on "Diarrhea". It appeared that nursing home staff desired a more action- and communication-oriented way of structuring information than is the case in current infection control guidelines. By employing a Card Sort Study, we tried to overcome problems with inadequate information structure. Since the categories' names were generated by the respondents themselves, usability problems caused by a mismatch in vocabulary and incomprehensible information were also prevented.

Table 4. Categories resulting from the Card Sort Study (n=18), each with an exemplary theme

Category	Example
Basic and hand hygiene	Am I allowed to wear nail polish during work hours?
Cleaning	Which products should I use in order to clean a client's po?
Definitions	What does the abbreviation PPM mean?
Diarrhea	How often should the toilet be cleaned in case a client has diarrhea?
How to act in case of an infection?	Which protective clothing should I wear when nursing a client with Anthony's fire (erysipelas)?
Laundry	Which precautions do I need to take with laundry of a client who has Methicillin Resistant *Staphylococcus aureus*?
Needles	Where should I dispose a used injection needle?
To work or not to work?	Am I allowed to work when I have weeping eczema?
Waste	Where to put paper and glass waste?
Wound care	Should I use sterile bandage in case of wound care?

3.3 Mock Up Prototyping (Lay-Out)

Our belief that a web-based format would improve the usability of the guidelines was strengthened by the findings of the traditional thinking aloud study. Although information quality problems (inaccuracy, incomprehensibility, and incompleteness) could have easily been prevented by solely improving the information and maintaining the paper-based format, the (1) mismatch and (2) "information structure" problems could be more optimally addressed via a website. (1) A content management system would enable the infection control nurse to add and delete keywords to the search engine's database that aid in matching system's with nursing home staff's vocabulary, and (2) a web-based format would allow the inclusion of combining several search options (search engine, categorical search, frequently asked questions) and could aid to enhance the clarity of the information structure, like a breadcrumb trail. We formulated three general principles for the improved communication of infection control guidelines, based on our understanding of nursing home staff's problems with the paper-based guidelines that resulted from the traditional thinking aloud:

1. Add practical, action oriented content (in order to avoid information quality problems), communicated in nursing home staff's vocabulary (to prevent matching problems);
2. Present guidelines in a multimodal way (in order to overcome information structure problems);
3. Consider different search strategies nursing home staff employ by incorporating three search options.

We applied these design principles next to usability guidelines when creating two non-working mock-ups [38]. The mock-ups each consisted of a homepage (see Figures 1 and 2). When asked to indicate their preference for one of the two mock-ups, 4 out of 5 respondents chose prototype 1, particularly because of "the convenient structure" (n=3), "the colors suit the theme of infection control" (n=4), and "the trustworthiness suggested by the logos of the involved organizations" (n=2). Prototype 2 was evaluated as "unattractive" (n=4) and "too gay (n=3)". Hence it was decided that the final lay-out of our website should be based on prototype 1. Asking users for subjective ratings of lay-out appeared useful. Even though respondents had different tastes and like and disliked different aspects of the mock-ups, one mock-up was disliked by four of five respondents. The constructive feedback given by the respondents was processed into the functional prototype of the website, which is depicted in Figure 3.

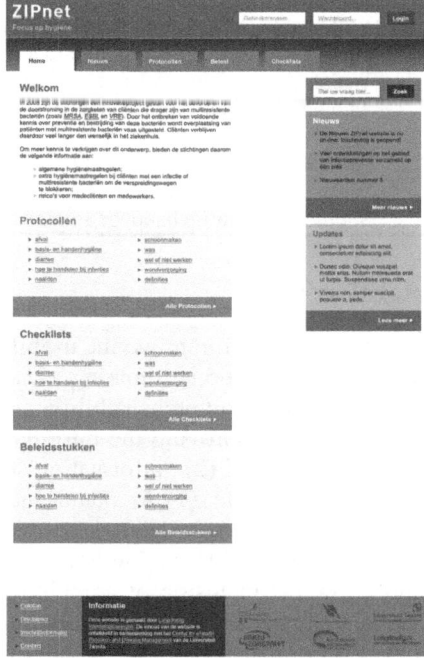

Fig. 1. Mock-up prototype 1

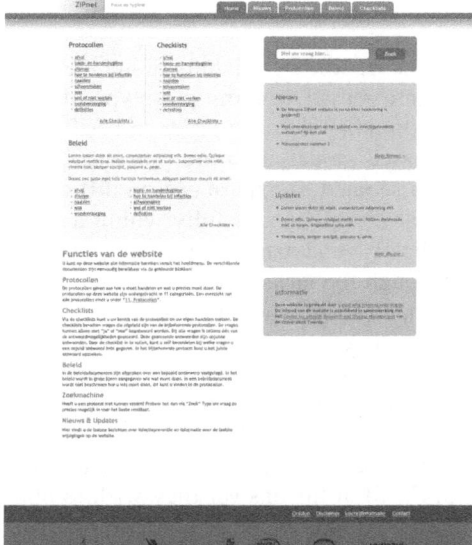

Fig. 2. Mock-up prototype 2

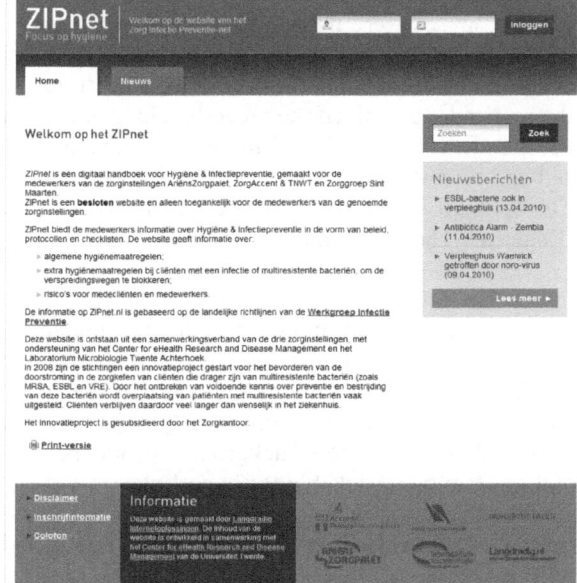

Fig. 3. Final version of the website's homepage (http://www.zipnet)

3.4 Simplified Thinking Aloud (Synergizing Content, Structure, and Lay-Out)

The results from each of the traditional thinking aloud, the Card Sorting, and the prototyping were integrated into a final working prototype of the website (see Figure 3). We undertook simplified thinking aloud in order to verify whether the problems that occurred with the paper-based guidelines were prevented with the web-based guidelines. All five respondents seemed to experience no difficulties when using the website. Almost every task was solved successfully within a time frame of 120 seconds. Each respondent immediately understood how the website had to be navigated through. They worked through the tasks quickly, and for the most part, determinedly. Respondents had little trouble understanding the guidelines and could translate the information to daily work practice.

It appeared that the amount of mismatch problems decreased due to the vocabulary that now matched nursing home staff's mental models. For the same reasons, information appeared to be more comprehensible compared to the paper-based guidelines. Information was perceived as complete, as the website allowed nursing home staff to decide upon the level of detail of the answer they wish to obtain, because next to the short answer, in-depth elaborations were provided, next to sources (e.g., scientific literature, newspaper articles, links to other websites for further reading, etc.). The multimedia examples (e.g., instruction movies and pictures of how to adequately apply personal protective equipment) were also highly appreciated. The respondents were enthusiastic about the information structure because important items were placed consistently at the top center, scroll stoppers were avoided as much as possible, and moderate white spaces were used. Also, information was not longer recognized as outdated: A dedicated content management system enabled the infection control nurse to add and delete information on the website at any time and location, which made that the respondents noticed the recently added news items.

The comments respondents made while thinking aloud, responses to the questions the researcher asked and remarks made during debriefing sessions, generated specific recommendations to optimally target the websites' content, structure, and lay-out to nursing home staff's needs. The most salient suggestions were:

Content. The mouse-overs, intended to be raised when nursing home staff moved the cursor over a difficult word, were not observed by the respondents. According to the respondents, the words to which a mouse-over was coupled had to be emphasized more explicitly. Furthermore, respondents mentioned that the risks involved in particular actions needed to be emphasized more clearly, e.g., through sparingly using underlines, bold, and italics. A colored background would be even better because underlining for emphasis can be mistakable for hyperlinks.

Structure. The order of the standardized structure (title, target, indication, when to use, location, definitions, responsibilities, materials needed, correct procedure, comments, references) according to which each guideline was presented, was not understood by every respondent. Respondents suggested that the order of the structural elements could better be changed: The main reason for using the website would be to look up the correct procedure. Therefore, the procedure should be placed on top of the page, followed by the remaining elements.

Lay-out. The news items, updates, and title were depicted in white text on a colored background (red, green, blue). However, respondents remarked that there was no sufficient contrast between text and its background and therefore, text was hard to read. Therefore, the background colors were set darker.

The recommendations suggested by the respondents were translated into practical design recommendations that the designer processed prior to website's final launch.

4   Discussion

4.1   Efficient, Effective, and Satisfying Process

The evaluation and usability methodology employed for discount user-centered e-health design proved to be both efficient and effective, and leading to high levels of satisfaction for the target group: nursing home staff [15, 39].

Efficient. The complete design process from the early beginning until the implementation of the websites took only 12 weeks and led to a rapid and consensual decision. The total cost of the process was less than 7200€ including the design and implementation of the application itself, the usability studies, and the project staff's fee. No additional equipment or room space was needed for the observations. Overall, time spent on planning, executing, reporting, and presenting the evaluation was approximately 229 hours.

Effective. Although we used a discount approach, the results proved to be very informative and efficiently supported the decision making process. Although our methods were fast and cheap, they still met the three principles of user-centered design: early focus on the user, empirical measurement, and iterative design [19]. The process led to a realistic choice for a website. The test report was sent to managers from participating wards of the various nursing homes. Several of them decided to invest in user-centered design for the design and implementation of other communication devices within the nursing home setting.

Satisfaction. The final choice of the website was strongly and positively by the results of the user-centered discount approach.

4.2   Benefits of Discount User-Centered e-Health Design

Based on our findings, we would advocate using this discount user-centered design approach for the design of e-health applications. The philosophy of involving end users and other relevant stakeholders rightly fits the concept of participatory health care. Effective health care requires productive interaction between activated patients and a prepared practice team [40]. In its landmark 2001 report on Crossing the Quality Chasm, the Institute of Medicine named "patient-centered care" as one of the fundamental aims of the health care system, to spearhead the concept that healthcare should be centered on the individual patient's needs, wants, and perspectives. Benefits of patient-centered care or patient participation include enhancing patient's knowledge about health concern, patients are helped to understand the decisions that health care providers make daily, collaboration between patient and provider frames discussions, and patients' empowerment to take action in their own healthcare process [41]. Several new concepts have risen, all with an identical meaning to patient-centered care such as "shared decision making" or "participatory medicine" [42]. When applying user-centered design for the development of e-health applications, stakeholder involvement might be enhanced, which creates ownership, fosters applicability of the application, and leads to a willingness to integrate the application into routine care. The intensive participation of the users in our test sessions greatly improved their knowledge of the project. At the end of the test weeks, a nursing home employee would have had to be deaf and blind not to know about the project and its content. Other scholars also emphasized this benefit. E.g., Petit Jones claims that "discount usability engineering results opened dialogue about usability issues (…) and helps secure more time to address usability on other projects. [43]"

Thus, user participation is increasingly recognized as a key element of the overall quality of healthcare, which might be supported by user-centered e-health design. However, involving relevant stakeholders in the design of health care applications has not become a standard procedure yet. Several barriers exist in realizing patient participation, such as financial constraints, fatigue and competing priorities, and a lack of tools to gauge and reward user-centered care. In other words: an efficient and effective mix of instruments and participants has not been identified yet. In here, discount user-centered design might serve as a solution. With our study, we identified a discount approach for user-centered design of a completely new e-health application within a time frame of three months, for cost lower than 7500€. The following factors enabled us to develop a user-centered website with infection control guidelines with such a restricted budget of time and money:

- Case-driven: No expensive laboratory had to be rented, nor had any expensive recording equipment to be purchased. A simple digital voicerecorder sufficed.
- Small sample size: Since the results did not have to be generalizable to the complete Dutch population, and five respondents were enough to detect at least 75% of user problems, we only needed to include few participants.
- Online, free software: Part of the analysis was conducted through online, free software: A trial version of WebSort^{TM}.
- Method of analysis: Data analysis of the second part of the study (prototyping, simplified thinking aloud) was solely based on the researcher's notes instead of data transcription, which saved time and thus money.

Our study was not the first attempt "to improve a system in the shortest time with the least effort" without performing extensive and formal usability evaluation, while at the same time preventing that results are completely worthless. Other researchers also discussed at what level discount usability methods are fast and cheap, but not so fast and cheap that they are no longer valid. E.g., Marty and Twidale [24] explored the value of discount usability engineering at extremes of times and tests, with conducting 36 entire evaluations in only thirty minutes. Kjeldskov, Skov and Stage [23] presented a data analysis technique which allows usability evaluations to be conducted, analyzed and documented in one day. Both Marty et al. and Kjeldskov et al. looked at the percentage of critical usability that the methods raised compared to standardized, formal usability evaluations. Our study however, was targeted not so much at comparing new discount methods to traditional usability engineering, but to identify a discount approach for user-centered design of a completely new e-health application (without a prototype being available). We achieved this by combining traditional thinking aloud and Card Sorting with the discount usability methods of prototyping and simplified thinking aloud, and by omitting heuristic evaluation. The findings of our study open a relatively unexplored area of the user testing continuum. Many usability evaluators make the rigid distinction between academic research on the one hand and pragmatic research on the other, with in between a huge gap [24]. Our study demonstrated that a compromise between the two is fairly possible, with the combination of traditional thinking aloud and Card Sorting on the one hand, and mock up prototyping and simplified thinking aloud on the other hand. Because the user has a more active role in our approach, we claim that our discount approach is more user-centered compared to the standardized discount approach suggested by Nielsen [19].

4.3 Study Limitations

The results gathered in this study need to be recognized as having a "real world application". In other words, the test results are not suited to test statistical significance. Certainly, for much research, one needs to have a high degree of confidence that the findings are not subject to chance. For the design of usable e-health applications however, one can be satisfied by less rigorous tests like those we conducted [19]. In other words, even tests that are not statistically significant are well worth doing since they will improve the quality of applications substantially. Although the methodology used in this study did not follow scientific standards, the results should be considered as relevant as scientific-based results and applicable in the real world [14].

Maybe, better results would have been achieved by applying more careful methodologies. However, more careful methodologies are also more expensive in terms of time and money, and also in terms of required expertise. For instance, a more extensive analysis of the data, particularly of the simplified thinking aloud tests with the website, would have produced a more detailed description of each of the identified usability problems. The simplified data analysis did not provide this detailed information but merely produced a list of shortly described problems. For the purpose of a scientific comparison between the paper-based and web-based infection control guidelines just like in Verhoeven et al [4], the thinking aloud data should have been recorded and transcribed verbatim. Previous research with traditional thinking aloud as a user test method of the website demonstrated the chosen approach (traditional thinking aloud, Card Sorting, mock-up prototyping) to be valid (see [4]). When we would have applied a more rigorous user evaluation of the website, the method could not have been called a discount method any longer.

Therefore, the simpler methods stand a much better chance of actually being used in practical design situations and they should therefore be viewed as a way of serving the user.

4.4 Future Research

In future research, it would be interesting to address the following issues:

Integrate methods of participatory design in discount usability engineering. In participatory experiences, the roles of the designer and the researcher blur and the user becomes a critical component of the process. The new rules call for new tools, by which users can express themselves and participate directly and proactively in the design process. Traditional design research methods were focused primarily on observational research (i.e., looking at what people do and use). Traditional market research methods, on the other hand, have been focused more on what people say and think (through focus groups, interviews, and questionnaires). New methods for participatory design should be more focused on what people make, i.e., what they create from the toolkits we provide for them to use in expressing their thoughts, feelings and dreams. Co-design methods such as probes, probe diaries, workshops, user sketching, low-tech prototyping, sticky-note feedback, and distributed collaboration might serve as a promising solution in here [45, 46]. For instance, a recent study showed that user sketching facilitated thinking, reflection, and discovery for respondents and resulted in receiving more reflective feedback. Tohidi et al therefore recommended the use of this practice as a quick and inexpensive addition to other commonly used practices. They believe that sketching has the potential to be developed into a light-weight form of usability testing, due to its relatively low cost in time demands for analysis [46]. Future studies should investigate the benefits of these creative co-design or participatory methods for discount usability engineering.

IntegrateWeb 2.0 research methods in discount usability engineering. Next to creative research methods, online research methods could also contribute to the feasibility of discount usability engineering. Studies conducted online are not only less error prone and labor intensive but also rapidly reach large numbers of diverse participants at a fraction of the cost of traditional methods. In addition to improving the efficiency and accuracy of data collection, online studies provide automatic data storage and deliver immediate personalized feedback to research participant; a major incentive that can exponentially expand participant pools. Furthermore, behavioral researchers can also track data on online behavioral phenomena, including Instant Messaging, social networking, and other social media [47]. Involving stakeholders and end users via social networking platforms creates new levels of participation. Web 2.0 tools such as social networking sites, blogs, podcasts, tagging and communication tools stimulate "apomediation", which is the phenomenon that users can help other users navigate through the wealth of information afforded by networked digital media, providing additional credibility cues and supplying further meta-information [42].

5 Conclusion

Our main research question was: Are the available, existing discount usability methods suitable for the design and development of new e-health applications, or do other research methods have to be incorporated? We claimed the latter to be true. For the case of this study, we adapted Nielsen's discount usability approach because (1) we deemed it less appropriate for the design of *new* applications (for which no prototype is yet available) and (2) heuristic expert evaluation, which is part of Nielsen's discount approach, will not play its full right given the fact that in our case, the expert-driven character of documentation is the major cause of usability problems. Therefore, we complemented Nielsen's methodology with traditional thinking aloud to make it suitable for new applications, and replaced the heuristic evaluation with a more user-centered method: Card Sorting. Together, the methods generated the optimal content, structure, and lay-out for a website with infection control guidelines for nursing homes. We intended to demonstrate that although our method is quick, it definitely is not dirty, since our methodology is based on scientific design principles and still enables data analysis at an academic level. Based on our findings, we would advocate using this discount user-centered design approach for the design of e-health applications. Next to this advice, we believe the design principles for web-based communication of infection control guidelines this study generated may also be helpful to others engaged in the infection control setting.

Acknowledgments. The authors thank Ria Hoentjen for selecting the respondents and Jessica Askamp, Marjolein Voskamp, and Els Koster for administering and transcribing the traditional thinking aloud tests. Finally, the authors would like to thank the respondents for their time and effort to participate in this study.

References

1. Pittet, D., Donaldson, L.: Challenging the world: patient safety and health care-associated infection. Int. J. Qual. Health Care 18, 4–8 (2006)
2. Berhe, M., Edmond, M.B., Mearman, G.M.: Practices and an assessment of health care workers perceptions of compliance with infection control knowledge of nosocomial infections. Am. J. Infect. Control 3, 55–57 (2005)
3. Verhoeven, F., Van Gemert-Pijnen, J.E.W.C., Friedrich, A.W., Daniels-Haardt, I., Hendrix, M.G.R., Steehouder, M.F.: The development of a web-based information tool for cross-border prevention and control of Methicillin Resistant Staphylococcus aureus. Int. J. Infect. Control 4, 1–11 (2008)
4. Verhoeven, F., Steehouder, M.F., Hendrix, M.G.R., Van Gemert-Pijnen, J.E.W.C.: From expert-driven to user-oriented communication of infection control guidelines. Int. J. Hum-Comput. Stud. 68, 328–343 (2010)
5. Verhoeven, F., Steehouder, M.F., Hendrix, M.G.R., Van Gemert-Pijnen, J.E.W.C.: Factors affecting health care workers' adoption of a website with infection control guidelines. Int. J. Med. Inform. 78, 663–678 (2009)
6. The AGREE Collaboration.: Development and validation of an international appraisal instrument for assessing the quality of clinical practice guidelines: the AGREE project. Qual. Saf. Health Care 12, 18–23 (2003)
7. Van Gemert-Pijnen, J.E.W.C., Hendrix, M.G.R., Van der Palen, J., Schellens, P.J.: Performance of methicillin-resistant Staphylococcus aureus protocols in Dutch hospitals. Am. J. Infect. Control 33, 377–384 (2005)
8. Fervers, B., Burgers, J.S., Haugh, M.C., Brouwers, M., Browman, G., Cluzeau, F., Philip, T.: Predictors of high quality clinical practice guidelines: examples in oncology. Int. J. Qual. Health Care 17, 123–132 (2005)

9. Thomas, C., Bevan, N. (eds.): Usability Context Analysis: A Practical Guide. NPL Usability Services, Teddington (1997)
10. Holzinger, A.: Usability Engineering for Software Developers. ACM Commun. 48, 71–74 (2005)
11. Hom, J.: The Usability Methods Toolbox. San José State University, San José (1998)
12. Nielsen, J.: Usability Engineering. Morgan Kaufmann, San Francisco (1993)
13. Jong, M., de Lentz, L.: Scenario evaluation of municipal websites. Development and use of an expert-focused evaluation tool. Gov't. Info. Q 23, 191–206 (2006)
14. Yao, P., Gorman, P.N.: Discount usability engineering applied to an interface for Web-based medical knowledge resources. In: Proceedings AMIA Annual Symposium, pp. 928–932 (2000)
15. Beuscart-Zéphir, M.C., Leroy, N., Alao, O., Darmoni, S.: Usability assessment study of a web site displaying medical resources on line: the CISMeF. Studies in Health Technology and Informatics 90, 133–137 (2002)
16. Kaplan, B.: Deriving Design Recommendations Through Discount Usability Engineering: Ethnographic Observation and Thinking-Aloud Protocol in Usability Testing for Computer-Based Teaching Cases. In: AMIA Annu. Symp. Proc., pp. 346–350 (2003)
17. Thursky, K.A., Mahemoff, M.: User-centered design techniques for a computerized antibiotic decision support system in an intensive care unit. Int. J. Med. Inform. 76, 760–768 (2007)
18. Elkin, P.L., Sorensen, B., De Palo, D., Poland, G., Bailey, K.R., Woord, D.L., LaRusso, N.F.: Optimization of a research web environment for academic internal medicine faculty. J. Am. Med. Inform. Ass. 9, 472–478 (2002)
19. Nielsen, J.: Guerrilla HCI: Using Discount Usability Engineering to Penetrate the Intimidation Barrier (1994),
    http://www.useit.com/papers/guerrilla_hci.html
20. Curtis, B., Nielsen, J.: Applying Discount Usability Engineering. IEEE Software 12, 98–100 (1995)
21. Dumas, J., Redish, J.: A practical guide to usability testing. Intellect, Bristol (1999)
22. Nielsen, J.: Report from a web usability study (1994),
    http://www.useit.com/papers/1994_web_usability_report.html
23. Kjeldsov, J., Skov, M.B., Stage, J.: Instant data analysis: conducting usability evaluations in a day. In: Proceedings of the Third Nordic Conference on Human-Computer Interaction, pp. 233–240 (2004)
24. Marty, P., Twidale, M.: Extreme Discount Usability Engineering, Technical Report ISRN UIUCLIS–2005/1+CSCW
25. APIC. Spreading knowledge.: Preventing Infection,
    http://www.apic.org/AM/Template.cfm?Section=Search&Template=
    /Search/SearchDisplay.cfm
26. Gutwin, C., Greenberg, S.: The Mechanics of Collaboration: Developing Low Cost Usability Evaluation Methods for Shared Workspaces. In: Proceedings of the 9th IEEE International Workshops on Enabling Technologies: Infrastructure for Collaborative Enterprises, pp. 98–103. IEEE Computer Society, Washington (2000)
27. Kane, D.: Finding a place for discount usability engineering in agile development: throwing down the gauntlet. In: Agile Development Conference, pp. 40–46. SRA Int., USA (2003)
28. Jaspers, M.W.M.: A Comparison of usability methods for testing interactive health technologies: Methodological aspects and empirical evidence. Int. J. Med. Inform. 78, 340–353 (2009)

29. Tullis, T.S.: Using Card-sorting Techniques to Organize your Intranet. J. Intranet Strat. Man 1, 1–9 (2003)
30. Spencer, D., Warfel, T.: Card sorting: a definitive guide, http://www.boxesandarrows.com/view/ card_sorting_a_definitive_guide
31. Walker, M., Takayama, L., Landay, J.A.: High-fidelity or low-fidelity, paper or computer? Choosing attributes when testing web prototypes. In: Proceedings of the Human Factors and Ergonomics Society 46th Annual Meeting, pp. 661–665. HFES, Santa Monica (2002)
32. Scriven, M.: Beyond Formative and Summative Evaluation. In: McLaughlin, M.W. (ed.) Evaluation and Education: A Quarter Century. University of Chicago Press, Chicago (1991)
33. Nielsen, J., Landauer, T.K.: A mathematical model of the finding of usability problems. In: Proceedings of INTERCHI, pp. 206–213. ACM, New York (1993)
34. Nielsen, J.: Why you only need to test with 5 users (2000), http://www.useit.com/alertbox/20000319.html
35. Virzi, R.A.: Refining the test phase of usability evaluation: how many subjects is enough? Human Factors 34, 457–468 (1992)
36. Lime & Chile Productions, LLC, http://websort.net/
37. Yu, H., Lee, M., Kaufman, D., Ely, J., Osheroff, J.A., Hripscsak, G., Cimino, J.: Development, implementation, and a cognitive evaluation of a definitional question answering system for physicians. J. Biomed. Inform. 40, 236–251 (2007)
38. Koyani, S.J., Bailey, R.W., Nall, J.R.: Research-Based Web Design & Usability Guidelines. U.S. Government Printing Office, Washington, DC (2006)
39. Kushniruk, A.: Evaluation in the design of health information systems: application of approaches emerging from usability engineering. Comp. Biol. Med. 32, 141–149 (2002)
40. Wagner, E.H.: Chronic disease care. Brit. Med. J. 7433, 177–178 (2004)
41. Wilson, E.V.: Patient centered e-health. Idea Group Publishing, New York (2009)
42. Eysenbach, G.: Medicine 2.0: Social Networking, Collaboration, Participation, Apomediation, and Openness. J. Med. Internet Res. 10 e22 (2008)
43. Petit Jones, C.: Lessons learned from Discount Usability Engineering for the Federal Government. Tech. Comm. 50, 232–246 (2003)
44. Sanders, E.B.M.: From user-centered to participatory design approaches. In: Frascara, J. (ed.) Design and the Social Sciences. Taylor & Francis Books Limited, Oxon (2002)
45. Westerlund, B., Lindqvist, S., Mackay, W., Sundblad, Y.: Co-design methods for designing with and for families. In: Proceedings for 5th European Academy of Design Conference in Barcelona, pp. 1–12. Techné, Barcelona (2003)
46. Tohidi, M., Buxton, W., Baecker, R., Sellen, A.: User Sketches: A Quick, Inexpensive, and Effective way to Elicit More Reflective User Feedback. In: NordiCHI, pp. 105–115. ACM, Oslo (2006)
47. Gosling, S.D., Johnson, J.A.: Advanced Methods for Conducting Online Behavioral Research. American Psychological Association, Washington DC (2010)

Towards a Pattern Language Approach to Sharing Experiences in Healthcare Technology Evaluations

Julie Doyle[1], Aaron Quigley[2], Paddy Nixon[3], and Brian Caulfield[1]

[1] CLARITY Centre for Sensor Web Technologies, University College Dublin,
Belfield, Dublin 4, Ireland
[2] School of Computer Science, North Haugh, University of St. Andrews, Fife, UK
[3] School of Computer Science and Informatics, University College Dublin, Ireland
julie.doyle@ucd.ie, aquigley@cs.st-andrews.ac.uk, paddy.nixon@ucd.ie,
b.caulfield@ucd.ie

Abstract. Healthcare technologies are becoming increasingly pervasive, moving from controlled clinical and laboratory settings, to real environments such as homes, acute care environments and residential care centres. As a consequence, new challenges arise in evaluating the impact of healthcare technologies and interactions in their context of use. In this paper we propose the use of a pattern language as a means of capturing experiences from researchers in the field of evaluating healthcare technologies. The potential benefits of such an approach include the availability of a centralised repository, or collaborative tool of past experiences which can contribute to the reuse of knowledge, which can encourage and improve communication between interdisciplinary members of the healthcare community and which is presented in a 'lay' language, understandable by all. We propose to structure the content of our pattern language along three stages of healthcare, namely home care, residential care and acute care and to organise evaluations across each of these stages in terms of physical, social, intellectual and purpose fitness.

1 Introduction

The recent developments and proliferation of unobtrusive and low-cost wireless sensor-based measurement technologies has resulted in an increased research interest in making healthcare technologies pervasive, moving from controlled clinical environments to 'real' environments, such as patient's homes [1] [2]. Pervasive healthcare technologies enable support for assisted living for older adults, that is, they facilitate this cohort in living healthy, independent lives in the place of their choice as they age. However, a consequence of the deployment of pervasive healthcare technologies to real contexts, such as homes, is that new challenges arise in the evaluation of the usability of these technologies and their impact on those who use them. Developing effective evaluation strategies is important for a number of reasons. Evaluation enables us to understand human behaviour and experience. It informs us as to whether a particular technology

G. Leitner, M. Hitz, and A. Holzinger (Eds.): USAB 2010, LNCS 6389, pp. 124–137, 2010.

is usable and receptive to user needs. It helps to ensure seamless integration of the technology with the user's environment. Furthermore, evaluation ensures optimal interaction and informs design.

Our research concerns the design, deployment and evaluation of home-based assisted living healthcare technologies for older adults. Throughout the deployment and evaluation cycle we have encountered many problems for which solutions had to be identified, typically by trial and error. We felt it would be of great benefit if we could learn from others' experiences of conducting in-home evaluations with older adults, reusing knowledge rather than (potentially) reinventing the wheel. Furthermore, we could assist other researchers by sharing our own experiences of problems encountered and solutions that solved these problems. As such, the motivation for this research resulted from the question 'How can we capture and share evaluator experiences and lessons learned?' The development of a pattern language appeared an ideal means of capturing such information.

The notion of some form of collaborative tool in evaluating non-lab environments has drawn much attention in recent years [2]. However, the idea of using a pattern language to help structure evaluations of healthcare technologies is unexplored, despite their success in other fields of research including architecture [3], software engineering [4] [5], e-learning [6] [7] and HCI [8] [9]. A pattern language is a structured method of describing best design practices within a field of expertise. In designing an evaluation, for example, the evaluator must make many decisions about how best to conduct the evaluation, or, how to solve evaluation 'problems'. A single evaluation problem, with a well documented solution of how this problem was solved in a particular context, constitutes a single pattern. A series of related patterns can, and should, be semantically linked to build an overall picture, or pattern language. Essentially, a pattern language is a conceptual tool to aid others in designing something, whether it is an evaluation, an online e-learning environment, or a house. Patterns provide an abstraction from any specific example, making them generalisable. The overall goal of this research is to contribute to the healthcare community's understanding of how to evaluate the use of healthcare technologies, as well as their impact on those who use them. As a first step in this process, this paper presents a pattern language framework and aims to discuss the concept of a pattern language for healthcare evaluations, to highlight the potential benefits for those researchers working within the field, as well as outlining how we plan to organise the content of our pattern repository.

2   Evaluating Healthcare Technologies in Real Environments

The movement of healthcare technologies to 'real' settings, such as homes or care settings, sees new challenges arise for evaluating usability, the feasibility of technology and user experiences 'in-situ' [2]. Laboratory evaluations are typically conducted in a controlled environment, where evaluators are present and can monitor, and control, proceedings. Participants typically carry out a scripted set of task scenarios and answer scripted questions based on each of these tasks, within a limited amount of time. Such settings are conducive to the collection of both qualitative and quantitative data.

However, it is vital to evaluate healthcare technologies in their environments of intended use. For example, while sensor networks for the collection of clinical data should, and typically are, validated prior to any home deployment, it is difficult to anticipate all the potential problems the home environment might create which could impact on the collection of healthcare-related data. While evaluating the living space prior to deployment, is one means of trying to predict potential obstacles, such environments are uncontrolled and when a technology is left 'in the wild' for long periods of time, any number of issues could arise that would not come to light in a lab-based study. This is particularly true when we consider that healthcare technologies might not only consist of one single piece of technology, but many integrated component parts, including hardware, software, sensor technology and interfaces, each of which is embedded within a real setting and each of which needs to be evaluated. Furthermore, participants of in-situ evaluations are real users who expect the deployed healthcare technology to meet their needs. Such real users will likely not always behave as we expect them to. Thus, observing the technology in use in real environments and by real users is highly beneficial. Another challenge in evaluating healthcare evaluations in real contexts of use, is that such evaluations need to be conducted over relatively long periods of time to ensure insightful data is collected. This creates further challenges as to the best methods for collecting quantitative and qualitative data. For example, how often, and at what stage of a home based evaluation should an evaluator meet with participants to collect qualitative data? How effective is self reporting of qualitative data, such as keeping a diary, over a long period of time? Evaluation challenges also arise in the recruitment and retention of participants for home-based long term studies of technology and in motivating continued usage of technology in the home after the initial 'novelty' factor has subsided. Each of these challenges are likely to affect other researchers interested in evaluating in-situ healthcare technologies. Many might seem simple, or unimportant in terms of a research contribution and hence may not have been documented in research papers. However, such experiences would be of benefit to other researchers in searching for solutions to similar evaluation problems.

We suggest a repository of documented problems relating to in-situ evaluation of healthcare technologies, including solutions to such problems as well as practicalities (for example is a particular evaluation too expensive/impractical to implement?) would be highly useful. Given the number of challenges associated with in-situ evaluations of healthcare technologies and the potentially significant costs of trial and error until effective evaluation techniques are found, we feel it is essential that some means of sharing and reusing solutions is necessary. Currently there is no such repository of others' findings within the field of healthcare technology evaluations. A pattern language essentially provides other evaluators with a resource to ensure they 'get things right' the first time round. While our particular research interests lie in evaluating healthcare technologies for older adults in the home, there are similar challenges faced in acute care and residential care settings. A pattern repository on evaluating healthcare technologies should thus also include experiences of evaluations conducted in settings other than homes, so as to appeal to the wider HCI/healthcare community who are interested in evaluating such technologies.

3   Pattern Languages

The concept of a pattern language was introduced by Christopher Alexander and was directed towards the field of architecture [3]. Entities called patterns combine to make up the language. Alexander described the central idea of a pattern language as a means to capture information about frequently encountered problems and how they are solved. More specifically, "each pattern describes a problem which occurs over and over again in our environment, and then describes the core of the solution to that problem, in such a way that you can use this solution a million times over, without ever doing it the same way twice" [3]. Pattern languages begin with a high level problem and work towards more detailed problems. While a single pattern can contribute to the reuse of knowledge, the biggest advantages are gained when a number of interconnected patterns are combined into a language. This connection among patterns is a crucial component to the overall language. Patterns do not live in isolation. Rather, they are similar to a network, whereby one pattern may link to another, one pattern may be a sub pattern of another etc. As such, a pattern language may be organised as a tree or a graph, enabling a top-down linear search of elements.

More recently, patterns have been used in fields including software design [5], interaction design [8], usability [9], [10], user interface design [11], ubiquitous computing [12] and e-learning [6]. What is evident among all the patterns research that exists, both within and across different research areas, is that many opinions exist on how best to organise the patterns within some structure. For example, Tidwell [11] organises content under the headings 'What', 'Use When', 'Why' and 'How'. In describing a pattern language for usability, Casaday [10] proposes structuring pattern content based on traditional usability attributes, including learnability, memorability, efficiency, reliability, flexibility, automation, understandability and subjective satisfaction. On the other hand, Mahemoff & Johnston [9] propose four categories of pattern languages for usability, based on tasks, users, the relationships that exist between user interface objects and finally patterns of entire systems. While there may be no one correct way to organise the content of a pattern language, there are certainly good ways which should reflect the application context that the pattern language will describe and which will help pattern users to locate patterns easily.

Surprisingly, given the success pattern languages have enjoyed in the research fields mentioned above, there has not yet been an investigation into the use of pattern languages as a means to gather information relating to experiences in evaluating healthcare technologies. While it might be argued that other methods of collating and sharing knowledge exist, such as standards and guidelines [13], for example, pattern languages offer a number of benefits over such methods and as such provide a much richer resource for healthcare evaluation designers:

- Foremost, having a centralised repository, or framework, in which knowledge and experience outlining others' findings in the field can be expressed, will vastly improve communication between interdisciplinary members of the healthcare community. Currently, such a facility does not exist.
- Information within a pattern language is presented in a 'lay' language, understandable by all types of users in the healthcare domain, including non-technical people. Healthcare is very much an interdisciplinary field and a pattern language should reflect this.
- A pattern language supports reuse of data and ideas. For example, pattern languages to describe usability have covered tasks, entire systems, user interface elements and users in deciding what should be stored and documenting what has previously worked, or not, reducing the costly trial and error cycle.
- Patterns represent an effective way to organise complex information and support navigation in a manner that guidelines or templates don't.
- Whole patterns are recorded. While guidelines typically record simple instructions, patterns provide meta-information surrounding this instruction, setting a context and highlighting the problem the pattern solves in addition to a workable solution.
- Patterns have a vocabulary specific to a particular field of research.
- They are simple to learn and use, they support a broad range of applications and are commonly accessible.
- Pattern languages are a collaborative effort - anyone can extend or evolve the language and this ensures that they are superior to guidelines or templates. A pattern language encourages communication.

There are a number of issues involved in developing a pattern language for structuring evaluations in healthcare technologies. For example, exactly what content should be stored? How do we structure this content? Where do we store this information? How do we ensure it is accessible by all community members? How do we ensure the patterns are applicable and easy to follow? The first two questions are the focus of this paper, while our current and future work is addressing the remainder.

4   Our Pattern Language Framework

We began the process of defining a pattern language for healthcare evaluations by considering the content it would likely contain and defining a structure for that content. Getting the structure of the framework right is crucial. To ensure the patterns are practically usable, they must be linked together logically to form a cohesive language that can be easily understood by interested users groups. As such, we adopted a top-down approach similar to that of Alexander, whereby the top level of the pattern language represents the highest level of abstraction and lower levels of sub-patterns represent more specific examples.

As we saw in the discussion of pattern languages above, there are many possible ways of structuring patterns within a repository. Given that we are interested in independent living technologies for older adults, particularly the evaluation of such technologies, we decided to structure our pattern language based on the Quality of Life versus Cost model which has been included in the EU project CAPSIL's roadmap [14]. This model, displayed in Figure 1, describes three stages of healthcare: 1) Home Care; 2) Residential Care; 3) Acute Care. The graph represents a 'shift-left' model, whereby we attempt to reduce the cost of care, while improving the quality of life of the patient. However, gaps (identified by CAPSIL [14]) exist in making this happen and it is a complex path to 'shift back' to a high quality of life, which ultimately might cost more with no actual guarantee of an improvement in the patient's quality of life. For example, for patients who have suffered a stroke, rehabilitation aims to improve physical and cognitive functionality [15]. Following a stroke, a patient may remain in acute care for any number of months. However, with rehabilitation there should be a progressive shift back to home care. As such, effective technology interventions are necessary in the home to monitor the patient through the remainder of their recovery.

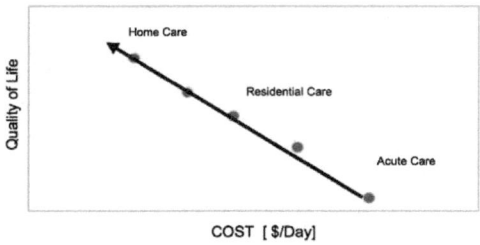

Fig. 1. Quality of Life versus Cost Model of Healthcare

At the centre of our framework is the 'patient'(Figure 2). While we use the term patient for our current purposes we expect that this will change or be refined in time. For example, with independent living technologies, technology in the home would ideally prevent the older adult from becoming a patient. Conversely, if a patient is moving along the shift-left model towards home-based care, in time they might no longer be a patient. We could also refine 'patient' to include different types of patients e.g. a patient with chronic heart disease, Parkinson's or Alzheimer's for example. A number of patterns might relate to the 'patient'. For example, how to overcome challenges in evaluating technologies with older adults, or those suffering from dementia. From the 'patient' extends the different environments where a patient might reside i.e. at home, in a residential care facility or in acute care. We further refine our pattern language by defining the types of 'fitness' we believe it is necessary to evaluate at each level of care. While many technologies are designed to monitor physical fitness, there are other aspects of ageing where technology can play a supporting role. These include promoting social fitness, intellectual and purpose fitness. Each of these play a crucial role in contributing to independent living for older adults, and as such evaluating technologies that promote each type of fitness are of interest to us for our research. Our proposed structure promotes evaluating physical, social, intellectual and purpose fitness at each stage of care - acute, residential and home. This is important as across each stage of care, different evaluation strategies are likely to be necessary to effectively assess these different levels of fitness. This is discussed further below.

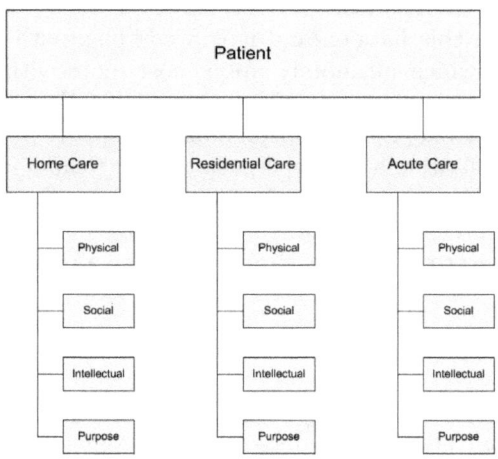

Fig. 2. Structure of our Pattern Language for Capturing Experiences in Healthcare Evaluations

4.1 Physical Fitness

With respect to this framework, we define physical fitness to mean a person's physical capacity to perform activities. Probably the most important aspect of physical fitness in relation to independent living for older adults is mobility. Mobility plays a vital role in ensuring older adults can remain active, helping them to age independently. Consequently, evaluating physical fitness might involve evaluating activities of daily living, an exercise regime for rehabilitation and falls prevention technologies. There exists much research regarding evaluating healthcare technologies to monitor activities of daily living. The majority of this research focuses on the feasibility of sensor systems in the home, that is, how effective different types of sensors placed in various locations throughout the home are in collecting clinical data. However, there may be certain challenges involved in the evaluation of sensor systems, many of which may not be reported in research papers as they do not constitute a major research contribution. Such challenges, and how they were overcome, may be very relevant to other researchers interested in installing sensor systems in the home. For example, consider a network of sensors placed in a person's home to monitor their mobility. Challenges in accurately measuring the older adult's mobility over a long period of time might include visitors to the home who may pass the sensors, thereby triggering them to record this person's activity, or pets who may also trigger sensors. Possible solutions to such problems may include having the subject keep a diary of all visitors, including times they arrived and left, or searching through the dataset for spurious data which evidently does not belong to the subject. A pattern language is an ideal means of recording such details, providing other interested researchers with details of 'what works' and 'what doesn't work' in different evaluation scenarios.

4.2   Intellectual Fitness

Cognitive impairment can affect an individual's ability to process and interpret information. It can have many negative consequences such as accident proneness, self-neglect, loss of initiative, diminished level of activities and low mood. In certain cases, serious cognitive decline can lead to dementia. Technology interventions for intellectual fitness have increased in recent years. They can generally be split into interventions to delay the onset of cognitive impairment and interventions to remediate those individuals who are currently suffering from cognitive deficiencies. Such interventions range from commercial products, such as Nintendo's brain training games, to more academic research oriented applications. Many studies have shown that cognitive training with older adults on a specific task improves subsequent performance of that task [16]. For example, researchers at Oregon Health & Science University have shown that the computer-based game FreeCell can be used to monitor subtle cognitive changes in older adults over time, and from within their own homes [16]. The benefits of this are that mild cognitive impairment could be detected before the onset of Alzheimer's disease, allowing doctors to plan treatments for the disease earlier. Evaluation of intellectual fitness in this unobtrusive and continuous manner may reveal more reliable information than yearly check-ups.

4.3   Social Fitness

Ageing, for many people, is a time of great change and transition and such changes may affect an individual's social fitness. A person's peer network begins to shrink, friends and family may be busy or living far away, and restricted physical mobility resulting from illness, injury, or as a consequence of ageing, may be restricted, inhibiting the level of social activities outside the home. Unfortunately, a lack of social interaction may lead to loneliness, depression and isolation for many individuals, effectively reducing their quality of life. However, research is examining how technologies can facilitate social interaction among older adults, by connecting them with family and friends [17], as well as with their peers. Evaluating such technologies may encompass both answering social questions in addition to assessing their usability.

4.4   Purpose Fitness

Purpose fitness is a topic of independent living research that is rarely considered. However, we believe it is equally important in ensuring an individual can lead a healthy, independent life. Purpose fitness relates to an individual's feelings of their purpose in life. For example, throughout the course of life, children, a spouse, or work might represent an individual's purpose. However, as a person ages their purpose will likely change as their children grow up and no longer require their care, they have retired from work and as the years go on the likelihood of losing a spouse increases. We believe it is vital for people to believe they have a purpose to ensure they don't isolate themselves or become depressed. Finding a new purpose might include looking after grandchildren, being part of a team or being a carer for a peer. Evaluating purpose fitness might not be as clear-cut as the above categories of fitness, but one might argue that ensuring someone is physically, intellectually and socially fit can certainly contribute to purpose fitness. Little research exists on this and it will be a topic of further investigation for us to define methods to evaluate the purpose fitness of older adults in their homes.

Physical, intellectual, social and purpose fitness are all somewhat interrelated. An older adult who has had a series of falls may develop a fear of falling, preventing him/her from leaving the house. This in turn negatively impacts on their social fitness. Despite this level of interrelatedness among the various levels of fitness, different evaluation techniques are necessary to evaluate/monitor each type of fitness across the different care settings outlined in our framework. For example, evaluating physical fitness in the home will most definitely require different evaluation methods to evaluating the physical fitness of someone in acute care, given the differences between home and hospital-based settings. In evaluating the effectiveness of interventions to aid stroke rehabilitation, an acute care setting is very much controlled. A medical professional will be present and will assess improvement in motor and cognitive functionality using observer-based, ordinal scale instruments, such as the Functional Independence Measure (FIM) [18]. However, as previously mentioned, there are many reasons for moving along the shift-left model of Figure 1 from acute or residential care, to home-based care. These include the cost of acute rehabilitation for both the patient and the healthcare system, as well as a patient's desire to be able to live independently in their home. As such, to remotely monitor and assess a patient's recovery in the home, a number of sensors are required, which in turn necessitates new evaluation techniques to evaluate the efficacy of data collected from sensors in addition to the impact of these sensors on the patient's day to day life. Furthermore, exercise-based rehabilitation programs in the home can extend the duration of rehabilitation, helping patients to continue with their rehabilitation and leading to greater improvements in motor and cognitive function. Similarly, a person's intellectual fitness could potentially be evaluated at home through games like Sudoku or techniques such as alertness training. On the other hand, if an individual is in the acute care stage of cognitive decline, evaluation techniques such as the use of memory aids or reminiscence to evoke emotions, are likely more suitable in such contexts [19].

4.5   Example Pattern

To put the topic of this paper into context, we provide an example of a pattern in this section. We outline pattern headings, provide an explanation of these headings, and elaborate with an example from our work.

- Name - The name should be intuitive, indicating the solution that the pattern offers.
- Pattern Location - This identifies whereabouts in the framework the pattern is located. For example, the pattern might be located under Home-based Care - Physical Fitness. The author of the pattern should indicate where they feel the pattern is best situated.
- Background - The background should provide the context and the scope of the pattern. If any other patterns (i.e. 'super-patterns') lead to this particular pattern it should be noted here. Super-pattern names should be highlighted in bold font.
- Problem - This should clearly identify the problem that the pattern is addressing.
- Solution - There may be one or more solutions to the problem described in the pattern that should be outlined here. The solution should also contain pointers to lower level patterns (sub-patterns) that might help to solve the problem. Sub-pattern names should be highlighted in bold font.
- Results - This heading is particularly relevant for patterns describing evaluations. It should provide a brief overview of evaluation results for the particular problem being described, essentially providing a basis for the solution provided. However, we have decided this will be an optional field, as pattern authors might have results under review for publication and thus may not want to include them here at the time of publishing the pattern.
- Additional Information - Any content that does not appear to fit in to any of the above categories could be placed here. Diagrams and examples might also be added to this field where they may serve as useful aids in describing any aspect of a pattern.

Name: Adapting the Microsoft Product Reaction Card Technique for Older Adults.

Pattern Location: Patient.

Background: Evaluation techniques for older adults. An issue we have faced in the past relates to how to gather useful and constructive feedback from older participants. At times we have found subjective feedback to be very positive, despite finding a number of usability problems through quantitative methods. This is particularly true of Irish older adults as many might consider it impolite to speak negatively of a technology, especially when they have struck up a relationship with the evaluator. The technique described in this pattern is benficial in drawing out negative as well as positive reactions. The original technique, developed by Microsoft [20] consists of a set of 118 cards containing adjectives, both positive and negative. Participants are asked to choose all the cards they feel describe the system. They are then asked to refine their choice by picking the top 5 cards. A semi-structured interview then proceeds between the participant and evaluator, whereby the participant explains the reason behind each of their choices. This is primarily a qualitative technique, with the main purpose to solicit a discussion on user opinions. However, it can also be quantified by counting positive and negative choices.

Problem: The Microsoft Product Reaction Card technique is an ideal method for collecting very useful qualitative data. However, in using this technique with older adults in their homes, we discovered that it didn't work very well in it's current structure. Firstly, there were too many words for the older adult to read through. While we have observed younger adults 'skimming' through the list of words and quickly choosing all words they felt applied to their experience, older adults tend to ponder over each word, read it aloud and maybe say a few words about it. Secondly, many of the words used were confusing to older adults, such as 'busy', 'consistent', 'integrated', 'responsive'. As such, many of the words had to be explained which lengthened the time to conduct the technique. It was important for us to minimise this time as the older adult would have already spent a significant amount of time using the technology being evaluated, so that we could observe their interaction. From past experience, we have found it is best to limit usability tests in the home to approximately one hour, as many participants might begin to feel fatigued after this amount of time. Finally, the home setting wasn't conducive to the original method of laying out 118 cards to be chosen. While there generally wasn't enough table space for this, we also noted that older adults preferred to sit in a comfortable armchair while we were 'interviewing' them, as this put them more at ease. As such, it was necessary to adapt this technique to suit our older cohort of participants.

Solution: We have found the following to be a good solution to the above problem. Our current solution has been used with around 40 older adults to date, across a number of projects, and has been very effective in providing us with useful feedback. We began adapting this technique for older adults by minimising the word set. This reduced set of 27 words (included in the pattern as a Table under 'Additional Information', but not in this paper for space purposes). It should be noted that this set may change, depending on the technology to be evaluated. We used words that not only would apply to the particular technology being tested, but which would be understandable to older adults. We also minimised the set by removing numerous synonyms. When using this technique in the home, we spread the words out over two sheets of A4 paper, in a font size that is clearly legible. If the participant is sitting at a table, we ask them to tick all words that apply to their experience and to then refine this list by circling their top five choices. If the participant prefers to sit in an armchair, we ask them to look through the words, read aloud any word they feel 'jumps out at them' regarding their interaction, and again to refine this to five words. On average, it takes no more than five minutes to complete this process, following which a semi-structured interview occurs, using the five chosen words as a basis.

5   Issues

A pattern repository provides an accessible place for researchers within the field of healthcare evaluations to pool their knowledge, share experiences and to search for tried and tested solutions to problems they might be facing. While the benefits of such a repository are many, there are a number of issues involved in its creation and maintenance which should be highlighted. A pattern repository is community dependent - writing the patterns that combine to form a cohesive language is a not insubstantial collaborative effort. As such, we may need to consider various means of motivating people to contribute. Providing author recognition for each pattern may be one way to achieve this.

To ensure that any patterns contributed are of a high quality, it is necessary to define a process for the submission and reviewing of pattern content, before they are added to the repository. For example, how do we ensure the submitted content is accurate? Enforcing pattern authors to register is one possible way of achieving some level of quality control. Also, any submitted patterns should undergo a review process, which ideally would be a collaborative effort among the pattern language community.

Pattern organisation is important as patterns need to be discoverable by interested readers. Patterns are submitted individually but need to be organised to develop a coherent pattern language. They should be grouped and linked appropriately. For example, it must be determined if patterns are sub-patterns of others etc. There are questions as to who should perform this task. Should pattern authors suggest where they feel their pattern fits in? Should the repository administrator make the final decision? As the number of patterns in our language expands, we will consider adding an index or a search feature. To this end, Yahoo have developed four vocabularies for classifying patterns. They note that these vocabularies were developed after studying initial pattern content that was submitted by authors [21]. Furthermore, there is a likelihood that pattern authors might feel that while they have a relevant pattern to submit, it doesn't quite fit into our existing structure, or it could fit into more than one category. For example, a pattern relating to usability testing of a touchscreen device doesn't appear at first glance to fit into any category, unless the device was used to evaluate social or cognitive fitness, for example. However, it is still relevant and as such new categories may have to be added or the overall structure reconsidered as the pattern language develops.

6   Conclusions and Future Work

The recent trends in pervasive healthcare technologies have seen the movement of healthcare technologies into real environments, such as homes, residential communities and acute care settings. This raises new challenges in the design of evaluations of such technologies, in terms of assessing usability, user experience and the feasibility of such technologies. The evaluation of pervasive healthcare technologies is still a relatively young research field. While some studies exist, there is no central repository of knowledge, detailing problems encountered by evaluation designers, and well-documented workable solutions to these problems. In this paper we propose a new concept in evaluating healthcare technologies, namely the creation of a pattern language. Single instances of evaluation problems, along with their solutions, are documented as single patterns. Each pattern can be semantically linked to other patterns to form a comprehensive and cohesive language. Pattern languages have enjoyed much success in various fields of research, from architecture to software engineering and human computer interaction. However, the idea of using a pattern language to capture experiences in evaluating healthcare technologies has never been explored, until now.

Deciding on the content that should be stored within a pattern language is important, as is how this content is structured, to ensure patterns are both easy to navigate and searchable. We have proposed to structure our pattern language such that patterns are organised based on whether they describe evaluations relating to home-based care, residential care, or acute care. This hierarchy is further refined by categorising patterns based on whether they relate to physical, social or intellectual fitness, as each of these are vital in contributing to a healthy, independent life. In organising patterns along this structure we wish to bring evaluators' focus beyond solely the traditional evaluation issues of usability, functionalities and cost-effectiveness concerns.

To support our hosting requirements for a pattern language, we have considered a number of different formal and informal solutions, such as a document repository system, a blog and a wiki. We ultimately decided to implement a wiki to act as our repository, as a wiki is relatively easy to implement and maintain and it meets each of our requirements, that is, it will ensure our pattern language is interactive, accessible, logical and searchable, it will support easy extensibility and it should be easy for contributors to add and update content. This wiki is currently under construction. Current and future work involves plans to make this a collaborative effort among the healthcare research community. Once a number of patterns have been added, we will design an evaluation process to assess the usefulness and usability of the repository, both in terms of its content and structure. Through a process of evaluation and refinement we believe this pattern language will be a much used resource for evaluation designers within the healthcare technology community.

Acknowledgements

CLARITY is a partnership between University College Dublin, Dublin City University and Tyndall National Institute (TNI) Cork. This work is supported by Science Foundation Ireland under grant 07/CE/I1147.

References

1. Bonato, P.: Advances in wearable technology and applications in physical medicine and rehabilitation. Journal of NeuroEngineering and Rehabilitation 2(2) (2005)
2. Neely, S., Stevenson, G., Kray, C., Mulder, I., Connelly, K., Siek, K.A.: Evaluating pervasive and ubiquitous systems. IEEE Pervasive Computing 7(3), 85–88 (2008)

3. Alexander, C., Ishikawa, S., Silverstein, M.: A pattern language - towns, buildings, construction (1977)
4. Gamma, E., Helm, R., Johnson, R., Vlissides, J.: Design patterns: Elements of reusable object-oriented software (1995)
5. Buschmann, F., Henney, K., Schmidt, D.C.: Past, present and future trends in software patterns. IEEE Software 24(4), 31–37 (2007)
6. Chen, C.-T., Cheng, Y.C., Hsieh, C.-Y.: Towards a pattern language approach to establishing personal authoring environments in e-learning. In: IASTED Conference on Web-based Education, pp. 13–18 (2007)
7. Chatteur, F., Carvalho, L., Dong, A.: Design for pedagogy patterns for e-learning. In: IEEE International Conference on Advanced Learning Technologies, pp. 341–343 (2008)
8. Borchers, J.: A pattern approach to interaction design (2001)
9. Mahemoff, M.J., Johnston, L.J.: Pattern languages for usability: An investigation of alternative approaches. In: APCHI, pp. 25–31 (1998)
10. Casaday, G.: Notes on a pattern language for interactive usability. In: CHI 1997 Extended Abstracts, pp. 289–290 (1997)
11. Tidwell, J.: Designing interfaces - patterns for effective interaction design (2005)
12. Landay, J., Borriello, G.: Design patterns for ubiquitous computing. IEEE Computer 36(8), 66–73 (2003)
13. Apple computer inc. macintosh human interface guidelines. Addison-Wesley, Reading (1992)
14. Capsil international support of a common awareness and knowledge platform for studying and enabling independent living (August 2010),
http://capsil.org/files/Integrated-Capsil-Roadmap-Slides.pdf
15. Eggleston, S., Axelrod, L., Nind, T., Wilkonson, A., et al.: A framework for a home-based stroke rehabilitation system. In: 3rd International Conference on Pervasive Computing Technologies for Healthcare (2009)
16. Jimison, H., Pavel, M., McKanna, J., Pavel, J.: Unobtrusive monitoring of computer interactions to detect cognitive status in elders. IEEE Transactions on Information Technology in Biomedicine 8(3), 248–252 (2004)
17. Kern, D., Stringer, M., Fitzpatrick, G., Schmidt, A.: Curball - a prototype tangible game for intergenerational play. In: 15th IEEE International Workshop on Enabling Technologies: Infrastructures for Collaborative Enterprises, pp. 412–418 (2006)
18. Hamilton, B.B., Granger, C.V., Sherwin, F.S., Zielzny, M., Tashman, J.S.: A uniform national data system for medical rehabilitation. In: Rehabilitation Outcomes: Analysis and Measurement, pp. 137–147 (2001)
19. West, D., Quigley, A., Kay, J.: Memento: A digital physical scrapbook for memory sharing. Personal and Ubiquitous Computing 11, 313–328 (2007)
20. Benedek, J., Miner, T.: Measuring desirability: New methods for evaluating desirability in a usability lab setting,
http://www.microsoft.com/usability/uepostings/desirabilitytooklit.doc
(retrieved 2009)
21. Leacock, M., Malone, E., Wheeler, C.: Implementing a pattern library in the real world: A yahoo! case study,
http://www.leacock.com/patterns/leacock_malone_wheeler.pdf
(accessed 2010)

Potential of e-Travel Assistants to Increase Older Adults' Mobility

Anne Kathrin Schaar and Martina Ziefle

Human Technology Centre (Humtec)
RWTH Aachen University, Aachen
Theaterplatz 14, 52062 Aachen
{Schaar,Ziefle}@humtec.rwth-aachen.de

Abstract. In this empirical study we examine the willingness of travelers to use small screen devices providing electronic travel ("e-travel") services. As in the near future increasingly more and older adults are travelling around, it is a basic question how we can support this wish for mobility. However, electronic travel services on mobile device are only accepted if it is understood in how far these devices meet the actual travel behavior on the one hand and user requirements respecting the usability of devices on the other. Yet, only little knowledge is prevalent regarding the individual reasons for the choice of means of transportation as well as the perceived needs when being supported by a device providing travel services. In order to get a broad insight into age-related mobility patterns, users of a wide age range (N = 151; 18-75 years of age) were questioned in a survey, in which the travel experience (frequency of using different means of transportation and their evaluation) as well as technical experience (Internet usage and handling of small screen devices) were explored. The findings show that age (but not gender) is a crucial factor regarding the acceptance of electronic travel assistants, and services. The crucial factor underlying age effects is the technical experience and travel expertise: The higher the familiarity with electronic services in general (Internet usage) and specifically (handling of mobile devices) and domain knowledge (travel experience), the higher is the perceived usefulness of future e-travel services. Outcomes might be helpful for the development of e-travel applications especially with for the intention to keep the elderly mobile and fit for travelling.

Keywords: e-travel, Aging, Mobility, social inclusion, tourism in the elderly.

1 Introduction

The demographical change is one of the dominating topics of our century. The public discussion asks for the influence of the aging process and its impact on future societies. Forecasts announce that we will have a contingent of 34% 65+ olds in Germany in 2060 [1], [2]. In comparison, in 2008, there was a proportion of 20% in the group of 65+ [3], [4]. This aging structure is not restricted to specific countries, but is valid for many nations. Thus, in the future we are confronted with more and older adults than ever before but in many respects this generation of seniors is different from former

G. Leitner, M. Hitz, and A. Holzinger (Eds.): USAB 2010, LNCS 6389, pp. 138–155, 2010.
© Springer-Verlag Berlin Heidelberg 2010

ones: In contrast to earlier times, the group of current and future older adults are - physically and mentally- much fitter than earlier generations were, due to a generally higher living standard. Basically, we can emanate from a cohort with sufficiently high nutrition status and health standards, accompanied by a higher longevity [5], a higher economic standard as well as a higher educational level [6]. Also, due to the higher economic independency, this generation is able to afford travelling and does have broad access to the achievement of mobility [6].

Studies show that travelling is an important if not the most important feature of an attractive life style for older adults [7], [8], [9], [10]. Keeping one's mobility is therefore an essential feature for older adults [11], in order to participate actively, self-determined and independently in social living. Interviews with older adults [8], [9] revealed that mobility is used as a synonym for freedom, life-control, societal status and self-worth. Traditionally, the car as traditional mean of transportation represents all these values. Thus, even though public transport facilities are advancing in many cities, still the automobile is the most important means of conveyance to access these services, especially in the view of older adults.

However, drivers aged 65 and older have the second highest accident rate and an increased crash risk [12], [13], [14]. From a cognitive point of view, driving is a complex multitasking demand, especially for older drivers. As drivers have to process information from multiple sources in order to maintain safe vehicle control [4], [15], [16], [17], and follow time-critical and context-adaptive traffic demand, older drivers and those with age-related disabilities are especially penalized as they are known to have limited cognitive resources to process complex and large amounts of information, to time-critically react and to cope with multitasking demands [14], [16], [17].

Public transports are therefore highly needed within modern societies. According to Burkhard (2000) [6] "we need non-auto-driver transportation alternatives. It is mandatory that these alternatives provide two features: the physical mobility to safely afford real connectedness with community opportunities and the consummately American psychic rewards now associated with auto-ownership- independence, self-reliance, and a sense of dignity and self-worth" (Burkhard, 2000, p. 120).

Public transportation is thus part of the answer to aging mobility. There is a need to redefine the traditional concept and to increase accessibility and availability of information within public transports. Recent developments in Information and Communication Technologies (ICT) in combination with high quality mobile devices, as well as an increased perceived value in public perception (e.g. iPhone) could represent a promising alternative concept of public transport in form of so-called e-travel assistants. E-Travel assistants are mobile portable devices which provide a wide range of travel information, e.g. trip planning, purchase of tickets, information about connecting trains/buses, potential delays and alternative routes. In addition, these devices provide city information, alternative routes and navigation aids, if the traveler gets lost. Those electronic travel services delivered by small screen devices are highly developed in the meanwhile [18], [19], and travel and mobile services can be retrieved at any time, at any place, with travel information being wirelessly delivered, continuously actualized, context-adaptive and even targeted to user profiles.

In combination with an increasing infrastructure of public transport and diverse means of transportations (rail, bus, underground) in many cities and countries, the cognitive concept of mobility could move into a new era, increasingly reducing the focus on auto mobility.

Especially for older adults, e-travelling has two prominent benefits: (1) the chance to actively and safely participate in public transportation without the burden to drive a car and risking an accident (2) the reliability to be instantaneously informed about the newest information about travel possibilities, or changes in connecting trains/buses during their journey by means of their smart phone.

The e-travel concept though requires three main prerequisites: (1) the broad acceptance of such a mobility concept, in combination with an understanding of the perceived benefits and barriers, which are associated with the different means of public transport (2) and the easy usage of small screen devices [18], [19], [20], [21]. In addition, (3), we need to understand, to which extent the experience with technical devices [22], [23], and the experience with travelling per se influences the acceptance of e-travel services, especially in the older group [18].

In this context not only age but also gender could be a relevant factor: Among the older adults of the future a large portion will be female [24], due to a shorter life expectancy among men [5]. In addition, at least in the current generation, still there is a high portion of (older) women, which do not have a driving license and which are therefore relying on using public transportation means. Furthermore, different societal (family) roles might also form a specific mobility pattern, which could be in line with electronically supported public transportation. Last but not least women show a reluctant usage and acceptance of technology and a comparably low self-competence when handling technical devices [25], [26], [27], [28], [29].

1.1 Aging and Mobility

Mobility is one of the main future topics in our society [9], [10]. The demographic change make it essential to explore the mobility needs and wants of the elderly. There will be more people with cognitive and physical handicaps who still have touristic plans or other needs for which mobility is necessary.

But even if mobility is not always a question of covering long distances, travelling becomes more and more and important role in the life of older people. The so-called "third age" means for many older people the time in one's life in which travelling is a central topic. After a long working life people have earned enough money to realize their individual dreams. Many older Germans target to an evening of life on the Canaries or Balearic islands. Others don't plan their emigration but also are delighted by the possibility of long voyages out of the busy season. But not only long distant trips play a role. Especially city trips are very popular in the elderly. Above all the elderly are intellectually interested and looking forward to make new cultural experiences in their retirement age.

In this context the demographic change confronts the tourist industry with a huge group of well-founded old people with special needs during their voyages. It is to figure out if mobility in the elderly could be supported by e-travel services delivered on portable mobile devices. In this context it is indispensable to look at the technical expertise of older users.

1.2 Aging and Technology

In order to make e-travel services in combination with small screen devices ("e-travel assistants") a true benefit for mobility in the elderly, interfaces have to be easy to use and to be perceived as useful. In this context it is essential to refer to the concept of technology acceptance.

The most popular model for acceptance analysis of ICT is the Technology Acceptance-Model (TAM). It is based on the theoretical ground of the Theory of Reasoned Action [28]. The TAM gives the option to link the technology acceptance and actual utilization behavior. The TAM assumes that users' decision to use a new technology is determined by their behavioral intention of using a special technical application [29]. The behavioral intention is formed by perceived ease of use and usefulness. The ease of use characterizes "the degree to which a person believes that using a particular system would be free from effort" the perceived ease of use is "the degree to which a person believes that using a particular system would enhance his or her job performance" [30]. According to studies older adults show to have a specific technology acceptance pattern in which especially the usefulness of technology is more strongly weighed over the ease of using a system [31], [32], [33], [34], [35].

In our context it is necessary to analyze the technical experience of people in different age groups, to find out if there are any correlations between the technical expertise and the acceptance of such services.

1.3 Question Addressed, Research Model and Hypotheses

This paper addresses two major points:

(1) On the one hand we want to explore older adults' travel patterns and their individual needs and wants for a comfortable travelling as well as the perceived barriers when using different means of transportation.
(2) On the other hand we want to identify the personal factors (their technical expertise and travel experience), which might influence the positive evaluation of e-travel systems.

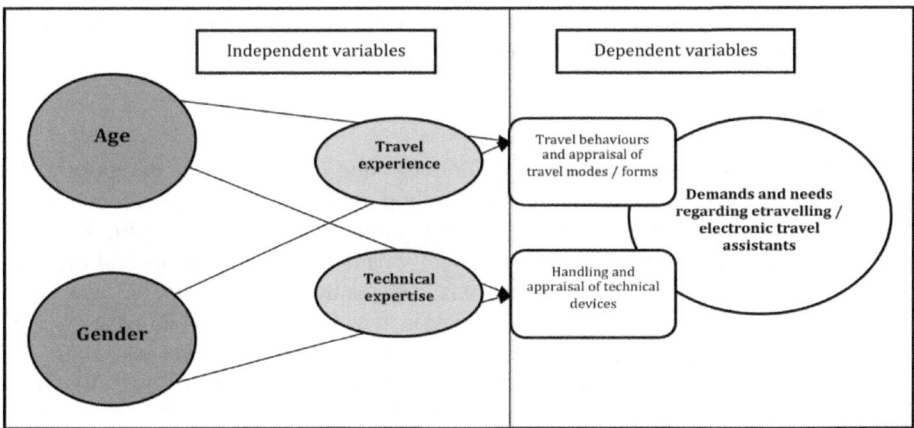

Fig. 1. Research model: Influence from personal factors and experience on travel behavior and technical expertise and its effects for an acceptance of an e-travel assistant

Our research model (see Figure 1) illustrates the theoretical approach and the assumed relation between and across variables. As independent variables we analyzed age and gender, and their impact on users' acceptance of e-travel assistants (H1). As moderating variables, we assumed the level of previous travel experience (H2) and the degree of technical expertise to influence the acceptance of e-travel assistants (H3).

H1:   The individual factors age and gender are related to users' acceptance (perceived benefits/barriers) of e-travel assistants.

H2:   Individuals with a high travel experience show a higher acceptance of e-travel assistants.

H3:   Individuals with a high technical expertise show a higher acceptance of e-travel assistants.

2   Method

2.1   Variables

Independent variables: Independent variables are age, gender as individual factors which influence the mobility behavior, and subsequently, the positive/negative attitude towards the usefulness of electronic travel assistants. Also, the extent of travel-experience and technical expertise are further independent variables, which are assumed to influence the acceptance of electronic travel assistants.

Dependent Variables: Dependent variables are the acceptance (positive and negative attitudes) towards the usefulness of e-travel assistants.

Respondents indicated the frequency of using different means of transportation (car and public transportation) in different travel contexts (business and leisure). To analyze the motives for the use of means of transport respondents marked the reason for using the one or other mean of transportation and to indicate the pleasantness of using them. Here, multiple-choice items had to be answered on six-point Likert scales ranging from 1 (do not agree at all) to 6 (fully agree).

2.2   The Questionnaire

In order to examine a large number of participants and to consider the diversity within the older age and group, the questionnaire-method was chosen. The questionnaire was designed to obtain information about (1) demographic data (age, sex, education), (2) travel experience (frequency of using different means of transportations and the comfort of using these means of transportations) (3) technical experience (frequency of using different information and communication technologies) and the ease of using these devices, (4) Perceived pros and cons of using an electronic travel assistant.

In the following, the different sections of the questionnaire and the respective items are detailed. Also answering modes and scales are explained.

Travel-behavior: Frequency, aim and evaluation
Participants were instructed to indicate the frequency of using different means of transportation (car, public transportation (trains, underground, bus), airplane, bike) in business contexts (commuting to work, business trips) and leisure (private tours;

visits; holiday). To analyze the motives for the use of special means of transport participants were asked to mark the reason for using the one or other mean of transportation and to indicate the pleasantness of using them.

Technical expertise: Frequency of usage and ease of use
Participants were requested to indicate the frequency of using different ICT devices (cell phone, PDA/Smartphone, PC, GPS, and digital camera) and ease of using these devices. Here the following usability items had to be answered:

Table 1. Ease of use items for handling of devices (1 = agree to 4 = disagree)

Typing on small keys is not easy for me
I often lose the orientation in the phones' menu
It is hard for me to recognize objects on small screens
On Web pages, I often lose the orientation
I have problems to maintain a high attention for a longer period of time
I have problems to remember key allocations of my cell phone

Table 2. Items for cell phone usage (1 = daily to 6 never)

I use the my cell phone for
... telephone calls
... short messages
... MMS
... ringtone/music downloads
... information services with costs
... mobile Internet account for pc or laptop
... emails check via cell phone
... writing emails

Experience with the Internet: Frequency and ease of use
In addition, we wanted to know which activities were accomplished by using the Internet, how frequent these activities were carried out and how easy to accomplish these activities are.

Table 3. Items for Internet usage (1 = daily to 6 never) and evaluation of the ease of using it (1 = very easy to 6 very difficult)

I use the Internet for
... browsing
... purchase items
... online banking
... travel arrangements (booking flights)
... emails
... chatting
... reading online (news)

E-travel

The last item set of the questionnaire was a set in which we asked questions about a still existing form of e-travel service in Germany. This is the Internet information platform of the Deutsche Bahn[1]. We asked respondents if and if so, which of the applications they would use, and how often. Also, the ease of using these applications was assessed. As highly frequented services on the Internet platform are planned to be available on the electronic travel assistants as well, the information about the handling of the Deutsche Bahn online services represents a good source for the acceptance of e-travel assistants.

Table 4. Items for the frequency (1 = daily to 6 never) and the ease of using of an e-travel application (1 = very easy to 6 very difficult)

How often do you use the DB Web page/ How easy is the usage of the following possibilities of the DB Web page
... to buy a ticket
... to search a train connection
... to check the punctuality of a train
... to get more information about new offers of the DB
... to book a city trip
... to rent a bike
... to get some inspirations for holiday
... to read the news

Evaluation of future e-travel assistants

The last section of our questionnaire includes an items set of pro using arguments of e-travel assistants and one of contra usage. Table 5 and 6 are giving an overview about the aspects, which were considered. All items had to be answered on a six-point scale (1- totally agree; 6 = totally disagree).

Table 5. Items for the pro using arguments of e-travel assistants

I would use an e-travel-assistant because...
... I hope to never miss a connecting train
... I want to be more flexible
... I do not want to rely on information delivered by the conductor
... I want to get more information about the stations passed and coming next
... I feel more relaxed during traveling
... the perceived disadvantages of rail travel could be balanced by the device support
... rail traveling would be less exhausting

---

[1] Deutsche Bahn is the German national travel company.

Table 6. Items for the con using arguments of e-travel assistants

I would not use an e-travel-assistant because...
... I do not want to be depending on a device
... I am not sure if a e-travel assistant is reliable
... I don not want to deal with an additional technical device
... I do not want to lose the contact with the conductor
... it is not necessary for me and my travel pattern
... I am afraid that third persons could get an insight in my travel plans
... I do not want to have such technical devices close to my body
... I have problems with technical applications anyway
... I fear that the data on my e-travel assistant could be interrupted by other electromagnetic fields

2.3 Participants

A total of 152 respondents participated, with an age range between 18 and 70 years of age (M = 34.3; SD = 13.6). Participants were recruited through the social network of authors. All participants volunteered to take part and showed a very high and personal interest in the topic. Participants were not gratified for their efforts.

The sample was allocated to three age and traveler groups, respectively, on the base of two criterions. One was to match different traveling profiles (using information provided by the Deutsche Bahn) and the other was to reach three groups of about the same size.

(1) *"Young travelers"* (N = 52), in an age range 18 to 25 (M = 23.1 ; SD = 1.8), 75% were female and 25% male. This group is characterized by being mainly in vocational training. The age of 26 marks a turning point, at which- statistically- switch into the professional life.

(2) *"Middle aged travelers"* (N = 52), in an age range of >26 - 40 years, (M = 29 SD = 3.3) 38.5% female; 61.5%. This group is characterized mainly by working and family life.

(3) *"Grown up travelers* (N = 46), in an age range of > 41 - 70 years of age, (M = 53.1; SD = 7.6). 63% were female, and 37% male).

All participants lived in or near urban areas in which a rich supply and offer regarding different transportation means (rail, bus, underground) is available.

3 Results

In order to learn to which extent people are willing to use public transportation means and Internet-based travel services, it is insightful to study

a) travel experience and mobility patterns (Section 3.1)
b) experience with small screen devices (Section 3.2)
c) Internet experience (Section 3.3) and
d) experiences with e-travel services (Section 3.4). Within all these analyzing contexts we differentiated effects of age and gender.

Data was analyzed by ANOVAs and nonparametric statistics (Mann-Whitney-Test and Kruskal-Wallis-Test), the level of significance was set at $\alpha = .05$.

3.1 Travel Experiences

Frequency of travelling for the factors age and gender
In order to obtain information about the travel experience, participants were asked to report the frequency, evaluation and aim of their usage of different means of transportation.

ANOVA analyses with the factors age and gender on usage of different means of transportation revealed that the three age groups differ significantly in their frequency of using tram, bus and underground and local/intercity traffic trains (F (12,252) = 4.84; p < 0.01). The young travelers are the group, which uses all forms of public means of transportation most often - about 1-3 times a week to every 1-2 times per month (M = 2.2 out of 6 points max; SD = 1.1). Middle-aged travelers use them also quite often (M = 2.7; SD = 2.6), less compared to the younger group, but more often than the oldest group, which uses public means of transportation (M = 3.7; SD = 1.4) significantly less frequent in comparison to both other age groups (Figure 2 tram, underground and bus, Figure 3 Local/intercity rail traffic).

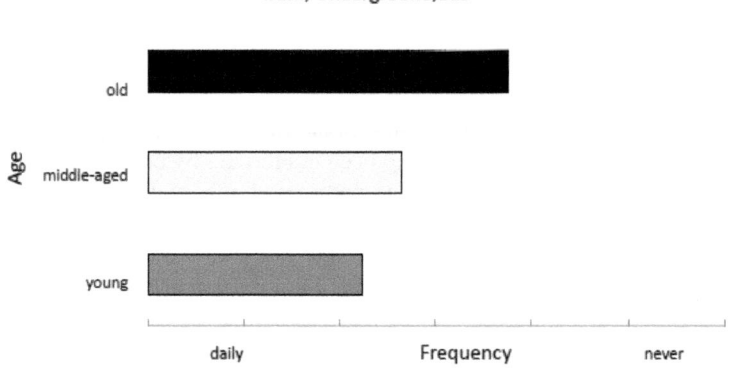

Fig. 2. Frequency of using tram, bus and underground: older travelers: 51-70 years; middle-aged travelers: 31-50 years; young traveler: 18-30 years

There were no significant gender effects in the context of the frequency of travelling and different means of transportation.

Evaluation of different means of transportation for the factors age and gender
When asked how the different means of transportation were evaluated (regarding comfort and performance), no differences between age and gender groups were revealed.

Furthermore we analyzed for which purpose travelers report to use the different means of transportation. As can be seen in Figure 4, there were different travel patterns within the different means of transportation across age groups. The tram, bus and underground are used especially for commuting to work by the younger and the middle-aged traveler group (young: 56.9 %; middle-aged: 48 %). Older traveler use tram, bus and underground equally for commuting to work (23.8 %), private every day travels (23.8 %), as well as for visits and leisure times (26.2 %).

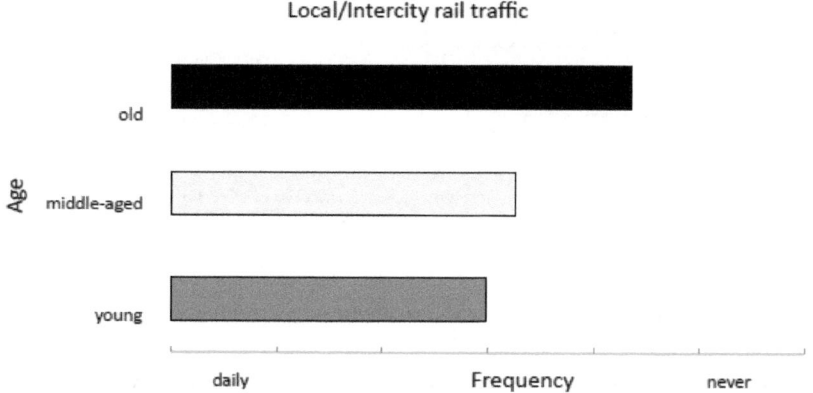

Fig. 3. Frequency of using the public rail traffic: older travelers: 51-70 years; middle-aged travelers: 31-50 years; young traveler: 18-30 years

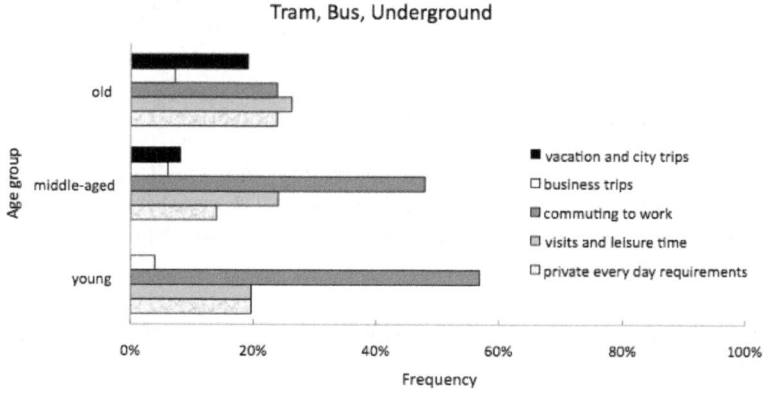

Fig. 4. Frequency of using Tram, Bus and Underground within the age groups: older travelers: 51-70 years; middle-aged travelers: 31-50 years; young traveler: 18-30 years

All respondents use the local rail traffic for visits and leisure time equally. The same applies for intercity rail traffic, which is used for vacation and city trips.

The car is the most central mean of transportation, which is used basically for private every day requirements by all age groups. Here gender differences were present showing that men in contrast to women more often use the car. All age groups use it mostly for vacation and city trips. The same applies to the bike which is - as a non-motor driven mean of transportation - equally used by all travelers, independently of

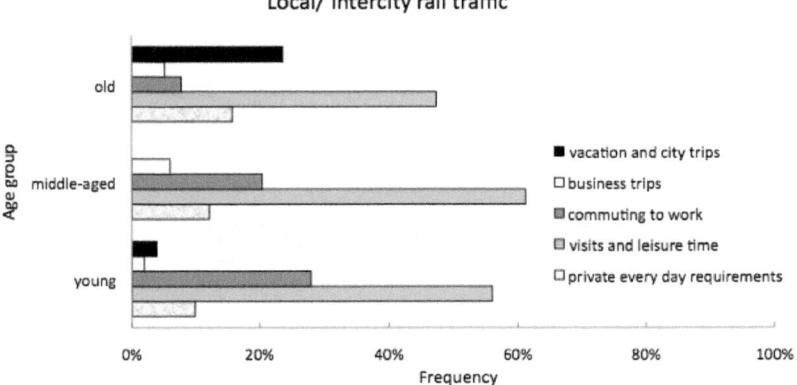

Fig. 5. Frequency of using the local/intercity rail traffic within the age groups: older travelers: 51-70 years; middle-aged travelers: 31-50 years; young traveler: 18-30 years

age and gender, mainly used for private every day requirements and visits and leisure time followed by commuting to work.

When summarizing this survey, we see a highly expected picture. The younger the travelers, the higher is the frequency of traveling in general, and the more diverse is the usage of different means. However, and this was the central focus here, we see that older adults still tend to use the car, but they do use the public transportation means for specific purposes (especially for leisure, city trips and excursions). Thus, respecting the tailoring of electronic travel services, this should be kept in mind.

3.2 Technical Experiences with Small Screen Devices

Regarding the technical experience when interacting with small screen devices significant differences between age groups ($F_{(12,278)} = 7.7$; $p < 0.001$) were identified, revealing a higher technical experience in the younger group, when compared to the middle-aged and older group.

Table 7. Means of age groups regarding the reported ease of use (N = 152). Older adults show the largest problems (grey shaded in Table 7).

	Young (18-30 years)		Middle-aged (31-50 years)		Old (51-70 years)	
	M	SD	M	SD	M	SD
Typing on small keys	3.3	.72	3.0	.85	2.1	.95
Disorientation in phones' menu	3.5	.67	3.4	.66	2.6	1.0
Readability and legibility problems	3.6	.63	3.5	.64	2.4	1.0
Disorientation within Web pages	3.4	.68	3.5	.64	3.1	.86
Problems to remember key allocations	3.6	.64	3.5	.7	2.9	.98

In Table 2 (Section 2.2), the evaluation regarding own competence and technical expertise is depicted, differentiated for age groups (1 = very difficult, 4 = very easy).

Table 7 reports that the older participants have more difficulties with typing on small keys, regarding the disorientation within the mobile phone menu, the disorientation on Web pages, and regarding the understanding and memory of key allocations. Within all these ergonomic issues, gender differences did not show up, revealing that a suboptimal interface design does equally affect male and female users when using small screen devices.

Frequency of using different small screen devices
Additionally, we analyzed the frequency of dealing with different types of mobile devices (e.g. cell phone, PDA, GPS, digital camera or mobile computer). In this context we found significant differences for cell phone, PDA and (F $(10,268) = 4.1$; p < .001) between the age groups. Throughout, the frequency of using the devices was higher in the younger group in comparison to the older group.

Though, also older adults show to have a sufficient experience using cell phones at least 1-2 times a week (young: M = 1.; SD = .19; middle-aged: M = 1.1; SD = .38; old: M = 1.7; SD = 1.0). Gender effects were found for cell phone and PDA usage (F $(5,134) = 5$; p < 0.001). Women use the cell phone more frequently (M = 1.2; SD = .44), with a nearly everyday usage. Men report to use their cell phones less frequently but still between everyday and 1-2 times a week (M = 1.4; SD = .89).

Comprising the outcomes, the usability of small screen devices is a serious barrier, especially for the older group. These barriers are not restricted to "hardware-design issues" (as the difficult usage of keys, and the low legibility of information delivered by the small display). More important, it regards the navigation efficiency in the menu, covering disorientation behavior, the not knowing where they are and where they have to navigate to within the menu structure. Also, the functions and keys' naming is a serious problem. When considering the time critical situations while traveling, we cannot expect a fast and trouble-free usage of small screen devices and the handling of complex menu structures. Respecting the tailoring of electronic travel services, this should be kept in mind, providing flat menu hierarchies and easy to reach navigation targets, which do not urge users to navigate through complex menus.

Frequency of using the Internet
The navigation in electronic travel assistant broadly relies on experience in using Internet platforms and applications. Therefore, it is essential to learn the Internet experience and the perceived ease of using it, especially in the older group.

ANOVA analyses revealed that there are significant age effects regarding the frequency of Internet usage (F $(14,262) = 3.7$; p < 0.001). For all Internet options we asked for browsing, purchase items, online banking, chatting and reading online (news) significant differences between the group of middle-aged and older users. In all cases significant group differences were revealed. Plus we found distinctions for the items browsing, online banking and reading online between the young and older users. Table 8 shows that – as expected- the young group shows basically the largest experience in Internet usage, followed by the middle-aged and older user group. But is becomes evident that there are also applications that are less used across all age groups (chatting and reading online).

Table 8. Means of age groups for the frequency of Internet usage (N = 152). Older adults show the lowest frequency of the respective Internet application (grey shaded in Table 8). Low values indicate high frequency (the six point scale complies 1 = daily to 6 = never).

	Young (18-30 years)		Middle-aged (31-50 years)		Older (51-70 years)	
I use the Internet for…	M	SD	M	SD	M	SD
…browsing	1.4	.63	1.2	.48	2.0	1.4
…purchase items	3.4	1.6	2.8	1.2	3.9	1.7
… online banking	3.9	1.4	3.3	1.2	4.0	1.6
…chatting	3.8	2.1	3.6	2.3	4.7	1.9
… reading online (news)	3.5	2.1	2.7	2.0	4.8	1.9

Evaluation of different Internet applications
We also asked for the preferences respectively dislikes within using different Internet applications. While gender differences were not detected throughout, age effects were present, showing that online banking, travel arrangements (booking flights) and chatting were not used within the older group. As taken from personal remarks data safety is a serious problem (online banking) in the perception of older adults and the fear that personal dates could be misused.

These results confirm -once again- that older people are not only more unfamiliar with using Internet applications, they also have higher demands on privacy and data security and safety, compared to other age groups. Future mobile travel services should consider this in order to include the seniors and in order to reach a high acceptance of these electronic services.

3.3   Experiences with e-Travel and Its Evaluation

Frequency of using e-travel services
To analyze the potential and benefit of an e-travel assistant we asked users whether they already have experience with any form of e-travel services. For the German

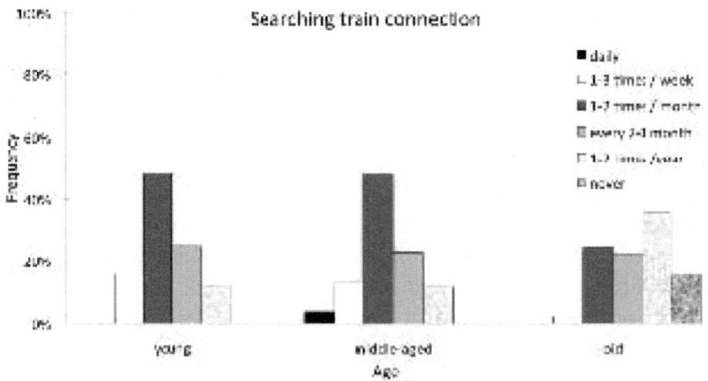

Fig. 6. Experience with e-travel: searching a train connection

context we analyzed the experience with the Deutsche Bahn Web presence as a free and popular e-travel service in Germany.

In this context we found significant differences between the age groups. Older adults report not to use the service regarding searching for a specific train connection. The young (M = 3.3; SD = .88) and the middle-aged travelers (M = 3.3; SD = .91) use this service about 1-2 times a month, in contrast to the older group, which reports to use this service about 2- 3 times per month (M = 4.4; SD = 1.0, Figure 6).

Furthermore, older adults reported mostly not to check the punctuality of a targeted train. The younger traveler group (M = 4.8; SD = 1.5) and the middle-aged users (M = 4.7; SD = 1.5) use this service every 2-3 months or 1-2 times a year, while older users use this service at best 1-2 times or, rather, never (M = 5.6; SD = .82, Figure 7).

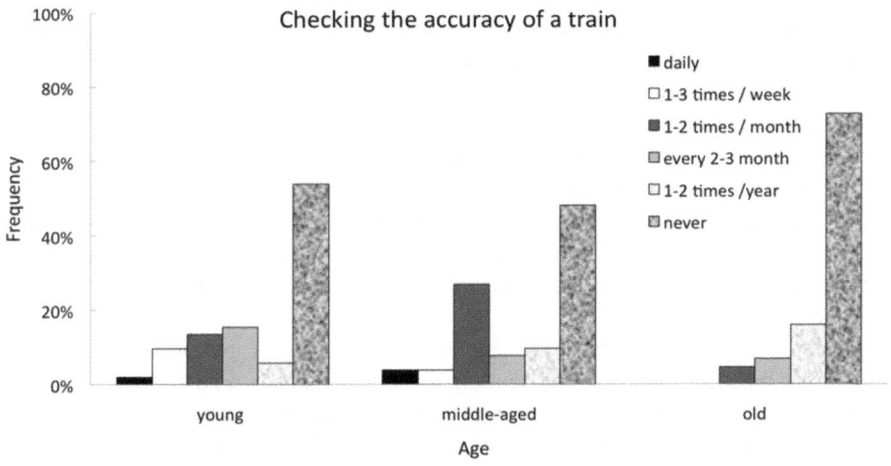

Fig. 7. Experience with e-travel: checking the punctuality of a train

Other offers of the DB Web presence, like searching for special offers and booking online tickets revealed no significant differences between the age groups.

Taken together, it can be roughly concluded that we have to assume age differences regarding travel behaviors, technical expertise, and the experience with e-travel services. All aspects are less pronounced in the older age group, therefore penalizing the senior group when it comes to the confrontation with modern electronic travel services. Gender, in contrast, did not affect the mentioned aspects. When looking into detail, young travelers show a frequent use of the public means of transportation (in contrast to the older group, which still uses predominately the car) In the context of the technical experience (especially with small screen devices) again the younger group shows the best performance, and the older group shows the largest usability barriers and also has the lowest technical experience. For the experience with Web services and Internet applications as well as with e-travel services, the picture is the very same. Younger adults can rely on a high experience, while older adults show basic shortcomings and seem not to be well prepared to use electronic travel services delivered by small screen devices.

In the next step we look for relations between the frequency of use and ease of using a) means of transportation, b) small screen devices and Internet as well as the attitude towards e-travel application. This is important to see the big picture, to identify the age-specific drivers for the sustainable usage of e-travel services and to isolate future research duties.

3.4 Age Drivers for the Evaluation of e-Travel Applications

To find out whether there are age specific drivers for the evaluation of e-travel assistants we correlated the positive[2] ("I would use it, if...") and negative[3] ("I would not use it, because") arguments with individual user characteristics (age, gender, technical expertise, travel experience).

Correlation outcomes confirmed age as a main factor for the travel experience, the technical expertise with small screen devices and experience with e-travel applications. It is an insightful finding that persons, which evaluated the benefit of e-travel applications as more negative, were predominately aged ($r = -.28$; $p < .001$) and have a lower technical experience. But also travel patterns and the preferred choice and high frequency of using a specific mean of transportation show correlations to the acceptance of e-travel assistants. It was found that persons, who report to not frequently use the local rail traffic, tend to negatively evaluate the availability of e-travel services ($r = .46$; $p < .000$) and show higher levels of confirming to barriers. As these persons are predominately young (Section 3.1), we can conclude that younger travelers do prefer e-travel services.

Regarding the experience with the single Internet applications (browsing, purchase items, online banking, chatting and reading online) there was a basic high correlation of Internet experience and the positive evaluation of electronic travel services. Also, people who report to have a high experience in existing electronic Travel services (searching for a train connection / checking the punctuality of a train) show higher pro-using motives for future e-travel assistants in comparison to person, which do not have any pronounced experience with electronic travel Web applications.

Summing up outcomes, we can state that the crucial acceptance mediating factor is experience and expertise, the more people are "unfamiliar" with electronic services in general (Internet usage) and specifically (handling of small screen devices) as well as regarding domain knowledge (travel experience), the more negative are attitudes to and the lower is the perceived usefulness of future innovate e-travel services.

4 The Revision of the Research Model and Discussion

We started this research with the question, how age and gender but also travel experience, the experience with the usage of electronic travel services as well as the technical experience (Internet and small screen devices) are interrelated and how these factors might impact the acceptance of e-travel services.

---

[2] To get an overall picture, for this analysis, all pro items were comprised.
[3] To get an overall picture, for this analysis, all pro items were comprised.

First, in contrast to expectations, gender did not play a significant role, neither within to the overall acceptance of e-travel services, nor to the choice of different means of transportations (contradicting hypothesis 1). But age revealed to be a key factor: Age effects were found within the travel behaviors experience with technical devices and the experience with e-travel services. All these age-specific attitudes impact the acceptance of e-travel services, which is currently quite low. It is noteworthy that age itself is not more than a mere carrier-variable. The prominent factor, which is underlying age effects, is the experience: experience with travel services and with technology (confirming H2).

It is an interesting finding that the positive attitudes towards e-travel services reveal no significant correlation with technical expertise, travel type and the experience with e-travel. It is exclusively the negative attitude and the reluctant behaviors towards the using of such systems, which shows significant relations. Thus, the hypothesis (H3) according to which a high technical expertise results in a higher acceptance of e-travel assistants is basically confirmed. However, here now confinements to this general assumption can be done. Technical expertise specifically influences the negative attitudes toward the usage of an electronic travel assistant, while there was no relation to the pro-using arguments. This means that a low technical expertise is connected to a strong confirmation of any arguments, which militate against the usage of such an electronic device (this is a typical age-specific cognitive model). But this means on the other hand, that if there would be enough experience in the older group, the negative evaluation could change and, then, could lead to a positive intention to use innovative future e-travel systems, whenever older users could rely on sufficient domain knowledge.

With our results in mind it might be interesting in future research to analyze specific traveler profiles and travel groups (e.g. families, professional travelers, handicapped travelers) and to learn more about the acceptance of e-travel services. Also, as there is always a gap between envisioned scenarios and real life experience, we will have to examine if acceptance increases when users really interact with travel assistance. In order to support the validity of the results and to complete the them with rich qualitative insights about key 'soft issues and needs' related to age that may influence their acceptance of e-travel (such as emotions and feelings elicited by distrust, frustration, etc.) this work should be complemented with an ethnographic study (e.g. including observation and in the field interviews).

Acknowledgements

Authors would like to thank all participants to patiently fill in the questionnaire. Many thanks also to Dina Barner and Christina Vedar for research assistance, as well as Patrick Sander, Christoph Päper, Jessica Kempa, Jasmin Geihe, Christoph Ptock, Sara Kleineheer, and Bela Brenger for their help collecting the data. Thanks also to three anonymous reviewers for their critical and helpful comments on an earlier version of this manuscript. This research was supported by the German Federal Ministry of Economics and Technology (Project CAIRO: context aware intermodal routing).

References

1. Bevölkerung Deutschlands bis 2060. 12. Koordinierte Bevölkerungsvorausberechnung. Statistisches Bundesamt, Wiesbaden (2009)
2. Wahrendorf, M., Siegrist, J.: Produktives Altern und informelle Arbeit in modernen Gesellschaften. Theoretische Perspektiven und empirische Befunde. VS Verlag für Sozialwissenschaften, Wiesbaden (2008)
3. HealthLink, Medical College of Wisconsin. Safe Driving for Older Adults (2002), http://healthlinkmcw.edu/article/1013707220.html
4. Ashley, S.: Driving the info highway. Scientific American 285(4), 52–58 (2001)
5. Leonhardt, S.: Personal Healthcare Devices. In: Mukherjee, S., et al. (eds.) Malware: Hardware Technology Drivers of Ambient Intelligence, pp. 349–370. Springer, Dordrecht (2006)
6. Burkardt, J.: Limitations of Mass Transportation and Individual Vehicle Systems for Older Persons. In: Schaie, K.W., Pietrucha, M. (eds.) Mobility and Transportation in the Elderly, pp. 97–124. Springer, New York (2000)
7. Jakobs, E.-M., Lehnen, K., Ziefle, M.: Alter und Technik. Eine Studie zur altersbezogenen Wahrnehmung und Gestaltung von Technik. Edition Wissenschaft. Aprimus, Aachen (2008)
8. Wirtz, S., Ziefle, M., Jakobs, E.-M.: Autopilot versus hearing aid – domain- and technology type-specific parameters of older people's technology acceptance. In: 9th International Conference on Work With Computer Systems, WWCS 2009, Beijing, China (2009)
9. Carp, F.M.: Significance of mobility for the well-being of the elderly. In: Transportation in an Aging Society: Improving Mobility and Safety for Older Persons, vol. II. Transportation Research Board, National Research Council, Washington (1998)
10. Liu, L., Park, D.: Technology and the Promise of Independent Living for Older Adults. A Cognitive Perspective. In: Charness, N., Warner Schaie, K. (eds.) Impact of Technology on Successful Aging, pp. 262–289. Springer, New York (2003)
11. Rosenbloom, S.: Transportation needs of the elderly population. Clinical Geriatric Medicine 9, 279–296 (1993)
12. Waller, P.F.: The older driver. Human Factors 33(5), 499–505 (1991)
13. Dingus, T.A.: Effects of age, system experience and navigation technique on driving with an advanced traveler information system. Human Factors 39(2), 177–199 (1997)
14. Maltz, M., Shinar, D.: Eye movements of younger and older drivers. Human Factors 41(1), 15–25 (1999)
15. Fozard, J.L.: Sensory and Cognitive Changes with Age. In: Schaie, K.W., Pietrucha, M. (eds.) Mobility and Transportation in the Elderly, pp. 31–45. Springer, New York (2000)
16. Ziefle, M., Pappachan, P., Jakobs, E.-M., Wallentowitz, H.: Future technology in the car. Visual and auditory interfaces of in-vehicle-technologies for older adults. In: Miesenberger, K., et al. (eds.) 10th International Conference on Computers Helping People with Special Needs. LNCS, vol. 5105, pp. 62–69. Springer, Berlin (2008)
17. Ziefle, M., Pappachan, P., Jakobs, E.-M., Christen, F., Wallentowitz, H.: Experimental evaluation of visual interfaces of In-Vehicle-Information Systems (IVIS) for older adults. In: Toomingas, A., Lantz, A. (eds.) Work with Computing Systems. Royal Institute of Technology, Stockholm (2007)
18. Arning, K., Ziefle, M.: What older user expect from mobile devices: An empirical survey. In: Pikaar, R.N., Konigsveld, E.A., Settels, P.J. (eds.) Proceedings of the 16th World Congress on Ergonomics (IEA). Elsevier, Maastricht, Amsterdam (2006)

19. Arning, K., Ziefle, M.: Effects of cognitive and personal factors on PDA menu navigation performance. Behaviour and Information Technology 28(3), 251–268 (2009)
20. Ziefle, M., Bay, S.: How older adults meet cognitive complexity: Aging effects on the usability of different cellular phones. Behaviour and Information Technology 24(5), 375–389 (2005)
21. Arning, K., Ziefle, M.: Barriers of information access in small screen devices. In: Stephanidis, C., Pieper, M. (eds.) Universal Access in Ambient Intelligence Environments, pp. 117–136. Springer, Berlin (2007)
22. Ziefle, M.: Modeling mobile devices for the elderly. In: Khalid, H., et al. (eds.) Advances in Ergonomics Modeling and Usability Evaluation. CRC Press, Boca Raton (2010)
23. Ziefle, M.: Information presentation in small screen devices: The trade-off between visual density and menu foresight. Applied Ergonomics 41, 719–730 (2010)
24. Baltes, M., Freund, A.M., Horgas, A.L.: Men and women in the Berlin aging study. In: Baltes, P.B., Mayer, K.U. (eds.) The Berlin Aging Study. Aging from 70 to 100, pp. 259–281. Academic Press, Oxford (1999)
25. Busch, T.: Gender differences in self-efficacy and attitudes toward computers. Journal of Educational Computing Research 12, 147–158 (1995)
26. Schumacher, P., Morahan-Martin, J.: Gender, Internet and computer attitudes and experiences. Computers in Human Behavior 17, 95–110 (2001)
27. Meelissen, M.R.M., Drent, M.: Gender differences in computer attitudes: Does the school matter? Computers in Human Behavior 24, 969–985 (2007)
28. Davis, F.D.: Perceived Usefulness, Perceived Ease of use, and User Acceptance of Information Technology. MIS Quarterly 13, 319–337 (1989)
29. Arning, K., Ziefle, M.: Different Perspectives on Technology Acceptance: The Role of Technology Type and Age. In: Holzinger, A., Miesenberger, K. (eds.) USAB 2009. LNCS, vol. 5889, pp. 20–41. Springer, Heidelberg (2009)
30. Venkatesh, V., Morris, M.G., Davis, G.B., Davis, F.D.: User acceptance of information technology: Toward a unified view. MIS Quarterly 27, 425–478 (2003)
31. Noyes, J.M., Sheard, M.C.A.: Designing for older adults - are they a special group? In: Universal Access in HCI: Inclusive Design in the Information Society, pp. 877–881. Lawrence Erlbaum, Mahwah (2003)
32. Melenhorst, A.S., Rogers, W.A., Caylor, E.C.: The use of communication technologies by older adults: Exploring the benefits from a users perspective. In: Proc. of the Human Factors and Ergonomics Society 45th Annual Meeting, pp. 221–225 (2001)
33. Ellis, D.R., Allaire, J.C.: Modelling computer interest in older adults: The role of age, education, computer knowledge and computer anxiety. Human Factors 41, 345–364 (1999)
34. Marcellini, F., Mollenkopf, H., Spazzafumo, L., Ruoppila, I.: Acceptance and Use of Technological Solutions by the Elderly in the Outdoor Environment: Findings from a European Survey. Zeitschrift für Gerontologie und Geriatrie 33, 169–177 (2000)
35. Ziefle, M.: Aging and Mobile Displays: Challenges and requirements for age-sensitive electronic information designs. In: 9th International Conference on Work With Computer Systems, WWCS 2009, Beijing, China (2009)

Making the Wii at Home: Game Play by Older People in Sheltered Housing

Dave Harley[1], Geraldine Fitzpatrick[2], Lesley Axelrod[3],
Gareth White[3], and Graham McAllister[3]

[1] School of Applied Social Science, University of Brighton
d.a.harley@brighton.ac.uk
[2] Vienna University of Technology
geraldine.fitzpatrick@tuwien.ac.at
[3] Interact Lab, University of Sussex
{l.axelrod,g.white,g.mcallister}@sussex.ac.uk

Abstract. Games such as the Nintendo Wii™ are being promoted for use by all ages but there is little experience with how groups of older people integrate Wii playing into their physical and social spaces. This paper focuses on Wii™ game play by older people in Sheltered Housing schemes, as part of an initiative to promote physical and social activity in these settings. Using participant observations, interviews and video analysis of sessions over a year we show *how* older people actively construct the sense of a meeting place as part of their Wii game play and the social processes that underlie this. Through the use of bounded regions and a sense of decorum older players create a 'sacred space' around the Wii where they can learn new technical literacies, make new social connections with peers and take ownership of the communal spaces in which they live. We conclude with guidelines for encouraging appropriation and empowerment for older people through game play in communal housing settings.

Keywords: Wii, elderly, older people, video games, digital hearth, appropriation.

1 Introduction

With populations ageing across the developed world [27] attention has recently turned to ways of maintaining a good quality of life for those experiencing an extended old age [30]. The experience of growing older in these societies is unfortunately tainted by increasing levels of social isolation and reduced community involvement with family and friends often living far away and older people choosing to live alone. Social isolation can negatively impact emotional well being when experienced as loneliness, increasing an older person's susceptibility to depression [6] as well as being linked to all causes of mortality and morbidity [18].

In the UK, some of the issues of social isolation have the potential to be addressed by Sheltered Housing schemes. Sheltered housing is an approach to elderly care services where residents are encouraged to maintain their independence in rented accommodation but where certain support is provided on site when necessary. The

G. Leitner, M. Hitz, and A. Holzinger (Eds.): USAB 2010, LNCS 6389, pp. 156–176, 2010.

presence of other peers in the scheme provides the potential for social interaction and support staff are on hand to initiate activities to promote interaction.

To date, technologies have rarely figured as part of these activities. More generally, computer-based information and communication technologies have been proposed as useful in offsetting the negative effects of physical, cognitive and social ageing [3] however the uptake of such technologies by older people is traditionally low. New forms of interaction with technologies such as the embodied gesture-based paradigm of the Nintendo Wii game have potential for changing this relationship with technology and helping to meet well being needs. We are still in the early stages however of understanding the potential of games such as the Nintendo Wii and *how* older people might integrate these into their lives, particularly in a peer-based community housing setting.

In this paper we document an initiative by a UK charity (Age Concern) using Nintendo Wii game consoles to promote social and physical activity amongst their members in Sheltered Housing. The philosophy behind this approach, often described as 'Active Ageing' [30], is heavily influenced by activity theory[1] [5,15] which sees the well-being of older people as intrinsically linked to ongoing participation in social roles beyond retirement. It is embedded in government policies for older people across Europe [8]. In the UK active ageing is evident in government health and social care policies aimed at promoting health and well-being in old age, through higher levels of physical activity in the older population and by reducing barriers to increased levels of physical activity, mental well-being and social engagement among excluded groups of older people [7].

The Age Concern Wii initiative also builds on a growing trend in games development and deployment that enlists the fun elements of game play to encourage more serious educational and therapeutic aims [e.g. 13] including initiatives involving use of the Wii [17]. In this more serious vein games have already been used to support the physical, mental [2], and socioemotional [11] well being of older adults. The adoption rate of computer-based technologies is not high amongst the older population [20, 10, 9] which makes the success of such initiatives intriguing. The Wii console in particular has been targeted at the older generation through specific advertising campaigns [14]. News reports herald its popularity with older players in the USA [29], UK [24] and global sales indicate similar trends in other developed nations. Studies looking at older people's use of the Wii suggest that it may mitigate against cognitive decline [20] and provide an important source of social contact for them as *computational meeting places* where they can engage with their peers and younger generations both within and beyond the game itself [28]. However it would be wrong to think that computational meeting places are the immediate result of merely introducing a Wii console or that such meeting places are easily established. As Voida and Greenberg [28] point out such meeting places can be highly contested and whilst their study describes them as *comfortable* places other studies have shown them to be quite problematic. Neufeldt [22] in a study of Wii introduction in a German retirement home found a number of obstacles to engaged and enjoyable game play with the Wii Sports Bowling game. These included usability problems associated with learning the appropriate button controls for the game and ergonomic difficulties associated with playing

---

[1] Not to be confused with activity theory from Vygotsky's work in the 1920s and used in HCI.

the game from an armchair. Developing a clear understanding of issues of functional accessibility in relation to older people's use of embodied [26] and mobile (non-desktop) applications is of course important [16]. However in this paper we focus more on the social aspects of access. Neufeldt [22] also found that the most problematic issues in his study were conflicts with activity organizers at the home who perceived the game as unwanted competition for their own activities. This suggests that the sociability of Wii gameplay and hence its ability to enhance the well being of older people is context-dependent. This paper therefore takes a closer look at the evolution of older people's use of the Wii over a period of time paying particular attention to the way in which the context is actively constructed by players and organizers to create the sense of a meeting place and the implications that this has for extended use.

The Wii console is different to other games consoles such as the popular Sony Playstation or Microsoft Xbox in its reliance on wireless movement capture as the central control feature of game play. This allows interactions with the game to take place in a physical space which is (relatively) independent of the console and display screen compared with previous consoles. This has the important consequence of allowing social interactions to continue during play which can add meaning to a purely physical activity. It is this juncture between game play and social meaning that is of interest to this study.

2   Methodology

Age Concern's initial idea was to create a Wii Bowling League across Brighton and Hove which would provide an engaging and fun physical and social activity for older people[2]. Initial trials with their existing members at Age Concern drop-in sessions suggested that the Wii was suitably accessible to this age group to make it a viable proposition. The league was set up in small districts around the city so that sheltered houses close to one another could play on a regular basis without having to arrange extra transport. The winners from these districts were then invited to compete in larger public events around the city. This study follows the Age Concern initiative over the first year of its life both at regular sessions and public events, looking at how the older players appropriated the Wii game play experience and incorporated it into their lives as a meaningful activity.

We used multiple methods over a period of one year to track evolving game play. Participant observations, interviews and video recorded sessions were all used to ascertain longitudinal changes in game play. Analysis was framed by this objective but was grounded in the data. Factors outside of the game play were included in the analysis to maintain the broader sense of context which existed outside of the game play but continued to support it. Initially the Age Concern staff responsible for running the Wii sessions were interviewed to clarify the rationale for its use, to gain an understanding of their support role and of what motivated older people to join in. Subsequently these Age Concern staff were accompanied to their weekly supported Wii sessions in the communal lounges of four sheltered houses and two 'Wii events'

---

[2] http://www.guardian.co.uk/society/2008/apr/30/health.longtermcare for report.

held in public venues across Brighton and Hove were observed. Over a period of 1 year, 10 sessions in Sheltered Housing settings were attended. Each session was about 2 hours long with a break in the middle for tea. Overall 30 older players were encountered aged between 60 and 94. The number of older players per session ranged from 2 to 13 with at least one Age Concern staff always present, one researcher and one Sheltered Housing scheme manager or staff member. Whilst the focus of the sessions was to engage older residents in the activity, others present were encouraged to join in and this allowed an element of participant observation to take place as part of the process. Notes were taken of participant observations and interviews were undertaken with the residents at appropriate intervals between games (recorded for later analysis). 3 sessions were also captured on video to establish the evolution of game play over time from initial use to that after 1 year. This was done using multimodal interactional analysis [23] which acknowledges the different ways in which meaning is conveyed in communication beyond the sole use of language. Examination of the video in this way therefore gave a fine grained, holistic account of interaction which incorporates not only language but also body posture, gestures, layout of the room, the sound qualities of speech, game elements, etc; in fact anything that was used to convey meaning whilst playing the Wii. Multimodal interactional analysis shows how those present through their actions, structure the awareness of one another by directing their attention towards particular aspects of the interaction and hence signify that which they deem to be *meaningful* within that context. After watching all three of the video sessions in full, five minute segments were chosen to illustrate the differences in game play and the evolution of players' engagement with the Wii. These segments were also chosen because they portray similar characteristics in terms of the expectations of the game, all showing the Wii Sports bowling game. Using these three segments allows us to compare the multimodal construction of meaning over different contexts and over time. Throughout the sessions players were observed playing a number of different games. The principle game and the one chosen by Age Concern to teach new players was the Wii Sports Bowling game, in particular a variant of the standard ten pin game called 'Power Throws' which involves knocking down increasing numbers of pins at each throw. Participants and organizers are identified throughout the paper by anonymised names.

3   Findings

3.1   Overview of Game Play Development

3.1.1   Game Choice

The Wii Sports Bowling game was chosen by the Age Concern organisers as an introductory game. From interviews with organisers it became apparent that older players were familiar with the bowling game concept likening it to lawn bowls or skittles and found the controls relatively easy to understand and operate. Similar usability issues were experienced in relation to button control as Neufeldt [22] found. This particular game leaves control of game play progression down to the current player which is helpful in terms of structuring the whole event, allowing breaks in play at any point and not dictating the overall pace of play.

3.1.2 Competition

Only a minority of residents in any given home volunteered to participate in the Wii initiative. Indeed communal activities in Sheltered Housing were generally not well attended. Age Concern recruited and trained teams from different sheltered houses and then got them to compete against one another as part of their league. The organisers saw team building and competition as important in engaging new players. At their public events two Wii consoles were set up side by side to give the impression of one team playing against another. In practice these early games were more about learning how to play the game rather than competing with others. Competition with oneself in terms of one's physical and mental capacity was seen to be just as important as a motivation for the players. Men tended to respond more to the competition element, with some practicing deliberately for competitions. As one player put it: "if you don't use your head you lose it" (Don).

3.1.3 Personal and Social Involvement

There were other reasons for joining in with the Wii initiative. Those with grandchildren were keen to keep up to date with them by learning about the Wii. They were aware that the Wii games console carried a lot of cultural capital with their grandchildren from family gatherings where it had been present. They were keen to share an appreciation of their grandchildren's enthusiasm and to be able to play with them at a later date. Particular elements of the Wii were also harnessed by the organisers to encourage personal and social involvement during game play. For instance the Wii uses on screen avatars called Mii's to represent individual players. These can be named and their appearance customized to suit each player. During Age Concern events players were encouraged to spend a good deal of time choosing their Mii and giving it a name that they could relate using *'nicknames they'd had as a child"* (Pamela). Mii's were also used to promote a group identity for competitions with a Mii being created specifically for the whole team and physical mascots being used to reinforce this group identity.

3.2 Playing on: Evolving Game Play

In order to understand the progression of how players made sense of and engaged with the Wii experience beyond these initial conceptions it was important to take a closer look at how people conducted themselves during the game play itself. Here multimodal interactional analysis [23] was used to understand both the verbal and non-verbal aspects of Wii game play. Each video captures use after a different time span: initial use; use after six months and use after one year, and is representative of other video and observation notes of game play at a similar stage. Each video is also showing a different sheltered home situation.

3.2.1 Video 1: Initial Use

This first video is at a point of initial use. It shows an 83 year old resident becoming acquainted with the 'increasing-pin' version of the bowling game on the Wii. Out of the group of players she is the only resident in this home and from the start is designated the captain of the group. The other players are visiting from another Sheltered

Housing scheme nearby and they all know one another. This is their second time playing the Wii and they are being instructed by a member of the Age Concern support team. Assistance is given when they encounter problems understanding game expectations or in using the Wii controller. This particular player has trouble working out when to press the B as also noted in previous studies [22]. Prior to playing the game, seating is arranged by the Age Concern staff in a semicircle around the game's display. During play the whole team sit around the display and are intently focused on the game, giving encouragement and advice to the person playing.

Table 1. Information about Wii game playing session in Sheltered Home 1

No. Residents	35 (Sheltered Home 1)
No. Older Players	5
Previous experience of playing Wii	Novices. Dependent on Age Concern to provide console and screen. Need support to set up and play.
Number of consoles	1
Others present	5 (1 member of Sheltered Housing staff (briefly), 2 Age support workers, 2 researchers)
Games played in session	Wii Sports – Bowling; Wii Fit – Ski Jump

Excerpt 1

Participants left to right:(off screen: Dee-Age Concern), Ben-researcher, Edna-player, Beryl-player, Pat-player, Ann-player, Jan-player.	
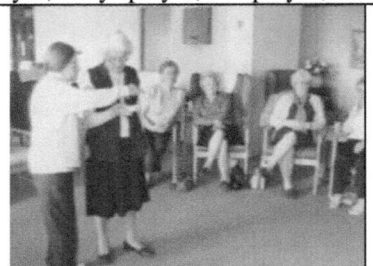	0.31.84 Dee: there's two buttons to remember my love. First press the button A. Edna: well it's not flashing. Dee: No you're all right press B then. Edna: Press B? Ann: Press B and play Dee: Press button B and put your arm back and you hold it like that.
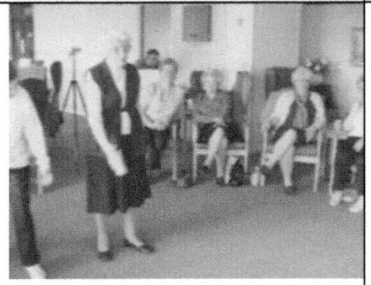	0.41.92 Dee: [demonstrates movement] 00.44.72 Edna: [successful throw] Dee: Hey that's a good one Ann: Cor that's a good one Edna Hurrah, one left Dee: Ha ha Beryl: Huhm Silence 9 seconds

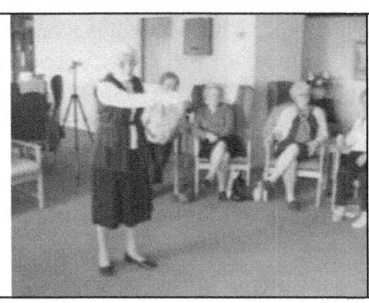

0.59.29
Edna: [swings without effect]

In excerpt 1 we see Edna trying to understand the action of button B in relation to throwing a ball down the alley and she starts off being quite impatient and irritated. Button A must be pressed briefly to place the Mii at the top of the alley (except the button has been covered with a piece of card by the Age Concern helper) and then button B must be pressed, held down whilst swinging and then released to let go of the ball. Whilst the Age Concern helper (Dee) is able to demonstrate the embodied throwing action easily she cannot describe the points in time necessary for pressing and releasing button B. With this first throw Edna gets the timing right with corresponding encouragement from the other players. Edna's subsequent attempts are not so successful. She continues to press button B and enact the throwing movement without success. Her fellow players offer suggestions which are plainly wrong and do not help. In the end she just keeps enacting the swinging motion repeatedly and pressing button B until it works.

Excerpt 2
The alternative to pressing button A to put the Mii at the top of the alley is to just wait until the game places the Mii there by itself. Eventually after a few multiple throws like the first one Edna decides to just wait. Whilst throwing her fifth ball a member of the Sheltered Housing staff enters the room.

Participants left to right:(off screen: Dee-Age Concern),Ben-researcher, E-player, A-player, Pat-player, Cath-housing staff, Ann-player, Jan-player	
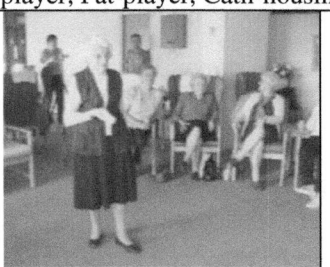	2.5.76 Cath: Hi yah [member of Sheltered Housing staff enters at far door] Jan: Hello Cath: Hi yah Dee: Yeah

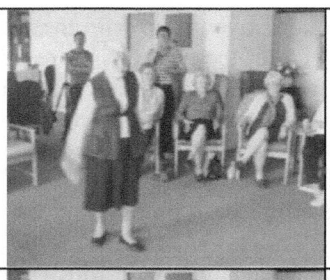	3.04.44 Edna: [Does a double swing, the second one being successful. She knocks all the pins down]
	    Ann:Very good
	    Jan: Oohoo

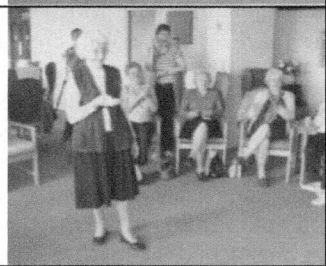	3.12.40 [Everyone except Cath applauds] Ann: Well done Edna 45 pins Dee: You see it doubles up when you get a strike you get double the points. Pat: 90 she's got there

During this throw there is intense silent concentration amongst all the players as Edna waits for the appropriate time to throw the ball. All the players are paying attention to Edna's mistakes and learning from them. The member of staff (Cath) interrupts the silence with her own greeting but is given minimal attention by everyone else as their attention is focussed on the game. With this throw Edna knocks down all the pins at once (a strike) with excited applause coming from all the other players and a big smile across her face. Cath does not join in the applause. The Age Concern demonstrator explains the scoring associated with a strike and player Pat reiterates this to the whole group as a way of confirming this new knowledge.

Excerpt 3
The member of staff continues to start conversation ignoring the game play.

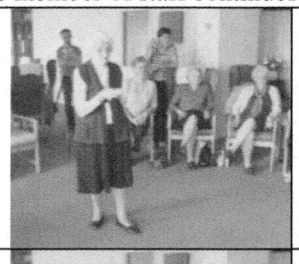	3.26.80 Cath: I thought they were doing skiing or something today
	    Beryl: We were doing that.
	    Cath: Oh you've done that have you. Yes.
	    Beryl: Failures
	    Cath: ha ha ha

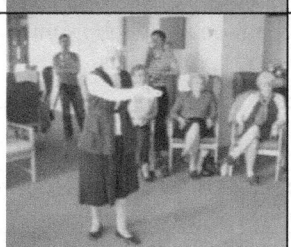	3.35.82 Edna: [Double Throws]
	    Cath: Where is everybody from our house then coz there's only Edna
	    Beryl:Go on
	    Jan: Ooh
	    Ann: It's a lot of pins in it. 54 pins
	    Silence 4 seconds
	    Beryl: No I don't know where they all are
	    Cath: I've only popped in I'm busy I can't stop. See ya later.

Despite the member of staff's attempts at initiating conversation with the players their attention remains focused on Edna and her playing of the game. Their responses to Cath are curt and do not invite extended conversation. Equally she makes it clear that she does not see their presence in the house as her responsibility, using a strange third person approach to talking to them as in *"I thought **they** were doing skiing or something today"*. She quickly defines her responsibilities as concerned with residents only and therefore not this mixed group, retreating from the room to continue with other duties.

Even at this early stage there is the sense of an inner gaming circle which emphasizes the importance of the collective activity taking place with the Wii, creating a 'sacred space' [12] around it. This seems to be at odds with the day to day working practices of this sheltered home. Goffman [12] talks about the ways in which people use conversation and body language to bound regions according to particular standards of behaviour or 'decorum'. In this setting consideration for the current player in terms of silence and appropriate encouragement are paramount as well as joint involvement in the ongoing game. The region of game play is bounded by the semicircle of chairs which creates a physical obstacle to outsiders. The staff member is excluded from the gaming circle in order to maintain the correct decorum for playing the game. Here we see the beginning of the creation of social meaning around the Wii, but at this early stage the mechanical aspects of the game play are foregrounded as the social focus.

3.2.2 Video 2: After 6 Months

Video 2 represents typical play after 6 months use. It shows an 81 year old lady (also designated as the captain) playing the standard ten-pin version of the bowling game. The players in this video are well acquainted with the Wii and have incorporated these sessions into their weekly routine. All the older players are residents of this particular home. The Age Concern support staff still give advice but are more focused on improving players' performances rather than teaching them how to use the

Table 2. Information about Wii game playing session in Sheltered Home 2

Number of Residents	27 (Sheltered Home 2)
Number of Older Players	3
Previous Experience of playing Wii	Accomplished players with 6 months experience. Played in the final of the Wii Bowling competition at a public venue. Dependent on Age Concern to provide console and screen. Can set up and need no support to play.
Number of consoles	1
Others present	6 (1 other older resident, 2 member of Sheltered Housing staffs, 2 Age Concern support workers, 1 researcher)
Games Played in Session	Wii Sports – Bowling; Wii Fit – Ski Jump

controls. The housing staff are present and join in with the games. The current player has just returned from a period in hospital and has not joined in with the Wii sessions for some weeks. The other resident present has difficulty playing standing up due to having had a stroke affecting his stability and joins in from his chair. She is fully conversant with the controls but has some trouble aiming her ball down the middle of the alley. The seating arrangements are not altered for the Wii and whilst those sitting around the game are supportive, their attention is not always focused on the game play with conversations about other topics taking place.

Excerpt 4

Participants left to right: Pedro-Age Concern, Mark-Age Concern, Irene-player, Julia-player, Pam-housing staff, (off screen: Pete-player, Liz-housing staff)	
00.20.00 Pedro:Famous strikes please	
00.22.86 Irene:[Pushes button with left hand to move across the alley]	
00.29.90 Irene: [Throws the ball –gets a strike]	
00.37.26 Pedro: [claps] Oooer Irene: Well I've had one so I'm happy Julia: You'll get more Pedro: That was the first one	

There are no problems with button B here and the A button is not covered by the Age Concern staff during this session. Irene uses advanced techniques to play the game such as moving her Mii character slightly to one side before throwing to compensate for her particular throwing style. Her control of the Mii at this point shows a degree of sophistication in terms of understanding what the Wii controller does and the way in which her physical actions affect her performance. The Age Concern demonstrator (Pedro) recognises Irene's abilities from past sessions as indicated by his first comment *"Famous strikes please"* but wants her to continue playing her best and improving. Initially he does not instruct her directly but there is an obvious shared understanding between himself and Irene evident in both their comments.

Excerpt 5
In excerpt 5, we see different members of the audience (Liz and Pedro) challenging Irene to recreate her best performances from the past. However the conversation surrounding the game starts to interfere with the silent shared concentration needed for playing. The conversation also starts to go off at tangents principally driven by the staff member Liz. Other members of the audience place their hands over their mouths to subtly indicate the need for silence whilst Irene is playing.

00.46.65 Liz: I want you to show me how this turkey's [3]done Irene Irene: You must be joking 'Liz' Liz: Nooo Pedro: Double get double Irene: [Pushes button with left hand to move across the alley, throws the ball]	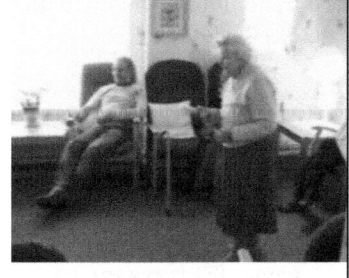
01.17.49 Irene: [Pushes button with left hand to move across the alley - throws the ball] Game: "Nice Spare" Pedro: Second try now	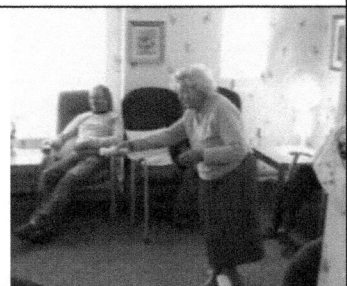

---

[3] A turkey in ten pin bowling is three strikes in a row.

01.31.67 Irene: [Pushes button with left hand to move across the alley - throws the ball] Liz: I didn't notice we've got a blue ball since we changed console, did we used to have a black ball or did we always have a blue ball? Pete: Can't remember Pedro: It changes. It changes. It depends. Liz: Maybe we'll always have this. Pedro: It was pink one before. Irene: Only one that time	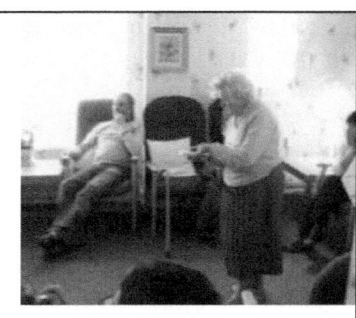

Excerpt 6

In excerpt 6 Pedro decides to give Irene some direct advice about how to correct her play seeing that her usual approach is not quite working. He recommends a subtle change to the positioning of her Mii character which Irene acknowledges and does. Unfortunately the conversation from the audience continues to interfere and becomes even more unrelated to the game. More of the audience start to cover their mouths with their hands as a way of reinforcing Liz's compliance in terms of being quiet and paying attention to the game.

Participants left to right: (off screen: Pedro-Age Concern), Mark-Age Concern, Irene-player, Julia-player, Pam-housing staff, (off screen: Pete-player, Liz-housing staff)	
04.03.00 Pedro:You're going too much to your right Irene: Yes I am aren't I. I noticed that. Pedro: If you go one less, you will get it right.	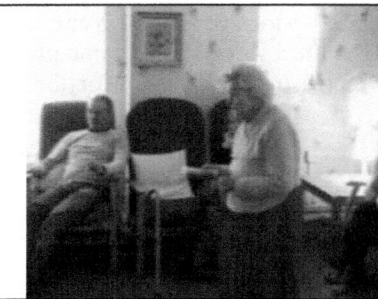
04.22.74 Irene: [pushes button to side - throws] Game: Nice spare Pete: Are they decorating the bedrooms? C: No, it will be the entire common area and Pedro: Try to be in the middle here Irene. Irene: in the middle there Pedro: Right in the middle there Liz: I'll ask for the wallpaper book Sunday	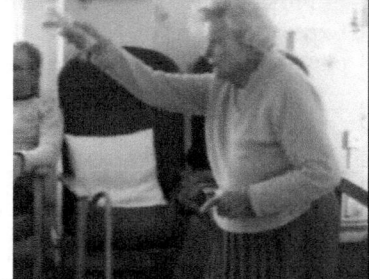

00.04.50 Liz: the majority will be like the paper of the hallway	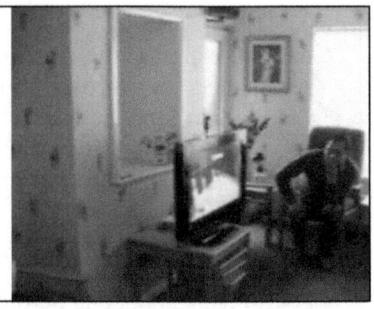

In this setting similar standards of behaviour or decorum are expected to those at Sheltered Home 1, i.e. consideration for the current player in terms of silence and appropriate encouragement as well as joint involvement during the game. In addition there is an expectation that players will challenge themselves and try to get the best scores. In this case the playing region is not bounded in space and instead is much more integrated into the existing spatial arrangement of the room. It is bounded in time and the rhythm of game play though such that the players and audience are expected to abide by the decorum of Wii game play during the sessions. In this case the staff member cannot be physically excluded from the gaming circle but cues are given to her that she should maintain the correct decorum during the game. Here we see the Wii becoming more integrated into social interaction more generally with the mechanics and usability aspects of game play starting to recede more into the background of play, enabling the social aspects to be more foregrounded.

3.2.3 Video 3: After 1 Year
The third video shows game play after 1 year. Here an 82 year old man is playing the 'increasing-pin' version of the bowling game with three other players. One of the

Table 3. Information about Wii game playing session in Sheltered Home 3

No. Residents	93 (Sheltered Home 3)
No. Older Players	13
Previous Experience of playing Wii	Accomplished players with 1 year's experience. Played in the final of the Wii Bowling competition at a public venue. Have their own console which they practice on regularly. Need no support to set up their own console and play.
Number of consoles	2 (Age Concern provide second console)
Others present	3 (1 member of Sheltered Housing staff from another home, 1 Age Concern support worker and 1 researcher)
Games Played in Session	Wii Sports – Bowling; Wii Play - Duck Hunt; Wii Sports – Golf; Wii Sports – Tennis

seated players (Sheila) is a newcomer to the Wii whilst the others are seasoned players. All of these players are resident of another sheltered home and have been invited to play by the residents (who are also present but not playing) at regular sessions every week for the last year. It is an established part of both houses' routines. This is a larger event than that shown in the preceding videos with 2 Wii consoles and 2 displays. This gives more of an atmosphere of an 'event'. The seating has been arranged in an extended semicircle around the displays and biscuits are placed out on tables adjacent to the seats before the visiting team arrives. This is all done by the residents of the sheltered home hosting the event rather than Age Concern and there are no housing staff present. The residents also greet people as they come in and make them cups of tea. Whilst people are playing the Wii they circulate amongst the players engaging in general conversation. Age Concern's input is minimal and focuses on keeping scores during games, keeping players focused on the game and informing everyone of city-wide Wii events that they could take part in. Seasoned players are responsible for passing on their Wii skills to newcomers.

Excerpt 7
Excerpt 7 shows how the game play has become a background element to a larger socialising event. There are multiple conversations taking place throughout the room, sometimes focussing on the game but shifting easily to all sorts of other unrelated topics. The volume of conversation drowns out the noises from the Wii console. Dee attempts to keep the focus on the game by pointing out the current state of affairs to others

Participants left to right: Peg-player, Sheila-player, Mary-player, Dee-Age Concern, Ron-player	
0.24.52 Ron: [throws] Mary: Oh nearly. Sheila: The trouble with me when I started doing that... Mary:Everybody does that. Sheila: I kept letting go of it	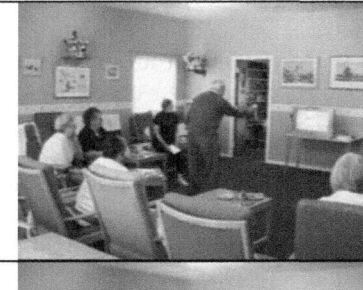
0.33.80 Sheila:[does action with the imaginary button in mid air] Peg: Yeah I keep doing that. Goes off the line don't it and I gotta go that way [does a jiggle] then I move over [points to playing area to show where] and then it starts going the right way.	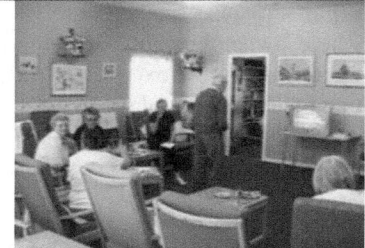

0.50.68 Ron: [successful throw] Mary: everybody does that Sheila Sheila: Do they? [picks up cup of tea and drinks] Dee: Do do da do [waves hand up and down] Mary: [picks up cup of tea and drinks] Peg: Oh it is hot in here isn't it	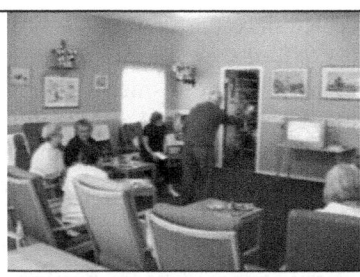
1.09.59 Peg: [picks up tea and drinks] Sheila: [puts tea down] Mary: [puts tea down] Sheila: Oh the supermarket down St James' Street Peg: Oh isn't it hard Sheila: I know I used to moan about it but I really miss it. Dee: [picks up cup of tea and drinks]	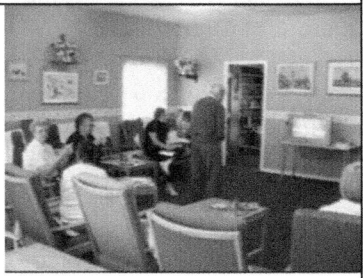

Here, the Age Concern demonstrator (Dee) is largely redundant in her role with existing players teaching new arrivals. For newcomers acquiring literacy with the Wii in this setting, the learning takes place in a more subtle manner to that seen in the other videos. It has become an aspect of communicating with one's peers, embedded in the process of getting to know one another. This contrasts with the situation in the other houses, who were at different points in the appropriation lifecycle, where learning was from a knowledgeable other (Age Concern demonstrator). The sense of decorum is also quite different with minimal consideration for the current player in terms of silence and encouragement. Expressions of joint involvement are still present but have shifted from an exclusive concentration on the game to sharing personal exchanges about their daily lives. The playing region is bounded in space in the same way as in video 1 with one important change, it now encompasses two sets of players (one for each console). Interestingly although this recreates a competitive setting, competition itself is absent from the game play with each console set up for completely different games. Players treatment of the playing region as a 'sacred space' is also less rigid with the providing of refreshments taking priority over game play. In summary, what we see here is the foregrounding of social meaning around the Wii, where ownership now lies clearly with the residents and where the Wii merely provides the context/excuse for their interactions, and where the space has meaning beyond purely game play.

4 Discussion

The focus of this paper is on understanding how older people in these Sheltered Housing situations have evolved their relationship with Wii game play over time. The fact that this is an active ongoing agenda across multiple Sheltered Homes more than a year after its introduction, and that the residents have clearly been able to actively construct socially meaningful engagement for themselves around using the Wii, is evident of a successful initiative by Age Concern. Undoubtedly too, their use of the Wii promotes physical, psychological and social activity. This is clear to see from the video excerpts. While an Active Ageing agenda [30] may assume that this kind of activity – Wii game play - is intrinsically beneficial, it is important to consider *how* it is that these older people actively define such activities as meaningful. To ignore this is to ignore the essence of what makes the initiative successful. The way in which the purpose of the Wii and the space around it have been negotiated and defined by the players and support staff is integral to understanding its success.

4.1 Creating a Sacred Space for Wii Game Play

Age Concern's role in the Wii initiative is pivotal, expressing an underlying empowerment principle towards players which encourages their independent mastery of technical literacies and a high degree of control over their living spaces. The redefinition of physical and social space which accompanies players' use of the Wii is also implicated in its successful integration into the daily life of these players. The physical movements which are a necessary part of playing the Wii help to define a 'sacred' space around the game console with its own sense of decorum. Players must step into this space in order to play the game and non-players are expected to be respectful of this space not entering it during play. Age Concern reinforce the sense of a sacred space with a chair circle around the Wii and define decorum in conjunction with players as being based on fun and friendly competition with patient consideration for new players but an expectation that players will challenge themselves to the best of their abilities. Engaging with this space players first acquire technical literacy with the Wii but soon start to take ownership of this space and the social potential that it offers.

4.2 Acquiring Technical Literacy

The sacred space of the Wii provides a safe place to learn about the new embodied gesture-based interactions of the Wii. Learning is also supported by the physical nature of play. Individual interactions with the Wii amplify older players' physical abilities allowing them to take part in activities (such as bowling) which they would not normally entertain. The embodied interaction metaphor that translates physical off screen movements into enhanced on screen activities (making participation in such activities possible) is quickly understood and appreciated by new players. Age Concern staff demonstrate these capacities very simply through miming of the necessary actions (see video 1). The transparency of Wii interactions (and their associated difficulties) make them available to other players providing socially-embedded opportunities for vicarious and shared learning, with non-players observing and offering advice. Age Concern maintain an empowering approach to teaching the Wii interactions using a scaffolding approach [4], reducing support as players' competence with them increases. What is interesting here is that once basic literacies have been acquired the game recedes as a focus of attention in its own right to becoming a context for other social purposes, and where the skills are taken for granted.

4.3   Taking Ownership of Communal and Social Space

Defining Wii game play areas as sacred space also encourages the older residents in these sheltered houses to take *ownership* of those spaces whilst playing. In videos 1 and 2 it was Age Concern support staff who were responsible for appropriating space though the repositioning chairs and tables and the placing of the Wii console and display screen to form circles. In video 3 it is the residents who take full control of their physical space rearranging it without Age Concern support and inviting guests into that space. Here we start to see the underlying social potential of the Wii being explored. Previously, residents were largely reliant on the Housing staff to organize social activities, and these were for residents only. Over time we also see the sacred space of these events being asserted in terms of time and social availability with their regular establishment in the diaries of players. The Wii in these settings has been used as a pivotal facilitator in both shifting the power and motivation for social organization to the residents themselves, and for widening the social participation to engage with other homes and with older residents in the neighbourhood, forging new social connections with peers that had not previously existed.

Such active participation in residential settings is acknowledged as important for the well being of Sheltered Housing residents although it can sometimes be at odds with the concerns of housing staff who are focused on managing an efficient working environment [1]. This appeared to be the case in Sheltered House 1 where ownership of space was contested. Wii game playing has allowed the older people in these homes to accomplish technical literacy with new technology, to express their own values in new and collective ways, expressing claims to ownership of communal space and time, defining new meeting places and providing opportunities for instigating new social connections with their peers. Together these contribute to the older people in these homes being able to frame what constitutes *meaningful use* of a technology for them.

4.4   Guideline for Appropriation and Empowerment

The Wii console is quickly being adopted as a panacea for ageing concerns with research showing its positive effects on physical health [2] and mental well being [11]. Other research has suggested that the Wii's ability to benefit older users in this way is due to its inherent sociability [28]. Undoubtedly the embodied aspects of game play do allow social interaction to continue during game play. However in this study we have highlighted the co-constructed and contested nature of Wii game play and the importance of older people themselves gaining control over the space as part of their appropriation of the Wii. It is their active performance within and surrounding game play that constructs it as a meaningful and beneficial engagement. Interventions for older people using the Wii should remain cognizant of the centrality of empowerment in promoting well being with appropriate decorum and control over their own space being important gauges of empowerment in such situations [19]. Here we present guidelines for encouraging empowerment as part of appropriating the Wii. This reflects a broader view of 'design implications' where any such intervention reflects not only the technical issues but designing for the broader context:

4.4.1 Identify Motivations

Determine older people's motivations for playing the Wii in the first place and try to support these. Where appropriate look to extend opportunities for social contact with peers and intergenerational connections through game play. Both this and previous studies [28] have highlighted potential for playing with younger generations and grandchildren. There are also opportunities to explore this through remote Internet-enabled game play that have so far not been explored.

4.4.2 Use Controllable Games

Choose games initially that allow older players to be in control of the pace and play rather than it being dictated by the game. This allows controlled engagement with the game which is particularly important for frail players and gives space for the 'in between' social interactions. There is a definite design opportunity here for more such games. Many of the games encountered during the study dictated the pace of game play too much for older players and were discounted by them (e.g. Ski jump).

4.4.3 Setting Up the Sacred Space: Physical Layout and Decorum

Physical layout: It is important to establish the layout of the room particularly in the early stages by arranging chairs and the display screen so that it creates a 'safe' enclosed circle for learning the embodied interactions of the Wii.

Decorum: The decorum surrounding game play is important to define as this creates expectations for what behaviour is appropriate, acceptable and/or encouraged. An initial attitude of friendly competition and self-challenge is important in that it motivates players to learn. Fostering a collective attitude towards learning and playing is important where joint involvement is encouraged. In this study this was promoted by the league element of Age Concern's approach. Previous studies have suggested downplaying the competitive element of Wii games [28] but it seemed to be a positive element here. Social interaction is the bedrock of the Wii's success and once players get to know one another they will start to define their own sense of decorum. This is to be encouraged. Tea breaks are one way of providing social 'openings' for players to start talking and getting experienced players to teach new ones in other homes is another.

4.4.4 Scaffold Learning

Training for basic skills acquisition should be adapted to account for the initial abilities of the player but should remain open to skillful development in the future. Basic embodied skills can be taught easily by the miming of embodied actions but more symbolic interactions which incorporate the use of buttons are more difficult to acquire for some older people. Engagement with the physical interface of the Wii controller should be managed (i.e. with the use of cardboard covers over buttons) so that only simple interactions are possible at first but can become more complex at a later date. Adaptivity of this sort is a common approach to accessible design for virtual interfaces [25]. A similar design approach could help here with the Wii controller's physical interface.

4.4.5 Manage Transition to Ownership

Plan explicitly for the transitioning of ownership by negotiating with other residents and staff within the home. Get everyone on board as much as possible from the start including them in sessions so that when support withdraws the physical and social space to play the Wii remains.

5 Conclusions

This longitudinal study of older people's use of the Wii in Sheltered Housing has shown how an initiative based upon competitive embodied gaming can address some of the ongoing issues related to growing older in a developed society. It introduced older players to new technical literacies in an inclusive non-threatening and fun way. It addressed social isolation by providing them with new social peer connections through community events. It provided new roles for older people within their local community as hosts of such events and encouraged their ownership of the communal spaces in which they lived. What also became clear in this study was the contested nature of these institutional settings and the way in which the Wii (with Age Concern's help) could empower older people living there to redefine these settings as community meeting places. The presentation of the key lessons as guidelines is intended to enable other groups of older people to realise the social value from games such as the Wii in sheltered housing settings whilst at the same time keeping an important grounding in empowerment issues. Whilst this study has focused exclusively on older people's appropriation of the Wii in Sheltered Housing it would be interesting to see whether similar processes of appropriation took place when other technologies were introduced into those same spaces.

References

1. Abbott, S., Fisk, M., Forward, L.: Social and democratic participation in residential settings for older people: realities and aspirations. Ageing and Society 20, 327–340 (2000)
2. Basak, C., Boot, W.R., Voss, M.W., Kramer, A.F.: Can training in a real-time strategy video game attenuate cognitive decline in older adults? Psychology and Aging 23(4), 756–777 (2008)
3. Bouwhuis, D.G.: Design for person-environment interaction in older age: a gerontechnological perspective. Gerontechnology 2(3), 232–246 (2003)
4. Bruner, J.: Actual Minds, Possible Worlds. Harvard University Press, Cambridge (1986)
5. Cavan, R.S., Burgess, E.W., Havighurst, R.J., Goldhamer, H.: Personal Adjustment in Old Age. Social Science Research Associates, Chicago (1949)
6. Choi, N.G., McDougall, G.J.: Comparison of Depressive Symptoms between homebound older adults and ambulatory older adults. Aging and Mental Health 11, 310–322 (2007)
7. Department of Health: Our health, our care, our say: a new direction for community services. Department of Health, UK Government (2006),
   http://www.dh.gov.uk/en/Publicationsandstatistics/
   Publications/PublicationsPolicyAndGuidance/DH_4127453?
   IdcService=GET_FILE&dID=456&Rendition=Web (accessed March 19, 2009)

8. European Commission: Green Paper Confronting demographic change: a new solidarity between the generations. European Commission (2005),
http://europa.eu/legislation_summaries/
employment_and_social_policy/situation_in_europe/
c10128_en.htm (accessed May 21, 2009)

9. European Commission: European i2010 initiative on e-Inclusion. To be part of the information society (2007),
http://ec.europa.eu/information_society/activities/
einclusion/docs/i2010_initiative/
comm_native_com_2007_0694_f_en_acte.pdf (accessed October 20, 2008)

10. Fox, S.: Older Americans and the Internet, Pew Internet & American Life Project (2004)

11. Goldstein, G.H., Cajko, L., Oosterbroek, M., Michielsen, M., Van Houten, O., Salverda, F.: Videogames and the elderly. Social Behavior and Personality: An International Journal 25(4), 345–353 (1997)

12. Goffman, E.: Presentation of Self in Everyday Life. Doubleday Anchor, New York (1959)

13. Griffiths, M.: The therapeutic value of video games. In: Raessens, J., Goldstein, J. (eds.) Handbook of Computer Games Studies, pp. 161–171. The MIT Press, Cambridge (2005)

14. Hall, K.: Nintendo: Wii Want To Expand Games' Appeal. Business Week (September 14, 2006),   http://www.businessweek.com/globalbiz/blog/eyeonasia/
archives/2006/09/nintendo_wii_wa.html (accessed July 15, 2009)

15. Havighurst, R.J., Albrecht, R.: Older People. Longman, London (1953)

16. Holzinger, A., Searle, G., Nischelwitzer, A.: On some Aspects of Improving Mobile Applications for the Elderly. In: Stephanidis, C. (ed.) HCI 2007. LNCS, vol. 4554, pp. 923–932. Springer, Heidelberg (2007)

17. Holzinger, A., Softic, S., Stickel, C., Ebner, M., Debevc, M.: Intuitive E-Teaching by Using Combined HCI Devices: Experiences with Wiimote Applications. In: Stephanidis, C. (ed.) HCII 2007 and EPCE 2007. LNCS, vol. 5616, pp. 44–52. Springer, Heidelberg (2009)

18. House, J.S., Landis, K.R., Umberson, D.: Social relationships and health. Science 241(4865), 540–545 (1988)

19. Light, A., Wright, P.C.: The Panopticon and the Performance Arena: HCI Reaches within. In: Gross, T., Gulliksen, J., Kotzé, P., Oestreicher, L., Palanque, P., Prates, R.O., Winckler, M. (eds.) INTERACT 2009. LNCS, vol. 5727, pp. 201–204. Springer, Heidelberg (2009)

20. Livingstone, S., Van Couvering, E., Thumim, M.: Adult media Literacy: A review of the research literature on behalf of Ofcom. Ofcom (2005),
http://www.ofcom.org.uk/advice/media_literacy/medlitpub/
medlitpubrss/aml.Pdf (accessed August 20, 2008)

21. McLaughlin, A., Allaire, J.: http://www.gainsthroughgaming.org/2009 (accessed July 10, 2009)

22. Neufeldt, C.: Wii play with elderly people. In: International Reports on Socio-informatics. Enhancing Interaction Spaces by Social Media for the Elderly: A Workshop Report 6(3), 50–59 (2009)

23. Norris, S.: Analyzing multimodal interaction: a methodological framework. Routledge, New York (2004)

24. Parker, A.: "OAPs say nurse, I need a Wii". The Sun (September 14, 2007),
http://www.thesun.co.uk/sol/homepage/news/article294579.ece (accessed July 15, 2009)

25. Stephanidis, C.: Adaptive techniques for universal access. User Modeling and User-Adapted Interaction 11(1-2), 159–179 (2001)

26. Stephanidis, C.: User Interfaces for All: New perspectives into Human-Computer Interaction. In: Stephanidis, C. (ed.) User Interfaces for All - Concepts, Methods, and Tools, pp. 3–17. Lawrence Erlbaum Associates, Mahwah (2001)
27. United Nations World Economic and Social Survey 2007: Development in an Ageing World. United Nations, New York (2007), http://www.un.org/esa/policy/wess/wess2007files/wess2007.pdf (accessed October 10, 2008)
28. Voida, A., Greenberg, S.: Wii All Play. The Console Game as a Computational Meeting Place. In: Proceedings of the ACM SIGCHI Conference on Human Factors in Computing Systems, pp. 1559–1568. ACM Press, New York (2009)
29. Wischnowsky, D.: Wii bowling knocks over retirement home. Chicago Tribune, (February 16, 2007), http://www.chicagotribune.com/news/local/chi-070216nintendo,0,2755896.story (accessed July 10, 2009)
30. World Health Organisation: Active Ageing: A Policy Framework (2002), http://whqlibdoc.who.int/hq/2002/WHO_NMH_NPH_02.8.pdf (accessed February 17, 2009)

Designing for Older People:
A Case Study in a Retirement Home

Benoît Otjacques[1], Marc Krier[1], Fernand Feltz[1],
Dieter Ferring[2], and Martine Hoffmann[2]

[1] Public Research Center – Gabriel Lippmann
Department ISC – Informatics, Systems and Collaboration
41, Rue du Brill
L-4422 Belvaux, Luxembourg
otjacque@lippmann.lu, krier@lippmann.lu, feltz@lippmann.lu
[2] University of Luxembourg
INSIDE Research Unit
Route de Diekirch, BP2
L-7220 Walferdange, Luxembourg
{dieter.ferring,martine.hoffmann}@uni.lu

Abstract. This paper discusses the design process of a system aiming to support daily life of older people in a retirement home. This system called Sammy was designed on a participatory basis by a multidisciplinary team. The main results are the importance of communicating with all the stakeholders regarding both strengths and weaknesses of the new system, the importance of the social factors in system acceptance, the need to combine various evaluation methods during the design process, the importance of contextual factors and the need to take into account the dynamics of population in a retirement home.

Keywords: Human Factors, Older People, Design Process.

1 Introduction

Older adults are becoming an increasing part of the population in many countries and it is nowadays acknowledged that this evolution will probably be one of the most important challenges in the coming decades. In this context it is of prime importance to study the design process of products and services targeting the older users. Indeed, it is still partly unknown what their involvement in the design process can bring and what are the limits of such an approach. This paper aims to contribute to a better understanding of this issue by discussing a field experience in a retirement home.

2 State-of-Art

2.1 ICT and Ageing

Information & Communication Technologies (ICT) are nowadays acknowledged as powerful means to tackle the challenges of an ageing population. The scope and

G. Leitner, M. Hitz, and A. Holzinger (Eds.): USAB 2010, LNCS 6389, pp. 177–194, 2010.

objective of the research projects in this domain are very large: to maintain older people at home and to tackle issues regarding quality of life or safety (e.g. [10], [14]); to counter the effects of the age-related physical or cognitive impairments (e.g. [5]) or to enhance the medical support to older users (e.g. [11]). A literature review has helped us to identify some valuable findings of this vast amount of research, which sometimes contradict some preconceived ideas.

- Many older adults are not basically reluctant to the use of ICT. Numbers shows that elderly people do use the Internet and are the fastest growing demographic of Web users [6]. ICT is also perceived by some older people as an important element for inclusion in the contemporary society [19]. This may motivate them to learn and to use new ICT devices and applications.
- Ageing is a universal but not a uniform phenomenon and there is no standard way of getting older [18]. Ageing concerns various dimensions (vision, dexterity, memory, social life, emotions…) and multiple combinations of impairments and living conditions can be encountered ([2], [3], [6]). Therefore, most of the results cannot easily be generalized to a hypothetical "older population". From a design view point, this make it almost impossible to design a device that can meet every combination of expectations and constraints that older people can exhibit. Consequently, design proposals should precisely describe the subgroup of the "older population" that is targeted, in order to delimit their scope of relevance.
- In general, older people want to remain (as long as possible) independent individuals, including in their use of computers ([13], [19], [20]). Therefore, designers should prefer (as much as possible) the ICT solutions that can be operated by older people with little or no help.
- Designing product and services for older people demands to go beyond tackling only physical and cognitive deficiencies. Interaction with technology involves emotions, values and social needs and it is influenced by socio-economic, cultural, linguistic or health constraints ([3], [8], [12]). The influence of some of these factors has been recently formalized in the Senior Technology Acceptance & Adoption Model [17].
- Age is not the unique factor to take into account to analyze ICT use by older people. Kang and Yoon [9] have shown that both age and background knowledge are important factors explaining differences in interaction behavior between younger and middle-aged adults. They discovered that age influences elements like the number of interaction steps or the subjective perception of performance. In contrast, background knowledge influences the trial-and-error behavior and the frustration level. On this basis, they suggest to designers targeting older users to identify the interaction features that depends on the age and those influenced by other factors (e.g. background knowledge). To sum up, they draw the attention to the fact that the "novice-expert" and "young-old" dimensions overlap each other.
- Older people do not want to be treated like deficient persons who need special assistance. To counter deficiencies, older users may sometimes prefer a strategy used by the whole population (e.g. wearing glasses) to an elderly-specific solution

(e.g. increased text police on a web site) [20]. From a design perspective, this means that it is important to avoid the features that might belittle the elderly persons or might be perceived as such. Including in the design process an evaluation of the social effects that can be generated by the use of the new system may lower this type of risk. It is clear that experiments in artificial environment cannot easily identify this threat for the acceptance of the new system.

- How ICT affect the well-being of older people is currently debated. A thorough review of research papers [2] has highlighted that the well-being of current older adults may not be negatively affected by digital exclusion. In fact, it is crucial to distinguish two phenomena. On one hand, ICT can indubitably support older adults in various aspects of their life (e.g. medical support, easier communications with relatives). On the other hand, the causal effect of the use of ICT on increased well-being of the individuals is yet to be scientifically proven. In an experiment trying to measure well-being, the social and psychological effects (e.g. training effect, richer social interactions or personal relationship with the evaluator) may produce completely biased results.

- Having a different behaviour does not mean being less efficient. Previous research has pointed out that older people behave differently than younger ones on the Web ([3], [6], [22]). Fairweather [3] stresses the fact that most of the comparative studies of performance between younger and older adults focus on local behaviors (i.e. atomized actions like "moving to the next page"). However, if the comparison is made at a higher level to consider purposeful behaviors (e.g. "retrieving weather information"), his experience did not demonstrate a significant influence of age on the rate of success. In fact, it simply showed that older people use different strategies that younger ones. They probably rely on skills and knowledge that are less affected by the ageing process and sometimes they use heuristics to compensate age-related limitations. Consequently, a sound understanding of which precise capacities decline with age is necessary to design efficient applications for older people.

- For older people, it seems that avoiding making mistakes is more important than being efficient [20]. According to Sayago and Blat [19], this effect originates in the fear to cause damages to the ICT system or to delete some data. These unwanted consequences have to be subsequently repaired or corrected, which generate frustration by making clear the lack of individual independence. This precedence of mistakes prevention on efficiency influences many design choices.

2.2 Design Methods for Older People

Newell [15] points out some limitations of the broad paradigm regrouping inclusive design, design-for-all and universal-design. He explains that a design whatever its quality cannot fit everyone needs and skills. He also suggests that research focuses on individual older and disabled users as people, rather than as simply a set of user characteristics. Dewsbury et al. [1] agree on this point and explain that *"Through treating participants as real people, designs reflect their own suggestions and idiosyncrasies."*

Design should address what the real people consider important and not what the designer thinks it is for a hypothetical representative older user.

For older and disabled users, Newell and Gregor [16] suggest to switch from the "Universal Design / Design for All" paradigm to a "User-Sensitive Inclusive Design" approach. They motivate this assertion by the fact that the high diversity of users may prevent to build a group of representative users as well as to design a product really accessible for all. In addition, they explain that *"User Sensitive Inclusive design needs to be an attitude of mind rather than simply mechanistically applying a set of "design for all" guidelines"*.

When designing for older people, Dewsbury et al. [1] emphasize the need to mix traditional technological approaches with detailed investigations into everyday life and user needs. Unfortunately, despite the growing awareness in the HCI community that the focus on cognitive aspects of single users performing tasks should move to the understanding of the social context and real-life experiences [19], few extended ethnographical study with older people are available.

The adequate level of social interaction between designers and (older) users is also debated in the literature. Some authors argue that the designers should develop empathy [15], trust or other types of social relationship [12] with the group of users. Dewsbury et al. [1] are less affirmative and simply claim that (in ethnomethodology) some form of empathy may appear but it is not a prerequisite for insightful research or design. They even explain that in some circumstance, empathy may limit the objectivity required to correctly understand a situation. Nevertheless, they acknowledge the importance to make a partnership agreement with the participants of the study.

Participatory design is often promoted as an appropriate methodology to imagine ICT systems for older users. Massimi et al. [12] identify three possible approaches in this context. The first one (*"Design for Me"*) relies on the capabilities of the individuals to create a system that best fits their personal needs. In the second paradigm (*"Design for Us"*) people take into account the abilities of the design team members but do not generalize to a larger population. The third one (*"Design for Them"*) aims to develop a system for a broader population whom members exhibit diverse abilities. Depending on the objective of the designers, any of the three methods may be adopted. The important point is to keep aware of the chosen paradigm and its consequences in terms of scope of validity.

Finally, the necessity for a relationship between design and evaluation activities is acknowledged in the literature but it still needs to be further investigated. For instance, it not very clear which evaluation method is the most appropriate in a given design paradigm. Wania et al. [23] explain that design and evaluation cannot be separated anymore but should be considered as one process.

3   Description of the Case

The research described in this paper was carried out in the context of a multidisciplinary project involving computer scientists and psychologists (experts in gerontology).

The purpose was to imagine an ICT application that can support older people ageing without severe impairments in their daily life. This ICT system is called "Sammy".

More precisely, the project team aims to study the context of a retirement home (later called "K") located in Luxembourg, a mid-sized city (~100.000 inhabitants) of Northern Europe. Around 120 persons were living there at the time of the study. It has been chosen because it is a specific context that differs from the home or hospital environments, which have both been well studied in the literature. To some extent, the "K" institution can be considered as an intermediate stage between those two contexts. Indeed, the residents live in autonomy in apartments located in the same building but common services are provided like catering, laundry or diverse social activities. People are free to use these services and to participate to those activities or to prefer individual initiatives. The "K" home policy imposes that health care of the residents must not exceed 12 hours per day. If this limit is reached, they must move to an institution that can provide the appropriate medical support. In our study, we focused on those of the residents having no or few cognitive or sensory impairments.

4   Sammy System

The core device of the Sammy system consists of an 8.4'' touch screen terminal with an integrated computer and an RFID reader (cf. Figure 1). These technologies were chosen for several reasons. First, like Dewsbury [1] our aim was to use a device that does not look like a computer in order to avoid the preconceptions that it entails for some older people. The system should also look and be robust. Indeed, Hanson [6] has pointed out that some older users may *"worry about breaking the computer"* and we wanted to avoid this effect. Finally, touch screen technology was conformed to findings from previous research [9] that has shown a preference, by older adults, for direct devices (like touch screen) over indirect devices.

The Java-based Sammy software enables the residents to subscribe to different activities organized by the "K" home or by fellow residents. Users log into the system by holding their personal RFID tag (which comes in different shapes like cards or key fobs) next to the terminal screen. The system then loads the personal profile of the user (e.g. preferred language) from a MySQL database. As the user navigates through the application by pressing buttons on the touch screen, the system gradually loads information to display via requests to the database. At the end of the process, users are given a ticket by a printer attached to the terminal. This ticket summarizes the choices the user has made.

Moreover, users have the possibility to subscribe to a personalized, weekly "Sammy Newspaper". This two-sided PDF document holds different categories such as weather forecast, news from Sammy, news from the world (RSS feeds), news of the "K" home, contribution of a resident, Quiz, crosswords, pictures of "K" newcomers. Some contents are different for each resident (e.g. news from Sammy) and others are identical for all (e.g. Weather forecast).

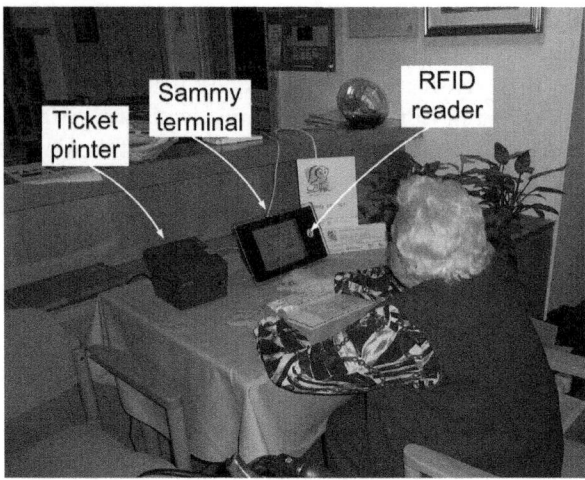

Fig. 1. Sammy System

5 Design Process

Identifying the real needs of users is always a challenge. Newell and Gregor [16] explain that *"users are not very good at explicitly stating what they need of a technology which does not yet exist."* Therefore, our design method was based on two successive stages. First, we identify a starting set of features without direct input from the real users. Then, we implement these initial features in a prototype in order to provide the real users with some tangible experience with the new system. This is the foundation that the older people can build upon to realize what is possible, what is useful and what should be added to the system. At that stage, we collect their feedback and associate them in an iterative co-design process for the next versions of the system.

5.1 Initial Data Collection from the Field

First, we have carried out several interviews with the manager of the "K" home. He described the general organization of the home. Among others, he explained that the residents can participate to various social activities organized by the institution. The proposals include daily activities (e.g. lunch at the "K" restaurant), regular but less frequent suggestions (e.g. shuttle to a shopping mall) and ad-hoc initiatives (e.g. movies sessions organized by a resident, painting exhibition in the entry hall). Before our intervention, the residents did register to those activities either via a paper form or verbally at the entry desk of the home.

We also carried out a study to have more information about the profile of the "K" home residents, especially regarding their skills and use of ICT. At that stage, we did not try to elicit specific needs of the interviewed persons. All in all, n=19 persons within the age range of 75 – 91 years were interviewed (thereof 68% were women). The results of the qualitative interviews elucidated no or very little overall experience with modern technologies (i.e. computers, internet, mobile phones) in the "K" home population. On the other hand, most respondents however showed a rather positive attitude towards modern ICT; only few persons reported negative experiences with modern technologies (especially with respect to ATM machines). When it came to factors determining the use of technologies, most arguments for not using these were related to *personal factors*, i.e. low self-esteem, low perceived self-efficacy and low ICT experience of elderly persons than to characteristics of the *technology itself* (especially its perceived applicability and usefulness). Since the interviewees belong to the so called "pre-computer generation" these findings may imply a low (perceived) level of technical skills and reluctance to learn new practices. Nonetheless, interviewees generally appreciated the idea of being involved in a scientific project and testing a newly developed technical device that should facilitate everyday life in the retirement home.

5.2 Identification of Initial Features

After those tasks, the members of our research team (computer scientists and gerontologists) carried out several brainstorming sessions. The purpose was to know what our ICT system should do in order to support the daily life of the "K" residents. The question was rapidly raised whether the social activities organized within the "K" home were a good case to study.

We realized that those activities are a significant part of what the "K" home offers to the residents beyond simply hosting them. Indeed, the common services and those social activities were the two main reasons why the residents could not be considered as living in separate apartments. Increasing the diversity and the quality of these social interactions might keep the residents more connected to each other, which might be a positive factor for the residents' well-being. However, what is not known is whether an ICT system is an adequate approach to maintain or increase the involvement of the residents in the social activities proposed by the "K" home. Despite the advantages that such a system may offer to the home management (e.g. optimization of orders, better planning), will it be accepted by the residents in their daily life? We also discussed which features should be implemented, in what order they should be developed and how the system should look like (cf. hardware).

The reservation of the menus at the "K" restaurant rapidly appeared as the appropriate initial feature to be implemented in the system. Indeed, for some residents lunch time is the only "social" event of the day and it can play a central role in their daily life. We were also told that there are frequent discussions about it among the residents. Another key advantage in favour of "lunch reservation" is the large involvement of the residents in general, which is not always true for other activities. For example, they are not equally motivated by visiting a painting exhibition. Starting by supporting very specific activities that few residents are interested in would have limited the potential group of users but we aimed to convince as many residents as possible to use our system. Two additional arguments were in favour of the "lunch reservation": it is a well known process for every resident and this process is operated on a regular basis. This means that it does not require a learning phase that would overlap with the discovery of the new system and that it naturally asks to be repeated often, which is a favourable factor for memorization.

Finally, the idea to implement first the reservation of the lunch menus at the "K" restaurant was discussed with the home manager. He was convinced by our arguments and decided to support this approach. This is also an important point because the participation of the home staff was therefore officially encouraged. It may be reminded from this perspective that previous research has emphasized the need to *"Make participation an institutional affair"* in participatory design methods with seniors [12].

5.3 Development of an Initial Version of Sammy

Wania et al. [23] reminds what many designers, including ourselves, have experienced on the field: *"It is very difficult, if not impossible to define all requirements before a system is actually used, to predict exactly how an information system will be used, and to predict how an environment will change after the implementation of an interactive system."* In order to tackle this challenge, they suggest *"to incrementally grow, not build, software systems"* [23]. Other researchers [20] have pointed out the difference (long recognized by social scientists) between what people say and what they do. Therefore, interviews of users are not sufficient to understand daily activities of people on the field. It is also well known that the field environment is influenced by numerous factors that cannot be reproduced in laboratory settings. We agree with those assertions. To take them into account, we have developed a first version of the Sammy system (later called Sammy 1.0) implementing the basic features that were identified as a good starting point during the initialization phase (login feature and lunch menu reservation at the "K" restaurant, cf. previous section). The purpose was to show to the residents how the system looks like, what it is intended for (in the initial stage) and how it can be operated.

This approach helps to overcome the major problem of shared concepts among the users and the designers. Indeed, the elicitation of needs of users having few (if any) previous experience with ICT (the study of the "K" residents profile during the initialization phase had showed that we were in this case) often faces the problem that basic ICT concepts are not known by the users. Moreover those users may encounter some difficulties to imagine what the designers are talking about or what a sketch may represent in reality. When an initial version of the prototype is available, some formative evaluation sessions can be organized with the older people and they can use their own words to express their comments. It is much easier for the designers to map this feedback to ICT concepts. The users (or their representative authority) also want very soon a concrete description of the new system. From this perspective, we have observed that our credibility has increased when the first working prototype was revealed. As a consequence, we received an increased support from the "K" manager who was then fully convinced that we can really deliver a system usable on the field. Nevertheless, deploying an early version of a system on the field with real users raises some challenges.

First, the overall physical aspect of the system must be firmly determined and should not vary too much otherwise the users may consider the subsequent versions as new systems. We could afford this approach because the design of the system for the "K" home was preceded by several months of investigation regarding candidate technologies (e.g. electronic paper, Wiimote, phidgets...). Therefore, we had gained a sufficient expertise regarding which hardware components were appropriate for our purposes.

Second, the software features must be developed while keeping in mind that this is not a "proof-of-concept" research prototype but an application dedicated to be deployed on the field. This demands to include significant code testing and debugging phases in the development process of the initial version. We also tackled this issue with a voluntary limitation of the features to what was explicitly needed. Indeed, the first impression is of prime importance for the acceptance of the new system and any problem may threat its future reputation.

It is nevertheless important that the designers do not work for months without any confrontation with the final users, even in the design phase of the initial version of the system. Despite the limitations in terms of scope of validity, some evaluations in artificial environment may help to avoid critical mistakes. Therefore, we involved a small subset of potential users from the "K" home (n=5) in formative evaluation sessions of this type. The purpose was to avoid any element that might generate fear or distrust in the new system due to reasons unexpected by the designers. However, it is important to keep in mind that those evaluation sessions were not valid from an ecological view point because they were not carried out in a real context. This limitation of the scope of validity is acknowledged in the literature [23] and some authors argue that evaluation should be situated in the context of use. We have followed this recommendation in the subsequent stages of our design process.

5.4 Final Validation of the Initial Version

5.4.1 Methodology

Before the official launch of the initial version of Sammy, we evaluated its acceptance by a subset of the residents. We undertook this operation in order to reassure ourselves concerning our design and development choices. Our primary goal was to avoid as much as possible any problem occurring when the system would be permanently available in the "K" home. From a methodological perspective, this step can be considered as a summative evaluation of Sammy 1.0 or as a formative evaluation in the design & development process of Sammy (all versions considered).

At this stage, our methodology combined an observational study and an evaluative post-test interview. Nineteen (n=19) residents were selected and recruited by the "K" home manager. In this sample, four (n=4) persons took part in the first evaluation. The participants were on average 84 years old, mainly female (68%), mostly widowed (84%), with low or no experience or interest in modern technologies. Participants were living in the "K" home for six years on average. None of them suffered from severe psycho-physical deficits or functional impairments.

In order to increase the ecological validity of the evaluation, the Sammy 1.0 system was brought to the "K" home and the personal profiles of the subjects were preloaded (e.g. real name, preferred language). This decision was taken to limit the potential biases due to unrealistic data loaded in the system to be evaluated (Genov et al. discuss this effect in [4]).

The subjects tested the Sammy system one by one. They were given some standardized information about its purpose and features. They also received standardized instructions to carry out some operations. They were asked to test Sammy during

20-minutes. Next, two trained researchers interviewed them regarding: (1) manage-ability, usability and overall acceptance; (2) design and features; (3) suggestions for improvement.

5.4.2 Results

Globally speaking, the observations showed that the subjects operate Sammy very confidently. Few persons exhibited nervousness, concentration difficulties or disinter-est. The interviews indicated a good acceptance, practicability and applicability. From a pure usability point of view, the subjects were asked to evaluate the font size, the font color, the background color, the display size, the graphic design of the screen for selecting the lunch menu, the graphic design of the calendar and the visibility of the reservations made. All these aspects were judged as "good" or "very good".

While the global results were positive, we identified some issues at the individual level. For instance, a small number of persons exhibit some difficulties to operate the tactile screen. They touch it several times at high frequency, which causes the naviga-tion to be too fast and prevents the users to actually see the intermediate screens. We solved this problem by adding a delay that disable the buttons for a short time after that they have been pressed for the first time. This problem typically illustrates what designers did not anticipate. However, this type of usability issue can be adequately identified in an evaluation session, even if it is not carried out in a context of real usage.

We were also surprised that some residents were trying to anticipate the potential problems that might appear in the deployment phase. For example, we collected some concerns from residents who were afraid of standing too long in a queue in front of the Sammy terminal. This type of feedback is also very important because it can help to avoid very pragmatic problems that the design team may have neglected but that may lower the acceptance of the new system. Indeed, if the designers are mainly fo-cused on the characteristics inherent to the ICT application (e.g. functional features, usability), they may underestimate some influential factors of the real environment where it will be deployed. For example, several weeks after the deployment of Sammy in the "K" home, a resident told us that she did not use the system because it was located in the entry hall which was too cold from her point of view. This example illustrates how difficult it may be to take care of every aspect of the real conditions of use. If the design is completely carried out with evaluations in artificial environments, some issues will never be identified. The latter example shows that even if some evaluations with a subset of users are carried out on the field before the deployment, some issues to be tackled afterwards will still appear. In this case, the diversity of older users (e.g. in terms of subjective heat perception) explained this unexpected issue. This example also demonstrates that diversity goes far beyond cognitive and sensory aspects.

We have also observed that some older people expressed fear concerning the ac-ceptance of the system by other residents. For example, they mentioned that some individuals have sensory or cognitive impairments that would prevent them to use Sammy. We acknowledged the limitations of our system from this perspective (see Description of the Case). However this comment shows that social factors may play a role in the acceptance of Sammy in the "K" home community. It seems that some residents consider the acceptance at the group level instead of at the individual one.

This information has helped us to adapt our communication strategy accompanying the deployment stage. In fact, it made us aware of the need to emphasize that the decision to use Sammy was clearly a personal one and that Sammy would not replace the traditional processes formerly used in the "K" home. By no means should Sammy be considered as a tool restricted to "valid residents" (which is moreover an inconsistent concept). This finding was also one of the motivations to add some paper-based features to the next versions of Sammy (e.g. Sammy newspaper described in a previous section). Indeed, we wanted to demonstrate that Sammy was potentially useful for any resident, even for those who do not use its ICT components at all.

During the interviews, it also appears that the process for choosing the lunch menus was implemented in the paper forms distributed by the "K" staff in a more rigid form than what really happens on the field. In fact, the residents were discussing informally with the waiter to compose their menu according to their personal preferences. A negotiation process was taking place and an agreement satisfying both the resident and the waiter was found most of the time. So much flexibility was not available in Sammy 1.0 because it was relying on the official process. In fact, this gap between the official process and the real one was a consequence of our design method based on producing an initial version without involving the real users. When we realized this limitation, it was too late to modify the initial version. Nevertheless, as this flaw was identified, we took care in our communication towards the resident and the home staff to stress the fact that this type of flexibility would be included in the next versions. In fact, identifying some limitations in Sammy 1.0 just before its official launch was not really critical providing that we knew them and that we had prepared an appropriate and coherent answer. The coherence of the researcher team answers was fundamental from this viewpoint. It is really important that every member provides the same answer to the same question otherwise the whole team can loose the older persons' trust.

Finally, another suggestion was to extend the scope of Sammy to other social activities than simply the reservation of lunch menus. This feedback was a very encouraging indicator for us because it confirmed the decisions taken in the initial phase of requirement elicitation with the "K" manager. From a technological view point, the system was designed to handle the registration process and the communication phase of any activity carried out in the "K" home. This example illustrates that older people can be creative and can imagine features that are not present yet. However, we think that the concrete manipulation of a real system is in many cases the fuel that feeds their imagination. From a design point of view, this means that co-designing a system with older people probably requires giving them an initial anchor in the form of an extensible working system. Experiencing this initial system may generate new ideas regarding how to extend or improve it that might never emerge from a sketch on a sheet of paper.

5.5 Deployment in the "K" Home

The deployment of Sammy 1.0 in the "K" home was carefully prepared from the technological, social and psychological points of view.

Some tests were carried out with the IT staff of the "K" home in order to validate that Sammy was working correctly in the real field settings (e.g. Internet access configuration, network security issues).

A strong communication plan was established to promote the system among all stakeholders. Some formation sessions were organized for the "K" employees working at the entry desk (i.e. where the Sammy terminal was located) and for the kitchen staff. The purpose was to demystify our initiative. We explained what the objectives of the project were and how the system works. We think this was a critical step because it was especially important that the "K" employees have a positive attitude towards Sammy. In fact, they became the ambassadors of the system when we were not present in the home.

A specific logo was designed for the Sammy system (i.e. a colored owl). Every item related to the system was marked with this logo. Our objective was to make visible to every stakeholder when an object belongs to the Sammy "ecosystem" (e.g. ICT terminal, ticket, poster). Rigid notices were placed to locate the emplacement of the Sammy terminal and to motivate the residents to use it. Some posters were put up in the lift and in the entry hall to promote the use of Sammy. These communication actions were keeping the residents consistently aware of the presence of Sammy. Those ambient reminders made almost impossible for the residents to forget its presence. Acting as memory aids these items were found to be quite useful to introduce Sammy in the "K" community. After a few weeks, the majority of the residents knew that Sammy was deployed in the home. However, we took a special care not to be intrusive. The challenge was to motivate the potential users of Sammy without offending those who do not use it. Indeed, Dickinson and Gregor [2] have stressed that we do not have any scientific demonstration of the positive effect of ICT on the older people well-being. Therefore, we must be very cautious when we introduce a new ICT system for them. The influence of social factors on the system acceptance is a second critical element. If some stakeholders feel offended by some communication actions, they may become fierce opponents to the system.

The staff members also received an account to use Sammy for their personal reservation of lunch menus. The residents could therefore see that they were using the same system as younger people (i.e. staff members). In fact, we wanted to take care of the effect observed by Sayago and Blat [19] that "*older people want to use the devices that other people normally use*". We did not want that the residents feel "assisted" in using a special version of Sammy.

We also decided to name our system. During the early design stages, we were simply talking about "*the prototype*" or "*the new system*". Before the final evaluation of the initial version, we adopted the name "Sammy". Our initial motivation was to ease the internal communication within the researcher team and between the team and the "K" staff. However, we were surprised during the early days of deployment that both the "K" staff and the residents were rapidly calling us the "Sammy Team". The importance of correctly naming the features of a new system for older users has already been pointed out ([12], [19], [20]). We observed that an easy-to-remember name also facilitates the diffusion of a new system within a community.

In order to make visible that our project was officially supported by the "K" institution, we organized a presentation meeting where the residents were all invited. After some presentations by the "K" manager and by the researcher team, a drink was offered and the residents were invited to try the new system. They were told that a permanent presence of the "Sammy team" was guaranteed from 8.00 until 18.30 during the first week of availability of the system. More than half of the residents accepted the invitation. This is really a high participation rate considering that some resident could not attend (e.g. medical reasons, holidays…). However, it is unknown whether the participation was motivated by the introduction of Sammy or by the wish to attend an unusual social event.

5.6 Iterative Co-design Process

During the first week after the official launch, we demonstrated how to use Sammy and collected the residents' first opinion about it. The researcher team adopted a *"suggest, convince but give choice"* strategy. When a resident showed some interest in Sammy (e.g. by directly asking how it works or more frequently by observing how another resident was using it), a member of the researcher team started to discuss with him/her. The researcher gave all information required by the resident and proposed him/her to try it for demystifying this new device but he never did more than suggesting. The resident was always choosing whether and when he/she will use Sammy.

During the next six months, Sammy was progressively improved on the basis of the users' feedback (i.e. residents and home staff). We consider it to be a co-design process because the users were not only involved in identifying flaws but also in suggesting improvements of existing features or proposing new ones. However, we acknowledge that the detailed description of the new or enhanced features was essentially made by ourselves. More precisely, the users did not tell much about how to improve the look-and-feel of the application (e.g. graphical design of screens) but they proposed enhanced solutions regarding the process of using Sammy (e.g. navigation, missing options in the succession of choices to choose a lunch menu). Two examples illustrate the input of users in this co-design phase: oversimplification and icons use.

Oversimplification is often claimed as a natural objective for systems targeting older users. Nevertheless, in a research project aiming to include seniors in the design of a mobile phone, Massimi et al. [12] found that contrary to common misconceptions, seniors desired a variety of applications. We observed a similar behaviour during the co-design process of the enhanced versions of Sammy (beyond Sammy 1.0). As previously explained, the very simple way to reserve the lunch menus at the "K" restaurant was judged too simplistic. The residents progressively proposed increasingly complex features to tackle the whole flexibility of the real process. What is unknown is the relative weight of "ease-of-use and simplicity" compared to "proximity to the real processes" in the adoption process of these older users. If a fully flexible application had been proposed since the beginning, it would have been much more complex to learn than Sammy 1.0. In this case, what would have been the residents' attitude? We do not know.

The navigation within the application is another example of oversimplified design that the users asked to be made more powerful. In Sammy 1.0, we aimed to minimize the number of clicks (i.e. touch on the tactile screen) needed to make a reservation of a lunch menu. The drawback was that the navigation through the reservation process was imposed by the application. The users requested more flexibility. For instance, they asked to be able to modify their choices whenever they want. The last versions of Sammy were much closer to classic IT applications than the initial one in terms of navigation. They were more powerful but also more difficult to use. Regarding design methodology, these examples illustrate how difficult it may be to find the right balance between "flexibility and complexity to cover all real cases" and "simplicity and ease-of-use to lower the entry barrier for non-expert users like many older people". This challenge has been previously identified by Dewsbury et al. [1] when they wonder "*how to provide greater configurability without making the system unnecessarily complex*".

The balance between graphics and text is also worth being discussed. Sayago and Blat [20] have pointed out that words are sometimes more appropriate than icons for older people because they are often used more consistently and because they convey the meaning of features more clearly. Consistency and clarity helps older people to remember how to operate the system. In Sammy 1.0 very few icons were used. As new features were added to the system, we introduced an initial screen to allow the user to select the type of activity he/she want to register to. At the time of writing, four options were available: reservation of a menu at the "K" home restaurant, trips to two different shopping malls and individual activities organized by residents. The buttons to select an option feature icons together with a text description. An interesting observation was made in this context. The "lunch menu" button featured a hamburger icon. It appeared that it was negatively perceived by the kitchen staff and some residents. We decided to change it for an icon featuring a chef. This example shows that icons by nature convey emotional and ambiguous information. While the designers may think that icons facilitate the use of a system, it seems that they may sometimes disturb the user. In the worst cases, using inappropriate icons may even be a curb on the system adoption. From a design point of view, it seems that only very neutral icons should be chosen to avoid frustration for some stakeholders of the system.

6 Adoption of Sammy

During the 6 months after the deployment of Sammy (June 2009 – December 2010) a longitudinal field study was conducted in the "K" home. Two personal interviews with selected users were planned as well as a continuous coaching and observation by two trained research students. Each Monday the research students assisted the residents in handling the device on demand. Right from the start of the project, the residents demonstrated a vivid interest. This was indicated by several indicators; one of them was certainly the large audience at the initial launching session of Sammy; furthermore, observations by students and feedback by the staff showed that Sammy also represented a main topic of discussion in the dining room. With regard to the overall acceptance of the system, it could be observed that participants, who made positive experiences in using Sammy from the start, contributed actively to motivating their co-residents to participate in the project. They encouraged them and also guided them physically to the device and provided assistance in its handling.

By the end of the first month of observation, a few tens of users had integrated Sammy into their daily routine to the extent that they didn't even consult the usual publication of weekly menus by paper anymore. These users also made constructive comments on how to further optimize the system and whether or not technical problems had emerged during the week.

Descriptive statistics of self-report data showed in general that the system was evaluated as a user-friendly and as a valuable device helping to facilitate the reservation and serving of the daily meals in the retirement home. The majority of the interviewees (89.4%; n=19) rated the operating instructions as rather "good" or "very good". A different profile of response frequencies emerged with respect to the self-reported motivation for using the system in the future: Half of the respondents (52.6%) rated the probability to use the system as "high" or "very high", a quarter (26.3%) seemed undecided and 21 percent of the participants rated the probability of using the system in the future as "low" or even "very low". Sammy is still in use at the time of writing (May 2010). Since it is available (June 2009 – April 2010), it was used so far by 17 staff members and 116 residents (be careful, due to newcomers, move to medical institutions and deaths, this does not mean that almost all of the 120 residents have used it). All in all the staff made 431 reservations and the residents used Sammy for a total of 5543 reservations. Descriptive analyses show a relatively stable users activity, ranging from 60 up to 200 reservations per week (mean = 122 reservations per week, st. deviation. = 30.21). Interestingly, so called "user peaks" can be observed on Mondays. Initially we thought that there is probably a relationship between this observation and the "nurse" or "researcher" effect previously reported in the literature ([2], [7]). Indeed, the trained students came every Monday to the "K" home to coach the residents with the handling of the device. The preference of older users for human support instead of proper documentation was also found by previous research [12]. However, we think that the presence of the trained students was a favorable factor but was not sufficient to completely determine the choice of some residents to use Sammy. Indeed, the Mondays' peaks are still currently present although the students do not come anymore. Moreover, Sammy is also significantly used during the rest of the week. A further peak of system use was observed in periods of Sammy-related events in the "K" home (i.e. launching session of optimized Sammy 2.0 in November 2009).

In a final evaluative step, qualitative interviews were carried out in November 2009 with a subsample of residents. Altogether twelve residents (aged between 78-92 years; 75% female) were selected by the home manager for evaluative follow-up interviews. A first subsample of these comprised six residents labeled as "*regular users*"; a second subsample regrouped two "*irregular users*" and a third subsample contained four persons who had stopped using the device during the test period ("*dropouts*"). One reason for an irregular use of the technology became evident when two irregular users who agreed on being interviewed dropped out due to hospitalization resp. massive cognitive decline over the six-month time period. Interviews addressed different issues related (a) to the device and its handling (i.e. gain/benefit, ease of use, reliability), and (b) to personal factors (i.e. motivational changes, changes in attitude towards technology, learning experience, changes in social contacts, miscellaneous).

Regular users consistently reported Sammy to be a timesaving, reliable and easy way to make menu reservations. Besides the positive evaluation of the technical aspects, regular users also consistently reported positive learning experiences and changes in their attitude towards modern technologies. These comprised: (1) increased feelings of self-worth and self-efficacy in using technical devices in general; (2) discovering of "unexpected" technical skills; (3) realizing that life-long learning is possible and not limited to a certain age.

Irregular users and *dropouts* cited several reasons why they did not use the device at all or on a rather irregular basis. Interestingly, these "inhibitory factors" were rather related to contextual aspects such as bad placement of the device in the retirement home lobby (too noisy, supply air, indiscreet, etc.) than to the device itself.

7 Conclusions and Perspectives

This paper discusses a design approach actively involving elderly persons in a retirement home. Various issues were identified during this process.

We have experienced that just one evaluation, whenever it is carried out in the design & development process, is insufficient. Different evaluation methods must be combined to identify as many problems as possible.

A good communication especially regarding the limitations of the system was found to be of prime importance in the acceptance of the system in the long term.

The social influence seems also to play a role for adopting the system because some resident think at the group level rather than only from their own perspective.

The progressive decline of physical and mental abilities (i.e. reduced mobility, dementia, etc.) of the users is another critical point. This dynamics must be taken into account as older users are obviously more likely to face this evolution than other categories of users.

The population of a retirement home permanently evolves due to death, move to medical institutions and newcomers. This factor implies that the users of the system continuously change and that nothing is ever gained in this context.

Regarding the user motivation and participation our findings recommend that a strong emphasis should be given to contextual factors (e.g. finding a comfortable and untroubled location for the emplacement of the device).

The formative evaluation showed that elderly persons are not technophobic per se, but rather reluctant towards technology that does not take account for age-related psycho physiological changes. Technology use may also reflect a life-long experience in education and learning meaning that those persons who already were acquainted with technology in various forms are more motivated to use new technology. This does however not exclude that users with no specific prior experiences can be encouraged and motivated by expert users which then will give rise to an increase in feelings of self-worth and autonomy. Furthermore, our experience showed that social interaction and exchange between residents was positively influenced by the implementation and the use of Sammy. Nevertheless, and despite all technical efforts some insurmountable neurophysiologic and physical limitations have to be acknowledged when designing ICT for the elderly. These age-related changes can make a system like Sammy only appropriate for relatively healthy senior users.

Acknowledgments

This research work was supported by a grant of the *Fonds National de la Recherche* of Luxembourg. We also thank the staff and residents of the "K" home.

References

1. Dewsbury, G., Rouncefield, M., Sommerville, I., Onditi, V., Bagnall, P.: Designing technology with older people. Universal Access in the Information Society 6(2), 207–217 (2007)
2. Dickinson, A., Gregor, P.: Computer use has no demonstrated impact on the well-being of older adults. International Journal of Human-Computer Studies 64(8), 744–753 (2006)
3. Fairweather, P.G.: How Older and Younger Adults Differ in their Approach to Problem Solving on a Complex Website. In: ACM SIGACCESS Conference on Computers and Accessibility (ASSETS 2008), pp. 67–72. ACM Press, New York (2008)
4. Genov, A., Keavney, M., Zazelenchuk, T.: Usability Testing with Real Data. Journal of Usability Studies 4(2), 85–92 (2009)
5. Hagen, I., Cahill, S., Begley, E., Macijauskiene, J., Gilliard, J., Jones, K., Topo, P., Sarikalle, K., Holthe, T., Duff, P.: Assessment of usefulness of assistive technologies for people with dementia. In: Association for the Advancement of Assistive Technology in Europe (AAATE), Lille, France (2005)
6. Hanson, V.L.: Age and Web Access: The Next Generation. In: International Cross-Disciplinary Conference on Web Accessibility (W4A 2009), pp. 7–15. ACM Press, New York (2009)
7. Hanson, E.J., Magnusson, L., Oscarsson, T., Nolan, M.: Case Study: benefits of IT for older people and their carers. British Journal of Nursing 11, 867–874 (2002)
8. Hirsch, T., Forlizzi, J., Hyder, E., Goetz, J., Stroback, J., Kurtz, C.: The ELDer Project: Social, Emotional, and Environmental Factors in the Design of Eldercare Technologies. In: ACM Conference on Universal Usability (CUU 2000), pp. 72–79. ACM Press, New York (2000)
9. Kang, N.E., Yoon, W.C.: Age- and experience-related user behavior differences in the use of complicated electronic devices. International Journal of Human-Computer Studies 66(8), 425–437 (2008)
10. Kientz, J., Patel, S., Jones, B., Price, E., Mynatt, E., Abowd, G.: The Georgia Tech Aware Home. In: ACM Conference on Human Factors in Computing Systems (CHI 2008), pp. 3675–3680. ACM Press, New York (2008)
11. Mamykina, L., Mynatt, E., Kaufman, D.: Investigating Health Management Practices of Individuals with Diabetes. In: ACM Conference on Human Factors in Computing Systems (CHI 2006), pp. 927–936. ACM Press, New York (2006)
12. Massimi, M., Baecker, R.M., Wu, M.: Using Participatory Activities with Seniors to Critique, Build, and Evaluate Mobile Phones. In: ACM SIGACCESS Conference on Computers and Accessibility (ASSETS 2007), pp. 155–162. ACM Press, New York (2007)
13. Mynatt, E.D., Essa, I., Rogers, W.: Increasing the opportunities for ageing in place. In: ACM Conference on Universal Usability (CUU 2000), pp. 65–71. ACM Press, New York (2000)
14. Mynatt, E., Rowan, J., Craighill, S., Jacobs, A.: Digital Family Portraits: Supporting Peace of Mind for Extended Family Members. In: ACM Conference on Human Factors in Computing Systems (CHI 2001), pp. 333–340. ACM Press, New York (2001)

15. Newell, A.F.: Accessible Computing – Past Trends and Future Suggestions. ACM TAC-CESS 1(2) (2008)
16. Newell, A.F., Gregor, P.: User Sensitive Inclusive Design – In search of a new paradigm. In: ACM Conference on Universal Usability (CUU 2000), pp. 39–44. ACM Press, New York (2000)
17. Renaud, K., van Biljon, J.: Predicting Technology Acceptance and Adoption by the Elderly: A Qualitative study. In: Annual Conference of the South African Institute of Computer Scientists and Information Technologists (SAICSIT 2008), pp. 210–219. ACM Press, New York (2008)
18. Rowe, J.W., Kahn, R.L.: Successful Aging. The Gerontologist 37(4), 433–440 (1997)
19. Sayago, S., Blat, J.: Telling the story of older people e-mailing: An ethnographical study. International Journal of Human-Computer Studies 68(1-2), 105–120 (2010)
20. Sayago, S., Blat, J.: About the relevance of accessibility barriers in the everyday interactions of older people with the web. In: International Cross-Disciplinary Conference on Web Accessibility (W4A 2009), pp. 104–113. ACM Press, NewYork (2009)
21. Struve, D., Wandke, H.: Video Modeling for Training Older Adults to Use New Technologies. ACM TACCESS 2(1) (2009)
22. Tullis, T.S.: Older Adults and the Web: Lessons Learned from Eye-Tracking. In: International Conference on Universal Access in Human-Computer Interaction, pp. 1030–1039. Springer, Heidelberg (2007)
23. Wania, C.E., Atwood, M.E., Mc Cain, K.W.: How do Design and Evaluation Interrelate in HCI Research? In: ACM Conference on Designing Interactive Systems (DIS 2006), pp. 90–98. ACM Press, New York (2006)
24. Wolters, M., Georgila, K., Moore, J.D., Mac Pherson, S.E.: Being Old Doesn't Mean Acting Old: How Older Users Interact with Spoken Dialog Systems. ACM TACCESS 2(1) (2009)

User Centered Interaction Design for Mobile Applications Focused on Visually Impaired and Blind People

Elmar Krajnc, Johannes Feiner, and Stefan Schmidt

FH JOANNEUM University of Applied Sciences, Werk-VI-Strasse 46, A-8605
Kapfenberg, Austria

Abstract. User centered design (UCD) is a key success argument for
modern software development. In this paper we present a case study on
developing a way finding application for mobile devices. The target users
are people with special needs such as visually impaired and blind people. It can be shown that user centered design is especially important
for "not mainstream" user groups and the resulting products have high
acceptance rates. This specialized development methodology combined
with customization leads to subjective satisfaction.

Keywords: User Centered Design, Visually Impaired, Mobile, Usability.

1 Introduction

*"Take your mobile Phone, use one of your favourite applications - but close your
eyes and imagine you are blind."*

Methods like Extreme Programming or Scrum are part of modern software
development[1][2][3]. Those agile and iterative methods are the flexible answers
to old and rigid methods where products were produced according to a given
specification. The ideas have gone mainstream in the last few years, but sel-
domly the needs of small, special groups are addressed. In this paper the focus
is on visually impaired – or even blind – people who need much more specialized
software applications.

1.1 Agile Development

Agile methods need a lot of communication within the developer team and also
with the customer to adopt the aims and features of the product. The customer
is also an important partner in the development process. The focus on the user
of a software product is part of the usability engineering too. User centered development starts with defining the adequate end user profiles, creates prototypes
fitting the expected users' need and finally evaluates the developed product with
tests or heuristics [4]. Usability engineering is an iterative process. The life-cycle

G. Leitner, M. Hitz, and A. Holzinger (Eds.): USAB 2010, LNCS 6389, pp. 195–202, 2010.

of designing, implementing and evaluating accompanies the whole software developing process. Excellent software products are a result of a tight connection of usability and software engineering [5].

1.2 Mobile Devices

Simple, everyday gadgets such as mobile phones are sometimes tricky. To use tasks like switching from one mobile to another is harder to do than one might believe [6]. Natural flick scrolling is compared to more difficult tilt scrolling in [7]. People without any disabilities have sometimes trouble when using smart devices. So it is clear, that users with special needs (e.g. visually impaired people) will need much more effort to use them. Mobile phones are one of many cost-effective assistive technologies for blind people [8], therefore the phones are used widely and suitable software is desperately needed.

1.3 Visually Impaired People

For visually impaired people much research has been done in medicine. For technical fields only few special surveys with blind people have been performed. See for example [9] for audio captchas which allow blind people to use this way of secure login, [10] for some aspects of improving mobile applications for elderly and [11] for an approach of navigation through audio-based virtual environments for blind people.

1.4 User Centered Design

It is well known since long that software production is ineffective [12]. So the importance of design is stressed again and again [13]. The impact of user centered design is on the single developer, the development team, but also on the whole organisation (see [14]). User centered design has been around for many years. The official reference for usability engineers is still [4], but a lot of additions and related fields are nowadays included. For example extreme usability (XU [15]) is an interessting approach, where extreme programming and usability are looked at in a combined way. Further comparison might be valuable within the field of "interaction design" [16]. In [17] extreme programming and user centered design are applied to build a mobile multi media application and in [18] agile software development and user centered design are discussed related to the software development life-cycle and the results of an online survey are presented.

1.5 Way Finding

The research project ways4all [19] tries to allow visually impaired and blind people barrier free travelling. Indoor and outdoor navigation, online schedules of the public traffic companies, information systems at railway stations and many other information sources help people to find their ways. To access these data on a trip we need a mobile application. One challenge of such a helpful appliance is to create a well-working user interface. As mentioned before, to fulfill this task methods of user centered design (see Section 1.4) are used.

Way finding for blind people is discussed in [20] who states that the missing human computer interaction requirements are important but underestimated aspects.

2   Designing for Visually Impaired

The development takes place in several iterative steps. The paradigm of iteration and repetition is important for fast and direct feedback (see Section 1.4 Agile Development).

One of the first steps in user centered design is the analysis of the user groups. If expected users are persons with disabilities or special needs, it is important to build applications which have a simple and intuitive user interface.

2.1   User Analysis

"Know Your User - Analyze Your User Group"

To build a suitable user interface for target users, one needs to know who the users are and what their previous knowledge is. That means that knowing their technical skilsl is as important as knowing their expectations. To gather this information a survey with blind people has been performed and the results are listed in Figure 1. The expert interviews made clear that basic textual information is the most important factor.

As a result of the survey and the interviews we have a lot of information about our expected users. Based on this information we create personas and for each persona we create a proper scenario. A Persona is a fictional character to define the expected user for the developer. Personas have a name, age, photo and some short background information to become a realistic user[12]. In this project we create three groups of primary personas - visually impaired people, blind people and people without visual restrains. One example persona can be found in Figure 2.

For every persona a goal and various scenarios are defined. A scenario shows the tasks of a persona within an application to reach this goal. With the help of a persona and scenario developers can start the user interface design.

2.2   Paper Prototypes

Before creating any type of real implementation it is crucial to create working paper prototypes. With help of the artifacts and tools "personas", "paper prototype" the interaction designer can imagine the actual end-user who will use the final product and gets knowledge about his/her tasks. The answers to critical questions like "why?", "what to do?" are added with some typical examples.

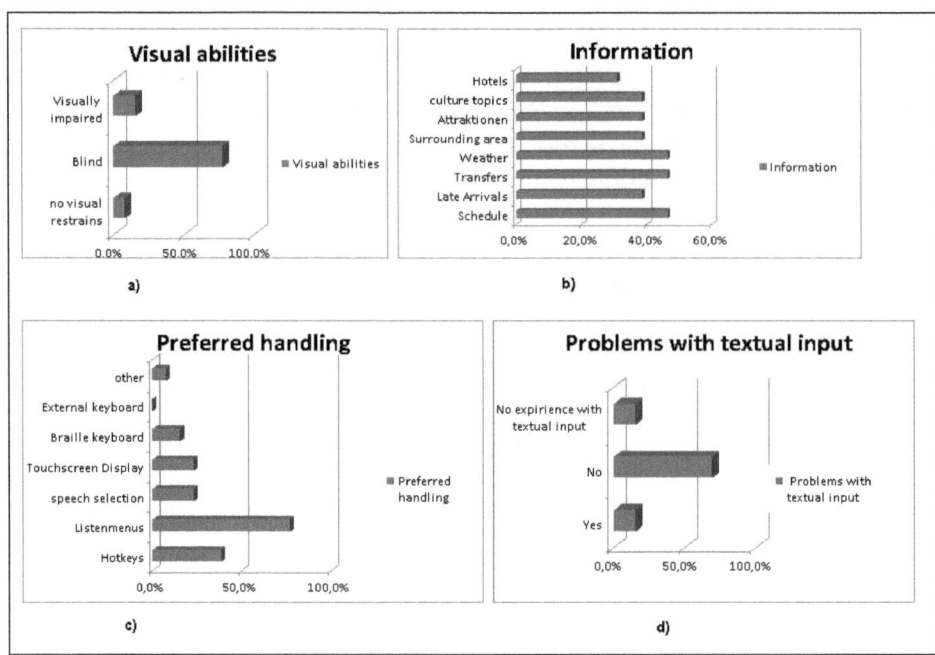

Fig. 1. This figure illustrates parts of the survey's results. Chart a) shows the percentage of blind, visually impaired and not visually impaired people. In chart b) the various kinds of information for travelling like the schedule, the transfers and the surrounding area are shown. In chart c) the usage of a mobile device is pointed out. Blind people need not always an extra device for input like a Braille keyboard, but often use list based menus, speech selection and hot keys. In the last chart d) it is illustrated that for most blind users a textual input is also no problem.

Name	Tamara Hill	
Age	20 years	
Job	Student	
Background	Tamara Hill is blind since her birth and lives with her parents in Graz. She likes to travel to meet her friends in Austria and she uses most of the time public transport. She has no experience with navigation systems but she would use one if it would be integrated in her mobile phone…	

Fig. 2. Sample persona ZG3P7 representing a blind user with selected attributes

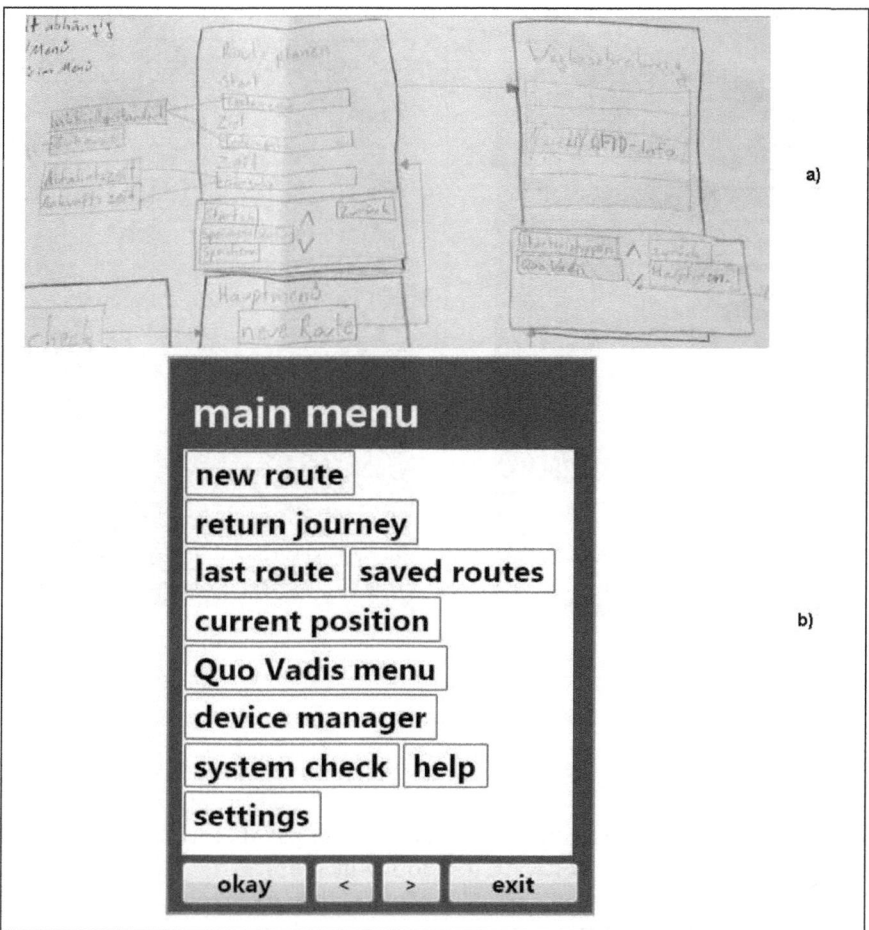

Fig. 3. a) A paper prototype showing parts of a typical graphical user interface. b) improvement of the first paper prototype with a sketch tool.

The resulting workflows [16] are the basis of development and will furthermore deliver criteria for feedback from experts.

The drafts of final paper prototypes and another prototype made with a sketch tool can be seen in Figure 3.

3   Ways4All Software Prototype

For the implementation of the user interface and the logic in software it is sensible to concentrate on the top prioritized features. Based on the conceptional work (see Section 2 for the User Centered Process) a working prototype has been implemented. The development started as soon as the first results of the

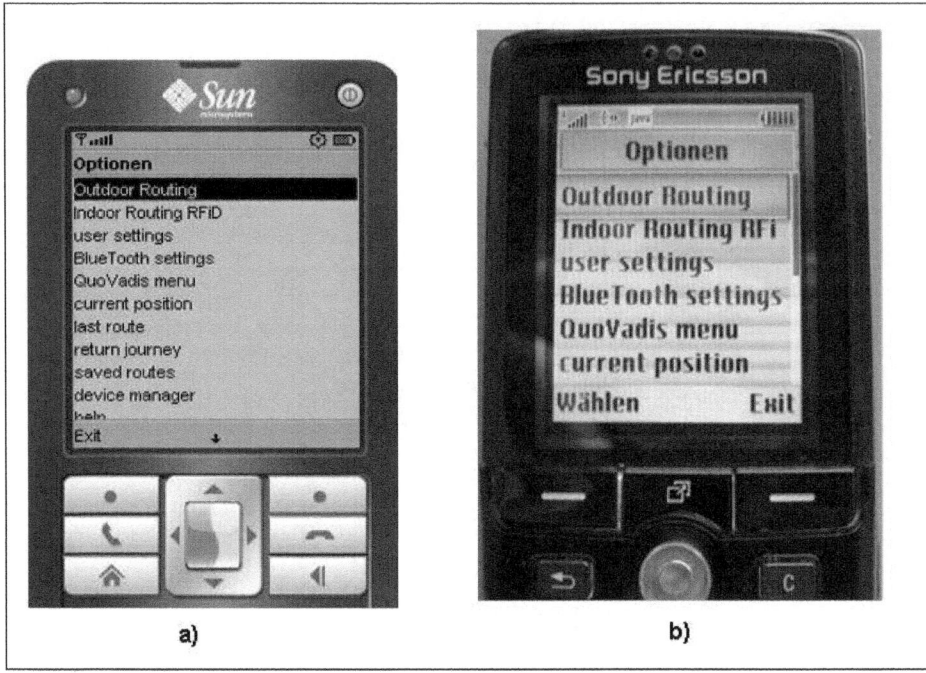

Fig. 4. The main menu of the implementation on a) the J2M emulator and b) on a Sony Ericsson mobile phone

paper prototype were available. This allowed the parallel work of the usability engineering team and the software development team.

The demo implementation uses the Model-View-Controller (MVC) pattern. This pattern allows separation of presentation and logic. The programming logic (the controller) can thereby easily be reused later on because it is independent from the data (the model).

One very important step during the development cycle is always to recheck the application with the needs and requirements stated for the different personas and scenarios. For compatibility reasons the application is implemented on the JME, the Java Mobile Edition. This application uses the more abstract High Level API. This API allows the usage of forms, textboxes and lists. To provide a simple text oriented user Interface a combination of various list-menus guide the blind user through the application. This list structure is very dynamic based on the users settings and the features of the mobile phone like GPS. One list contains at most eight items and the depth of the levels is at most three. The user always gets help from the application, which options are now and next available. Various user settings like home address or favourite public transport are stored on a mobile database to avoid text input for standard usage. At this time no speech output is built-in, because most of the blind persons in the survey wanted to use their own customized screen reader.

4   Summary and Outlook

Although the development is still in progress it is obvious, that choosing agile development methods for user groups with special needs is really important. The separation of programming logic and presentation helps the software developer and the usability developer to work in parallel without loosing too much time on recoding. The different viewpoints brought together generate an end product with higher quality. In the case of this study it was a user interface for way finding for visually impaired people which worked out to be well-prepared for everyday situations.

Further usability engineering is necessary such as tests with a large group of real users. We plan to perform for example a thinking aloud (TA) test later this year.

Acknowledgements

The authors want to thank the team of ways4all, especially Mr. Werner Bishof and Martijn Kiers. Further thank to Jurgen Schwingshandel for always helpful cooperation during the interviews and.tests.

References

1. Beck, K., Andres, C.: Extreme Programming Explained – Embrace Change. Addison-Wesley Professional, Reading (November 2004)
2. Schwaber, K., Beedle, M.: Agile Software Development With Scrum. Prentice-Hall, Englewood Cliffs (2002)
3. Memmel, T., Reiterer, H., Holzinger, A.: Agile methods and visual specification in software development: A chance to ensure universal access. In: Proc. 4th International Conference on Universal Access in Human Computer Interaction (UAHCI 2007), pp. 453–462. Springer, Heidelberg (2007)
4. Nielsen, J.: Usability Engineering. Morgan Kaufmann, San Francisco (September 1993)
5. Holzinger, A., Miesenberger, K. (eds.): USAB 2009. LNCS, vol. 5889. Springer, Heidelberg (2009)
6. Yamashita, A.F., Barendregt, W., Fjeld, M.: Exploring potential usability gaps when switching mobile phones: An empirical study. In: Proc. 21st British CHI Group Annual Conference on HCI (BCS-HCI 2007), British Computer Society, pp. 109–116 (2007)
7. Fitchett, S., Cockburn, A.: Evaluating reading and analysis tasks on mobile devices: A case study of tilt and flick scrolling. In: Proc. 21st Annual Conference of the Australian Computer-Human Interaction Special Interest Group (OZCHI 2009), pp. 225–232. ACM, New York (2009)
8. Narasimhan, P., Gandhi, R., Rossi, D.: Smartphone-based assistive technologies for the blind. In: Proc. 2009 International Conference on Compilers, Architecture, and Synthesis for Embedded Systems (CASES 2009), pp. 223–232. ACM, New York (2009)

9. Bigham, J.P., Cavender, A.C.: Evaluating existing audio CAPTCHAs and an interface optimized for non-visual use. In: Proc. 27th International Conference on Human Factors in Computing Systems (CHI 2009), pp. 1829–1838. ACM, New York (2009)

10. Searle, A.H.G., Nischelwitzer, A.: On some aspects of improving mobile applications for the elderly. In: Proc. 4th International Conference on Universal Access in Human Computer Interaction (UAHCI 2007), pp. 923–932. Springer, Heidelberg (2007)

11. Sánchez, J., Sáenz, M., Pascual-Leone, A., Merabet, L.: Navigation for the blind through audio-based virtual environments. In: CHI EA 2010: Proceedings of the 28th of the International Conference Extended Abstracts on Human Factors in Computing Systems, pp. 3409–3414. ACM, New York (2010)

12. Cooper, A.: The Inmates Are Running the Asylum. Macmillan Publishing Co., Inc, Basingstoke (1999); Foreword By-Saffo, Paul

13. Terstiege, G.: The Making of Design: From the First Model to the Final Product. Birkhäuser Architecture (July 2009)

14. Brown, T.: Change by Design: How Design Thinking Transforms Organizations and Inspires Innovation. HarperBusiness (September 2009)

15. Holzinger, A., Slany, W.: XP + UE → XU. Praktische Erfahrungen Mit eXtreme Usability. Informatik Spektrum 29(2), 91–98 (2006)

16. Cooper, A., Reimann, R., Cronin, D.: About Face 3: The Essentials of Interaction Design. John Wiley & Sons, Inc., Chichester (2007)

17. Hussain, Z., Lechner, M., Milchrahm, H., Shahzad, S., Slany, W., Umgeher, M., Wolkerstorfer, P.: Agile user-centered design applied to a mobile multimedia streaming application. In: Holzinger, A. (ed.) USAB 2008. LNCS, vol. 5298, pp. 313–330. Springer, Heidelberg (2008)

18. Hussain, Z., Slany, W., Holzinger, A.: Current state of agile user-centered design: A survey. In: Holzinger, A., Miesenberger, K. (eds.) USAB 2009. LNCS, vol. 5889, pp. 416–427. Springer, Heidelberg (2009)

19. Bischof, W.: Ways4all (2008), http://www.ways4all.at/

20. Bradley, N.A., Dunlop, M.D.: An experimental investigation into wayfinding directions for visually impaired people. Personal Ubiquitous Computing 9(6), 395–403 (2005)

E-Learning Accessibility for the Deaf and Hard of Hearing - Practical Examples and Experiences

Matjaž Debevc[1], Primož Kosec[1], and Andreas Holzinger[2]

[1] University of Maribor, Faculty of Electrical Engineering and Computer Sciences,
Smetanova ulica 17, 2000 Maribor, Slovenia
{matjaz.debevc,pkosec}@uni-mb.si
[2] Medical University Graz, Institute of Medical Informatics, Statistics and Documentation,
Research Unit HCI4MED, 8010 Graz, Austria
andreas.holzinger@meduni-graz.at

Abstract. Development of information and communication technology has offered new horizons to the deaf and hard of hearing for their integration into working, social and economic environment. Despite the positive attitude of international guidelines, the lack of accessibility of e-learning material is still noticeable for these users. The process of adapting the e-learning materials for deaf and hard of hearing required different approach and guidelines to properly displaying sign language video. Paper presents basic e-learning accessibility guidelines for deaf and hard of hearing and basic directions for suitable design of e-learning sites accessibility. E-learning course (European Computer Driving License Course – ECDL) for deaf, automated video recording system and the transparent presentation of a sign language interpreter within the e-learning material are used as examples of good practice. Evaluations of these examples show high degree of satisfaction, ease of use and comprehension.

Keywords: E-learning, accessibility, usability, user interfaces, video streaming, human-computer interaction, deaf and hard of hearing.

1 Introduction

The development and subsequent wide availability of e-learning systems have caused significant changes in education and everyday business and also home activities for a large number of end users. The end user target group dealt with in this paper, consists of both deaf and hard of hearing people. Based on the data collected by the World Health Organization (WHO), there are 600 million people with disabilities in the world, representing roughly 10% of whole population. The World Federation of the Deaf (WFD) estimates about 70 million deaf people, approximately 80% of whom have deficient education and/or literacy problems, low speech abilities and often disordered living conditions [1]. Other studies show that the members of our target group, referred to in this paper as end users, are often confronted with a problem when acquiring the meaning of new words and notions [2].

G. Leitner, M. Hitz, and A. Holzinger (Eds.): USAB 2010, LNCS 6389, pp. 203–213, 2010.
© Springer-Verlag Berlin Heidelberg 2010

The increasing application of technology in educational environments, from junior schools to university, necessitates special steps to uphold the right of people with disabilities to equal participation in this technological environment.

The additional requirements of this group make it difficult to integrate them into society. The difficulties and functional barriers of people with special needs mean that they require an adapted environment for education, work and communication, which can be either of a technical or an interpersonal nature. This is often the reason for them failing to complete their education at an appropriate level. As a result, the number of people in this group obtaining any level of university degree and integrated into society and the working environment, is still low.

According to Hanson [3], for any deaf or hard of hearing individual, language experience cannot be assumed, since the individuals have diverse knowledge and skills, such as sign language, speaking clearly, lip-reading and textual reading. This knowledge has implications for designers who seek to address the needs of deaf and hard of hearing users.

Some of the key problems of using videos of sign language interpreters on web pages are already recognized. The existing solutions on the Web, for example AILB [4], which also gives support for forum contributions, SMILE [5], ShowSounds [6], Signing Web [7], SignOn [8], History of the Deaf [9] and Signing Savvy for American Sign Language [10] demand additionally placed space for the video of the sign language interpreter, which unfortunately reduces the area available for regular positioning of the website's content with text and images.

Further, it has been noted that, to date, natural video is more widely welcomed and accepted than signing avatars and synthetic gestures [11]. Due to this fact, a higher value has been set on the quality of the video of a natural sign language interpreter, integrated into e-learning materials.

2   Overview of Policies and Guidelines

Deaf and hard of hearing users have limited options for additional education; such as learning a foreign language, and for the use of online tools at all levels of education. This aspect shows the high demand for enabling appropriate access to information, professional development and contextual integration of information and telecommunication technologies into educational and social process for deaf and hard of hearing persons.

The most important worldwide document, improving the status of this area, is the Convention on the Rights of Persons with Disabilities, adopted on December 13th, 2006 [12]. This is the first legally binding document by the United Nations in the area of disability and ensures the promotion of human rights and the principle of equal opportunities and equal treatment, as well as prevention of discrimination as experienced by disabled people in various walks of life. In 50 articles of the Convention, accessibility, education, health, training, rehabilitation and other similar issues are discussed.

The European Union follows the trends of the United Nations. With their "Disability Action Plan", they want to establish equal treatment for people with disabilities, in working, social and private life. In the European context, European guidelines are defined, such as the Resolution to foster the integration of information and communication technologies (ICTs) in educational systems in Europe, adopted on May 11th, 2004 and the action plan by the European Commission for the support of equal rights for persons with disabilities, adopted on October 30th, 2003 and the European initiative "eEurope: An Information Society For All" adopted on 19th June, 2000. The European Commission wants to broaden the usage of World Wide Web and to grant access to Internet and distance education in every education institution, household and office.

In the Riga declaration, adopted on 11th June, 2006 [14], the European Union, among others, also defines accessibility of all public websites until 2010. However, the review from 2008 ("Measuring progress of eAccessibility in Europe" (MeAC) study) [13] reveals slow progress towards achieving this goal that should have been fostered.

Thus, on 31st March, 2009, the European Council adopted conclusions with the support of the European Communication "Towards an accessible information society" COM (2008) 804. Moreover, WCAG 2.0 [15] was included in the development of standard 376, which will offer new aspects for accessibility of web sites to public ICT intermediaries [16].

3 E-Learning Web Design Guidelines

This paper will focus on a limited number of guidelines and instructions for the design of e-learning sites, suitable for our special target end user group: the deaf and hard of hearing. Further, three examples of good practice developed by University of Maribor, Faculty of Electrical Engineering and Computer Science (UM FERI), Slovenia, will be presented.

These users are characterized by their particular need for visually supported information, as opposed to that of blind and visually impaired people. These students can listen to a certain extent with the help of technical equipment; such as hearing aids, induction coil or FM systems with wireless microphones for hearing aids and cochlear implants for the deaf [17]. This requires them to ensure maximum use of all channels in order to receive the information (auditory, visual, tactile and other channels), and as far as possible, to reduce verbalization and abstraction. To enable this, sounds must be visualized for the students: subtitles, translation of text into sign language (especially for the deaf) and the classrooms equipped with wireless devices to listen to the professor or assistant.

According to WebAIM (Web Accessibility in Mind) [18], the following current basic additional recommendations for web design are especially suitable for this user group:

- Enable subtitles or transcripts for other media. Videos must be subtitled or the transcript (written copy of speech) must be enclosed.
- Verify that the text is clear and easily readable. Text on the web should be written in a clear, simple form with titles and appropriate lists.

- Use standard forms. Accessible websites in HTML language are more robust and offer an easier implementation of search mechanisms. Cascading Style Sheets (CSS) allow distribution of content from the presentation of information, thereby offering greater flexibility and accessibility of online content.

The list does not contain all the aspects of accessibility for deaf and hard of hearing persons, however, by using these basic guidelines, we can achieve significantly higher accessibility of our websites. Further guidelines can be found in WCAG - Web Content Accessibility Guidelines [15].

4   E-Learning Examples for Deaf and Hard of Hearing

4.1   ECDL Educational Site for Deaf

European Computer Driving License (ECDL) is a European certification in end-user computer skills. In the European Union, ECDL is the standard for certifying/*determining* individual computer skills and verifying knowledge of use of specific software using practical examples.

An ECDL e-learning site has been constructed to fulfil the needs of teaching the skills required to obtain ECDL certificate to the target group. Here, the learning material has been prepared in advance with an added sign language interpreter video [19].

For the management of the material, the course management system Moodle, which is a free, open-source system for managing e-materials, was selected. Although there are many different open source systems for the management of teaching materials, we decided to use Moodle since it is user friendly, it supports installation on various platforms, and particularly because it includes the most important pedagogical principles.

The e-learning materials were made according to the plan for the ECDL 4.0 and were adjusted and updated for the target group. In the Moodle system, the content was organized into four modules or thematic sections, namely: Introduction to Information Technologies, Computer use and file management, Word processing, and Information and communication. In addition to media content, each of the modules included the following basic activities: forum, dictionary and the initial and final examinations to monitor progress of participants. Figure 1 shows an example of the material with an interpreter within the module.

From experience in working with the users less experienced in ICT in other projects and following usability guidelines [21], we have highlighted some additional guidelines and have taken them into account in adjusting ECDL materials:

- User interface should be simple and clear, without too many additional options.
- User interface should be simple in design.
- Navigation should be placed in the same (clearly visible) position throughout the site.
- No new windows should be opened automatically, as this may confuse the beginner user.
- Language and interpretations should be relatively simple; use of simple technical computer terms is recommended.

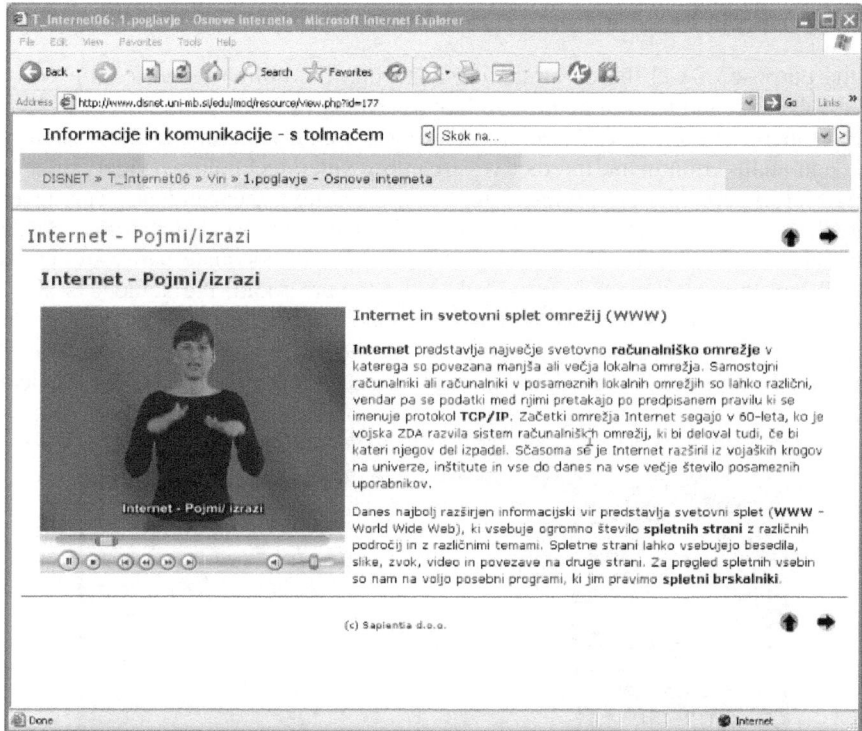

Fig. 1. ECDL material with a sign language interpreter in Moodle

After considering various video installations with an interpreter and based on the recommendations, we decided to permanently position the box with an interpreter in the relevant modules on the left side in the browser window.

Video and subtitles should be especially underlined in the above guidelines, since other solutions, such as the project AILB [4] or SignOn [8], do not include subtitles into the sign language video. Specifically, the sign language video for a translation of the spoken text into sign language must be of appropriate quality, without any additional information and continually present without interrupting.

Evaluation study. Usability evaluation, using Software Usability Measurement Inventory (SUMI) method [22], with unemployed deaf and hard of hearing adults with a knowledge of Slovene sign language who had taken part in the education process, shows global usability acceptance [23]. SUMI "global" usability sub-scale was 54, which is slightly above the positive limit of 50.

On the other hand, the usability sub-scale "efficiency" and "learnability" shows greater disagreement among users on this matter. After investigation of the problem, we found that it was based in the Moodle functionality and not in the ECDL e-learning content. After removing the left and right part of the typical Moodle design and after interviewing three deaf people, the acceptance of the new design was higher.

4.2   Hypermedia Based Virtual Lecture Room

For the purpose of web based streaming lecturing, the online video lecture was created for the deaf and hard of hearing in live streaming or on demand.

Our Video Supported Web Lecture incorporates a portable interactive system with video and audio equipment, interactive streaming video technology (video streaming) and virtual hypermedia environment into a new learning environment. The development of such an interactive system along with the appropriate furniture and audio equipment in lecture halls also requires the purchase of adequate hardware and software. When this equipment is provided in the lecture room, the student is able not only to listen to lectures live, but also has the opportunity to listen to the lectures later. The difference is that the subtitles are added to the video and other media if needed, such as audio subtitles for the blind and sign language interpreter video for the deaf.

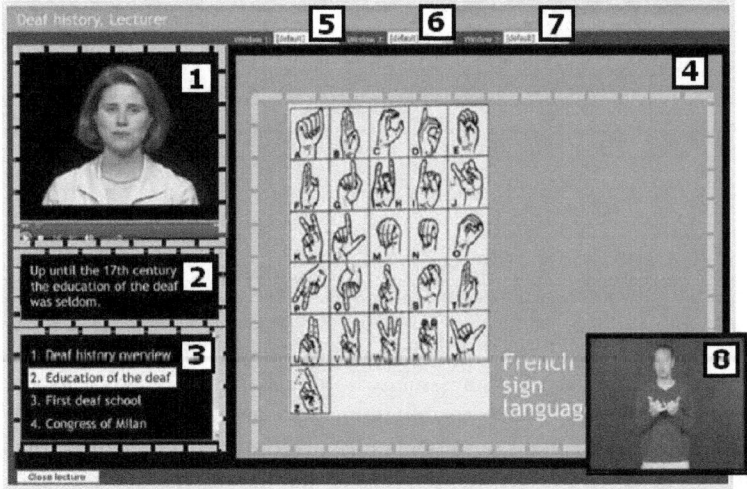

Fig. 2. A typical web based video lecture for deaf and hard of hearing people

The result of this process is the e-lecture, designed for our target group, demonstrated in Figure 2. It consists of the following media elements: video (1), audio (1), visual subtitles (2), a table of contents (3) (for content navigation) and presentation slides (4), as well as three media switches (5, 6, 7). The media switches are dropdown lists. In this way, the user can control the screen layout by selecting their own custom viewing preferences. The third switch (7) triggers a pop up window (8) with alternative streams (for instance, a sign language interpreter). This can be placed on any part of the screen over the e-lecture.

Evaluation study. There were 11 deaf and 2 severe hard of hearing participants in the experiment, whereby 23% were female and 77% were male. Participants ranged from 34 to 72 years of age, with a mean age of 52. 61% of the participants had no previous Internet browsing experience, while 8% had browsed only a couple of times and 31% had excellent skills.

As the main purpose of the Web portal is to deliver Web lectures, we tested basic tasks in online participation for both groups. Users were asked to complete six tasks that were read out to them one at a time: log in to the user account, find profile settings, find a specific lecture, change the video in Window 1, quit the lecture and log out of the system. A gestural think-aloud protocol was used in the evaluation to gather rich information [24]. The main focus with the subjects was the Web lecture experience; therefore there were 30 seconds available for each mode shown in Table 1. During each mode, the evaluator observed the participant's reactions. The communication among evaluator participants was established with a sign language interpreter, where he asked questions about e-lecture interface.

Table 1. Web lecture GUI modes for deaf

	Window 1	Window 2	Window 3 (pop-up)
Mode 1	Lecturer	PPT slides	Nothing
Mode 2	Lecturer	SL interpreter	Nothing
Mode 3	SL interpreter	PPT slides	Nothing
Mode 4	Lecturer	PPT slides	SL interpreter

The results from the experiment revealed that 69% needed help when performing tasks, basically due to their lack of browsing experience. They received additional instructions from the evaluator (assistance in completing the task was given). 77% of our test subjects confirmed that the most appropriate configuration for the e-lecture was provided by mode 3, where the sign language video is in top-left corner (Window 1), presentation slides are on the right (Window 2), and the third window was hidden. With this, we conclude that deaf persons do not prefer two different videos, streaming simultaneously (one video of a lecturer and one of a sign language interpreter) [25].

4.3 Sign Language Interpreter Video

Transparent video for deaf and hard of hearing users has been developed within the framework of the DEAFVOC 2 [20] project, enabling interactive lectures with sign language interpreter videos embedded on the websites. We named the system the Sign Language Module (SLIM). A practical example of the transparent sign language is visible at http://www.slimodule.com/.

When designing the system, we took into account linguistic specifics and bilingualism, both characteristics of substantial proportion of our target population. In the system, we wanted to focus first on sign language and emphasize the importance of adopting knowledge and delivery of information in this language. A system which offers the display of transparent (translucent) video, on the users' request, anywhere on the existing Web page has been developed. This offers users, whose primary language is sign language, a previously prepared translation of certain words, text, pictures, photos, animation or any other video clip.

The innovation of the system is reflected in the fact that the display on the site combines video, audio, subtitles and navigation links over the existing site as a transparent video and at the user's request. (Figure 3). When the short video clip is finished or manually terminated, a standard web site is displayed.

Research done by Debevc and Peljhan [9] has shown that deaf students perform better when they have an online system with a sign language interpreter video available than with traditional forms of teaching. Having materials in sign language also increases their daily exposure to sign language and enables students to use the material for independent study at home and for repetition of the material.

With an increasing number of similar materials in Slovenian sign language, we expect the users to become much more literate in their Slovenian mother tongue. It will then be easier for them to integrate into the larger social group, while maintaining their own identity, improving their self-esteem and developing their culture and language.

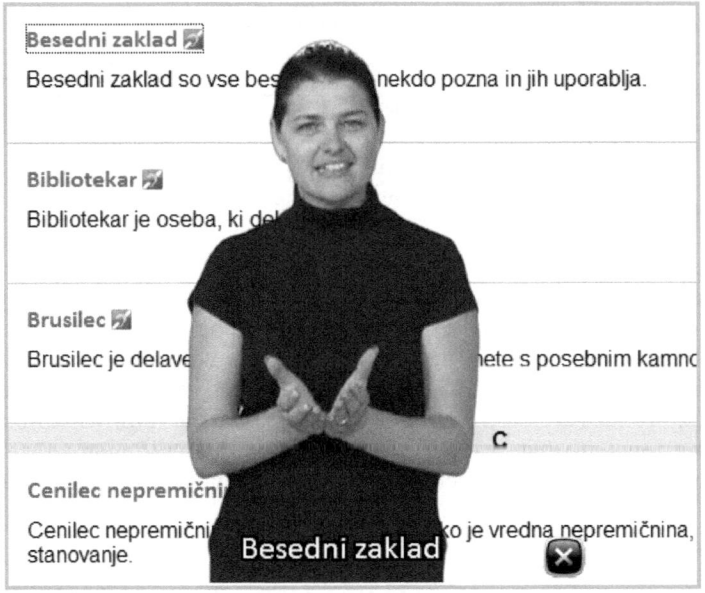

Fig. 3. Transparent sign language interpreter video for deaf and hard of hearing persons

This system also offers a contribution to the Slovenian Act on the use of Slovenian sign language. This Act gives deaf people the opportunity to use the Slovenian sign language as a language of communication with each other and as a natural means of communication, as well as the right to receive information in adopted techniques.

Evaluation study. There were two evaluation studies conducted with deaf and hard of hearing users. The first evaluation included 14 participants who use sign language as their first language, and were aged from 18 to 72. In the second evaluation 31 deaf and hard of hearing participants were involved, and were aged from 15-21. The aim of the first evaluation was to gather first impressions about the first prototype. We applied the gestural thinking method [24]. The communication between the evaluator and the participant was carried out with the help of a sign language interpreter. At the end of the evaluation, the user had to fill out the questionnaire with three basic questions about user experience.

The second evaluation combined several methodologies: pre-test questionnaire for the participant's demographic profile, post-test questionnaire for evaluating usability (5-point Likert scale), and an open debate to determine positive/negative or missing functionalities of the prototype.

Results from the first evaluation showed a high degree of users' satisfaction; 92% of the participants thought that the system was useful, while 8% were undecided. Based on results gathered throughout the evaluation studies in [26], we have provided further suggestions for the development of the transparent video for the next prototypes: providing a clearer and more easily recognizable icon for the sign language video, providing an additional button for closing the video, displaying the video appearance and disappearance in a slow rather than a sudden action, providing video playback controls (play, pause and stop) for longer videos.

The second evaluation, done by Kosec, Debevc and Holzinger [27] of the prototype confirmed a high degree of evaluated usability metrics, such as satisfaction (80%), ease of use (77%), comprehension (83%). The most interesting information that we received was revealed by a group debate, which confirmed some missing functionalities in the prototype. Some of the participants found that the video of the sign language interpreter was too fast; therefore they would needed a functionality for slowing down the video playback. Moreover, a few participants wanted to move the video around the screen. These features were taken into consideration for the implementation of the next prototype.

5   Conclusion

The use of Information and Communication Technology is, with appropriate adaptation to enable accessibility, even more suitable for deaf and hard of hearing people, as it offers better options for equal integration into a working, social and educational environment.

International documents and action plans, such as the United Nations' Convention on the Rights of Persons with Disabilities, the European Action plan, the Riga Declaration and the Slovenian Action Plan for Persons with Disabilities are all legal documents, which explicitly specify that web sites must be accessible to everybody, irrespective of the degree of their handicap. It is therefore necessary to invest more effort in raising awareness of appropriate technological options and the requirements and needs of deaf and hard of hearing people.

In examples of good practice, such as ECDL e-materials, we have examined, among other things, the appearance on the screen for the visually impaired, as well as for the deaf and hard of hearing. The text must be short, concise, with clear navigation links in the top right hand corner of the screen, with images having text in the background and sign language interpreters in a video window, located on the left side.

For the needs of monitoring and storage of lectures, a system for the automatic recording of lectures has been arranged, allowing simultaneous capturing of speaker, slides, subtitles, sign language interpreter and text typing. Immediately after the lecture, which may also be broadcasted live, all elements are combined together and immediately placed on an appropriate web site where the video can be retrieved later. The system is designed to take into account the needs of the deaf and hard of hearing.

The people who use sign language as their first language are unfortunately the most vulnerable population due to the low educational level, needing a translation of the text on the website. One option is through a continuous window, as we built it in the ECDL e-materials, but it cannot be added to existing and established websites. In this case, it turned out to be the right solution for the sign language interpreter to appear over the existing site, in terms of implementation of the additional web layer (the CPC Web Layer), while keeping the existing form of web pages. We named this approach a transparent sign language video or sign language module (SLIM).

With these instructions and practical examples of good practice, other web designers are provided with appropriate ideas and solutions for the implementation of more accessible web sites for the disabled and elderly, to enhance opportunities for increasing self-esteem and more active integration of this target population in an educational and social environment.

Acknowledgment. The project is partially supported by the European commission within the framework of the Leonardo da Vinci program, project DEAFVOC 2. It is also partially supported by the Slovenian Research Agency in the framework of the Science to Youth program, financial support for young researchers. Special thanks go to the Association of the deaf and hard of hearing people of Podravje for their help in the evaluation of the application and to Milan Rotovnik from University of Maribor for his help at designing transparent sign language video.

References

1. Haualand, H., Allen, C.: Deaf People and Human Rights. World Federation of the Deaf and Swedish National Association of the Deaf (2009), http://www.wfdeaf.org [accessed January 12, 2010]
2. Marschark, M., Convertino, C., McEvoy, C., Masteller, A.: Organization and use of the mental lexicon by deaf and hearing individuals. American Annals of the Deaf 149, 51–61 (2004)
3. Hanson, V.L.: Computing Technologies for Deaf and Hard of Hearing Users. In: Sears, A., Jacko, J.A. (eds.) Human-Computer Interaction Handbook: Fundamentals, Evolving Technologies and Emerging Applications, 2nd edn., pp. 885–893. Lawrence Erlbaum Associates, NJ (2008)
4. Straetz, K., Kaibel, A., Raithel, V., Specht, M., Grote, K., Kramer, F.: An e-Learning Environment for Deaf Adults. In: Conference Proceedings 8th ERCIM Workshop "User Interfaces for All", Vienna, Austria (2004)
5. Kronreif, G., Dotter, F., Bergmeister, E., Krammer, K., Hilzensauer, M., Okorn, I., Skant, A., Orter, R., Rezzonico, S., Barreto, B.: SMILE: demonstration of a cognitively oriented solution to the improvement of written language competence of deaf people. In: 7th International Conference on Computers Helping People with Special Needs (ICCHP 2000), Karlsruhe, Germany, July 17-21 (2000)
6. Vanderheiden, G.C.: Full Visual Annotation of Auditorially Presented Information for Users Who Are Deaf: ShowSounds. In: RESNA International Conference, Toronto, Canada, June 6-11 (1992)
7. Fels, D.I., Richards, J., Hardman, J.L., Daniel, G.: Sign Language Web Pages. American Annals of the Deaf 151, 423–433 (2006)
8. Hilzensauer, M.: Information Technology for Deaf People, pp. 183–206. Springer, Heidelberg (2006)
9. Debevc, M., Peljhan, Z.: The role of video technology in on-line lectures for the deaf. Disability and Rehabilitation 26, 1048–1059 (2004)

10. Signing Savvy (2010), `http://www.signingsavvy.com` (accessed January 12, 2010)
11. Olivrin, G.J.-L.: Is Video on the Web for Sign Languages. In: W3C Video on the Web Workshop, San Jose, California and Brussels, Belgium, December 12-13 (2007), `http://www.w3.org/2007/08/video` (accessed January 12, 2010)
12. United Nations: Convention on the rights of persons with disabilities. United Nations (2006), `http://www.un.org` (accessed January 12, 2010)
13. Olsen, M.G.: How Accessible is the Public European Web? (2010), `http://www.mortengoodwin.net/publicationfiles/how_accessible_is_the_european_web.pdf` (accessed January 12, 2010)
14. European Commission: Ministerial Declaration. European Commision, Riga (June 11, 2006), `http://ec.europa.eu/information_society/events/ict_riga_2006/doc/declaration_riga.pdf` (accessed January 12, 2010)
15. Caldwell, B., Cooper, M., Reid, L.G., Vanderheiden, G. (eds.): WCAG 2.0 - Web Content Accesssibility Guidelines: W3C Recommendation (December 11, 2008), `http://www.w3.org/TR/WCAG20/` (accessed January 12, 2010)
16. European Commision: Web Accessibility. European Comission (September 15, 2009), `http://ec.europa.eu/information_society/activities/einclusion/policy/accessibility/web_access/index_en.htm` (accessed January 12, 2010]
17. Moores, D.F.: Cochlear implants: A Perspective. American Annals of the Deaf 154, 415–416 (2010)
18. WebAIM: The WebAIM Guide to Web Accessibility. WebAIM (2009), `http://www.webaim.org` (accessed January 12, 2010)
19. Debevc, M., Stjepanovič, Z., Povalej, P., Verlič, M., Kokol, P.: Accessible and Adaptive e-Learning Materials: Considerations for Design and Development. In: Stephanidis, C. (ed.) HCI 2007. LNCS, vol. 4556, pp. 549–558. Springer, Heidelberg (2007)
20. Sign Languages and European Written Languages in Virtual Vocational Education for the Deaf (January 2010), `http://www.deafvoc.fi/` (accessed January 12, 2010)
21. Holzinger, A.: Usability Engineering for Software Developers. Communications of the ACM 48, 71–74 (2005)
22. Kirakowski, J., Corbett, M.: SUMI: The Software Usability Measurement Inventory. British Journal of Educational Technology 24, 210–212 (1993)
23. Debevc, M., Lapuh Bele, J.: Usability testing of e-learning content as used in two learning management systems. EURODL (Oslo) (2008), `http://www.eurodl.org/materials/contrib/2008/Debevc_Bele.htm` (accessed January 12, 2010)
24. Roberts, V.L., Fels, D.I.: Methods for inclusion: Employing think aloud protocols in software usability studies with individuals who are deaf. International Journal of Human-Computer Interaction 64, 489–501 (2006)
25. Kosec, P., Debevc, M., Holzinger, A.: Towards equal opportunities in computer engineering education: design, development and evaluation of videobased e lectures. Int. J. Eng. Educ. 25, 763–771 (2009)
26. Debevc, M., Kosec, P., Holzinger, A.: Improving multimodal web accessibility for deaf people: sign language interpreter module. Multimedia Tools and Applications (April 15, 2010), doi:10.1007/s11042-010-0529-8
27. Kosec, P., Debevc, M., Holzinger, A.: E-learning accessibility for the deaf and hard of hearing – practical examples and experiences. In: Miesenberger, K., Klaus, J., Zagler, W., Karshmer, A. (eds.) 12th International Conference, Computers Helping People with Special Needs, ICCHP 2010, Vienna, Austria, July 14-16 (2010)

Enhancing Digital Inclusion with an English Pseudo-syllabic Keyboard

Francesco Curatelli[1] and Chiara Martinengo[2]

[1] Università di Genova, Dept. of Electronics (DIBE), Italy
curatelli@unige.it
[2] Università di Genova, Dept. of Mathematics (DIMA), Italy
martinen@dima.unige.it

Abstract. The capability to efficiently input texts with hardware or soft keyboards is a major achievement to improve the digital inclusion of motor-impaired users in the modern ICT world. One way to obtain this capability is the use of multi-character keyboards that make it possible to significantly reduce the number of selected keystrokes. To this aim, in this paper we propose the orthogonal pseudo-syllabic layout for an English keyboard with high keystroke savings. Since English is characterised by a large number of frequent monosyllabic words, the careful design of the consonant and vowel graphemes that compose the pseudo-syllables makes it possible to directly select the most frequent multi-character units of the language. Therefore, the frequency statistics of English have been carefully analysed to select a suitable set of pseudo-syllables and to choose their placement on the orthogonal layout. The keyboard layout has then been tested with the automatic acquisition of a set of English texts. The obtained keystroke savings are comparable with those obtained with other languages which, in contrast with English, are characterised by very regular orthographies.

Keywords: Human-computer interaction, assistive technology, pseudo-syllabic keyboard, digital inclusion.

1 Introduction

According to a document written within the European i2010 initiative on e-inclusion: *"It is conservatively estimated that currently some 30% to 40% of the population does not fully benefit from the information society"* and *"As our everyday and work lives are increasingly entangled in activities and relations enabled by ICT, growth depends from ICT use to a large extent, and will increasingly continue to do so in the future. Therefore, the goal of broad-based growth is dependent also on the number of digitally included and digitally empowered individuals"* [1]. In this context, ICT itself can and should fill this gap by providing suitable hardware and software tools which allow impaired user groups, such as elder and disabled people, to enhance their active participation in work, learning, communication and leisure activities.

G. Leitner, M. Hitz, and A. Holzinger (Eds.): USAB 2010, LNCS 6389, pp. 214–227, 2010.

In particular, the capability to efficiently input texts with hardware or soft keyboards is a major achievement for motor-impaired users, because it allows them to improve both the interaction with the computer toools and the communication with other people. Moreover, this capability can also help impaired children with cerebral palsy to improve their cognitive abilities and e-inclusion [2]. Unfortunately, although expert and trained users can reach high text entry speed by simply using hardware or soft standard keyboards, this is not the case for motor-impaired users. For example, by typing letter-by-letter, most AAC (*Augmentative and Alternative Communication*) users are not able to input more than a few words per minute, and for some users the scores are as low as one word per minute, or even less [3].

The use of optimised hardware or soft keyboards, where letters are optimally allocated, is not a universal solution. In fact, although the use of these keyboards can increase typing speed [4,5], only expert users are able to fully exploit the advantage given by an optimised layout, because their movements are fast and they are able to access keys without the need of a visual search on the keyboard. This is not the case for non-expert users, who need a visual exploration of the keyboard to access the keys, and, mainly, for motor-impaired users, whose movements may be very slow. The times required for performing the visual search and the movement to the target key can be estimated quite carefully. The visual search time can be modelled by the Hick-Hyman law for choice reaction time [6]: $T_v = a' + b' \log_2(n)$, where n is the number of the keys, a' is the response time and $1/b'$ is the bandwidth, expressed in bits per second. The latency time, needed to move the cursor or the finger from the current key to the following one, can be carefully characterised by the Fitts' law model for movement plus reaction time [7]: $T_l = a + b \log_2\left(\frac{d}{w} + 1\right)$, where d is the distance between the two keys, w is the width of the keys, and a, b are empirical constants which depend on the device and on the user. It is worth noting that, while for non-expert users T_l is typically lower than T_v, this is not the case for most motor-impaired users, because their low typing speeds (which are often less than one character per second) are mainly due to their movement difficulties.

Another unsuitable (in our case) way to increase typing speed is to use chord keyboards, in which the user selects more keys concurrently [8]. In fact, even more than optimised keyboards, chord keyboards can be fully exploited only by expert users and after a long training period. Moreover, many motor-impaired people cannot easily use these devices because they may find it difficult to concurrently select more keys. Finally, another limitation of chord keyboards is that they are natively hardware devices; indeed, the implementation of a soft chord keyboard is possible, but this strictly requires the use of a multi-touch screen.

Instead, a suitable strategy to improve text entry for all users is to reduce the number of keys (*NKeys*) the user has to select to input a text. If *NChars* is the total number of input characters, this reduction can be measured in terms of $KSPC = NKeys/NChars$ (*keystrokes per character*), which is the mean number of key selections to input a single character, and $KSR = 100 \times (NChars - NKeys)/NChars$ (*keystroke saving rate*), which is the percentage of keys selections saved with respect to typing one character at the time [9]. In fact, $KSPC = 1$ or $KSR = 0\%$ mean that there has not been any keystroke saving, whereas $KSPC = 0.5$ or $KSR = 50\%$ mean that only half of the keys selections were required, and $KSPC = 0$ or $KSR = 100\%$ mean that no key selection was required at all (obviously the latter is a purely hypothetical limit).

Text prediction software tools [10,11,12,13,14] are very effective in increasing KSR, but high values are obtained only with 5 or more suggested words, whereas with one suggestion only 37.1% is obtained for English [15] and 35% for inflected languages, such as Dutch, French, German and Swedish [12]. This is a significant limitation, because all the predictive methods with selection intrinsically involve a significant cognitive load to perform word choice and selection; the more are the provided suggestions the more is the cognitive load needed. This fact affects the final communication rates, in spite of the high KSR values obtainable with prediction tools, although the increased cognitive load do not overcome the advantages of good word prediction systems [3].

Another way to improve the KSR values is to adopt multi-character hardware or soft keyboards, in which the keys hold a suitable set of the syllabic or subsyllabic units of the target language. To this aim, we have proposed a novel *orthogonal keyboard* paradigm which is based on the use of *pseudo-syllables* (*p-syllables*) as basic text entry units [16]. The hardware or soft keyboard is defined as a two-dimensional array of keys, where the user can introduce, in a direct and intuitive way, pseudo-syllables or single characters. The orthogonal paradigm, initially applied to Italian and Spanish, has been recently applied to Croatian, which is another language with a very regular orthography [17].

This paper describes the application of the orthogonal approach to English, which is one of the less transparent languages in the world. To this aim, the frequency statistics of English have been carefully analysed to select the set of pseudo-syllables and to choose their placement on the orthogonal layout. Then, the target KSR values have been simulated on a set of English texts. The obtained results are comparable with those obtained with languages with very regular orthographies. The paper is organised as follows. Section 2 describes the use of pseudo-syllables as text entry units, and briefly outlines the orthogonal paradigm. Section 3 describes the statistical analysis of English and outlines the design of the English orthogonal keyboard layout. Section 4 contais the results and conclusions.

2   The Orthogonal Keyboard Model

The orthogonal text entry paradigm [16] is based on the definition, for the target language, of a certain number of different keyboard *layers*, of which only one is active at any given time, where the pseudo-syllabic units are accessible by the orthogonal composition of vowel and consonant graphemes. In fact, in each specific keyboard layer, each column is assigned to a specific *consonant grapheme* $\hat{C}$, which can be a single consonant or a sequence of consonants (e.g. *tt*, *sh* or *ch*); analogously, each row is assigned to a specific *vowel grapheme* $\hat{V}$, which can be a single vowel or semi-vowel or a sequence of them (e.g. *ee*, *ee*, or *oy*). This means that in the current keyboard layer the key at (x, y) position contains both the vowel grapheme of row x and the consonant grapheme of column y; so, cognetively the two coordinates are orthogonally (i.e., independently) accessible.

The *dominant p-syllables* are those belonging to the basic layer and can be selected without using any additional key. Instead, the *subordinate p-syllables* belong to the other layers, which are activated by selecting specific shift hardware or soft keys. According to the residual motor capabilities of the user, the shift keys may be selected concurrently with the p-syllable keys, or must be selected before them; obviously, in the latter case the shift keys are implemented as sticky keys. It is worth noting that when a shift key is selected concurrently with the p-syllable key, the two selections actually occur at the same time, so that they can be considered parts of a unique action. Therefore, in this case only the selections of the p-syllable keys must be counted.

The syllabic or pseudo-syllabic entities that cannot be built according to the orthogonal scheme are not allocated to the orthogonal keyboard; so, they must be selected with a sequence of dominant or subordinate p-syllables. It is worth noting that the orthogonal pseudo-syllabic paradigm is conceptually very different from the method to input syllables that is present in the literature, which is based on the selection of more single-letter keys to build syllabic entities belonging to Abugida scripts [18]. Moreover, the significant improvement with respect to all other syllabic keyboards is that the independent composition of consonant and vowel graphemes intrinsically reduces the cognitive load needed to look for the p-syllables in the current keyboard layer.

For a given language L the first step consists in defining the two sets $\widehat{CS_L}$ (*complete consonant set*) and $\widehat{VW_L}$ (*complete vowel set*) which contain all the most used consonant graphemes $\widehat{C_i}$ and vowel graphemes $\widehat{V_i}$ of language L ($n_{\widehat{CS_L}} = |\widehat{CS_L}|$ and $n_{\widehat{VW_L}} = |\widehat{VW_L}|$ are the cardinalities of the two sets); both sets also contain the empty grapheme ϵ The orthogonal composition of the graphemes belonging to $\widehat{CS_L}$ and $\widehat{VW_L}$ defines a first, non-optimised, set of p-syllables PS_L (*complete p-syllable set*), which then contains any possible string $\widehat{C_i}\widehat{V_i}$ and $\widehat{V_i}\widehat{C_i}$, with $\widehat{C_i} \in \widehat{CS_L}$ and $\widehat{V_i} \in \widehat{VW_L}$. PS_L is mapped onto the 2-D non-optimised *complete keyboard array* ($x \in [1, n_x], y \in [1, n_y]$), in which $\widehat{C_i}\widehat{V_i}$'s are the dominant p-syllables, and $\widehat{V_i}\widehat{C_i}$'s are subordinate p-syllables which are selectable by using a specific *FR-Sh* forward/reverse shift key. Since this array is typically too large to be implemented in a real hardware or soft keyboard, some of the following optimisation steps must be applied: (another possible optimisation step, *column merging*, has not been used in the implementation of the English keyboard):

1. *Column deletion (CD):* elimination of columns whose p-syllables have low marginal frequencies in the target language.
2. *Row deletion (RD):* elimination of rows whose p-syllables have low marginal frequencies in the target language.

3. *Column folding (CF):* columns containing p-syllables with low marginal frequencies are folded with other columns. The selection of the subordinate keys is done through a *CF-Sh* shift key (unique for all the folded columns).
4. *Row folding (RF):* - rows containing p-syllables with low marginal frequencies are folded with other rows. The selection of the subordinate keys is done through an *RF-Sh* shift key (unique for all the folded rows).

At the end of the optimisation, there will be $n_{SK} \in \{1, 2, 3\}$ used shift keys; *FR-Sh* is always present, while *CF-Sh* is present only if column folding has been applied, and *RF-Sh* is presens only if row folding has been applied. The elimination of some consonant and/or vowel graphemes yields the two *optimised consonant and vowel set sets* $\widehat{CS}_L^o$ and $\widehat{VW}_L^o$ ($n_{\widehat{CS}_L^o} = |\widehat{CS}_L^o|$ and $n_{\widehat{VW}_L^o} = |\widehat{VW}_L^o|$ are the cardinalities of the two sets).

Finally, the *optimised p-syllable set* PS_L^o is built by the orthogonal composition of graphemes belonging to $\widehat{CS}_L^o$ and $\widehat{VW}_L^o$, which is mapped onto the final 2-D *optimised keyboard array* ($x \in [1, n_x^o], y \in [1, n_y^o]$). The cardinality of PS_L^o depends on how the selection of the shift keys are managed in the keyboard design. In particular, if all the n_{SK} used shift keys can be freely and independently selected, the graphemes composition can be complete and PS_L^o will contain, any possible string $\widehat{C_i V_i}$ and $\widehat{V_i C_i}$, with $\widehat{C_i} \in \widehat{CS}_L^o$ and $\widehat{V_i} \in \widehat{VW}_L^o$. However, in this case, the design must give the possibility to use more shift keys to select a subordinate p-syllable or the definition of $2^{n_{SK}} - 1$ composed shift keys to access directly the $2^{n_{SK}} - 1$ subordinate layers. Instead, a more easily usable design solution (mainly for impaired users) allows, for each p-syllable selection, the use of only one key shift to access directly n_{SK} subordinate layers, so defining a reduced PS_L^o. For this reason, this has been the solution adopted for the English keyboard.

3   The English Orthogonal Keyboard

The orthogonal paradigm has been initially studied and implemented for languages with regular (or transparent) orthographies, where there is an almost one-to-one correspondence between phonemes and graphemes, i.e., a sequence of phonemes can be directly translated into a unique syllable, and vice versa, without the need to capture the overall word meaning. In fact, the almost univocal and non-ambiguous phonemes to graphemes associations make it easier the direct and efficient use of the orthogonal paradigm. While Italian, Spanish and Croatian have very regular orthographies, this is not the case for English, which has one of the less regular orthography in the world. Incidentally, this is the main reason why it is much more difficult to learn to read in English and why so many dyslexic people are detected in English speaking countries [19]. Moreover, English has much more syllables and syllable structures than most languages, and typically a specific phonemic sequence can be associated to different graphemic sequences and vice versa. This means that a complete implementation of the orthogonal paradigm, which is based on the almost direct phoneme to grapheme association, would require the definition of a huge and unmanageable number of p-syllables. On the other hand, the most important feature of the proposed paradigm (i.e., the orthogonal and deterministic composition of the graphemes associated to rows and columns, which makes easier the access to the target keys) holds for any language. This argument has suggested that the orthogonal keyboard could be an efficient text entry paradigm also for English.

In English, all the 26 one-letter graphemes of the extended Latin alphabet are used. Moreover, most consonants can be doubled and some consonants can be followed by a h to denote a single sound, namely ch, gh, ph, sh, wh, while the grapheme qu is present in almost all the words that contain the consonant q. These graphemes constitutes, with the empty grapheme ϵ, the complete consonant set:

$$\widehat{CS}_{en} = \{ \ \epsilon, b, bb, c, cc, ch, cch, d, dd, f, ff, g, gg, gh, ggh, h, hh, j, jj,$$
$$k, kk, l, ll, m, mm, n, nn, p, pp, ph, pph, qu, cqu, r, rr, s, ss, sh,$$
$$ssh, t, tt, th, tth, v, vv, w, ww, wh, wwh, x, xx, y, yy, z, zz \ \}.$$

Concerning the vowel graphemes, in addition to the 5 vovels of the Latin alphabet, also the consonant y has been included in the complete vowel set because in English it often act (after a consonant) as a vowel. Moreover, English has a large number of different two-letter vowel graphemes where also the consonants y and w can be present as second vowel, Therefore, as all the unused and less used graphemes will be discarded during the optimisation steps, at this point it is convenient to include in the complete vowel set all the two-letter vowel combinations $\hat{V} = V_1V_2$, where $V_1 \in \{a, e, i, o, u, y\}$ and $V_2 \in \{a, e, i, o, u, y, w\}$. By adding the empty grapheme ϵ, the complete vowel set is:

$$\widehat{VW}_{en} = \{ \ \epsilon, a, e, i, o, u, y, V_1V_2 \ , \ \text{where} \ V_1 \in \{a, e, i, o, u, y\},$$
$$V_2 \in \{a, e, i, o, u, y, w\} \ \}.$$

Since, $n_{\widehat{CS}_{en}} = 55$ and $n_{\widehat{VW}_{en}} = 49$, the complete orthogonal keyboard cannot be directly implemented because it would require $n_x \times n_y = 55 \times 49$ keys; so, the size must be reduced through the application of some optimisation steps. In doing this it must be considered that the final keyboard (either hardware or soft) should have, for usability, a limited y size, while x size can be quite larger. As the folding optimisation steps CF and RF could at most halve the x and y sizes, this means that the CF and RF steps must be preceded by an RD step that significantly reduce the number of vowel graphemes.

To reduce the keyboard width and height, two reduced optimised consonant and vowel sets $\widehat{CS}_{en}^{o}$ and $\widehat{VW}_{en}^{o}$ must be built by eliminating the less frequently used graphemes. To this aim, we have used the data available from the *British National Corpus*, which contains texts for about 100,000,000 words [20].

Table 1 outlines the number of occurrences for all the 54 non-empty elements of $\widehat{CS}_{en}$. We can note that few non-doubled consonant graphemes have frequencies less than 1,000,000, namely, z, ph, qu, j, x, gh, and that all the doubled consonant graphemes, except ll, have frequencies less than 1,000,000; moreover,

Table 1. Consonant frequencies in English, sorted: (a) alphabetically; (b) by frequency [20]

$\widehat{C}$	$\#\widehat{C}$	$\widehat{C}$	$\#\widehat{C}$	$\widehat{C}$	$\#\widehat{C}$	$\widehat{C}$	$\#\widehat{C}$
b	4,103,323	ph	142,824	bb	41,259	pph	257
c	3,522,690	qu	432,793	cc	230,427	cqu	15,855
ch	1,413,984	r	7,812,539	cch	863	rr	287,115
d	7,175,060	s	9,529,616	dd	141,111	ss	714,927
f	6,594,283	sh	1,275,208	ff	492,119	ssh	780
g	2,981,068	t	20,310,660	gg	92,069	tt	477,605
gh	836,170	th	11,659,448	ggh	52	tth	3,429
h	17,481,123	v	2,444,348	hh	2,093	vv	861
j	567,557	w	6,700,716	jj	353	ww	814
k	1,893,935	wh	1,449,537	kk	1,506	wwh	2
l	4,691,073	x	588,819	ll	1,717,772	xx	860
m	4,887,799	y	4,753,186	mm	304,710	yy	342
n	11,956,620	z	134,147	nn	197,923	zz	13,045
p	2,468,086			pp	413,109		

(a)

$\widehat{C}$	$\#\widehat{C}$	$\widehat{C}$	$\#\widehat{C}$	$\widehat{C}$	$\#\widehat{C}$	$\widehat{C}$	$\#\widehat{C}$
z	134,147	b	4,103,323	wwh	2	cqu	15,855
ph	142,824	l	4,691,073	ggh	52	bb	41,259
qu	432,793	y	4,753,186	pph	257	gg	92,069
j	567,557	m	4,887,799	yy	342	dd	141,111
x	588,819	f	6,594,283	jj	353	nn	197,923
gh	836,170	w	6,700,716	ssh	780	cc	230,427
sh	1,275,208	d	7,175,060	ww	814	rr	287,115
ch	1,413,984	r	7,812,539	xx	860	mm	304,710
wh	1,449,537	s	9,529,616	vv	861	pp	413,109
k	1,893,935	th	11,659,448	cch	863	tt	477,605
v	2,444,348	n	11,956,620	kk	1,506	ff	492,119
p	2,468,086	h	17,481,123	hh	2,093	ss	714,927
g	2,981,068	t	20,310,660	tth	3,429	ll	1,717,772
c	3,522,690			zz	13,045		

(b)

ll is more frequent than *z*, *ph*, *qu*, *j*, *x*, *gh*, *sh*, *ch*, *wh*. Therefore, a significant reduction of n_x can be obtained by discarding the doubled consonants with low frequencies. As outlined in Table 1(b), 15 graphemes have frequencies lower than 20,000 and are rarely used in English. For this reason the deleted graphemes are: *cch*, *ggh*, *hh*, *jj*, *kk*, *pph*, *cqu*, *ssh*, *tth*, *vv*, *ww*, *wwh*, *xx*, *yy*, *zz*.

Concerning the vowel set, the 6 single vowels *a*, *e*, *i*, *o*, *u*, and *y* have been defined as dominant graphemes and placed in different rows of the orthogonal keyboard. Therefore, since 7 (i.e., 6 rows for the vowels plus 1 row for the empty grapheme) is a reasonable height for the orthogonal keyboard, the number of the other vowel graphemes should be reduced from 42 to 6. To obtain this reduction, the BNC frequency data have been used in a more detailed way, according to 3 statistics: Statistic St_1 concerns the global frequencies of the $V_1 V_2$ graphemes independently of the position in the words, and is outlined in Table 2(a). The data have been used to select the 20 most frequent graphemes discarding the other ones. The second and final selection has been done according to the statistics St_2,

Table 2. V_1V_2 frequencies in English - (a) statistic St_1; (b) statistics St_2 and St_3 [20]

V_1	$\#V_1a$	$\#V_1e$	$\#V_1i$	$\#V_1o$	$\#V_1u$	$\#V_1y$	$\#V_1w$
a	8,550	36,756	959,685	10,588	345,464	895,388	214,204
e	624,275	306,832	542,283	237,023	75,152	605,452	378,032
i	484,604	729,930	19,088	990,771	31,448	1,963	2,589
o	183,055	128,307	311,193	742,596	182,599	135,918	154,004
u	338,840	363,181	298,046	23,804	3,447	29,403	2,999
y	51,649	515,937	120,971	934,121	5,702	342	24,545

(a)

V_1V_2	O_2	St_2	O_3	St_3	V_1V_2	O_2	St_2	O_3	St_3
ou	1	2,163,202	1	670,268	ew	11	233,852	5	169,143
ee	2	894,969	6	126,841	ui	12	182,164	17	463
ow	3	643,943	4	284,798	ie	13	161,734	9	14,715
oo	4	607,849	7	70,098	au	14	129,615	18	409
ay	5	548,330	3	389,112	ue	15	103,805	10	11,659
ai	6	517,507	13	1,529	ua	16	71,296	19	262
ea	7	514,800	8	23,852	ye	17	51,529	12	3,080
ey	8	457,304	2	435,137	ia	18	50,577	11	6,168
ei	9	419,379	16	699	io	19	34,718	15	749
oi	10	257,539	14	943	yo	20	2,232	20	21

(b)

which concerns the frequencies of the V_1V_2 graphemes that are at the beginning
of words, and St_3, which concerns the frequencies of the V_1V_2 graphemes that
constitute a complete word. Both statistics are outlined in Table 2(b), where,
the 20 remaining V_1V_2 graphemes are sorted according to St_2 (O_2 is its ordinal
position), but also St_3 is outlined (O_3 is its ordinal position). From the values in
the two columns the following V_1V_2 graphemes have been chosen: *ou, ee, ow, oo,
ay, ea*. The first 5 elements have been selected because they have high values in
both statistics, the 6th element (*ea*) has been selected because: a) the preceding
element in the list (*ai*) has a very small figure concerning statistic St_3; and b)
although the following element in the list (*ey*) has a very high figure concerning
statistic St_3, almost all its occurrences (420,413 of 435,137) are due to the single
word *they*, so that it is not a good choice to allocate a whole row to the grapheme
ey. So, after the above optimisation steps the optimised consonant and vowel
sets are:

$$\widehat{CS}^{\,o}_{en} = \{\ \epsilon,\ b,\ bb,\ c,\ cc,\ ch,\ d,\ dd,\ f,\ ff,\ g,\ gg,\ gh,\ h,\ j,\ k,\ l,\ ll,\ m,\ mm,$$
$$n,\ nn,\ p,\ pp,\ ph,\ qu,\ r,\ rr,\ s,\ ss,\ sh,\ t,\ tt,\ th,\ v,\ w,\ wh,\ x,\ y,\ z\ \}$$

$$\widehat{VW}^{\,o}_{en} = \{\ \epsilon,\ a,\ e,\ i,\ o,\ u,\ y,\ ay,\ ea,\ ee,\ oo,\ ou,\ ow\ \}$$

Finally, the CF and RF optimisations are applied and define the 4 layers, 1 for
the dominant and 3 for the subordinate p-syllables (whose selection requires that
one of the shift keys *FR-Sh*, *CF-Sh* or *RF-Sh* be *on*). According to the already
presented frequence statistics, the dominant p-syllables are built by the 6 single

vowels and/or by the 21 non-doubled consonants with higher frequencies (i.e., with frequencies higher than 1,000,000); both the consonants and vowels sets are ordered lexicographically along the x and y coordinates, respectively. This fixes the size of the final orthogonal keyboard to $(n_x^o \times n_y^o) = (22 \times 7)$.

The subordinate p-syllables that are selected by *CF-Sh* are built by the 6 single vowels, and/or by all the doubled consonants belonging to the optimised consonant set and the 6 non-doubled consonants that have not been allocated yet. The doubled consonants are allocated to the same columns of the related single consonant; in this way, the cognitive task of the user is made much easier because both the single and doubled consonants share the same horizontal position in the keyboard. This is the basic reason why the doubled consonant *ll* belongs to subordinate p-syllables, despite the fact that its frequency is higher than those of some single consonants. The remaining non-doubled consonants are allocated to 6 of the 9 free columns, ordered lexicographically each other. The subordinate p-syllables that are selected by *RF-Sh* are built by the 6 two-letter vowels belonging to the optimised vowel set and/or by the dominant consonants; along the rows the two-letter vowels are ordered lexicographically.

As *CF* optimisation assigned only 18 columns, the 3 remaining columns have been used for the allocation of $3 \times 7 = 21$ additional strings (*added words*). The added words has been allocated at the x coordinates of the dominant graphemes *th*, *wh* and *y*; in each column there are 7 complete words beginning with the dominant consonant grapheme of that column. This has been done because, although the added words do not strictly belong to the basic orthogonal paradigm, it is anyway convenient to use strings that be somehow coherent with the orthogonal structure, so that the visual search of the added words by the user be made much easier. Since most words in a text are actually followed by a space, a space character is automatically inserted at the end of each added word; this is done to obtain an additional reduction of the number of keystrokes. The added words have been selected among the most frequent words beginning with the dominant consonant grapheme of the related column. According to the BNC Corpus, in decreasing order of frequency for each consonant we have: (*the*, that, this, they, there, their, them); (which, what, when, *who*, where, while, *why*); (*you*, your, year(s), yes, yet, young).

Table 3 outlines the layer of the English orthogonal keyboard for the dominant p-syllables and the reverse subordinate p-syllables (*FR-Sh* = *on*), while Table 4 outlines the layers for subordinate p-syllables with *CF-Sh* = *on* and *RF-Sh* = *on*. Each added word in the *CF-Sh* = *on* layer is followed by an underscore which visually denotes the presence of the added space. As can be seen, the orthogonal keyboard layout contains a large set of p-syllables which constitute whole English words, so that only one action is needed to select them also for subordinate p-syllables (provided that the shift key can be selected concurrently with the p-syllable key). This is a very significant characteristics of the language, which derives from the fact that English has a very large number of monosyllabic words.

Table 3. English orthogonal keyboard for: (a) dominant p-syllables; (b) subordinate p-syllables (*FR-Sh = on*)

	b	c	ch	d	f	g	h	k	l	m	n	p	r	s	sh	t	th	v	w	wh	y
a	ba	ca	cha	da	fa	ga	ha	ka	la	ma	na	pa	ra	sa	sha	ta	tha	va	wa	wha	ya
e	be	ce	che	de	fe	ge	he	ke	le	me	ne	pe	re	se	she	te	the	ve	we	whe	ye
i	bi	ci	chi	di	fi	gi	hi	ki	li	mi	ni	pi	ri	si	shi	ti	thi	vi	wi	whi	yi
o	bo	co	cho	do	fo	go	ho	ko	lo	mo	no	po	ro	so	sho	to	tho	vo	wo	who	yo
u	bu	cu	chu	du	fu	gu	hu	ku	lu	mu	nu	pu	ru	su	shu	tu	thu	vu	wu	whu	yu
y	by	cy	chy	dy	fy	gy	hy	ky	ly	my	ny	py	ry	sy	shy	ty	thy	vy	wy	why	yy

(a)

	b	c	ch	d	f	g	h	k	l	m	n	p	r	s	sh	t	th	v	w	wh	y
a	ab	ac	ach	ad	af	ag	ah	ak	al	am	an	ap	ar	as	ash	at	ath	av	aw	awh	ay
e	eb	ec	ech	ed	ef	eg	eh	ek	el	em	en	ep	er	es	esh	et	eth	ev	ew	ewh	ey
i	ib	ic	ich	id	if	ig	ih	ik	il	im	in	ip	ir	is	ish	it	ith	iv	iw	iwh	iy
o	ob	oc	och	od	of	og	oh	ok	ol	om	on	op	or	os	osh	ot	oth	ov	ow	owh	oy
u	ub	uc	uch	ud	uf	ug	uh	uk	ul	um	un	up	ur	us	ush	ut	uth	uv	uw	uwh	uy
y	yb	yc	ych	yd	yf	yg	yh	yk	yl	ym	yn	yp	yr	ys	ysh	yt	yth	yv	yw	ywh	yy

(b)

Table 4. English orthogonal keyboard for subordinate p-syllables: (a) *CF-Sh = on*; (b) *RF-Sh = on*

	bb	cc	gh	dd	ff	gg	j	ph	ll	mm	nn	pp	rr	ss	qu	tt	the_	x	z	which_	you_
a	bba	cca	gha	dda	ffa	gga	ja	pha	lla	mma	nna	ppa	rra	ssa	qua	tta	that_	xa	za	what_	year_
e	bbe	cce	ghe	dde	ffe	gge	je	phe	lle	mme	nne	ppe	rre	sse	que	tte	their_	xe	ze	when_	years_
i	bbi	cci	ghi	ddi	ffi	ggi	ji	phi	lli	mmi	nni	ppi	rri	ssi	qui	tti	them_	xi	zi	where_	yes_
o	bbo	cco	gho	ddo	ffo	ggo	jo	pho	llo	mmo	nno	ppo	rro	sso	quo	tto	there_	xo	zo	while_	yet_
u	bbu	ccu	ghu	ddu	ffu	ggu	ju	phu	llu	mmu	nnu	ppu	rru	ssu	quu	ttu	they_	xu	zu	who_	young_
y	bby	ccy	ghy	ddy	ffy	ggy	jy	phy	lly	mmy	nny	ppy	rry	ssy	quy	tty	this_	xy	zy	why_	your_

(a)

	b	c	ch	d	f	g	h	k	l	m	n	p	r	s	sh	t	th	v	w	wh	y
ay	bay	cay	chay	day	fay	gay	hay	kay	lay	may	nay	pay	ray	say	shay	tay	thay	vay	way	whay	yay
ea	bea	cea	chea	dea	fea	gea	hea	kea	lea	mea	nea	pea	rea	sea	shea	tea	thea	vea	wea	whea	yea
ee	bee	cee	chee	dee	fee	gee	hee	kee	lee	mee	nee	pee	ree	see	shee	tee	thee	vee	wee	whee	yee
oo	boo	coo	choo	doo	foo	goo	hoo	koo	loo	moo	noo	poo	roo	soo	shoo	too	thoo	voo	woo	whoo	yoo
ou	bou	cou	chou	dou	fou	gou	hou	kou	lou	mou	nou	pou	rou	sou	shou	tou	thou	vou	wou	whou	you
ow	bow	cow	chow	dow	fow	gow	how	kow	low	mow	now	pow	row	sow	show	tow	thow	vow	wow	whow	yow

(b)

4 Results and Conclusions

The suitability of the proposed layout to obtain significant keystrokes savings has been evaluated with the automatic acquisition of 18 medium-length English texts. Each text is part of 4 famous English Speeches of the last century [21]. The related data statistics are outlined in Table 5, where N_α, N_O and N_{Sp} are the number of alphanumeric, non-alphanumeric, and space characters in the text; $N_C = N_\alpha + N_O$ is the total number of characters in the text. For each text acquisition, the following statistics have been obtained:

K_α : number of selected alphanumeric keys,
K_O : number of selected non-alphanumeric keys,
$K_T = K_\alpha + K_O$: number of selected keys,

which concern the number of key selections, belonging or not to the orthogonal layout, that are needed to cover the text (it has been assumed that any selection requires one single action, i.e., that the shift keys are selectable concurrently with the p-syllable keys). The above data have been used to compute the following performance parameters:

$KSPC_\alpha = K_\alpha/N_\alpha$: *alphanumeric keystrokes per character;*
$KSPC_\gamma = K_T/N_C$: *keystrokes per character;*
$KSR_\alpha = 100 \times (N_\alpha - K_\alpha)/N_\alpha$: *alphanumeric keystroke saving rate;*
$KSR_\gamma = 100 \times (N_C - K_T)/N_C$: *keystroke saving rate.*

Table 5. Test files statistics

Text	N_α	N_O	N_C	N_{Sp}	Text	N_α	N_O	N_C	N_{Sp}
T1	1415	328	1743	298	T10	1361	309	1670	271
T2	1336	376	1712	327	T11	1317	313	1630	270
T3	1351	330	1681	290	T12	1239	278	1517	247
T4	1316	320	1636	285	T13	1457	332	1789	295
T5	1294	329	1623	285	T14	1450	342	1792	301
T6	1321	329	1650	292	T15	1401	303	1704	280
T7	978	249	1227	224	T16	1153	272	1425	251
T8	953	257	1210	229	T17	1082	252	1334	235
T9	914	248	1162	218	T18	1231	315	1546	282

Table 6(a) outlines the $KSPC$ and KSR values that have been obtained with the full English orthogonal keyboard layout, i.e., with the presence of the added words. KSR_α's show a nearly double improvement, with values that are greater than 44.1% and *mean* = 45.20, SD = 0.84. This is a significant result, taking also into account that the English orthogonal keyboard contains only alphabetical strings, whereas N_α and K_α also take into account all the digits. But significant improvements are also shown by the KSR_γ values, which are greater than 36.9% and *mean* = 38.51, SD = 0.99. Instead, Table 6(b) outlines the $KSPC$ and KSR values that have been obtained with a reduced English orthogonal keyboard layout, in which all the added words have been discarded. In this case, the KSR_α values are anyway greater than 43.2% with *mean* = 43.98, SD = 0.46; the KSR_γ values are greater than 34.1% with *mean* = 35.36, SD = 0.60. This means that the gain is only slightly lower than in case (a): namely, 1.22 for KSR_α and 3.15 for KSR_γ.

The performance figures of the second test are directly comparable with those obtained with the Italian, Spanish and Croatian orthogonal keyboards, in which there are not any added words [16,17]. From this point of view the values obtained with the basic English orthogonal paradigm (i.e., without the added words) are quite similar to those obtained with the other languages. More precisely, the results are slightly worse for Spanish and Croatian, and slightly better with

Table 6. $KSPC$ and KSR statistics: (a) with added words; (b) without added words

Text	$KSPC_\alpha$	$KSPC_\gamma$	KSR_α	KSR_γ	Text	$KSPC_\alpha$	$KSPC_\gamma$	KSR_α	KSR_γ
T1	0.5561	0.6144	44.38	38.55	T10	0.5540	0.6197	44.59	38.02
T2	0.5516	0.6308	44.83	36.91	T11	0.5504	0.6122	44.95	38.77
T3	0.5588	0.6258	44.11	37.41	T12	0.5488	0.6150	45.11	38.49
T4	0.5463	0.6130	45.36	38.69	T13	0.5525	0.6215	44.74	37.84
T5	0.5571	0.6284	44.28	37.15	T14	0.5496	0.6155	45.03	38.44
T6	0.5314	0.5987	46.85	40.12	T15	0.5517	0.6144	44.82	38.55
T7	0.5347	0.5957	46.52	40.42	T16	0.5576	0.6266	44.23	37.33
T8	0.5456	0.6157	45.43	38.42	T17	0.5406	0.6034	45.93	39.65
T9	0.5350	0.6041	46.49	39.58	T18	0.5402	0.6112	45.97	38.87

(a)

Text	$KSPC_\alpha$	$KSPC_\gamma$	KSR_α	KSR_γ	Text	$KSPC_\alpha$	$KSPC_\gamma$	KSR_α	KSR_γ
T1	0.5660	0.6477	43.39	35.22	T10	0.5613	0.6425	43.86	35.74
T2	0.5621	0.6582	43.78	34.17	T11	0.5618	0.6460	43.81	35.39
T3	0.5647	0.6502	43.52	34.97	T12	0.5609	0.6413	43.90	35.86
T4	0.5607	0.6466	43.92	35.33	T13	0.5600	0.6416	43.99	35.83
T5	0.5672	0.6549	43.27	34.50	T14	0.5586	0.6428	44.13	35.71
T6	0.5473	0.6375	45.26	36.24	T15	0.5574	0.6361	44.25	36.38
T7	0.5572	0.6471	44.27	35.28	T16	0.5646	0.6477	43.53	35.22
T8	0.5603	0.6537	43.96	34.62	T17	0.5582	0.6416	44.17	35.83
T9	0.5579	0.6523	44.20	34.76	T18	0.5548	0.6455	44.51	35.44

(b)

Italian. This is a significant result taking into account that all these three language have very regular orthographies, whereas this is not the case for English. What has made it possible to obtain similar or better keystroke savings is the careful choice of the p-syllable set, which makes it possible to directly input many monosyllabic English words. Therefore, we can argue that the orthogonal paradigm, although initially conceived for transparent languages, is well suited for obtaining high keystroke savings for a highly non-transparent language such as English, which has a large number of frequent monosyllabic words. Moreover, we can observe that word completion and prediction techniques, space addition tools, and phrase understanding methods can be directly applied on the text produced through the orthogonal keyboard, so yielding further additional keystroke savings.

In conclusion, the obtained results suggest that the English orthogonal keyboard can be a viable solution to allow motor-impaired users to improve their text entry performances. In fact, for these users the speed of movemements is severely contrained, so that each single action typically requires seconds to be done and cannot be significantly augmented with training. As a consequence, text entry speed can be improved only by reducing the number of actions that are needed to input the text, and this is just what is obtained with the orthogonal keyboard. In particular, the presented results refer to the keystroke savings that can be obtained when, as it is often the case, the motor-impaired users are able to perform, although slowly because of their disability, the concurrent selection of the shift keys and the p-syllable keys. However, as already stated, the use of the proposed layout does non at all need this ability. In fact, even when the degree of disability limits the user to select the keys sequentially, the proposed paradigm can be applied by using sticky shift keys, obviously at the expense of a reduction of the keystroke savings.

In any case, an intrinsic advantage of the orthogonal keyboard is that it allows the user to access the target text entry units by thinking in terms of syllabic entities rather than in terms of mere sequence of letters. Since this is a more natural way to segment the words to be input, it is arguable that the proposed paradigm can also help, in their cognitive effort, users who are affected by learning disabilities such as dyslexia and dysgraphia. This is one of the further issues of the present research, which also concerns the extension of the p-syllable model to significantly extend the pseudo-syllabic structures that can be selected on the orthogonal keyboard. Instead, the implementation of a soft English orthogonal keyboard and its on-field evaluation is the aim of an ongoing experimental research which will be presented in a forthcoming paper.

References

1. UE Impact Assessment Document: European i2010 Initiative on e-Inclusion "No One Left Behind in the Information Society", Brussels (2006),
   http://ec.europa.eu/information_society/activities/einclusion/docs/
2. Martinengo, C., Curatelli, F.: Improving Cognitive Abilities and e-Inclusion in Children with Cerebral Palsy. In: Holzinger, A., Miesenberger, K. (eds.) USAB 2009. LNCS, vol. 5889, pp. 55–68. Springer, Heidelberg (2009)
3. Trnka, K., McCaw, J., Yarrington, D., McCoy, K.F.: User Interaction with Word Prediction: the Effects of Prediction Quality. ACM Trans. on Accessible Computing 1(3), 17,1–34 (2009)
4. Lesher, G.W., Moulton, B.J., Higginbotham, D.J.: Optimal Character Arrangements for Ambiguous Keyboards. IEEE Trans. on Rehabilitation Engineering 6(4), 415–423 (1998)
5. MacKenzie, I.S., Zhang, S.X.: The Design and Evaluation of a High-Performance Soft Keyboard. In: Proc. of CHI 1999, Pittsburgh, pp. 25–31 (1999)
6. Soukoreff, R.W.: Text Entry for Mobile Systems: Models, Measures, and Analyses for Text Entry Research. M.Sc. Thesis York University, Canada (2002)
7. Zhai, S.: Characterizing Computer Input with Fitts' Law Parameters - the Information and Non-Information Aspects of Pointing. Int. J. of Human-Computer Studies 61(6), 791–809 (2004)
8. Gopher, D., Raij, D.: Typing on a Two-Handed Chord Keyboard: Will QWERTY Become Obsolete? IEEE Trans. on Systems, Man, and Cybernetics 18, 601–609 (1988)
9. MacKenzie, I.S., Soukoreff, R.W.: Text Entry for Mobile Computing: Models and Methods, Theory and Practice. Human-Computer Interaction 17(2-3), 147–198 (2002)
10. Darragh, J.J., Witten, I.H.: Adaptive Predictive Text Generation and the Reactive Keyboard. Interacting with Computers 3(1), 27–50 (1991)
11. Rosenfeld, R.: A Maximum Entropy Approach to Adaptive Statistical Language Modelling. Computer, Speech and Language 10, 187–228 (1996)

12. Matiasek, J., Baroni, M., Trost, H.: FASTY: a Multi-Lingual Approach to Text Prediction. In: Miesenberger, K., Klaus, J., Zagler, W.L. (eds.) ICCHP 2002. LNCS, vol. 2398, pp. 243–250. Springer, Heidelberg (2002)
13. Wandmacher, T., Antoine, J.Y., Poirier, F.: SIBYLLE: A System for Alternative Communication Adapting to the Context and its User. In: Proc. ASSETS 2007, pp. 203–210 (2007)
14. Ward, D.J., Blackwell, A.F., MacKay, D.J.: Dasher: a Gesture-Driven Data Entry Interface for Mobile Computing. Human-Computer Interaction 17(2-3), 199–228 (2002)
15. Trnka, K., McCoy, K.F.: Evaluating Word Prediction: Framing Keystroke Savings. In: Proc. of ACL 2008, pp. 261–264 (2008)
16. Curatelli, F., Martinengo, C.: A Powerful Pseudo-Syllabic Text Entry Paradigm. Int. J. of Human-Computer Studies 64(5), 475–488 (2006)
17. Curatelli, F., Martinengo, C.: Keystroke Saving in a Language with Highly Transparent Orthography. J. of Computing and Information Technology 18(3), 275–283 (2010)
18. Joshi, A., et al.: Keylekh: a Keyboard for Text Entry in Indic Scripts. In: Proc. of CHI 2004, Vienna, Austria, pp. 928–942 (2004)
19. Paulesu, E., et al.: Dyslexia: Cultural Diversity and Biological Unity. Science 291, 2165–2167 (2001)
20. Davies, M.: BYU-BNC: The British National Corpus (2004), http://corpus.byu.edu/bnc
21. The Speech Site: Famous Speeches by Famous Speakers (2004), http://thespeechsite.com/en/famous/Churchill-Blood.shtml

LDS:
Computer-Based Lesson Development System for Teaching Computer Science

Daniel Safta and Dorian Gorgan

Tehnical University of Cluj Napoca, Computer Science Department,
Baritiu. 25, Cluj-Napoca, Romania
davonkeep@yahoo.com,
dorian.gorgan@cs.utcluj.ro
http://cs.utcluj.ro/

Abstract. In this article we present a new approach to teaching computer science - the evaluation and visual modeling of algorithms based on metaphorical forms - applied within the core of a virtual education system, the development module for computer-based lessons (LDS). We reveal the structure and characteristics of the teaching process that we implemented in the proposed system, students and their roles, applied teaching methods, solutions for evaluation and a case study on a lesson model. We presented the state of the art in this domain highlighting the advantages of the described solution set, and also possible extensions.

Keywords: Computer assisted instruction, visual modeling, teaching process, algorithmic thinking, programming language.

1 Introduction

Currently there is a strong concern in the field of Informatics didactics to familiarize students with computer science from an early age. In this regard there are well-known efforts from Massachusetts Institute of Technology, where through Lifelong Kindergarten [1] they develop and maintain educational projects aimed at school children and preschoolers. Their motto, "Sowing the seeds for a more creative society" indicates the importance of developing children's inclinations toward programming since primary school. Besides literacy itself, it must also be achieved a so-called computer-use literacy. To this end, visual programming and programming by example is used, involving children in educational projects such as the Intel Computer Clubhouse Network, or Scratch.

Scratch [2] is addressed to children aged 6-16 and encourages three lines: imagine, program, share with others. Here's how a programming language is hidden in a fun educational background, an environment in which students interactively create and share with the rest of the online community their stories, games, music, fine arts etc. Currently there are thousands of active projects on the Scratch website and the importance of the project is supported by advocates such as the

G. Leitner, M. Hitz, and A. Holzinger (Eds.): USAB 2010, LNCS 6389, pp. 228–243, 2010.

National Science Foundation, Microsoft, Intel Foundation, Nokia, Iomega and the research consortium at MIT Media Lab.

Other environments that promote computer science among young people are the so called Computer Clubhouses like Intel Computer Clubhouse Network [3], Lego Mindstorms [4], PicoCrickets [5] etc. In these online communities students share their own ideas and experience in the field of visual programming applied on practical areas such as communication networks, programmable Lego robots, and even art (music, sculpture, dance, jewelry shops etc).

Starting from the premise that they are already familiar with computers and have minimal programming skills, young high school students can develop their thinking and programming by using systems based on visual programming like Visual Basic Game Programming for Teens [6], Macromedia Authorware [7].

However, familiarizing young people with the IT environment does not mean that they will know how to develop an algorithm or that they will be able to master a programming language. There is a very high barrier between student and programmer status [8]. There are many attempts to help the student in its way but most encounter the same obstacle, how to clearly establish, in human thinking, the connection between visually modeling a solution and its description in a programming language. Particularly very young students, accustomed to that introductory "fun programming" fail to adjust to a new approach to algorithms, to synthesize visual modeling into abstract concepts and translate them further into words. It takes a certain level of intelligence and maturity of thought in the individual in order to make this leap.

Computer programming was always considered by many authors the cornerstone of developing young minds [9]. As such, it was assumed that learning how to program, students will develop their problem solving skills. Indeed, experience in developing algorithms orientates the individual's thinking toward a more effective questioning and abstraction, a better problem analysis and improved decision making. But to get here, there is a new problem, perhaps even more costly for some than the benefits it brings - the shift from the user status to programmer.

Motivation. In teaching computer science - especially for beginners - there is a major shortcoming in the interaction between the student and the programming language: the approach. The novice's thinking is not sufficiently structured to develop an algorithm constrained by rules of a pseudo or even a programming language and also has shortcomings in describing the logical path to solving a problem. We notice two simultaneous major needs: the need to develop a logically structured way of thinking, able to translate abstract ideas into an algorithm and the need to master the rigors of a programming language [10].

The current approach in teaching computer programming is that the student has to change his way of thinking in order "to think like a computer", which is a big mistake. In fact, algorithms are made by the human mind and shaped after human thinking and therefore we construct the whole system described further on that idea: the student writes source code through actions and not through instructions!

2   The Computer-Based Lesson Development System

A computer-based lesson development module stands as the core of a virtual education system currently under development, a system, accessible both locally and remote, that offers a different approach to computer science, especially in the study of algorithms and programming languages. LD provides lessons based on a new concept in teaching computer science, focusing on the student's approach: his interaction with the programming environment is through an interface that is oriented on the algorithm's visual and interactive modeling, and not on simple editing of source code, the latter being accomplished automatically.

The novelty lies in the teaching strategy used in developing the lessons package, in the assessment and interpretation of results: the emphasis is on the final form of the described model and not on the intermediate steps. Thus:

- the student is not restricted in the choice of solutions, but is free to create his own path in solving the problem, to visually shape the algorithm to his own ideas;
- the focus is not on the states diagram, but on the result;
- only after the solution's validation will we be proceeded to the analysis of the covered steps;
- if the answer is right, the trail of described actions is retained as a new method to solve the problem;
- if the answer does not coincide with the expected metaphorical form, the system follows the trail of events and indicates the first deviation from known routes.

This concept underpins the development of a package of lessons with practical application in the study of algorithms and programming techniques, customized by age levels, capacity of understanding and not least on the basis of prior knowledge.

2.1   The Educational Process

Combining the advantages of visual programming with structured programming principles, the following alternative in student-algorithm interaction is being highlighted: initially the student is not forced to use a programming language, but is inclined to visually model a possible solution, eliminating any apparent connection with editing source code. This way the student doesn't stumble any more in the particularities of the used language, but distributes his full attention to the logical component in determining the solution of the problem, focusing solely on the required algorithm's development.

Therefore, during the lessons from our application the student uses - initially without being aware of - elements that are hardly accessible in the classical teaching ways, models algorithms by his own logic, freely and unrestricted by the rigors of a programming language, but at the same time, through his actions, he "dictates" executable source code. Afterwards, by using graphical annotations, he can write his own source code corresponding to each action and submit it to automatic evaluation by the LDS.

In selecting and generating lessons, we take into account not only the knowledge level, but also each student's level of understanding. Lessons can also be customized based on the age group.

In terms of beginners, the learning process has two components (Figure 1.a):

- the modeling space, in which the student receives the necessary theoretical knowledge and solves problems by modeling solutions;
- the command interpreter.

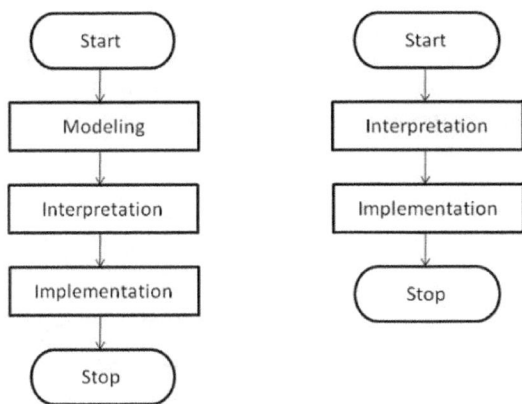

Fig. 1. The educational process in terms of the beginner (a) and the advanced learner (b)

The modeling space is "the classroom" in which the student works, the scene where he uses visual and interactive techniques to build the requested algorithm's metaphorical form. After this stage, according to the teacher's predefined templates, the interpreter establishes connections between the described actions and instructions. The interpreter then transforms the actions into instructions that further on lead to the writing of executable source code.

Advanced students are able to interact directly with the interpreter, describing actions in pseudo code, skipping the solution's visual modeling phase and getting closer to source code editing in a programming language (Figure 1.b).

2.2 Roles

In order to achieve its purpose, the system will interact with three actors, the roles in LD being: administrator, teacher (professor) and student.

The administrator ensures resources integrity and oversees the teaching process from a technical point of view, authentication, student's level of access to the application's core, maintains databases etc. Based on the teachers' suggestion, the administrator adds new tools to the application, creates new modeling environments and interaction techniques between the student and the system.

The teacher (professor) does not disappear from the educational process, but his role is even more significant. He has the specific documents based on which will the entire application work; creates, uploads and assures the lesson's synchronization with the current school curriculum.

The professor uses LD tools to manage the entire educational process: creates the set of lessons drawn up in accordance with current school documents and establishes the theoretical concepts and practical applications that will be addressed in each lesson in hand.

In order to generate problems, the teacher creates objects for which he associates possible actions, describes metaphorical shapes and identifies the connection between student actions and instructions. Thus, in order to achieve the applicative context of the lesson, the teacher creates metaphorical forms, from simple to complex, represented by a wide range of predefined objects or created using the tools made available by the LD (Figure 2).

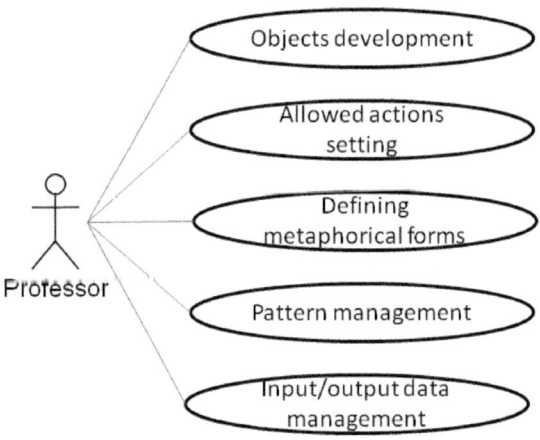

Fig. 2. The teacher's role

The teacher also defines test data used to validate the solution and templates regarding:

- the relationship between pseudo-instructions and the events described by the student;
- specifying the appropriate data structures for the used metaphors;
- constants in the metaphorical form that will be replaced with variables.

Based on such templates predefined by the teacher, the resulted pseudo code is converted to executable source code.

The target user, the learner (pupil or student), attends classes based on his level of training and predefined educational path.

During a lesson, the student studies the necessary theoretical concepts and solves relevant problems, either by interacting through visual modeling, or, if the more advanced, by describing the solution in pseudo code. In the first case, the student visualizes a scene that contains a set of objects predefined by the teacher, characterized by specific attributes and permitted actions, with which he interacts and uses them to model a solution in solving the problem (Figure 3).

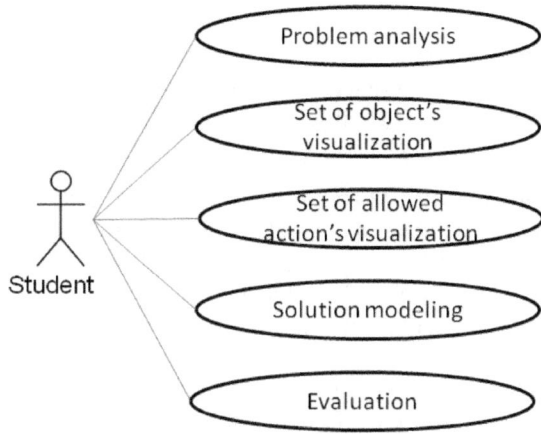

Fig. 3. The student's role

2.3   Characteristics of the Teaching Process

Ease in the Algorithm'S Description. By visually modeling the solution, beginners' thinking is not limited by their lack of experience in using a certain programming language. In addition to this student - environment interaction technique that is already well known and implemented in familiarizing beginners with computer science, our proposed teaching strategy is distinguished by the evaluation process and the feedback analysis based training.

Freedom in Choosing a Solution. The student is not required to use a particular problem solving method; there is no predefined template that describes the object-action couple's sequence of states. If, in the end, the described metaphorical shape matches the expected, then the maximum score is obtained.

Although there may be many alternative routes to model a possible solution, there is only one final metaphorical form, therefore the evaluation process cannot fail. Whatever the chosen path is, the destination remains the same. For example, consider the classic problem of sorting an array of elements in an ascending way. There are many sorting methods that can be applied, yet the input and output remain the same: the given array and the ordered array.

Regardless of the algorithm being implemented, while not seeking efficiency - makes no sense for beginners - but only the correctness of the solution, the evaluation process will not fail.

Handling Judgment Errors. Since we develop algorithms through visual modeling, we have eliminated the possibility of syntax errors, therefore incorrect answers can only appear due to judgment errors. Their identification takes place as it follows: the set of solutions is being searched to find the closest available solution in terms of the described actions' effect. Afterwards, a step by step comparison takes place between the states described by the student and their corresponding in the solution. This way the student is shown alternative ways to the logical path followed in modeling the requested algorithm.

Identifying False Solutions. Through his interaction with the solution modeling space, the student can obtain a correct result, a metaphorical form identical to the predefined one, but built by a series of actions describing a particular case and that the effect of which cannot be generalized.

For example, ascending sorting the elements of a vector can be described by the following metaphor: a constant number of barrels is given, each containing a specific quantity of powder (the set of objects). The barrels can be interchanged between any two of them (set of actions). Let us assume that according to the model shaped by the student, such an alignment of the barrels is obtained so that every barrel of the array contains at least as much powder as a neighbor on the left and up as much dust as the right neighbor. This solution can be valid, the student's actions describing a generally valid sorting method or a false one, in which arranging the barrels is made randomly and so the sorting process' description is impossible to generalize. In this case it will be proceeded to guide the student towards the correct solution using programming by examples.

The identification of such situations occurs when the switch is made to executable code, when the algorithm is tested based on the input data set and the expected output data is not achieved in all cases.

Enriching the Data Base. Each validated description of the algorithm that does not exist in the system's library will be added to the set of corresponding solutions for the given problem. The set of solutions is used in the feedback process in which the student is guided, as appropriate, to the nearest correct answer or to the optimal one.

Efficiency and Solution Optimization. If the student obtains a valid solution, the system displays the algorithm's efficiency relative to the maximum possible and, where appropriate, compares the student's solution and optimal one. This way the student is directed toward tracking performance in computer programming.

3   The Lesson

Teaching computer programming is oriented on problem solving, using through the visual-interactive component active-participatory methods, focusing on the problem analysis stage. The lesson has two components:

1.Theory in which the transmission of new knowledge takes place;
2.Practice based on problem solving.

The lesson is generated according to the student's school route, the previously acquired knowledge and not least, the syllabus in force. The lessons are aimed at carrying out a series of learning activities [11] such as:

- using informatics tools to model daily activities;
- obtaining, depending on the intended purpose, complex processing by combining elementary operations (steps);
- describing an algorithm by using metaphors as natural as possible;
- detailed description of the problem solving steps, in terms of algorithm modeling;
- comparing various algorithms used to solve a certain problem in order to emphasize efficiency, advantages and disadvantages of each solution at hand;
- modeling problems encountered in daily life or in the study of other disciplines (interdisciplinary applications);
- familiarizing with a programming language by viewing the actions of corresponding instructions, the steps of an algorithm and specific control structures;
- design, modeling and implementation of an algorithm;
- using feedback to debug programs;
- studying the behavior of programs for different inputs.

New knowledge is thought especially using programming by example or demonstration. The fundamental concepts are illustrated and exemplified on a small number of objects. Then, by generalization, the algorithm's abstract form is outlined.

Evaluation is performed in the second stage of the lesson, the problem solving step, in each of its moments:

- description of the metaphorical shape;
- process description;
- pseudo code description;
- the final source code;
- the final, executable result.

For beginners, who exclusively apply visual solution modeling in problem solving, assessing the response will focus on the comparison with a metaphorical form predefined by the teacher, that is being built as the unique solution or one of the possible solutions. The evaluation process includes the analysis of student actions and the comparing of the obtained results with the expected return.

3.1   The Teaching Process

The LD functions as a link between the educational system's main actors, the teacher and the student, and provides the educational context for the acquisition and practice of structured programming principles.

In solving problems, especially for beginners, the emphasis is on the student's thinking ways. Through the LD we seek to train the student toward an algorithmic approach, to develop the capacity to analyze problems so they can retrieve from context the input and output data, to write and especially to tailor a solution to their own ideas, describing the process as a metaphorical shape, without worrying about writing source code in a programming language. Their actions describe pseudo instructions that are then transcribed, based on teacher predefined templates in executable source code.

After acquiring the theoretical concepts, passing on to the practical part of the lesson, the student studies the problem to be solved, visualizes the set of available objects and, through his actions, he builds a metaphorical form. The system draws it up according to the process described by the student's actions and compares the obtained response with the existing solutions in the database.

If the answer is correct and the route specified by the participant in the action-based shaping process does not exist in the database, then this solution will be retained, contributing to the complexity of the solution analyzer. Associating each action with appropriate instructions, the process described by the student is then transformed into pseudo code and further, coupling with existing source code templates results the executable source code.

If the student's final solution is not correct, then he is indicated the encountered logic errors and is shown clues for obtaining the expected model.

Feedback is a fundamental element in education. For each student, a set of features is created and updated after each lesson, features that are highlighted during the teaching process; the set also stores information about the student's ability to assimilate and apply new knowledge into practice, working speed in modeling certain solutions, types of encountered errors and their frequency.

3.2   Case Study

Lesson Plan. Unit: Algorithms' description.

Content: The alternative structure (decision).

Specific skills: Problem analysis. Input/output data identification, setting the proper problem-solving steps. Algorithms modeling and representation. The principles of structured programming in developing algorithms.

Learning activities: The implementation of the alternative instruction. Examples of use in everyday life. Tracking the execution of the instruction step by step. Applications: determination of the minimum and maximum between two numbers, a number's parity check, solving I and II degree equations, divisibility etc.

3.3   The Lesson Components

Theoretical considerations: defining and describing the alternative structure.

Practical application: selecting the maximum between two numbers.

Metaphorical form: comparison of two quantities and selection of the heaviest. Filling two buckets of water, comparing them by using a scale and thus selecting the heaviest.

Set of objects: tap, water, buckets, scales.

Possible actions: opening/closing valve, filling buckets with water, placing buckets on the scale, selecting a bucket.

3.4   Lesson Conduct

The student models a solution for the given problem by using the set of available objects and the actions that are allowed in the lesson. He can obtain metaphorical forms accepted as solutions, taking alternative routes however, leading to the expected result. In that case, the system's solutions database will be added a new algorithm.

If the student fails to reach a final form, he is able to visualize intermediate metaphorical forms in order to break the deadlock and can also follow a step by step tracing of a correct solution's modeling.

Based on a deterministic problem-solving approach, the LD associates the objects and actions used in the visual modeling with a programming language's variables and instructions.

Even from this very simple example it shows that the student apparently controls the entire solution modeling process in a visual, interactive way, without having any connection with source code editing. The control is just apparent, because this is one of the big problems in programming, particularly for novice students - they become lost between solutions. To avoid sinking into the sea of false solutions and to prevent as much as possible the occurrence of logical errors, the student is constrained in using only a predefined set of objects.

The lesson presented above can be interpreted according to Table 1.

Visually modeling the solution through actions	Equivalent data and instructions	C++ source code
visualization of available items (two buckets and a scale) and allowed actions	two variables and an alternative structure	float x,y;
filling the buckets with water	reading the values of two variables	$cin >> x >> y;$
weighing the buckets	if-then-else logical test	if $(x < y)$ max=x; else max=y;
selecting the heaviest bucket	display solution	$cout << max;$

We adopted this deterministic approach to lead the beginner toward finding a correct solution by limiting his possibilities and so reducing the risk of judgment error occurence. The teacher's role is even more important as he is responsible to load into the database, according to each proposed problem, sets of objects and actions that allow the development of as many solutions as possible, while at the same time anticipating each move and guiding the student to shape the optimal solution.

4   Implementation Details

4.1   Lesson Environment

The LDS is mainly implemented in Visual C++ [12]. The lesson environment can be either 2D or a 3D scene. For each lesson, objects are defined by their attributes and behavior. Because for future usability purposes the LDS object database stores all available objects, it is possible to edit the available actions are permitted in a certain lesson.

Objects Generation. The 3D scene is created by using OpenGL [13]. In this case, should the teacher posses the necessary skills, he can create 3D objects in a modeling environment of his choosing and export them as an .obj file [14]. Otherwise, if not so familiar with 3D modeling, teachers can load predefined objects or can instruct the LDS administrators to the creation of new ones.

In a 2D environment, the teacher can create objects by themselves using a graphics tablet for the more talented, a drawing environment or they can simply load predefined objects from the LDS database.

Both created and selected objects are then loaded into the lesson. The next step is for the teacher to edit their behavior by setting specific actions and customize the interaction between them.

4.2   Case Studies

Custom 2D Objects. The objects are in a 2D environment and have been created by the teacher using a graphics tablet. For the previously presented problem of finding the maximum between two given numbers, the modeling process takes place as follows:

The student views the available objects and the set of permitted actions (Figure 4).

Buckets are characterized by a content level indicator called "quantity indicator" and a "grab" action that allows the student to move them around the scene. The tap is handled through the ON/OFF action switch. After input from the "measure" button, the scale indicates the maximum weight positioned on its trays.

He then proceeds at modeling a possible solution. The first step is to read the input data, meaning to fill the two buckets with water levels corresponding to the two given numbers. This is achieved by placing each bucket under the water tap and handling the ON/OFF switch (Figure 5.a).

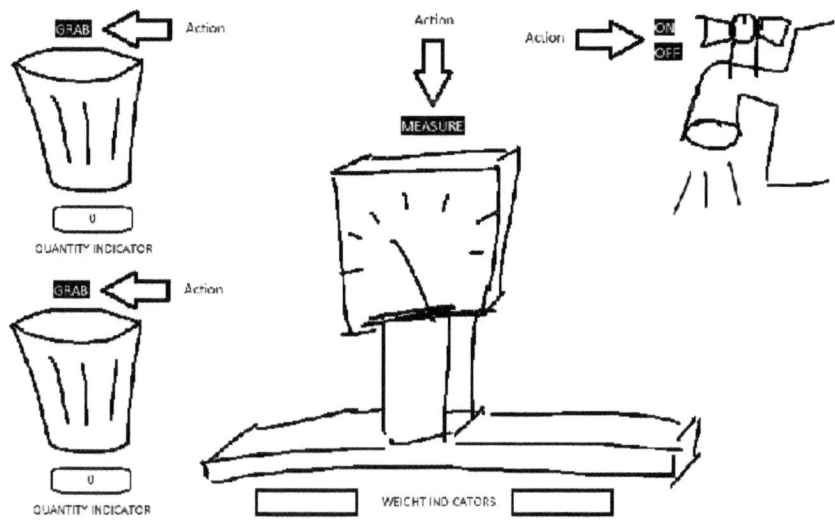

Fig. 4. The set of objects and corresponding behavior

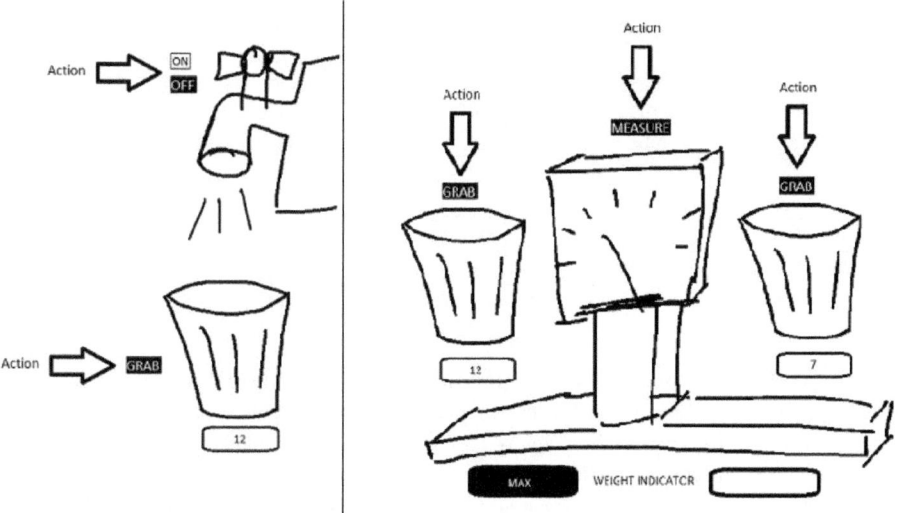

Fig. 5. Reading the input data (a) and The output - the solution (b)

After both buckets have been filled appropriately, the student places them on the scale trays and presses the "measure" button. He is now shown the result of the problem, the heaviest of the two buckets, meaning the maximum of the two numbers (Figure 5.b).

3D Objects. The objects are created using 3D Studio Max [15] at the teacher's request, either by the administrator or by the teacher himself should he possess the necessary skills to do so. They are exported as .obj files and can be loaded either in a 2D scene or a 3D environment. For the array sorting problem previously mentioned in the "Identifying false solutions" chapter, we will consider a 2D scene in which the modeling process takes place as follows:

A constant number o barrels (five) is given representing an array of elements. The student views the available objects and the set of permitted actions (Figure 6). Barrels are characterized by their size and position in the scene. He is allowed to "grab" the objects just like in the previous example and move them around the scene, interacting with the environment and other objects.

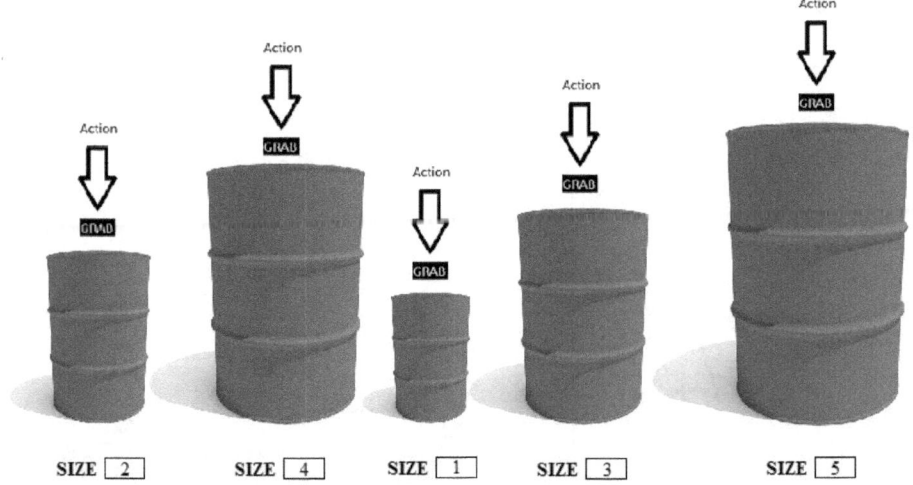

Fig. 6. The set of objects and corresponding behavior

The purpose is to obtain an arrangement of the given objects in a descending order. The model described by the student must match exactly the expected metaphorical form shown in Figure 7. To do so, the student can now apply several sorting methods that have been taught to him in the proceeding part of lesson regarding new knowledge assessment. He is also free to try and arrange the barrels using his own method; however in this case, false solutions are likely to occur. Such situations take place, as we mentioned earlier, when the solution modeled by the student works for the given example, but cannot be generalized to a valid algorithm.

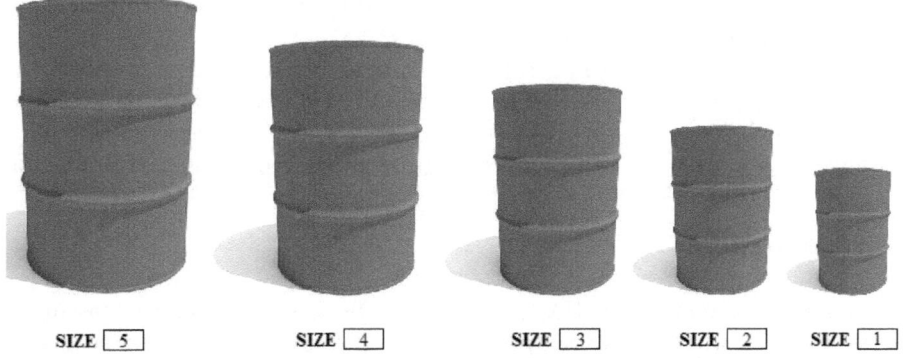

SIZE 5   SIZE 4   SIZE 3   SIZE 2   SIZE 1

Fig. 7. The solution: a descending array of elements

The system stores predefined sorting methods such as: Bubble sort, Insertion sort, Shell sort, Merge sort, Heapsort, Quicksort, Counting Sort, Bucket sort, Radix sort and Distribution sort [16], [17]. This is due to multiple reasons:

1. To teach the methods above using programming by example;
2. To follow the path modeled by the student and confront it with valid solutions;
3. To offer clues, should students require, based on the most similar valid solution.

4.3   Generalization

In the same way that these simple examples were described above, there can be shaped any programming lesson, the base principle being generally the same: the student writes source code through his actions and not through instructions. Based on the action-instruction relationship, the LD generates pseudo-instructions and then, matching with templates from the database, provides executable source code. The code is then viewed by the student, a point where each action's being annotated one or more instructions.

This approach can be extended to any lesson in the study of computer programming or programming techniques. There can be explained programming concepts such as: data types, control structures, structured types, pointers, trees, graphs, lists, routines, you can study programming techniques, properties etc. For instance, the following metaphorical form: the student creates circles of various sizes through graphic modeling, illustrating various properties such as object instantiation (circle class), duplication, encapsulation, inheritance, multiple inheritance, etc.

For the more advanced, since the student is already familiar with handling objects, the level of detail increases and the lesson contains more objects which are now seen as the equivalent variables in a programming environment. He can continue to model, as preferred, visually or in pseudo code, but in an increasingly nondeterministic way. The LD still contains one or more solutions and will analyze the result of student's sequence of actions. It will thus obtain new solutions that will be saved for the next lesson.

Since in this approach the solution is seen as a particular state of objects, any solution given by the student can be tested in the same way. If the student does not find his way toward the expected results, he can access full or partial guidance toward possible solutions through step by step graphical annotations.

5   Conclusions

The approach presented in this paper would be a step closer to crossing the barrier between users and developers, compared to the methods currently available, especially in our country, in teaching computer science. We focused on the introductory aspect, on familiarizing novices with computer programming, on the components that build the interface between untrained users and the programming environment.

The application is characterized by its tools easily usable by teachers in lesson development and an engine that automatically evaluates the learners' solutions. Students are trained in an accessible learning system, which stimulates algorithmic thinking and keeps away from the constraints of a programming language. At the same time the association between visual modeling and code editing takes place, in the end achieving executable source code.

5.1   Extensions of the Proposed Model

The deterministic approach, suitable for beginners, is to be replaced as the student evolves, by one going toward no determinism; as an expert the student does not need to visually shape the algorithm, as he possesses the necessary skills to write source code directly in a programming environment.

Switching from a particular problem to a general algorithm, for example, in the case studies presented above, the generalization is to determine the maximum from a set of given numbers or sorting a given number of elements in an array.

Expanding the devices used in achieving the educational environment to 3D scenes, interaction via keyboard, mouse and/or graphics tablet to design an entire 3D virtual learning environment and controlled by glove.

Incorporating the lessons generated by the LD in an eLearning platform, facilitating distance learning, offering the possibility to attain algorithms development capacity to students everywhere and yet maintaining feedback and linear evolution control.

References

1. The Lifelong Kindergarten group, http://llk.media.mit.edu/index.php
2. MIT Media Lab, http://www.media.mit.edu
3. The Intel Computer Clubhouse Network, http://www.computerclubhouse.org
4. Lego Mindstorms NXT, http://mindstorms.lego.com/en-us/default.aspx

5. PicoCricket computers, http://www.picocricket.com
6. Harbour, J.S.: Microsoft Visual Basic Game Programming for Teens, 2nd edn. Course Technology PTR (2007) ISBN-13: 978-1598633900
7. Adobe Authorware 7, http://www.adobe.com/products/authorware
8. Ko, A.J., Abraham, R., Beckwith, L., Blackwell, A., Burnett, M., Erwig, M., Lawrance, J., Lieberman, H., Myers, B., Rosson, M.B., Rothermel, G., Scaffidi, C., Shaw, M., Wiedenbeck, S.: The State of the Art in End-User Software Engineering. ACM Computing Surveys, http://faculty.washington.edu/ajko/papers/Ko2010EndUserSoftwareEngineering.pdf (accepted for publication)
9. Gretschel, M., Pulleyblank, W.R.: Mathematics of Operations Research. In: INFORMS, Linthicum, Maryland, USA, vol. 11(4), pp. 537–569 (1986) ISSN:0364-765X
10. Safta, D., Gorgan, D.: Recommendations For E-Learning Solutions Development And Evaluation. ICID: 900899, Revista Romana de Interactiune Om-Calculator (2), 105–110 (2009)
11. Curriculum for High school, Year I - Intensive informatics, http://www.edu.ro/index.php/articles/curriculum/c556+559+580+
12. Visual C++ Developer Center, http://msdn.microsoft.com/en-us/visualc/default.aspx
13. Open Graphics Library - The Industry's Foundation for High Performance Graphics, http://www.opengl.org
14. OBJ Files - A 3D Object Format, http://people.sc.fsu.edu/~burkardt/data/obj/obj.html
15. Autodesk 3ds Max Products, http://usa.autodesk.com/adsk/servlet/pc/index?siteID=123112&id=13567426
16. Knuth, D.: The Art of Computer Programming, 3rd edn. Sorting and Searching, vol. 3. Addison-Wesley, Reading (1997) ISBN 0-201-89685-0
17. Cormen, T.H., Leiserson, C.E., Rivest, R.L., Stein, C.: Introduction to Algorithms, 2nd edn. MIT Press and McGraw-Hill (2001) ISBN 0-262-03293-7

Enhancing Virtual Reality Learning Environments with Adaptivity: Lessons Learned

Olga De Troyer, Frederic Kleinermann, and Ahmed Ewais

Vrije Universiteit Brussel, WISE Research Group, Pleinlaan 2,
1050 Brussel, Belgium
{Olga.DeTroyer,Frederic.Kleinermann,Ahmed.Ewais}@vub.ac.be

Abstract. Virtual Reality (VR) is gaining in popularity and its added value for learning is being recognized. However, its richness in representation and manipulation possibilities may also become one of its weaknesses, as some learners may be overwhelmed and be easily lost in a virtual environment. Others may spend all their time on exploring features not relevant for their learning tasks. Therefore, being able to dynamically adapt the virtual environment to the personal preferences, prior knowledge, skills and competences, learning goals and the personal or social context in which the learning takes place becomes important. In this paper, we discuss possible adaptations and adaptation strategies for virtual learning environments. We also report on a prototype implementation of an adaptive Web-based virtual learning environment and the lessons learned from this.

Keywords: E-Learning, Virtual Reality, Adaptivity, Virtual World Learning Environment.

1 Introduction

Some material is easier to learn when it is visualized and when the learner can interact with it. Virtual Reality (VR) provides ways to use 3D visualizations with which the user can interact. For some learning situations and topics, VR may be of great value because the physical counterpart may not be available, too dangerous or too expensive. The most famous example is the flight simulator that pilots safely teach how to fly a plane in various circumstances. Another example where VR has been used successfully is the domain of medicines, e.g., to simulate operations or to study the human body. Virtual worlds (such as Second Life [1] and Active Worlds [2]) are complete 3D computer environments containing 3D (and possible also 2D) objects in which the user can navigate and interact with the objects. Usually, the objects may have different behaviors and users are presented by means of avatars. These virtual worlds are also called Virtual Environments (VE). In collaborative environments, such as Second Life, users can also meet each other and socialize.

G. Leitner, M. Hitz, and A. Holzinger (Eds.): USAB 2010, LNCS 6389, pp. 244–265, 2010.

For certain subjects and for certain types of learners using such a VE may be much more appealing and motivating that the use of classical learning material, e.g., to simulate the effect of physical laws (e.g. [3]); to simulate social environments and allow people to practice social skills; or to learn about history (e.g. [5], [6]).

However, the richness of such a Virtual Reality Learning Environment (VLE) can also become its weakness. The learner may be overwhelmed or get lost in the VLE [7], not knowing what to do first or next, or may be distracted too much and not be able to focus on the actual learning task. For people not familiar with VEs (novice users), the time required to get acquaint with such a VLE (i.e. learnability) may be long and therefore their short-term satisfaction may be low. On the other hand, youngsters used to play video games, may spend their time in activities not very much related to the learning activities, especially if they have low motivation for learning. This then results in a low effectiveness. These concerns are confirmed in [8]. The authors reported "novice student-players made quite a lot of navigational effort. This means that on average they had wasted quite a lot of their time trying to find their way in the virtual reality worlds and thus they had been left less time for reading the theory and answering questions that would help them extend and consolidate their knowledge", "virtual reality distractions were observed in many students' protocols but not to a great extent. The distractions occurred when users behaved as if they had forgotten what their ultimate goal was... Instead, they repeated actions without any particular meaning" and "one important finding is that the first two kinds of usability problem (user interface acquaintance and navigational effort) affect mostly the less experienced whereas the third kind of usability problem (virtual reality distractions) affects mostly the more experienced users". The authors concluded: "these findings show that all categories of user may benefit less than they could from the educational content of a VR-educational game due to usability problems. Thus the design of VR-game interfaces has to attract a lot of attention for the elimination or improvement of these three kinds of problem". Although, these results were obtained in the context of a VR-educational game (which is a special type of VLE) Dede et al. [6] made similar statements. They noted that students exhibit noticeable individual differences in their interaction styles, and abilities to interact with the 3-D environment. Furthermore, they observed that usability and learning are two goals that may conflict. Optimizing for usability may impede learning if it requires changes to the interface that rely on interactions or representations that are inappropriate for the learning task.

One way to solve these problems it by providing the VLE in an adaptive way, e.g., adapted to the individual learner and to the progress that he makes during the learning. Augmenting a VLE with adaptive capabilities has many advantages [9]. It could solve the difference between novice and more experienced used, but also adapt the VLE to other individual differences. For instance, it may be more effective to guide a learner through the VE according to his/her background and learning goals, or only show him/her the objects that are relevant for his/her current knowledge level, or adapt the environment to his/her learning style. It is also well known that cultural aspects influence the learning process [10], so adapting the VLE to the culture of the learner can also be important.

In this paper, we explain how a VLE can be dynamically adapted to an individual learner to better support the actual learning process and increase the usability. The actual creation of the VR learning material is not in the scope of the research.

With the success of application such as Second Life, Active Worlds, more and more VR material becomes available for free on the Web (e.g., in Google's 3D Warehouse [11]) and easy to use tools are available to create such material (e.g., Google SketchUp [12], 3D Studio Max [13]).

The rest of the paper is structured as follows. In section 2, we consider related work. Section 3 deals with possible adaptations in a VLE. In section 4, we give some adaptation strategies that can be used in an adaptive VLE to enhance usability. Section 5 presents the different approaches that can be used for an adaptive virtual reality learning system and the different components needed. In section 6, we report on a prototype adaptive virtual reality learning system implemented and on the lessons learned from this. Finally, section 7 presents conclusions and future work.

2 Related Work

In general, little research has been done in the context of usability of VLEs. Some work deals with the development of methods to investigate the usability of VEs (e.g., [14], [15]), which is not directly relevant for this paper. Other work investigated the usability of some individual VE, such as [6], [4], [7], [8]. No work has been found on investigating the usability of adaptive VR environments, neither on guidelines for using adaptive techniques in the context of VR learning environments. Some work deals with adaptation in 3D environments. We will review this work without being limited to the domain of E-learning.

Brusilovsky et al. [16] have integrated some adaptive hypermedia methods into virtual environments by developing an approach that supports different navigation techniques in the context of 3D E-Commerce. It matches the user needs for shopping by supporting different navigation techniques. This work is interesting because it has extended some of the adaptive hypermedia methods (such as direct guidance, hiding, sorting) to 3D environments.

Chittaro and Ranon have done quite some work in the context of adaptive VR. In 2000 [17], they have described how to introduce adaptation inside e-commerce. Their approach is called ADVIRT. A set of personalization rules exploits a model of the customer to adapt features of the VR store, such as the display of products through the concept of shelf, display spots and banners. They have also customized and personalized the navigation and different layouts of the store. In 2002 [18], they have introduced a software architecture for adaptive 3D web sites called Awe3D (Adaptive Web 3D) which can generate and deliver adaptive Virtual Reality Modeling language (VRML). This work targeted E-commerce and not E-learning. However it shows how 3D content can be personalized according to the user. In 2007 [19], the same authors has explained that adaptation can happen for navigation and interaction in order to help the users in finding and using information more efficiently. For navigation and interaction, they proposed direct guidance, hiding, sorting and annotation based on the work of Brusilovsky et al. [16].

The adaptations they propose, are derived by making an analogy with adaptive web-based hypermedia. We take a different approach. The types of adaptation what we propose are based on the different components that make up a VR environment. This results in a more elaborated set of adaptation types. Furthermore, Chittaro and Ranon suggested an alternative approach for sorting and annotation by using virtual characters that act as navigation guides to show users the path to an object of interest, and to provide annotations in the form of additional information on navigation and interaction possibilities. Finally, and based on their previous work [20], Chittaro and Ranon have extended the E-learning platform EVE [21]. They introduced Adaptive EVE that is tailored to the knowledge level of a student and to their preferred style of learning. To achieve adaptivity in the context of EVE, they have used the AHA! engine which was originally developed for adaptive hypermedia applications [22].

Santos and Osorio [23] have introduced another approach for adaptation in VR. Their approach is called AdapTIVE (Adaptive Three-dimensional Intelligent and Virtual Environment) and is based on agents, called Interactive and Virtual Agents that assist the users and help them to interact with the environment. They have applied their approach to E-commerce and Distance Learning systems.

Celentano and Pittarello [24] have developed an approach for adaptive navigation and interaction where a user's behavior is monitored in order to exploit the acquired knowledge for anticipating user's needs in forthcoming interactions. The approach uses "sensors" that tells when an object has been interacted with. These software sensors collect usage data and compare them with previous patterns of interaction. These patterns represent sequences of activities that users perform in some specific situation. Whenever the system detects that the user is entering a recurrent pattern of interaction, it may perform some activities of that pattern on behalf of the user.

Daschelt et al. [25] have developed an approach that provides adaptation to the user's device. Their approach suggests different alternatives with respect to the screen space usage for the same 3D interface element and information presented. Furthermore, 3D content is also considered in media adaptation. For instance, they describe a showcase where the seat capacity of a conference room can be adapted. This work is more on adapting the content for large audience.

In the ELEKTRA project [26], an EU-project aiming to bridge the gap between cognitive theory, pedagogy and gaming practices, a framework for adaptive interventions in educational games was introduced. They introduce a difference between macro- and microadapativity. Macroadapativity refers to traditional techniques of adaptation such as adaptive presentation and adaptive navigation. Microadaptivity is adaptation within learning tasks. Microadaptivity affects only the presentation of a learning object or a learning situation. It is achieved without compromising the learner's gaming experience. For this they use an adaptation system that provides recommendations to the game engine, but it is the ultimate decision of the game engine to whether or not to enact a recommendation. This approach was also followed in the 80Days project, the successor of ELEKTRA. Pedagogically, this project is grounded in the framework of self-regulated personalized learning which propagates the importance of self-regulation [27].

3 Adaptation in Virtual Reality Environments

There are many definitions of Virtual Environments (VE) or Virtual Reality (VR) [28]. In the context of this research, we focus on desktop VR, which can be defined as a three-dimensional computer representation of a space, displayed on screen, in which users can move their viewpoints freely in real time and perform several actions.

Before we discuss how a VE (and more in particular a Virtual Learning Environment VLE) can be adapted, we first discuss the different components of a VE:

1. The scene and the objects

The scene corresponds to the 3D space in which the objects are located. It contains lights, viewpoints and cameras. Furthermore, it has also some properties that apply to all the objects being located inside the 3D space. For instance, gravity can be a property that applies to all its objects. The objects are usually 3D, but there can also be 2D objects in the 3D space. They have a visual representation with color and material properties, a size, a position in the world, and an orientation. Special objects, so-called avatars, are used to represent the user(s) in the 3D space. The user's avatar can be represented explicitly (by an object) or implicitly in which case the viewpoint of the camera is used to show the user's position.

2. **Behaviors**

The objects may have behaviors. Behaviors may reflect real life behaviors. For instance, objects may be able to move, rotate, change size, transform, and so on. An avatar is an object with behavior. Usually, avatars can walk, run, and sometimes even fly through the 3D space. Navigation trough the 3D space is achieved by the behavior of the user's avatar. In general, the 3D space also contains objects without behavior.

3. User Interaction

In a VE, the user is able to interact with the objects. For example, a user may pick up an object and drag it to some other place in the space (if the object is moveable). User interaction can also trigger behavior, e.g., clicking on an object may start a behavior. User interaction may be achieved by means of a regular mouse and keyboard or through special hardware such as a 3D mouse or data gloves [30].

4. Communication

Nowadays, more and more VEs are also collaborative environments in which remote users can interact with each other, e.g., talk or chat to each other or perform activities together. For some learning situations, e.g., practicing social skills, this can be an important requirement.

5. Sound

A VE usually also involves sound. Sound can be important in simulations, to enhance the feeling of reality or simply to simulate some sound. Sound/speech can also be used as an instruction and feedback mechanism during the learning process.

A VE can be adapted in many different ways. In principle, adaptation can happen for each of the components of a VE. An adaptation can be limited to a single component of the VE, but it can also involve many different components. We will first describe adaptations that apply on single component, i.e. on objects, behaviors, interaction, and for avatars. We call these *adaptation types*. For the moment, we didn't consider any adaptations types yet for the scene or for sound. Communication is also not considered because we focus on single-user VLEs. Next, in section 4, we will consider more high-level adaptations that involve more than one component. These we called *adaptation strategies*. In this paper, we particular focus on adaptation strategies for VLEs. To express the adaptation types and adaptation strategies, formal instructions have been developed but they are omitted here; we only describe them informally.

3.1 Adaptation Types for Objects

Objects populating the VLE have a visual appearance in terms of a geometry (shape) and material properties (colors and textures). To enhance the usability of a VLE for a learner, it may be advisable to change the visual appearance of an object during the lifetime of the VLE. We illustrate this with some examples. To visually indicate that an object has not yet been studied we may want to highlight it, make it smaller or even hide it. When a student is learning about an object being represented in the VLE, the visual appearance of the object could change according to the aspects being studied, for instance when studying a planet, it would be interesting to adapt the representation of the planet to the aspect considered, like its internal composition, or its atmosphere. It may also be useful that the visual representation of an object becomes more detailed while more and more knowledge is acquired. For instance, the planet Saturn can be shown first with its rings. Once the user has read enough on Saturn and its satellites, the satellites inside the rings of Saturn can be shown as well.

Therefore, a first set of adaptation types for objects is concerned with the adaptation of the visualization of an object, i.e. how to display it and how to hide it:

- *semiDisplay* is used to display the object in a semi-manner, by having a semi-transparent bounding box around it. See figure 1(a) for an example: the Sun has been semi-hided.
- *changeSize* is used to change the size of an object.
- *changeMaterialProperties* is used to change the material properties (color or texture) of an object. Figure 1(b) shows the sun with a different texture than in figure 1(a).
- *changeVRRepresentation* is used to change the visual representation of an object completely; its current visualization will be replaced by a different one.

- *semiHide* allows to make the visual appearance of objects semi-hidden. This is similar as the semiDisplay but the purpose is slightly different, i.e. hiding instead of displaying.
- *hide* allows hiding an object visually.
- *display* allows displaying an object that has been hidden before.

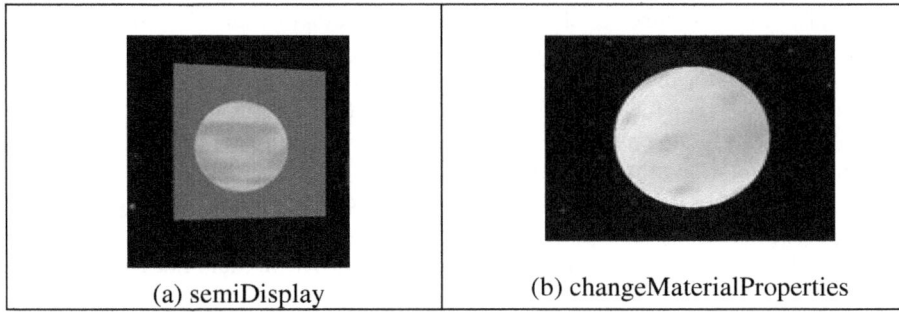

(a) semiDisplay   (b) changeMaterialProperties

Fig. 1.

Furthermore, like in classical textual learning material, it may be useful to mark objects. A reason for marking an object is for instance to draw the attention of the learner that the material associated with the object has (or has not yet) been studied or to indicate the importance of the object. In a VLE, marking an object can be done in different ways. We distinguish two different adaptation types for marking because they are essentially different:

- *spotlight* allows to mark an object by putting a spotlight on it; in this way the object becomes more visible and can be used to draw the attention to this object. Figure 2(a) shows an illustration of the planet earth with a red spotlight.

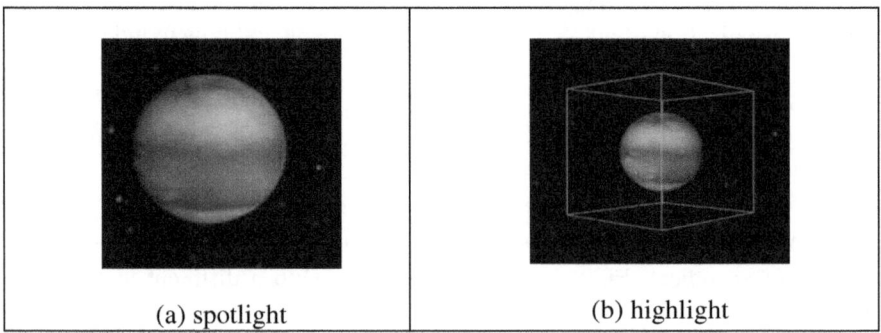

(a) spotlight   (b) highlight

Fig. 2.

- *highlight* allows to mark an object by drawing a box around the object where only the edges of the box are displayed. Figure 2(b) shows the planet earth being highlighted. The size of the box and the color of the edges can be specified.

Note that marking is considered different from changing the material properties (like the color) of an object, as by marking we don't change any property of the object. Also note that adding a title or a name to a VR object is not considered as marking, but as annotation. In general, annotations can be used to attach explanations, comments or names to objects. Annotations should only be shown when appropriate for the learning process as otherwise it might clutter the VLE too much. In addition, it may be necessary to adapt the annotations to the profile of the learner. Therefore, adaptation types are defined for adding and hiding annotations:

- *displayAnnotation* allows displaying an annotation with an object. An example is show in figure 3.
- *hideAnnotation* allows hiding an annotation associated with an object.

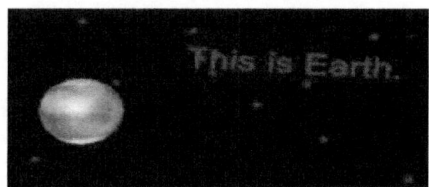

Fig. 3. DisplayAnnotation

3.2   Adaptation Types for Behaviors

Behaviors are used to make the VLE dynamic, i.e. to create environments where objects are active by performing some behaviors. For instance, in a VLE for the solar system we can have planets that are rotating and comets that move through the universe. However, to guide the learning process it may be useful to disable and enable behaviors when appropriate, e.g., a solar system where all planets are rotating at the same time may be confusing for a beginner. It may also be useful to adapt the parameters of a behavior, for instance to show the behavior of the sun with a different value for its temperature. Possible adaptation types for behaviors are:

- *enableBehavior* allows enabling a behavior associated with an object.
- *disableBehavior* allows disabling a behavior associated with an object.
- *changeBehavior* allows changing a behavior by modifying the values of its parameters.

3.3 Adaptation Types for User Interactions

In a VE, there are different ways to interact with an object, e.g., by clicking on it, by touching it, by passing closed. Furthermore, interaction (e.g., clicking) can trigger the start (or end) of a behavior. In the context of a VLE, it may be useful to control the user interaction. For example, to not overload the learner, we may want to prohibit interaction with an object as long as the learner has not obtained a certain level of knowledge. The enabling of an interaction possibility could also be used as a kind of reward after some successful study, and disabling interaction after some time could avoid spending too much time with some appealing feature.

Adapting interaction comes down to *enabling* or *disabling* some type(s) of interaction provided for an object. Possible interaction types considered for objects are: touching, clicking, and passing by.

3.4 Adaptation Types for Avatars

Avatars play a special role in a VLE. The avatar of the user is used to provide the view of the user inside the VLE. The avatar can have the look of a person, but other types of representation are also possible. As already explained, sometimes the avatar does not have a representation. Furthermore, an avatar has behaviors that allow the avatar to progress inside the VLE (i.e. navigate), for instance, jumping and walking. *Jumping* means going from one point to the next by making jumps. *Walking* means going from one point to the next smoothly and by following a certain path. Note that other behaviors are also possible like *flying*. An adaptation type *adaptAvatar* is defined to change the representation and/or the behavior for an avatar.

4 Adaptation Strategies for VR Learning Environments

In the previous section, we have discussed possible adaptations for individual components (object, behavior, interaction, …) of a VE. In this section, we deal with adaptations that go beyond the adaptation of a single component. These adaptations can have an impact on several components of the VE or on a part of the VE. We call them *adaptation strategies*, as they can be used as pre-defined strategies to adapt a VE. We focus in particular on adaptation strategies for learning purposes.

A first group of adaptation strategies defined are those that will have an impact on how the learner can navigate through the VLE:

- *restrictedNavigation* allows restricting the navigation of the learner to some of the objects in the scene. In other words, the learner will only be able to navigate from one object to the next object in a given list of objects. Furthermore, the navigation can be restricted to a particular navigation behavior, e.g., junping or waking. To specify the objects allowed to navigate to, different selection criteria can be used. For instance, it could be useful to select objects based on the learner's knowledge, or based on pre-requisite relations between objects. In general, this adaptation strategy can be used to force a learner to visit only a pre-defined number of objects.

- *navigationWithRestrictedBehavior* allows restricting the possible behaviors of objects while navigating. The restricted behavior can apply on all objects (in the VLE) or on a specified list of objects. This strategy is for instance useful to allow a learner to first explore a VLE (or a part of it) without being annoyed by objects showing all kinds of behavior; afterwards when he is more familiar with the VLE behavior can be enabled (using another adaption strategy).
- *navigationWithRestrictedInteraction* allows restricting the possible interactions with some objects while navigating. Similar as for navigationWithRestrictedBehavior, this adaptation strategy can be used to allow a learner to first explore the VLE (or a part of it) without being able to fully interact with the objects in the scene.
- *TourGuide* provides a tour guide to the learner. A tour guide takes the learner through a tour in a VLE. Like in real life, a tour guide can provide an easy and efficient way to learn quickly some essential facts about objects in a large and unknown VLE.
- The following adaptation strategies allow specifying that the learner can navigate freely in the VLE, with or without suggestions (*freeWithSuggestions* and *completelyFree*). Suggesting is done by using marking (i.e. spotlight or highlight). This strategy can be used to give the learner a lot of freedom but still provide some guidance.

A second group of adaptation strategies allow adapting a group of objects:

- *filterObjects* allows to filter the objects that should be available (visible) in the VLE. This strategy can be used to avoid that the learner doesn't know on which objects to focus first. It also allows gradually building the VLE; the more knowledge the learner obtains the more objects become visible.
- *markObjects* allows to mark (i.e. by highlight or spotlight) a number of objects in the VLE. This adaptation strategy can be used as an alternative to the filterObjects. In some situations it may not be possible (or not desirable) to hide objects (e.g., if we want to show the connections and dependencies of a complex system). Also, some learners may find it annoying that not all objects are visible or may perceive the VLE not attractive anymore. The strategy can also be used to mark the objects already studied.

A next group of adaptation strategies are strategies to specify some conditions for displaying objects:

- *displayAtMost* allows to specify when some objects should not be displayed anymore. The condition can be some pedagogical criteria like the knowledge level the learner currently has for the object or a limit on the number of times that the object should be displayed. This strategy can for instance be useful if the purpose is to perform some tests without having the subject(s) of the study visible.

- *displayAfter* allows to specify the condition(s) that need to be satisfied for objects to be displayed. This adaptation strategy can for instance be used to keep the VLE appealing by dynamically changing the objects in the scene. This can avoid that the learner gets bored.

The next group of adaptation strategies consists of strategies for adapting the behavior of some objects conditionally:

- *behaviorAtMost* allows to specify when a behavior should be disabled. This adaptation strategy can for instance be used to avoid that the learner keeps "playing" with an object or a number of objects having the same behavior.
- *behaviorAfter* allows to indicate when a certain behavior of an object (or some objects) should be executed. This adaptation strategy can for instance be use to state that the behavior for some specific objects should only start when the knowledge level of the learner for these objects is above a certain threshold.
- *behaviorSpeed* allows to specify the speed of a behavior. This is in particular useful when the behavior simulates a real world behavior. Being able to slow down the behavior will allow the learner to better observe what is happing, especially for behaviors that are happing very fast in real time (e.g., an explosion, or the trajectory followed by a bullet).

The last group of adaptation strategies contains strategies for limiting the interaction with some objects by means of a condition: *interactionAtMost* and *interactionAfter*.

The adaptation strategies presented here are only a subset of possible adaptation strategies. It is not our aim (and it would also not be possible) to define all possible adaptation strategies, but to provide a set of adaptation strategies that is useful in adaptive VLEs. It is of course possible to define a new adaptation strategy if there is a need for.

5   Driving the Adaptation in a VR Learning Environment

In the previous two sections we have provide the ingredients for making VLEs adaptive. In this section, we discuss how to actually drive the adaptation process and how this differs from the adaptation process of a regular learning environment. Similar as for an adaptive learning system, there are three different approaches: an author-driven approach, a teacher-driven approach and a model-driven approach.

In the *author-driven approach*, the author of the course is given full control over the adaptation process. During the design of the course, the author needs to specify the adaptations explicitly, e.g., through rules. This gives the control to the author but also requires that the author keeps track, at design time, of all possible adaptation scenarios, which may be hard. The alternative is to have some kind of automatic adaptation. This is what we call a *model-driven approach*, as the adaptation process is then driven at run-time by means of adaptation models and/or intelligent algorithms. The models and algorithms can be engineered in advance or be based on advanced AI techniques [29, 30, 31]. This approach is used in so-called intelligent tutoring systems [32]. Although, it relieves the work of the author, it inevitably also introduces intransparency. The author does not know in advance how the VLE will be adapted. The last approach, the *teacher-driven approach*, is similar to the author-driven approach in the sense that it is human-driven but the specification of the required adaptation is done at run-time, i.e. while the learner is in action. This has the advantage that the teacher can respond to the particular situation of the learner and don't need to preview all possible adaptation scenario's, but it has the big disadvantage that the learning need to be supervised by a teacher which is in general too time consuming. This approach is therefore not used a lot.

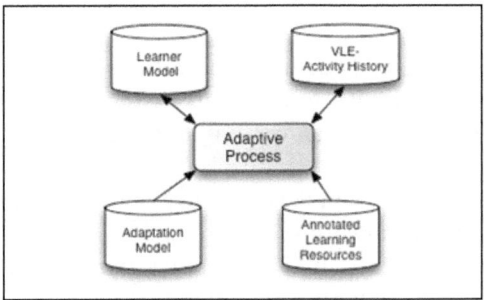

Fig. 4. Adaptation Models

What every approach is used, it requires a set of models to drive the adaptation process [33]. The models needed to drive the adaptive process in case of VR are illustrated in figure 4. First of all, it is necessary to assign attributes to the learning content, such as the level of difficulty, pre-requisites, learning time required (see e.g., the IEEE 1484.12.1 – 2002 Standard for Learning Object Metadata (LOM) for an elaborated set of such meta data). This information is needed to be able to adapt the content to the learning goals and to the learner. To adapt content to the learner, it is also necessary to have information about the learner (personal preferences, background knowledge, etc) and to keep track of his/her learning progress at runtime. This is usually done through the use of a *user-profile*, a *user model*, or *learner model*. In general, meta data for learning objects and user data are the two main models required for driving the adaptation process. However, in case of a VLE, it is also necessary to keep track at runtime of what is happing in the virtual world. For instance, to be able to use some of the adaptation strategies mentioned in section 4, it is necessary to keep track of the objects with which the learner has interacted, or which behaviors have been performed, or the time spent with a certain object or in a certain part of the VLE. For example, to be able to perform the adaptations associated with the adaptation strategy *displayAtMost*, the system needs to keep track of how often the object has already been displayed to the learner. We call this information *VLE activity history*. The more information is kept about the activities of the learner in the VLE, the more it can be taken into account to adapt the VLE to the individual learner. Note that some data from this VLE activity history will also impact the state of the learner model, for instance activities performed in the VLE by the learner may raise his knowledge level of a certain topic.

6   Prototype and Lessons Learned

To be able to experiment with the adaptive VLEs, we developed a prototype implementation for the approach. This prototype implementation is based on an existing Web-based adaptive learning environment [34], developed in the context of an EU FP7 STREP called GRAPPLE. GRAPPLE is using an author-driven approach for specifying the adaptations.

Therefore, we have also followed this approach in our prototype. As the learning environment is Web-based, the VR format supported is X3D [36]. The actual delivery of the adaptive VE is done using an existing VR player Vivaty [37] inside a Web browser.

We will now briefly elaborate on the different components of this prototype and on lessons learned in developing and using this prototype.

The two main components of GRAPPLE are the *Authoring Tool* and the *Adaptive Delivery Environment*. The Authoring Tool allows a course author to define a course. Therefore, the author needs to define a *Domain Model* and a *Conceptual Adaptation Model* [35]. The Domain Model describes the concepts that should be considered in the course. Learning resources are associated with these learning concepts. The Conceptual Adaptation Model expresses at a high-level how the content and structure needs to be adapted at runtime. The kernel of the Adaptive Delivery Environment is the *Adaptive Engine*. Based on the state of the learner's profile (captured in the *User Model*) and the specifications given in the Authoring Tool, the Adaptive Engine will select the proper learning resources and deliver the required navigation structure and content to a Web browser. Also note that the Adaptive Engine can keep track of the progress of the learner and will inform the User Model of this. Updates in the User Model may trigger new adaptation rules specified in the Conceptual Adaptation Model and in this way the course will be adapted at run-time. In GRAPPLE, the control over de User Model is left to the author, i.e. the author can decided which information to maintain in the User Model and how and which learning activities should update that information. GRAPPLE also allows importing information about the learner from external learning management systems (see [34]).

In order to support adaptive VR, it was necessary to extent GRAPPLE. GRAPPLE is a web-based learning environment using XML for the learning resources. Therefore, for displaying VR inside a browser, X3D [36] (which is XML-based) can be used. However, to support adaptive VR, two extensions were necessary. To be able to allow authors to specify how adaptation should happen inside a VLE an adapted authoring tool was necessary. Next, an extension of the adaptive delivery environment was needed to allow for the actual adaptive delivery of the VE, i.e. adapting the presentation of the objects, enabling and disabling behaviors and interaction, including objects conditionally, and/or providing dedicated navigation possibilities in the virtual world. We will not discuss the extension of the adaptive delivery, as this was rather a technical issue, but we do mention difficulties encountered when extending the authoring tool, as they are more at the level of usability. We also discuss an example adaptive VLE elaborated with the prototype. We end this section with some conclusions.

6.1 Authoring the Adaptation

For the authoring tool, we started by following the authoring approach of GRAPPLE. Let us start by briefly explaining this approach (more information can be found in [35]). GRAPPLE allows an author to specify the required adaptation using *pedagogical based adaptation rules*. We illustrate this concept with an example, a "prerequisite" adaptation rule. This adaptation rule is based on the pedagogical relationship "prerequisite" that may exist between topics (concepts) in a course. This adaptation rule specifies that if concept A is a prerequisite for concept B, the course material for concept B should be hidden as long as the knowledge level for concept A is not above a certain threshold (details are omitted).

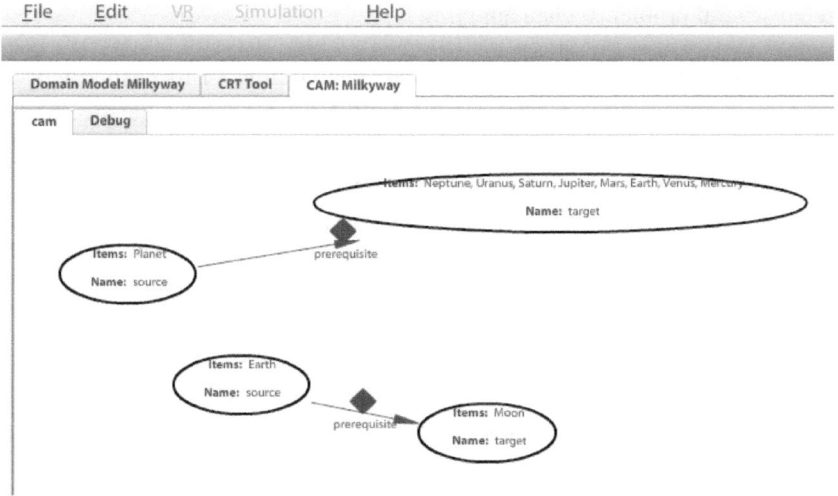

Fig. 5. GRAPPLE Adaptation Rules Examples

Important to know is that those rules are predefined. To be reusable in different courses, they are defined in a generic way, i.e. using placeholders for the different concepts.

In the Conceptual Adaptation Model, the author can then use (i.e. instantiate) such an adaptation rule by filling in the placeholders with concrete concepts (from the Domain Model). For instance, the author can specify that the learning material for concept "Earth" should be hidden as long as the learner doesn't have enough knowledge about the concept "Planet" by using this "prerequisite" adaptation rule. In this case, the author instantiate this adaptation rule by replacing the placeholders by the concepts "Planet" and "Earth". Figure 5 shows an example. It is a screenshot of the GRAPPLE authoring tool. In this tool, a graphical notation is used for the adaptation rules. On the canvas, we see two applications of the "prerequisite" rule. The upper one states that the concept Planet is prerequisite for the concepts Neptune, Uranus, Saturn, Jupiter, Mars, Earth, Venus, and Mercury. The lower one states that the concept Earth is a prerequisite for the concept Moon.

In the Conceptual Adaptation Model, the adaptation rules are given in an order-independent way. It is actually GRAPPLE's adaptive engine that will figure out when to use which adaptation rule (based on the conditions in the rules). In addition, it is also the adaptation engine that selects the most appropriate learning resource for a concept. For instance, a learner with no or low knowledge of the concept "Planet" should be given an "introductory" learning resource for the concept "Planet". The selection is done by matching the meta data of the learning objects with the ones required by the adaptation rules. Actually the exact content of the course is composed on the fly by the adaptation engine. So, GRAPPLE is using a declarative approach for specifying an adaptive course. This is a powerful approach, as the author of a course only needs to specify the desired results and not how this needs to be achieved. Although, at first sight this declarative approach looked applicable for VLEs, we encountered several problems when applying it:

1. The first problem that we encounter is that adaptation in VLEs cannot be specified at the level of concepts (as done in GRAPPLE) but needs to be specified at the level of individual concepts, behaviors, and so on. While in a classical text-oriented learning environment it is easy to compose a page by combining different pieces of text or adapt a page by replacing one piece of text by another, this is not straightforward in a VLE. Indeed, let's go back to the example of the planets. There may be different 3D representations of Earth (being possible learning resources for the concept "Earth"), however they may not all fit in a given VLE. They may be too large or too small or the texture used may not be appropriate. The same applies for behaviors. It is not always possible to replace one behavior by another. Therefore it is not possible to let the adaptive engine autonomous replaces VR resources, and it is certainly not possible to let the adaptive engine compose the actual VLE as all 3D objects should fit together and need to be positioned and oriented in the 3D space with care. It is even not possible to leave the selection of the appropriate learning resources to the adaptive engine as currently the meta data used for the learning objects is not capable to specify 3D specific issues (such as size, texture, etc.) needed to be able to do an appropriate selection. This forced us to adapt the format of the adaptations rules to make it possible to use them at the

level of the individual resources. More in particular, instead of having placeholders for concepts, we need placeholders for the combination concept, resource.

2. Next, there are much more possibilities for adapting a VLE (see section 3) than for adapting a text-based course. To be able to allow authors to fully exploit all these possibilities, it would be necessary to predefine a large set of pedagogical based adaptation rules. Actually, a rule needs to be predefined for each possible combination of pedagogical situation and adaptation technique. While for text or figures, there are only a few adaptation techniques for indicating a pre-requisite relation (i.e. hiding or make it inaccessible), there are plenty of possibilities in a VLE (hiding, semi-hiding, changing size, disabling behaviors, disabling interaction, using marking, etc.). This means that while for text-based adaption, there will only be two adaptation rule associated with the pre-requisite relation, there can be many more adaptations rules associate with this pre-requisite relation in case of VLEs. It is easy to see, that already for only a few pedagogical situations, providing a generic adaptation rule for each possible combination would result in a large and unwieldy set of predefined adaptation rules.

3. Another important obstacle was the fact that in the Conceptual Adaptation Model, the adaptation rules are specified in an order independent way. This was confusing for authors of a VLE as they usually have a certain storyline in mind that they want the learner to follow. For instance, in case of a course about the solar system (see section 6.3 for this example), an author wanted to start by taking the learner on a tour though the VLE representing the solar system, then he wanted to allow the learner to study the generic concepts Sun, Planet and Satellite. During that phase, all behavior and interaction would be disabled. While studying such a concept (e.g., Planet), examples of the concept (Earth, Mars, Venus, …) would be marked. Next, he wanted the student to study about the inner solar system and then he would remove all objects not belonging to this inner solar system. In a similar way, he would allow to learner to study the outer solar system, and so on. Unfortunately, it was rather impossible for the author to specify this scenario using the approach used in GRAPPLE because it doesn't allow to specify adaptations in an order dependent way. Complex and artificial conditions were needed to realize this.

6.2 Example VLE

To test the prototype, an example adaptive VLE has been developed. The VLE is part of a course on the solar system. The course is a combination of textual learning material about the solar system and a VLE of the solar system where the sun and different planets are displayed in 3D. The textual material is displayed in one frame of the browser where the learner can navigate through the textual material using standard

navigation, i.e. a menu and hyperlinks. He is also able to navigate (using VR navigation techniques) through the VLE displayed in another frame (see figure 6). Using the
Conceptual Adaptation Model, the author has specified how the VLE should adapt
according to the learner's knowledge level.

As already explained in section 6.1, the authoring of the adaptation was not easy.
However, we were able to show that the VLE could be adapted dynamically based on
the User Model, the VLE-activity history and the Conceptual Adaptation Model. For
instance, we specified that at the start the names of the planets familiar to the learner
should be in green, and the names of the planets that the learner still needs to study
should be in red. Then the learner can start the course and he will be presented with a
classical menu in the left panel of the browser window and an empty VLE (complete
black). If he clicks on the Sun-link, a textual explanation of the sun will be displayed
in the text frame. It was specified in the Conceptual Adaptation Model that the text
describing the sun should be extended each time the learner visit the Sun-page, and
once the learner has seen the complete textual explanation, a 3D model of the sun will
be displayed inside the VLE (see figure 6). The other planets will appear in the same
way. Furthermore, planets that are studied completely will stop rotating. When all
planets have been studied, the learner will see the complete solar system in the VLE
and is able to explore it freely.

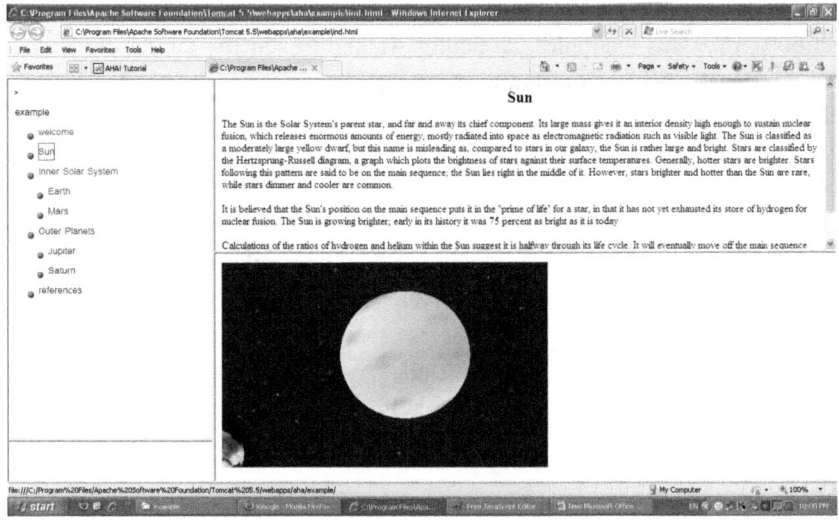

Fig. 6. Example Course

Below are some examples of adaptation rules used in the prototype. To make it
easier for the reader, we are not using the format of GRAPPLE, but we have expressed the rules as if-then rules.

The first example is a rule that specifies that if the user's knowledge for the concept Earth is above the minimal required level (which is expressed by means of an integer value), then the VR object Earth should be highlighted in the VLE. The goal of this adaptation is to draw the attention of the learner to the fact that he reached the required minimal level of knowledge for Earth.

Example adaptation rules:
if (user_knowledge (Earth) > min_required)
then { highlight(Earth)}

if ((user_knowledge(Earth) > min_required)
*   AND (hasInteractedWith(Earth) > 3)*
*   then { spotlight(Mars), Annotate(Mars), behaviour(AroundOrbit, Mars)}*

The second rule is to state that if the user's knowledge for the concept Earth is above the minimal required level and he has interacted with the planet Earth more than 3 times, then a spotlight should be set on the VR-object Mars, a certain annotation should be displayed with it, and it should start to move around the sun. The goal of this adaptation is to draw the attention to the next subject to study.

6.3   Conclusions for the Prototype

Because the adaptations that we could specify with the current authoring approach are limited and also cumbersome to achieve (see section 6.1), we decide to postpone the planned evaluation of the adaptive VLE itself. We found it not useful to set up an elaborated experiment with end-users to validate the usability of an adaptive VLE when we are not satisfied with the type of adaptations that can be specified (and therefore achieved). Therefore we decided to first work on an improve approach for authoring the adaptation. In that approach, it will be possible for the author to compose a time-based storyline. Furthermore, we will opt for adaptation rules that are easier to understand by an author by untangle the pedagogical aspects (the conditions) from the adaptation effects, and which the authors themselves can compose (hence removing the need for predefined adaptation rules). Figure 7 shows a screenshot of this new authoring tool. The scenario modeled in this figure is as follows. The course starts by marking the VR object Earth, and then it will start rotating around its axis. Once this VR object is rotating and the user has interacted with it by clicking on it, the VR object Earth will start to move around its orbit. If now, the user interacts again with Earth it will be unmarked and instead the VR object Mars will be marked and the viewpoint of the user will be moved towards Mars. Note that this scenario doesn't have any pedagogical meaning but was only created to verify the feasibility of the authoring approach. The squares with the letters AB denote Adaptations Blocks. They are used to specify the adaptations required for the different VR objects.

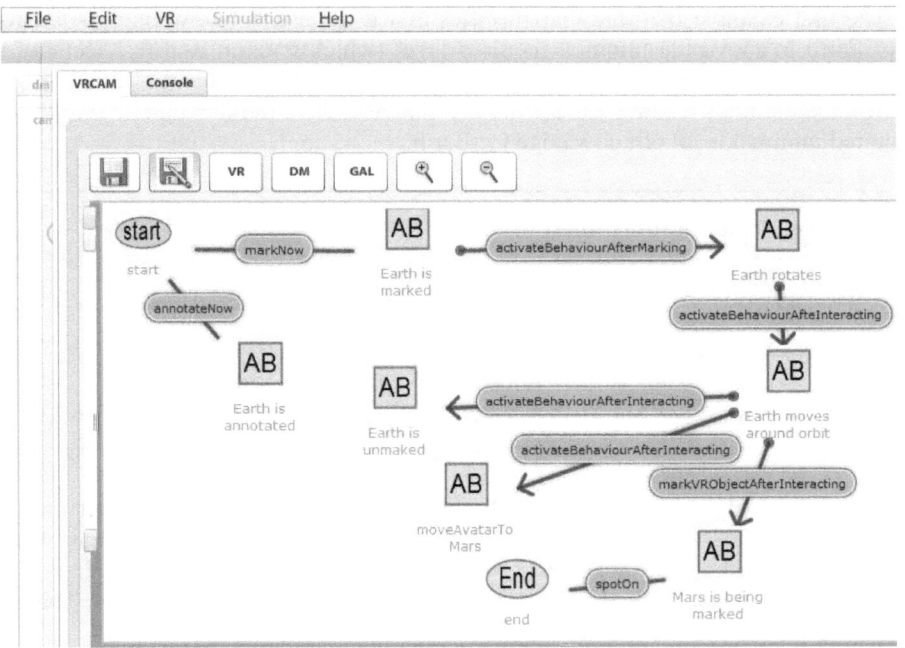

Fig. 7. Time-based Authoring Approach

Once we have finished the prototype for this authoring approach, we will perform an empirical evaluation to study the usability both of the author tools and an actual virtual learning environment. In a first phase, the evaluation will be rather exploratory with the aim of identifying weaknesses and gathering ideas for recommendations for improvement. Later, an explicit, experimental comparison will be performed to measure user acceptance and the impact of adaptively on the actual learning process.

7   Conclusions and Future Work

We have discussed the potential of adaptivity for VR learning environments. As in classical, text-based learning environments, adaptivity could be used to adapt a VR learning environment to the individual characteristics and preferences of the learners, their background, learning goals etc. However, the richness of Virtual Reality allows much more possibilities for adaptations than possible in a classical text-based learning environment. Therefore, we introduced a set of adaptation types for VR, as well as a set of adaptation strategies specific for VR learning environments. Next, we presented the different models needed for the adaptive process. We also discussed a prototype implementation of an adaptive VR learning system. The prototype is based on an existing Web-based adaptive learning environment that is author-driven (meaning that the author of a course specifies at design time the required adaptations) and its authoring tool uses a declarative approach, based on pedagogical-based adaptation rules. This turned out to be quite difficult for authors of virtual learning environments. First of all, it was difficult to realize a storyline (often used in the virtual environments). Next, the richness of the adaptations possibilities for VR resulted in a large and unmanageable set of pedagogical-based adaptation rules. This was due to the fact that in the approach used, the pedagogical issues and adaptations types are entangled in a single adaptation rule. Therefore, we are currently working on a different authoring approach using a time-based storyline and adaptation rules that are easier to express. Next, an empirical evaluation will be performed to study the usability both of the author tools and an actual virtual learning environment.

Acknowledgments. The work described in this paper is realized in the context of the EU FP7 project GRAPPLE (215434).

References

1. Second Life, http://secondlife.com
2. Active Worlds, http://www.activeworlds.com/
3. Dede, C., Salzman, M., Loftin, B.: The Development of a Virtual World for Learning Newtonian Mechanics. In: Brusilovsky, P., Kommers, P., Streitz, N. (eds.) MHVR 1994. LNCS, vol. 1077, pp. 87–106. Springer, Heidelberg (1996)
4. Cobb, S.V.G., Neale, H.R., Reynolds, H.: Evaluation of virtual learning environments. In: Proceedings of the 2nd European Conference on Disability, Virtual Reality & Assoc. Tech., Skövde, Sweden, ECDVRAT and University of Reading, UK, pp. 17–23 (1998)
5. Di Blas, N., Paolini, P., Poggi, C.: SEE (Shrine Educational Experience): an Online Cooperative 3D Environment Supporting Innovative Educational Activities. In: Lassner, D., McNaught, C. (eds.) Proceedings of Educational Multimedia, Hypermedia and Telecommunications 2003, pp. 1527–1534. AACE, Chesapeake (2003)
6. Dede, C., Ketelhut, D.J., Ruess, K.: Motivation, usability, and learning outcomes in a prototype museum-based multi-user virtual environment. In: Bell, P., Stevens, R., Satwicz, T. (eds.) Keeping Learning Complex: The proceedings of the Fifth International Conference of the Learning Sciences. Erlbaum, Mahwah (2002)
7. Bricken, M., Byrne, C.M.: Summer students in virtual reality: A Pilot Study on Educational Applications of Virtual Reality Technology. In: Wexelblat, A. (ed.) Virtual Reality: Applications and Exploration, pp. 199–218. Academic Press, Inc., New York (1993)
8. Virvou, M., Katsionis, G.: On the usability and likeability of virtual reality games for education: The case of VR-ENGAGE. Computers & Education 50(1), 154–178 (2008)
9. Chittaro, L., Ranon, R.: Adaptive Hypermedia Techniques for 3D Educational Virtual Environments. IEEE Intelligent Systems 22(4), 31–37 (2007)
10. Mushtaha, A., De Troyer, O.: Cross-cultural understanding of content and interface in the context of e-learning systems. In: Aykin, N.M. (ed.) HCII 2007. LNCS, vol. 4559, pp. 164–173. Springer, Heidelberg (2007)
11. Google 3D Warehouse, http://sketchup.google.com/3dwarehouse
12. Google SketchUp, http://sketchup.google.com
13. Murdock, K.L.: 3ds max 5 bible. Wiley Publishing, Chichester (2003)
14. Bowman, D., Gabbard, J., Hix, D.: A Survey of Usability Evaluation in Virtual Environments: Classification and Comparison of Methods. Presence: Teleoperators and Virtual Environments 11(4), 404–424 (2002)
15. Tromp, J.G., Steed, A., Wilson, J.R.: Systematic Usability Evaluation and Design Issues for Collaborative Virtual Environments. Presence 12(3), 241–267 (2003)

16. Brusilovsky, P., Hughes, S., Lewis, M.: Adaptive Navigation Support in 3-D E-Commerce Activities. In: Proceedings of Workshop on Recommendation and Personalization in eCommerce at the 2nd International Conference on Adaptive Hypermedia and Adaptive Web-Based Systems (AH 2002), Malaga, Spain, pp. 132–139 (2002)
17. Chittaro, L., Ranon, R.: Adding Adaptive Features to Virtual Reality Interfaces for E-Commerce. In: Brusilovsky, P., Stock, O., Strapparava, C. (eds.) AH 2000. LNCS, vol. 1892, pp. 86–97. Springer, Heidelberg (2000)
18. Chitttaro, L., Ranon, R.: Dynamic Generation of Personalized VRML Content: a General Approach and its Application to 3D E-Commerce. In: Proceedings of 7th International Conference on 3D Web Technology, Web3D 2002, pp. 145–154. ACM Press, New York (2002)
19. Chittaro, L., Ranon, R.: Adaptive 3D Web Sites. In: Brusilovsky, P., Kobsa, A., Nejdl, W. (eds.) Adaptive Web 2007. LNCS, vol. 4321, pp. 433–464. Springer, Heidelberg (2007)
20. Chittaro, L., Ranon, R.: Using the X3D Language for Adaptive Manipulation of 3D Web Content. In: De Bra, P.M.E., Nejdl, W. (eds.) AH 2004. LNCS, vol. 3137, pp. 287–290. Springer, Heidelberg (2004)
21. Chittaro, L., Ranon, R.: Adaptive Hypermedia Techniques for 3D Educational Virtual Environments. IEEE Intelligent Systems 22(4), 31–37 (2007)
22. Chittaro, L., Ranon, R.: An Adaptive 3D Virtual Environment for Learning the X3D Language. In: Proceedings of the 2008 International Conference on Intelligent User Interfaces (IUI 2008), pp. 419–420. ACM Press, New York (2008)
23. dos Santos, C.T., Osorio, F.S.: AdapTIVE: An Intelligent Virtual Environment and Its Application in E-Commerce. In: Proceedings of 28th Annual International Computer Software and Applications Conference (COMPSAC 2004), pp. 468–473 (2004)
24. Celentano, A., Pittarello, F.: Observing and Adapting User Behaviour in Navigational 3D interface. In: Proceedings of 7th International Conference on Advanced Visual Interfaces (AVI 2004), pp. 275–282. ACM Press, New York (2004)
25. Dachselt, R., Hanz, M., Meissner, K.: Contigra: an XML-based architecture for component-oriented 3D application. In: Proceedings of the 7th International Conference on 3D Web Technology, pp. 155–163. ACM Press, New York (2002)
26. Kickmeier-Rust, M.D., Peirce, N., Conclan, O., Schwarz, D., Verpoorten, D., Albert, D.: Immersive Digital Games: The Interfaces for Next-Generation E-Learning? In: Stephanidis, C. (ed.) HCI 2007. LNCS, vol. 4556, pp. 647–656. Springer, Heidelberg (2007)
27. Law, E.L.-C., Kickmeier-Rust, M.D.: 80Days: Immersive digital educational games with adaptive storytelling. In: Klamma, R., et al. (eds.) Proceedings of the First International Workshop on Story-Telling and Educational Games (STEG 2008) - The Power of Narration and Imagination in Technology Enhanced Learning (2008)
28. Gutierrez, M.A., Vexo, F., Thalmann, D.: Stepping into Virtual Reality: A Practical Approach. Springer, Heidelberg (2008)
29. Manslow, J.: Using Reinforcement Learning to solve AI Control Problems. In: Rabin, S. (ed.) AI Game Programming Wisdom, 2nd edn., pp. 591–603. Charles River Media, Inc., Hingham (2004)
30. Manslow, J.: Learning and Adaptation. In: Rabin, S. (ed.) AI Game Programming Wisdom, pp. 557–566. Charles River Media, Inc., Hingham (2002)
31. Funge, J.D.: AI for Games and Animation: A cognitive Modeling Approach. A K Peters, Ltd., Wellesley (1999)
32. Sleeman, D., Brown, J.S. (eds.): Intelligent Tutoring Systems. Academic Press, London (1982)

33. Paramythis, A., Loidl-Reisinger, S.: Adaptive Learning Environments and e-Learning Standards. Electronic Journal of e-Learning 2(1), 181–194 (2003)
34. De Bra, P., Smits, D., van der Sluijs, K., Christea, A., Hendrix, M.: GRAPPLE, Personalization and Adaptation in Learning Management Systems. In: ED-MEDIA, World Conference on Educational Multimedia, Hypermedia & Telecommunication (2010)
35. Hendrix, M., De Bra, P., Pechenizkiy, M., Smits, D., Cristea, A.: Defining adaptation in a generic multi layer model: CAM: The GRAPPLE Conceptual Adaptation Model. In: Dillenbourg, P., Specht, M. (eds.) EC-TEL 2008. LNCS, vol. 5192, pp. 132–143. Springer, Heidelberg (2008)
36. Brutzman, D., Daly, L.: X3D: Extensible 3D graphics for Web Authors. The Morgan Kaufmann Series in Interactive 3D Technology (2008)
37. Vivaty, http://www.vivaty.com/

Mobile Learning and Commuting: Contextual Interview and Design of Mobile Scenarios

Eva Patricia Gil-Rodríguez and Pablo Rebaque-Rivas

Learning Technologies Office
Universitat Oberta de Catalunya. Av. Tibidabo 39-43, 08035, Barcelona, Spain
{egilrod,prebaque}@uoc.edu

Abstract. This paper presents a case study on the design of mobile applications for on-line learning, based on the needs of its potential users. From the User-Centered Design (UCD) perspective and based on a qualitative approach, in-depth interviews have been held with students who carry out learning-related tasks in a commuting context, together with ethnographic observations of this context. The objective of this research was to understand the needs and requirements of students who learn on-line and who take advantage of their travel time to study or to carry out study-related tasks. Through the content analysis of the data gathered, the tasks carried out by students in a mobile context are contemplated, detecting their inconveniences and needs. From this analysis m-learning application scenarios have been built based on the potential users' requirements.

Keywords: UCD, m-learning, commuting, user studies, contextual inquiry, scenarios.

1 Introduction

In a setting where society is becoming more and more mobile and connected, m-learning has emerged over the last few years as a natural evolution of e-learning. Indeed, in recent times we have seen a profusion and availability of mobile devices on the market, together with the possibility of using these devices in contexts not confined to on-site classrooms, such as waiting time or travel.

In this sense, the main challenge of m-learning stems from the enormous potential that taking advantage of the combination "other contexts - mobile connection" for learning implies. The question is therefore to bring this potential closer to the reality of students and their study contexts.

Definitions of m-learning found in literature [1, 2, 3, 4, 5] attach importance to different aspects, such as: communication and conversation, type of device, context, availability, portability, learning process... among others. For example, in Lee and Chan [6, based on 7] we find attributes that mobile learning should have, specifically: spontaneous, personal, informal, contextual, portable, ubiquitous and pervasive. In Geddes [8] the advantages of mobile learning are given with regard to other learning methods, such as access, context, collaboration and appeal.

G. Leitner, M. Hitz, and A. Holzinger (Eds.): USAB 2010, LNCS 6389, pp. 266–277, 2010.
© Springer-Verlag Berlin Heidelberg 2010

These advantages have been compared in several studies, however, few were carried out in a pure e-learning context, or in other words, in a context in which all learning is carried out on-line. When looking through the bibliography the absence of research that relates the use of m-learning with an exclusively on-line education is notable and, more importantly, what its use could be in a commuting context.

The majority of research includes experiences of cases which study the suitability and possibilities of a mobile device (mobile or e-book) and/or a content used in an on-line context, but as part of or complementary to on-site learning [9, 10, 11, 12, 13]. Only in Lee and Chan [6] and Ramírez-Montoya [14] have we found experiences of the use of m-learning in exclusively on-line contexts. We maintain that, given its extreme characteristics, these entirely on-line learning contexts could be exemplary with regard to new technological m-learning uses.

On the other hand, and as stated in Ramírez-Montoya [14], one of the mobile learning challenges is the configuration of resources content. There has been a consensus in recent literature that m-learning should not substitute e-learning or traditional learning methods, but should expand and/or complete it [6, 15, 16, 17]. In addition, this content configuration should take into account contexts of mobile device use, and the requirements of users on a day-to-day basis. We agree with Rodríguez and Constantine [12] in that currently students are demanding more and more content that can be studied while commuting, waiting for someone or at the gym, however, there is also a lack of research that relates m-learning with the commuting context. We have only found references of this relation in de Jong [9] and Gil-Rodríguez and Planella-Ribera [18], where the use of e-books by students is researched and one of the positive evaluations made was the ability to use e-books when travelling.

The in-depth exploration of this relationship between commuting and m-learning is the main purpose of this paper, whose specific objectives and methodology are detailed below.

2 Study Objectives

The purpose of this case study [19] is to explore the relationship between m-learning and commuting, with a student profile that takes advantage of his/her travel time for activities related to his/her university learning. Therefore, the objective of this investigation was to understand the needs and requirements of these students who study and/or carry out study-related tasks whilst commuting. This objective means understanding the current behavioural patterns of students in their mobile contexts and discovering how new devices and materials used, such as e-reader devices, audios and mobile internet, can help support their studies. On the basis of these requirements, it is possible to define m-learning scenarios in a commuting context with a view to developing new applications for mobile devices.

Applying a user-centered design perspective [20], based on a description of personas [21] and student focus groups, it could be observed how the commuting context was a potential opportunity for reading (thanks to e-readers, tablets, etc) and for connecting to the virtual campus (thanks to mobile internet). This opened up the possibility of interviewing students as they commuted so as to explore and analyse these scenarios [20].

Therefore, the aim of interviewing students in their habitual commuting context was to discover what the study pattern of these students is in general and in particular during travel. In other words, how they organise their studies and what type of materials they use for studying in each one of their study contexts, at the same time as exploring the difficulties they currently encounter when carrying out a learning activity whilst travelling and how they think these can be resolved.

In addition, their opinion of e-reader devices, the possibility of having their teaching materials available on audio and the possibility of having internet connection on a mobile device is also sought after, as well as how they believe that all these options could affect or condition their current form of study and of carrying out their academic activities.

The purpose of doing the interviews on public transport was also to observe this context in-depth, to determine how the interviewee interacts with it and also to detect variables that could influence the student, such as the number of people, availability of seats, noise, etc, when carrying out a learning activity.

Once all this information was gathered, the ultimate objective was to describe a series of scenarios for m-learning applications in order to contribute to the design and development of mobile device-related solutions.

2.1 Methodology

Therefore, to gather the data, 7 in-depth interviews were carried out with students of the Open University of Catalonia (UOC) -a fully on-line, higher education institution- during their daily commute by train, metro or bus. The students interviewed were those who normally performed some kind of academic activity when commuting, mainly reading learning materials. Students who take advantage of travel to read or perform other activities associated with study are very typical in the UOC (internal document).

Using the "contextual inquiry" methodology [22] the student, in his/her travel context, is able to reflect and communicate more easily the daily nature, thus achieving more involvement, truthfulness and recall from the student. In addition, from the interviewer's point of view, an immersion in the natural situation in which the student develops his/her activities, is achieved. Therefore, they have access to their speech, practices and daily tasks, in situ, as well as other important aspects of the context which could be crucial to the design of applications.

We contacted students to ask if we could accompany them on a typical journey and interview them. We arranged to meet the students, for example, at an underground station, and conducted the interview as we accompanied them to their destination. The 7 journeys were as follows: 4 longer journeys (40-45 minutes) and 3 shorter journeys (20-30 minutes), of which 2 took place in the morning (on the way to work or an activity) and 5 in the evening (on the way home from work or an activity). In general, the interviews were held on transport that was fairly uncrowded, with travel by metro being the most crowded situation encountered and where the students stated they had no problem studying standing up.

A semi-structured interview was designed for the contextual interviews, which were conducted as a conversation, with the points listed in the interview protocol incorporated in a natural way in the conversation. The most important points of the interview focused on: general study organisation, study patterns and behaviour during the journeys, teaching materials and forms of use and on how students perceived the usefulness, for their academic studies, of e-readers, mobile internet and audio content used when commuting. Additional observations of the characteristics of the context, such as passenger numbers, the availability of seating, noise, etc, were also noted in a field log.

Transcriptions of the interviews and field log observations have been subjected to a content analysis [23], described in section 3 of the main results.

2.2 Sample

The sample comprised 5 men and 2 women, between 23 and 42 years of age, who use their commuting time to carry out tasks related to their UOC studies. All have prior studies (mostly diplomas or degrees) and work full-time until 6pm or 6:30pm and arrive home between 7pm and 7:30pm. A characteristic of the sample worth noting is that 6 students stated that they study to improve professionally and 1 studies as a hobby.

3 General Results

As background for the study, it is also worth noting that the students described themselves as constant, not leaving everything until the last minute and trying to do something each day. It is important to point out that this perseverance stems above all from the fact that the subject assessment at the university is continual. Assessment activities are carried out every 2-3 weeks for each one of the enrolled subjects (normally 3 to 5), which as a result requires a steady working pace. Therefore, the learning activity deliverables and group work is what sets the study pace. Also, as all the students work full-time they do not have much free time, therefore it is normal that, as commented by one student, they *"get on with something each day"*. A common trait among the students is that *"doing something each day"* means at least accessing the UOC to consult the subject forums, discuss group work, view email or messages from lecturers, which creates a certain sensation of stress and urgency. E4 said: *"I access the campus at least everyday, if not I worry, there are always new messages"*.

These circumstances cause the students, a part from tasks they carry out at home, to use every moment or situation to *"get ahead with work"*. Therefore all of the students study UOC activities at home and whilst commuting and some also during waiting time and at work.

In general, the UOC students interviewed organise their studies in a regular way. First they read the theory material before reading the learning activity questions, although they say that if they don't have much time this order could vary, in which case they read the learning activity questions and then read the material focusing more on what is going to be assessed. When they finish a learning activity, they start the next one, trying not to mix them.

3.1 How They Study Whilst Commuting

Focusing on how UOC students carry out their study activities whilst commuting, it is worth noting that the students read on all types of transport they use during the day. The only time when they do not read is during short trips (5 minutes) or if they have to start a new section and they won't have time to finish it during the remainder of the journey. Also, some students don't read if they can't sit down, although in general they state that normally they are able to sit on public transport. Therefore, to make the most of any travel time they always carry notes on them, either in a briefcase, backpack or folder. E6: *"I am me and my folder"*. They also say that they can concentrate easily during the journey unless there are children or people talking close by. Finally, all of the students underline using one colour and mark, make notes and brief outlines.

3.2 New Formats and Devices

With regard to the students' expectations of new formats and devices to use during their journey (e-reader devices, audio material and mobile internet), even before the interviewer asked any questions on this matter, 2 students mentioned e-book readers, pointing out the advantages that having one would contribute to studying during their commute. For instance, E3 said: *"having seen e-books I hope they'll bring out a super-e-book that lets you connect directly and do everything from it"*.

After asking about the possibilities of e-books all of the students were enthusiastic about the advantages they could provide for studying and said that they are part of what would be their ideal study conditions in a commuting context, provided that they have a series of specific characteristics for studying. These characteristics include:

- being able to underline and write
- having internet connection
- having materials provided by the university that are compatible with the device
- being able to work with more than one document at a time
- being able to search in the text
- having basic editing functions such as copy, paste, etc.

With regard to audio format, it is not considered useful given the ease of losing concentration and because it is not the best way to study. Therefore, they would only use it if the audio were adapted to short commutes, on journeys where they cannot sit down or for learning languages.

Finally, the possibility of having internet on their mobile for on-line learning activities was highly valued, above all for the fact that whilst travelling they could search the internet and consult forums and emails, and especially when they are tired and do not feel like reading, for example, after a day's work. In fact, one of the complaints made by the students was that the daily enquiry on forums and study groups and the search for information on the internet takes up too much time.

4 Discussion

As a notable result and contrary to what is shown on some forums [24], is the fact that the students interviewed consider commuting to be a study context [20]. This means that they study both whilst travelling as well as at home, and therefore always carry learning content on hard copy with them. Therefore, organisation and planning of studies takes into account both studying contexts, including of course mobile contexts. What differentiates the mobile context from the fixed context, are the tasks carried out and the variety of materials and devices that they could use to carry out these tasks in each context [20]. Thus, at home they have access to hard-copy materials for reading (although several students said that they don't read at home) and to the computer and/or laptop and netbook with internet connection for learning activities, accessing the virtual campus, doing searches and consulting digital formats. Whereas, during the commute they only have access to hard copies, therefore they only read materials, underline and make notes (E3 said: *"I have read all the subjects on the metro. I've become used to this time, to doing it this way and it works well for me"*), read the assessment activity questions, and some write down their initial ideas for the activities. Only one student carries a netbook when he/she has to revise or prepare a presentation and to write the initial ideas for the activities. Finally, at work the students use their computer to access the campus, and during waiting time they use paper to read and write up their initial ideas about the assessment activity.

These study behaviour patterns whilst commuting correspond perfectly to the possible use that students would make of an e-book device, of audio format materials and of mobile internet. Table 1 shows the unresolved situations and/or needs that arose during the commute and how an e-book, mobile internet and audio materials could solve them.

During travel time, students request the possibility of connecting to the internet to access the university's virtual campus and to be able to consult emails, classroom communication spaces and study groups, either to work in these spaces or to consult their queries. Apart from this, the possibility of having internet would enable them to carry out searches relating to the assessment activity they are working on. Having a mobile device with internet connection would cover the requirement of accessing the UOC campus and carrying out these tasks. Also, these two tasks could be carried out at moments of mental and physical tiredness, such as after work, or when there are no free seats, as they are tasks easily and comfortably done whilst standing, compared to reading study material.

Table 1. Unresolved situation or need arisen during commuting and proposal or solution

Unresolved situation or need that has arisen	Proposal or solution
Connection to email, classroom and group communication spaces	Mobile device with internet
Search for information relating to the assessment activity on the internet	Mobile device with internet
Resolving queries	Consult forums, lecturer and other current and past subjects
Tiredness or no available seats	Consult internet (virtual campus or information search) instead of reading
Read and select different teaching contents without being loaded down	E-book
Underline and take notes	Options available on an e-book
More than one document at a time	Option available on an e-book
Feel like a student	e-book with UOC logo
Noise	Listen to audio and video
No seats available	Listen to audio and video
Short journeys	Listen to audio

As previously mentioned the students use their commute to read and to work on the reading material, underlining, making notes, using more than one document at a time. These tasks could easily be carried out using an e-book. In addition, all the study material could be uploaded onto the e-book, therefore making it unnecessary to carry a folder or briefcase. Furthermore, bearing in mind that these students had previous studies and always bring their notes with them (some in the typical UOC folder), it appears that they are proud to be students again, so branding the e-reader with the university logo would reinforce their social identity as students.

In some situations, such as excess noise on public transport, or short journeys, the possibility of listening to audio material adapted to these needs would also serve as a form of making the most of their time for studying.

From this information, we conclude with the creation of two scenarios. A scenario [25] is an account describing an event and a person carrying out a series of actions using technology or an application. These actions and events are related to a setting which includes the objectives, plans and reactions of people who participate in this episode.

The two scenarios created are based on the information gathered from the interviews and on the observations made within the same context. The first scenario takes place during a short, 20-minute journey, and the second during a long, 45-minute journey. The scenarios include how the students could use mobile internet, as well as electronic ink devices, for their studies and academic activities.

4.1 Scenario 1: Short Journey (20 Minutes)

Xavi is 35 and lives with his partner in Sant Cugat. To get to work he takes a train for 20 minutes from Sant Cugat to Diagonal. He is studying a Business Administration and Management degree to improve professionally. He is in his third semester and is studying 3 subjects. Whilst he waits for the train he accesses the virtual campus from his mobile to check the calendar and to find out what he needs to do for the next activity because he handed one in the night before. He listens to the introduction audio that is on his classroom with the summary and key words and concepts. The lecturer asks students to search for news in the papers relating to the economic crisis and to prepare a group project. He doesn't understand the information very well, so he writes a message to the lecturer to resolve his doubts. The train arrives, he gets on the middle carriage because it's normally emptier and there are more seats free. He doesn't find an empty seat so he leans against the doors which don't open to continue looking at the campus. He looks at the forums of other subjects he is enrolled on, email, study group messages and takes part in a discussion. Later he puts his headphones on and watches a video that the subject lecturer has uploaded. At work, at lunch-time and after eating, he accesses the campus from his work computer. The lecturer has responded to his query. During the journey home in the evening, from his mobile he connects to internet to search for the news article. He finds a suitable one, downloads it and sends it to his study group. As there is still time before he arrives home, he answers a self-assessment, multiple-choice activity. When he arrives home at 7 o'clock, he reads the theory module he has pending, he begins the assessment activity and discusses the news article with his group.

4.2 Scenario 2: Long Journey (45 Minutes)

Imma is 28 and lives with her partner in Mataró. To get to work she takes a train for 45 minutes from Mataró to Sants. She is studying a bachelor's degree in Humanities as a hobby. She is in her third semester and has enrolled on 3 subjects. She arrives at the station and 2 minutes later the train arrives. The train is normally fairly empty so she can sit down. She gets out her e-book, which she always puts in her briefcase the night before. She has downloaded all the open content on UOC, the materials of subjects she is enrolled on this year and subjects from previous semesters. Using the e-book she connects to the internet and checks the schedule for a subject. She downloads the questions for the assessment activity and starts to read them. She opens the subject to read it (whilst she underlines, makes notes and marks the points which will be useful for the assessed activity) and at the same time has a blank document open for making brief outlines. A concept comes up that she doesn't understand and she searches on the e-book for a subject from the previous semester. Another query comes up and she consults the forum to see if they can solve it for her. During the return journey she also finds an empty seat although the carriage is fuller. She is tired so instead of reading she searches the internet. For the new assessment activity she needs to consult more bibliography and searches the UOC's open content to see if the bibliography is there. She also searches on Google scholar. She finds 3 documents that will be useful and downloads them to be able to read them the following day on her morning commute. She does a self-assessment test. When she arrives home, thanks to what she has read in the morning she can begin to do the assessment activity following the outline she prepared during the journey.

5 Conclusions

The potential of m-learning for on-line education in a mobile context is evident: students plan their studies taking into account all the moments and places where they can possibly study. One of these moments and places is whilst commuting. For example, it is common to see students reading material on regional train and metro journeys. Therefore, commutes form another context of studying (E4: "*I think I get a lot out of studying during the commute*"), which is basically used for reading. Therefore the introduction of devices such as e-books would cover these needs. However, so that the e-book is really useful in a commuting context, students request that they be able to underline, make notes and connect to the internet.

The internet connection, either using an e-book or a mobile, is also a basic element for students during their commute, as the possibility of connecting to the internet to carry out learning activities on the virtual campus and consult forums, enables students to spend their travel time doing this.

Therefore, a student profile exists that is characterised by people who work full-time with little free time for studying and who use their commuting time to read or do learning activities. Using mobile devices such as the e-book or a mobile, these students can meet their needs as students, as well as opting for new learning content given the technological and application potential of an e-book and a mobile, above all if they have internet connection. However, this learning content must be created based on the student profile it is designed for. In the introduction to this article we emphasised that the majority of research mentions cases in which a mobile device is used for providing complementary on-line content to on-site education. What is clear in the case of the UOC student profile, where education is exclusively on-line, is that there is no place for providing complementary educational content for use in a commuting context.

Therefore, what type of content and mobile application devices should be provided to this type of student? Is the possibility of reading and consulting community spaces on the virtual campus enough? For example, Ramírez-Montoya [14] explains the experience of the Virtual University of the Monterrey Institute of Technology, where m-learning is carried out in an exclusively on-line context and where students are offered various applications, such as access to User Services, case studies, class reinforcement cases, exercises, simulations, illustrations, co-assessments and self-assessments, consult qualifications, messages, calendars, consult study groups, mobile radio chat, live channel, audio and video resources using podcasting technology, Really Simple Syndication technology (RSS) and mobile telephone.

However, again it is worth asking if this content and these applications would be valid in a commuting context and if they are of use to students who work full-time and who have little free time to spend on learning activities.

The possibilities are infinite and we hope that new research will shed more light on this subject.

Finally, thanks to these scenarios it has been possible to make progress in redesigning and adapting the UOC Virtual Campus to different mobile devices (mobiles, e-readers and iPad).

The design and architecture of the information for each case was defined bearing in mind the properties of the different devices, while maintaining the services and contents of the website of the UOC Virtual Campus and, in some cases, adding new services. For example, a mobile adaptation for UOC Virtual Campus mobiles (HTC and iPhone) and an email, teacher and forum update alert system (Fig. 1) have been developed and tested with users.

The adaptation of content and the OUC Virtual Campus to e-readers (Fig. 2) has commenced. The OUC Virtual Campus has also been adapted to iPad (Fig. 3) and is ready for evaluation by users.

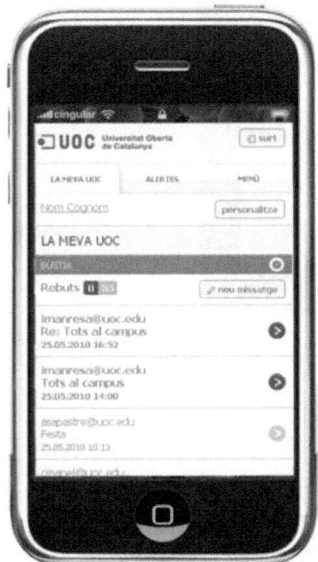 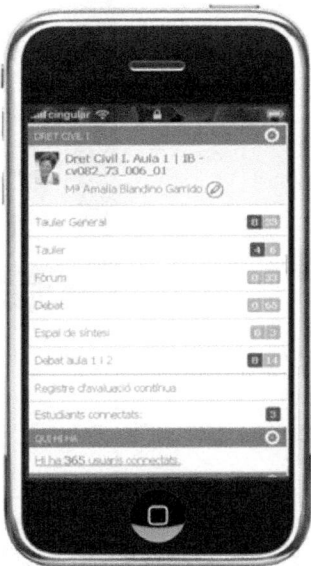

Fig. 1. UOC Virtual Campus adapted to the iPhone

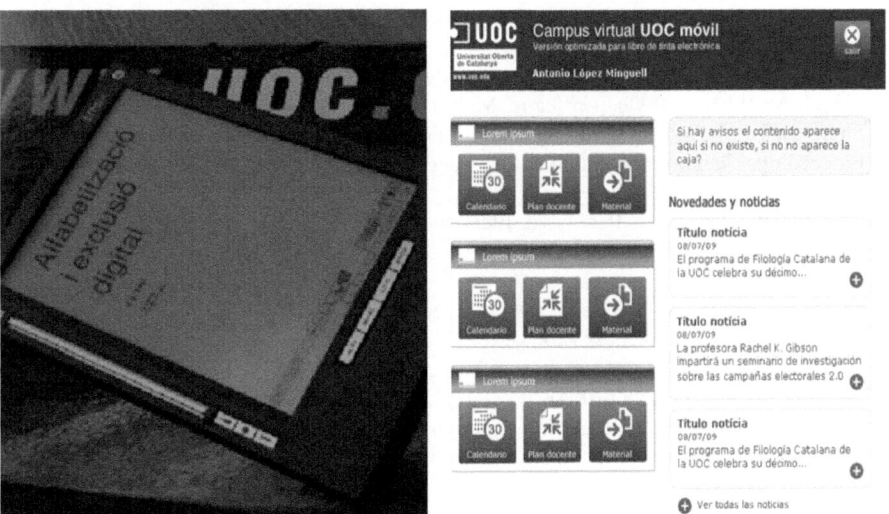

Fig. 2. Content and UOC Virtual Campus adapted to an e-reader

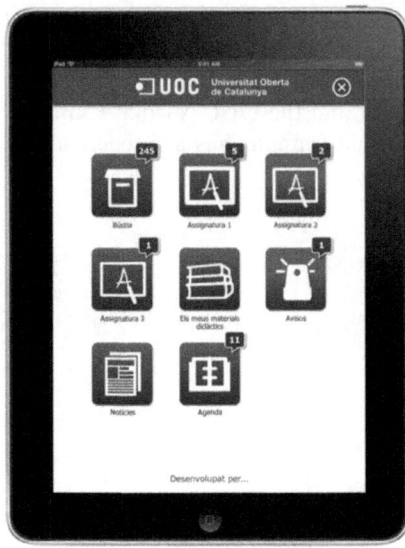

Fig. 3. UOC Virtual Campus adapted to the iPad

References

1. Laouris, Y., Eteokleous, N.: We need an Educationally Relevant Definition of Mobile Learning. In: 4th World conference on mLearning, mLearn 2005, Conference theme: Mobile technology: The future of learning in your hands (2005), http://www.mlearn.org.za/CD/papers/Laouris%20&%20Eteokleous.pdf (retrieved October 17 2008)
2. Pinkwart, N., Hoppe, H.U., Milrad, M., Perez, J.: Educational scenarios for the cooperative use of Personal Digital Assistant. Journal of Computer Assisted Learning 19(3), 383–391 (2003)
3. Quinn, C.: mLearning: Mobile, wireless, in your-pocket learning. LiNE Zine. Fall (2000)
4. Salz, P.A.: When will we ever learn? Mobile Communications International 1, 129 (2005)
5. Sharples, M.: Learning as conversation: Transforming education in the mobile age. In: Proceedings Seeing understanding, learning in the mobile age. Budapest, April 28-30, pp. 147–152 (2005)
6. Lee, M.J.W., Chan, A.: Pervasive, lifestyle-integrated mobile learning for distance learners: an analysis and unexpected results from a podcasting study. Open Learning 22(3), 201–218 (2007)
7. Kukulska-Hulme, A., Traxler, J.: Mobile learning: a handbook for educators and trainers. Taylor & Francis, New York (2005)
8. Geddes, S.J.: Mobile learning in the 21st century: benefit for learners. Knowledge Tree e-journal 30(3), 214–228 (2004)
9. de Jong, P.: Anyplace and anytime learning using mobile technologies: the use of e-book readers in undergraduate medical education. In: Proc. of OnlineEduca. 2009, Berlin, December 2-4 (2009)
10. Frydenberg, M.: Podcasting in the classroom: student-created media for mobile learning. In: IADIS International Conference on Mobile Learning 2007 (July 73-80, 2007)

11. Holzinger, A., Nischelwitzer, A., Meisenberger, M.: Lifelong-learning support by m-learning: example scenarios. eLearn, 2005(11) (November 2005)
12. Rodríguez, M., Constantine, M.: Going Mobile: a practical guide for faculty. In: Proc. of OnlineEduca 2009, Berlin (December 2-4, 2009)
13. Veelo, K.: Anyplace and anytime learning using, mobile technologies_4 examples. In: Proc. of OnlineEduca 2009, Berlin (December 2-4, 2009)
14. Ramírez-Montoya, M.S.: Mobile learning –mlearning- technology resources and their relationship with distance learning environments: applications and research studies. RIED. Ibero-American Review of Distance Education, 12.2, México (May 2009) ISSN:1138-2783
15. Metcalf, D.: Stolen moments for learning. eLearning Developers' Journal (March 18-20, 2002), http://www.elearningguild.com/pdf/2/March02-Metcalf-H.pdf (retrieved February 9, 2010)
16. Son, C., Lee, Y., Park, S.: Toward a new definition of m-learning. In: Proceedings of E-Learn 2004, Washington, DC, November 1-5, pp. 2137–2140 (2004)
17. Yuen, S., Wang, S.: M-learning: mobility in learning. In: Proceedings of E-Learn 2004, Washington, DC, November 1-5, pp. 2248–2252 (2004)
18. Gil-Rodríguez, E.P., Planella-Ribera, J.: Educational Uses of the e-Book: An Experience in a Virtual University Context. In: Holzinger, A. (ed.) USAB 2008. LNCS, vol. 5298, pp. 55–62. Springer, Heidelberg (2008)
19. Eisenhardt, K.M.: Building Theories from Case Study Research. Academy of Management Review 14(4), 532–550 (1989)
20. Rebaque-Rivas, P., Gil-Rodríguez, E.P., Manresa-Mallol, I.: Mobile Learning Scenarios from a UCD Perspective. In: Proceedings of Mobile HCI 2010: a mobile world for all, Lisboa, September 7-10 (in press, 2010)
21. Pruitt, A.: The Persona Lifecycle. Elsevier, San Francisco (2006)
22. Beyer, H., Holtzblatt, K.: Contextual Design: Defining Customer-Centered Systems. Morgan Kaufmann, San Francisco (1998) ISBN: 1-55860-411-1
23. Krippendorff, K.: Content Analysis: An Introduction to Its Methodology, 2nd edn. Sage, Thousand Oaks (2004)
24. Schank, R.C.: Predictions for the 2010. Elearn Magazine (2010), http://www.elearnmag.org/subpage.cfm?section=articles&article=106-1 (retrieved February 8, 2010)
25. Rosson, M.B., Carroll, J.M.: Usability engineering: scenario-based development of human-computer interaction. Morgan Kaufmann Publishers Inc., San Francisco (2001)

The XAOS Metric – Understanding Visual Complexity as Measure of Usability

Christian Stickel[1], Martin Ebner[1], and Andreas Holzinger[2]

[1] Department of Social Learning
Graz University of Technology
Steyrergasse 30/I, A-8010 Graz
stickel@tugraz.at,
martin.ebner@tugraz.at
[2] Research Unit HCI4MED,
Institute for Medical Informatics, Statistics and Documentation
Medical University Graz
Auenbruggerplatz 2/V, A-8036 Graz
andreas.holzinger@medunigraz.at

Abstract. The visual complexity of an interface is a crucial factor for usability, since it influences the cognitive load and forms expectations about the subjacent software or system. In this paper we propose a novel method that uses entropy, structure and functions, to calculate the visual complexity of a website. Our method is evaluated against a well known approach of using the file size of color jpeg images for determining visual complexity. Both methods were applied on a dataset consisting of images of 30 different websites. These websites were also evaluated with a web survey. We found a strong correlation for both methods on subjective ratings of visual complexity and structure. This suggests both methods to be reliable for determination of visual complexity.

Keywords: Visual Complexity, Entropy, User Experience, Usability.

1 Introduction

Defining and measuring 'Visual simplicity' and its opposite 'Visual complexity' is originally one of the main goals of psychologists working in gestalt tradition. The 'principle of simplicity' or 'maximum homogeneity' goes back to Hochberg [1] who states that a gestalt good organization is a simple organization. The Gestalt theorists followed the basic principle that the whole is greater than the sum of its parts, which means that the whole carries a different and bigger meaning than individual parts.

Individual parts can be considered as design elements and both the construction and the perception of any bigger object, respectively interface, will involve several of them (e. g. planes, fonts, lines, color, etc.) as well as the principles how to apply and combine them best.

These principles include unity, contrast, balance, proportion, etc. [24]. Consequently, the design elements are the individual parts that make up an interface, while the design principles are general rules of perception that describe and suggest the

G. Leitner, M. Hitz, and A. Holzinger (Eds.): USAB 2010, LNCS 6389, pp. 278–290, 2010.

optimal relationships between parts of an interface. An example for this may be the principle of unity, which refers to a congruity among the single parts. Unity describes that they are perceived as if they belong together, respectively the viewer senses some kind of visual connection beyond mere chance which causes the parts to come together [24].

When components are comprehended as a 'whole', an elementary cognitive process takes place. This process is the attempt to visually and psychologically generate order out of chaos. The creation of harmony and structure from apparently disconnected bits of information. It is obvious that this process depends in many ways on the visual complexity of a stimulus. Consequently by being able to shape and adapt visual complexity of a stimulus means to shape and adapt the mental effort of the user.

Harper et al. investigated the visual complexity of websites and proposed using the measure of visual complexity as implicit marker of cognitive load [2]. Used this way measures of visual complexity will ultimately support the design of interfaces which are easier to interact with. A further work on

Interaction with computers relies on human perception and cognition [3]. The perception of a website is the determining factor for the emotions evoked in the user, which will evidently affect the extent of the pleasure. According to Berlyne's theory of aesthetic response [4], viewers' pleasure in response to an object is connected to the complexity of this object. Taking this into account, measures of visual complexity can support shaping the user experience of a website.

In this paper we propose a novel method for measuring the visual complexity of websites. Different to existing approaches for measuring visual complexity, like using the size of compressed images, the structure of our formula reveals the real issues of high visual complexity. The revelation of these issues and the principles they are based on, will support designers to increase the usability of interfaces.

2 Theoretical Background

This chapter describes Berlyne's theory of aesthetic response and gives an overview on some measures of visual complexity.

2.1 Berlyne's Theory of Aesthetic Response

The word "aesthetics," is used in reference to something beautiful, as well as to a branch of philosophy that deals with the nature of beauty, fine arts, taste and also with the appreciation and creation of beauty. Aesthetics is derived from the Greek word "aisthetikos" which means "pertaining to sense perception" or "perceive, sense, feel". The German philosopher Alexander Baumgarten was the first who introduced the term in the 17th century.

He chose the word in order to express the experience of beauty and art as a field of concrete knowledge communicated in sensory form, compared to the strict reasoning or logical knowledge [4].

Human perception is unconsciously sensitive to such things as proportions or unity of elements. An example is the "golden section" which describes a special ratio of length to height (1.6:1) that can be found very often in nature. It is said that this proportion is visually pleasing for the viewer. So far it played a prominent role in art and architecture throughout history [4]. The golden section provides a good example of how a design principle is unconsciously acquired through mere exposure to the environment. As people encounter this principle in nature very often, they find it appealing and so it works also in arts and designed artifacts [4]. This also applies to other design rules. Consequently the users have subjective views of aesthetics as a result of personal, social and cultural development.

Berlyne's (1971) theory of aesthetics proposed a Wundt-curve function, which linked the preference for a stimulus with the level of arousal. He suggests that only moderate increments in the arousal potential of a stimulus are perceived pleasurable, while sharp rises in arousal are experienced as being unpleasant and punishment. Fig. 1 depicts the proposed relationship.

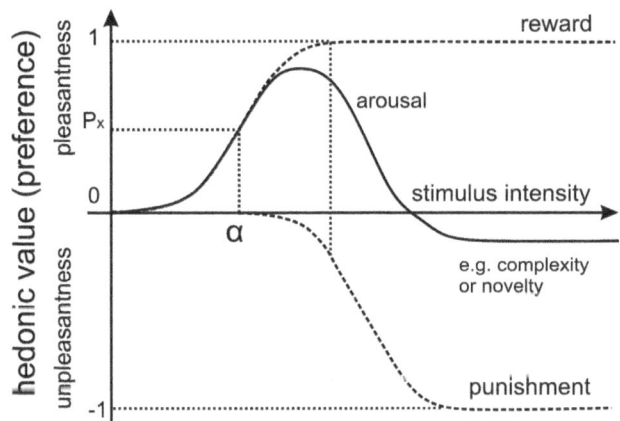

Fig. 1. Berlyne's proposed Wundt-curve function

'. . .aesthetic patterns produce their hedonic effects by acting on arousal. . . positive hedonic values can come about in either of two ways, namely through a moderate increase in arousal. . . or through a decrease in arousal when arousal reached an uncomfortably high level. . .' [4].

In software development, aesthetics has to be considered in regard of interface design and fortunately there are empirically measurable benefits of the application of principles of aesthetics [27, 28]. The sense of aesthetic is said to be influenced by visual complexity [9]. The visual complexity of an object depends on the amount of constituent elements and the diversity of these elements. This means the more single elements are perceived on an interface e.g. a website, the more increases the subjective impression of complexity of this site.

Berlyne considered visual complexity as subjective and also objective. Subjectivity comes from afore mentioned process of individual development resulting in relative views on complexity from subject to subject. Objectivity takes the physical constraints of the objects into account, as they are all the same for all subjects. He described complexity as an objective property of an object and defined relative complexity according to the number of elements within the objects [11].

The theory of aesthetic response states that a viewers' pleasure in response to an object will increase with increased complexity, to an optimal level. With further increasing complexity, pleasure begins to decline. So users don't like objects that are either too simple or too complicated. Consequently users will prefer objects, respectively websites that are moderately familiar and will be averse to the novel and the over familiar. The theory is expressed in an inverted U-shaped curve for pleasure, with a linearly increasing line for complexity, as can be seen in fig. 2.

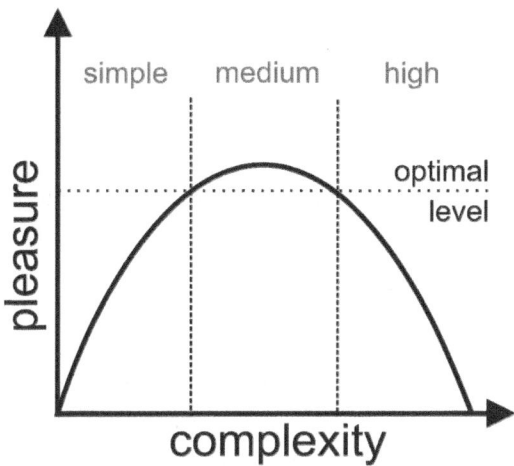

Fig. 2. Curve depicting the theoretical relationship between the hedonic value and visual complexity

The curve predicts that by adjusting visual complexity to an optimal level, viewers' pleasure of an object will increase. The influence of website complexity on user attitudes is supported by several recent studies [6],[7]. Some support Berlyne's theory, such as Geisser et al. who found that consumers responded more positive towards websites which fell within a moderate range of perceived complexity [8]. Others did not directly support it [9],[10], as they found a negative correlation between visual complexity and website perception.

2.2 Aesthetic Measures

Birkhoff was early to publish on measures of aesthetic. He aimed at determining the aesthetic effect of different objects e.g. vases, tiles or polygons.

Therefore he proposed that different classes of objects could not be compared and thus limited the range of objects. Birkhoff found out that also the aesthetic effect was subjectively dependent and thus he also limited the number of observers and conducted his experiments on a restricted group of subjects [29]. The model for aesthetic measures proposed by Birkhoff is based on three steps of perception.

The first step is the effort needed to focus the attention on an object, which relates proportional to the objects complexity, denoted as (C). In the second phase the reward for this effort is a feeling of value, which Birkhoff denotes as aesthetic measure (M).

Finally in the third step the aesthetic measure is verified and influenced by a harmony metric, describing symmetries and order. From this Birkhoff derived the following formula:

$$M = O/C$$

The relationship of the components can be interpreted such that a rising complexity (C) in combination with disorder (O) creates an unpleasant reaction of the subject, thus the aesthetic measure (M) variable will be low. On the opposite a higher level of order, respectively symmetry will result in a more pleasant experience for the subject, respectively in a higher value of aesthetic measure. However recent studies suggest the perceived aesthetic value of users is curvilinear related to Birkhoffs aesthetic measure (M), peaking at a moderate M value [26].

The aesthetic measure seems to be useful for interface designers; however questions remain how to effectively measure metrics like order and complexity. Some input to this question comes from the field of algorithmic information theory (AIT), which will be covered in the next chapter.

2.3 Algorithmic Information Theory (AIT)

A recent approach to the measurement of visual complexity comes from algorithmic information theory (AIT). AIT provides a mathematical link between distributional rules used to produce a set of forms and the complexity code for a single form. This is done by measuring the probability of a string of symbols and linking it to the probability of the complexity of this symbol string. The string of symbols is generated by translating the form e.g. scanning and identifying the pixels that reproduce the form [13].

AIT provides a direct connection between the concepts of simplicity, respectively complexity and probabilistic measures. It thereby connects two principles about the organization of visual perception, namely the "likelihood principle" and the "simplicity principle".

The likelihood principle describes that a given visual sensory input will lead to the perception of the most likely distal object, which puts visual perception into a hypothesis-testing framework. Thereby the "hypotheses" are the possible distal objects representing the input, while the "data" is the actual visual input. This allows formulating the visual perception as a Bayesian probability decision [13]:

$$p(H/D) = p(D/H) \cdot p(H) / p(D)$$

H denotes the perceptual hypothesis; D is the sensory input data. The visual system then fixes as the percept generated by sensory input D and maximizes the perceptual hypothesis H. In order to calculate this, the visual system needs probabilities for H, D/H and D. Thereby H is the probability of possible perceptual hypothesis, D is the probability of the current visual input and D/H are the probabilities of the data D given each hypothesis H.

The "simplicity principle" in AIT assumes that the human visual system chooses a perception based on Bayes' theorem, where the complexity of a possible perception (H), given the sensory input (D), will equal the complexity of the perception (H) added to the conditional complexity of the data (D) given the percept (H), minus the complexity of the data D.

$$I(H/D) = I(H) + I(D/H) - I(D)$$

The perceptual hypothesis to be chosen has to minimize the complexity function. To solve the equation one will need the complexities of H, D and D/H.

The likelihood principle and the simplicity principle are connected as probability and complexity are directly linked. Thus the most probable perception is the least complex, and the least probable perception is the most complex. AIT shows that, given the input, the visual system either minimizes the complexity of a perception or maximizes the probability of the perception [13].

Another promising approach of using information measures to describe visual complexity was done by Klinger & Salingaros [16]. They propose two pragmatic measures, termed temperature (T) and harmony (H). The temperature describes symbol variation, whereby harmony measures the correlations of subunits via symmetries. Interestingly they link the results of their measure to Russel's circumplex Model of affect [17], which supports Berlyne's theory on the relationship between complexity and arousal.

2.4 Visual Complexity Measures

Visual complexity can be determined either by subjective user ratings, or by objective measurements. Subjective user ratings can be obtained by questionnaires or web surveys. Objective measurements can be the number of elements, dissimilarity of elements, or the degree to which several elements are responded to as a unit [11].

A present-day approach from Harper et al., which is applicable for websites, is using the number of each structural element on the page (density), the number (variety) of different structural elements and information presented (diversity) and the layout of the structural elements (position) [2].

A really easy and reliable way to assess the visual complexity is the utilization of digitized image compression. The File sizes of digital images after compression (e.g. JPEG, TIFF, GIF) can provide a measure of complexity. Thereby larger files indicate a higher complexity. In the same way complexity can be measured as the number of bytes preserved after compression [12]. There is strong evidence that the file size measure predicts the subjective complexity rating of images [14, 15]. Although digital image compression is not directly linked to theories of visual perception, it is connected to information theory. From the previous mentioned ideas and studies we derived our own measure of visual complexity, which was used in the present study. Our formula for visual complexity (X) consists of three factors:

1. Number of possible interactions, which can be considered as functional elements or just actions (A)
2. Number of higher level structures or gestalt groups, in short organizational elements (O)
3. Summed Entropy of RGB values (S).

$$X = A \cdot O \cdot S$$

As functional elements we consider all kind of links and active GUI elements like buttons, drop boxes, checkboxes etc. Organizational elements are all kind of binding boxes, pictures, in short everything that fulfills the gestalt laws for grouping. The entropy measure should provide us with information on contrast.

3   Methods and Materials

This chapter covers the used dataset, methods and results. It describes the experiment as well as the analysis.

3.1   Hypothesis and Research Question

Due to the possible affective impact of visual complexity on users, this study strived at investigating the elements of website complexity by generating a novel measure called XAOS metric. The XAOS metric had to be tested against established objective measurements and also against subjective user ratings. For this test we expected to find high correlations between the user ratings, traditional measures and the XAOS metric (H1).

Taking into account the idea of compressed images, expressing visual complexity, we were interested in testing this against uncompressed images. Following the suggestions of Donderi, we expected to find no or just weak correlations between the user rating item complexity and the file size of uncompressed (PNG) images (H2).

With Berlyne's theory in mind we expected to find correlations between the objective measures of visual complexity and subjective valence ratings (H3).

3.2   Dataset

The dataset for the present experiment consisted of 30 different screenshots of website landing pages. Coming from an e-learning context, we chose start pages of different Learning Management Systems (LMS). Real websites were chosen in order to ensure ecological validity.

All screenshots were taken in uncompressed PNG format, with a resolution of 1024x768 pixels. They showed just the website without the browser interface. The interface elements would have influenced the perception of the users, as they had to be embedded in the web-survey. Thus a replication of the browsers navigational elements would have biased the results.

3.3   Methods

For the comparison with the XAOS metric we chose the JPEG file size method for determination of visual complexity [14][15], as it seemed to be the fastest and most reliable. For the JPEG files a compression ratio of 70% was used. The file sizes of the JPEG and PNG files of the dataset were collected.

3.3.1   XAOS Metric

The generation of the XAOS metric was a little more exhaustive as we had to calculate the entropy of the screenshots, which was done with a MatLab script. The number of actions and organizational elements of each website was elaborated empirically, following the gestalt laws. However for a website this could also be done automatically with a parser for functions and computer vision techniques for analyzing the structure.

3.3.2 Websurvey

Finally a web-survey was implemented, which showed one screenshot at a time. This can be considered a typical passive viewing test. In a pilot study we used iFrames linking to the real websites, however this proved to be distracting and error-prone. The participants were asked to rate their first impression of the shown website, concerning complexity, structure, color, contrast and valence. The dimensions were arranged on a seven point semantic differential, whereof an example can be seen in fig. 3. The scores for each dimension ranged from 1 to 7.

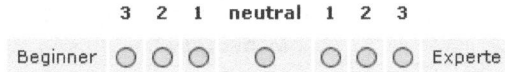

Fig. 3. Example for used seven point semantic differential

The semantic differentials were expressed as shown in following table 1. Although it was tested, we disclaimed using a more elaborative questionnaire. Due to the voluntary nature and the amount of tested websites, we didn't want to risk participants aborting the survey.

Table 1. Shows the used semantic differentials for describing first impression

color	dreary	colorful
complexity	simple	complex
structure	Empty	overloaded
contrast	low-contrast	high-contrast
valence	Pleasant	unpleasant

A22 participants took part in the web survey, with the age ranging from 19 to 42 (mean ~ 28). 12 of them were familiar with the concept of Learning Management Systems (LMS). 11 out of 22 had already used an LMS. The Internet expertise of the participants ranged from 4 to 7 (mean ~ 5,86), which suggests that there were lots of experts.

3.4 Analysis

For the subjective user rating the results for each webpage and item were averaged over participants, so that every page finally had five averaged scores of subjective measures (complexity, structure, color, contrast and valence). The objective metrics were calculated, so that every page had three objective scores. These were 'PNG file size', 'JPEG file size' and XAOS metric.

3.5   Results

The first hypothesis asked for a comparison of a reliable traditional method with our novel proposed XAOS metric and with the subjective user rating. Therefore the results of the three metrics were normalized in order to make it comparable. For visual simplicity reasons we just show the trend lines of the metrics in fig. 4. The trend line of the XAOS metric matches the JPEG file size method and both objective methods almost match the subjective user rating of visual complexity. Table 2 shows the correlations between the compared metrics.

For testing hypothesis H2, the PNG file size and the JPG file size were compared against the user rating of visual complexity. As expected the JPG measure correlated much higher (r=.79) with the user score, than the PNG measure (r=.33). That data can be seen in fig. 4 and tab. 2.

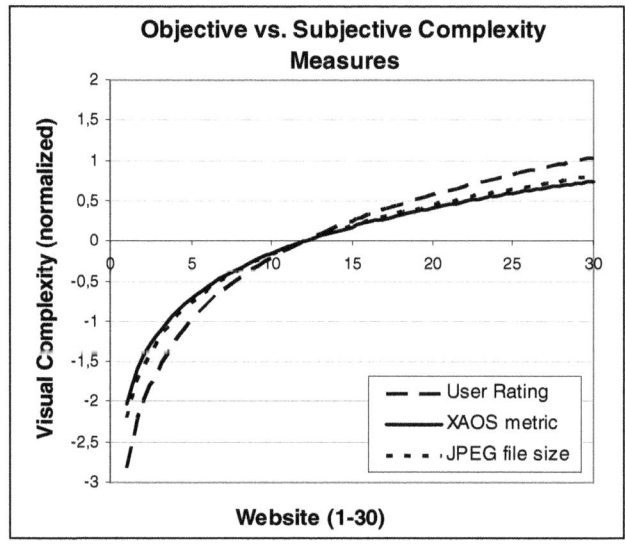

Fig. 4. The XAOS metric matches the JPEG file size method and user ratings

Table 2. Shows the correlations between the complexity metrics

	User rating	JPEG file size	XAOS metric	PNG file size
User rating	1,00	0,79	0,77	0,33
JPEG file size	0,79	1,00	0,68	0,51
XAOS metric	0,77	0,68	1,00	0,31
PNG file size	0,33	0,51	0,31	1,00

For testing hypothesis H3, the objective and subjective measures of complexity were first compared to the subjective valence score. As tab. 3 shows there are no significant correlations. So far this study does not support Berlyne's theory.

Table 3. Color Harmony of best vs. worst

	User rating	JPEG file size	XAOS metric	PNG file size
Valence	0,25	0,21	0,27	0,50

Mentionable at this point may be that the most influencing factors on the valence score were the subjective ratings on contrast (r = .68) and color (r = .69). So far color variables can be considered as an important factor for valence.

4 Discussion

The XAOS metric has proven to be reliable, also the JPEG method showed good performance for predicting subjective user ratings of the visual complexity of websites. However JPEG prediction does not work with uncompressed images, as this method depends on the compression algorithm.

4.1 Validation of the XAOS Metric

Based on the results of this study the proposed XAOS metric is applicable as a measure of visual complexity for websites. The underlying factors, namely number of interactions, organizational elements and the entropy of the image are influenced by the ideas of the Gestalt psychology and algorithmic information theory and have proven to be reliable. The metric could be enhanced, taking into account variables like size and position of objects, or by other measures of color and contrast. Further development should include the complete automatic derivation of all factors of the formula. Testing should include different kind of software interfaces.

The XAOS metric can be used directly in the design process, by just simple multiplication of functional elements with organizational elements. We found that the entropy part of the formula is not necessary for the prediction of visual complexity. However it raises the correlation of the result for valence (r+.24) and contrast (r+.20). With this simplification and Berlyne's theory in mind it should be possible to systematically develop an applicable scale for visual complexity with a connection to valence.

4.2 Validation of JPEG Method

The JPEG file size method can be considered as reliable, as the present study replicated a high correlation (r = .79) between JPEG file size and subjective user ratings of complexity. The technical background on this phenomenon is that the JPEG compression algorithm cause larger compressions depending on image features like details, contrast, color and redundancies [21]. In addition other research has found the file size of images like charts, web images and photos to correlate highly and significantly (0.82) with human judgments of visual complexity [15][22]. This makes file size a suitable general measures of the visual complexity of images.

4.3 Validation of Berlyne's Theory

The outcome of the present study does not support Berlyne's theory of an inverted U-shaped relationship between pleasure and a linearly increasing complexity. None of the applied methods was able to reproduce the proposed relationship. This may be due to the limited variance in visual complexity of the shown websites. An artificially constructed dataset with sufficient variance is able to reproduce the theory of aesthetic response [8].

4.4 Limitations

The limited variance in complexity resulted from choosing the dataset out of real–life websites. Furthermore the uncontrolled real life setting of the web survey may bias the results. The last shortcoming is the small number of 22 participants as base for the subjective ratings.

5   Conclusion and Future Research

Visual complexity analysis provides a quick way to review a visualization design before any user study can be conducted. It's also applicable in the design cycle.

Although our data does not support the theory of aesthetic response, there is evidence that visual complexity should be considered as important metric for usability and user experience [8] [18], as it is indeed influencing emotions [20]. Further more it can be considered as extraneous load [19], influencing the cognitive load and mental effort of the user [2], [30], [31].

Further work may want to investigate the idea of Wolfram, that the perceived complexity of an image is a function of the most complex structure in the image, detectable by humans [23]. Finally, using visual complexity as metric offers the challenge of integrating it into design cycles of software engineering. It seems likely that understanding and application of shaping the visual complexity of information systems will improve usability and user experience. Ultimately it is a tool for cognitive performance support.

Acknowledgements

We express our sincere gratitude to all participants of our web survey for spending their valuable time for our research.

References

1. Hochberg, J.: Effects of the gestalt Revolution: The Cornell symposium on perception. Psychological Review 64(2), 73–84 (1957)
2. Harper, S., Michailidou, E., Stevens, R.: Toward a definition of visual complexity as an implicit measure of cognitive load. ACM Transactions on Applied Perception (TAP) 6(2), 1–18 (2009)
3. Card, S.K., Moran, T.P., Newell, A. (eds.): The psychology of human-computer interaction. Lawrence Erlbaum, Hillsdale (1983)
4. Berlyne, D.E.: Studies in the New Experimental Aesthetics. John Wiley and Sons, New York (1974)
5. Berlyne, D.E.: Aesthetics and Psychobiology. Appleton-Century-Crofts, Educational Division, Meredith Corporation, New York (1971)
6. Bruner, G.C., Kumar, A.: Webcommercials and advertising hierarchy of effects. Journal of Advertising Research 40(1), 35–42 (2000)
7. Stevenson, J.S., Bruner, G.C., Kumar, A.: Webpagebackground and viewer attitudes. Journal of Advertising Research 40(1), 29–34 (2000)
8. Geissler, G.L., Zinkhan, G.M., Watson, R.T.: The influence of homepage complexity on consumer attention, attitudes, and purchase intent. Journal of Advertising 35(2), 69–80 (2006)
9. Pandir, M., Knight, J.: Homepage aesthetics: the search for preference factors and the challenges of subjectivity. Interacting with Computers 18, 1351–1370 (2006)
10. Tuch, A.N., Bargas-Avila, J.A., Opwis, K., Wilhelm, F.H.: Visual complexity of websites: Effects on users experience, physiology, performance, and memory. International Journal of Human-Computer Studies 67, 703–715 (2009)
11. Berlyne, D.E.: Conflict, Arousal and Curiosity. McGraw-Hill Book Company, New York (1960)
12. Riglis, E.: Modeling visual complexity in image architectures. Technical Report, Heriot – Watt University (1998)
13. Donderi, D.C.: Visual complexity: A review. Psychological Bulletin 132(1), 73–97 (2006)
14. Donderi, D., McFadden, S.: Compressed file length predicts search time and errors on visual displays. Displays 26, 71–78 (2005)
15. Donderi, D.C.: An information theory analysis of visual complexity and dissimilarity. Perception 35, 823–835 (2006)
16. Klinger, A., Salingaros, N.A.: A pattern measure. Environment and Planning B: Planning and Design 27(4), 537–547 (2000)
17. Russell, J.A.: A circumplex model of affect. Journal of Personality and Social Psychology 39, 1161–1178 (1980)
18. Comber, T., Maltby, J.R.: Layout complexity: does it measure usability? In: Howard, S., Hammond, J., Lindgaard, G. (eds.) Human-computer interaction: Interact 1997, International Conference on Human-computer Interaction, Sydney, Australia, July 14-18, pp. 623–626. Chapman Hall, London (1997)
19. Schmutz, P., Heinz, S., Métrailler, Y., Opwis, K.: Cognitive Load in eCommerce Applications—Measurement and Effects on User Satisfaction, Advances in Human-Computer Interaction, Article ID 121494 (2009)
20. Tsai, T.W., Chang, T.C., Chuang, M.C., Wang, D.M.: Exploration in emotion and visual information uncertainty of websites in culture relations. International Journal of Design 2(2), 55–66 (2008)

21. Sprott, J.C., Bolliger, J., Mladenoff, D.J.: Self-organized criticality in forest landscape evolution. Physics Letters A 297(3-4), 267–271 (2002)
22. Calvo, M.G., Lang, P.J.: Gaze patterns when looking at emotional pictures: Motivationally biased attention. Motivation & Emotion 28, 221–243 (2004)
23. Wolfram, S.: A new kind of science. Wolfram Research, Champaign (2002)
24. Lauer, D.A.: Design Basics. Holt, Rinehart, and Winston, New York (1979)
25. Rigau, J., Feixas, M., Sbert, M.: Informational aesthetics measures. IEEE Comput. Graph. Appl. 28(2), 24–34 (2008)
26. Tateosian, L.G., Healey, C.G., Enns, J.T.: Engaging viewers through nonphotorealistic visualizations. In: Proceedings of the 5th international symposium on Nonphotorealistic animation and rendering, pp. 93–102. ACM Press, New York (2007)
27. Cawthon, N., Moere, A.V.: The Effect of Aesthetic on the Usability of Data Visualization. In: Proceedings of the 11th International Conference Information Visualization, pp. 637–648. IEEE Computer Society, Washington (2007)
28. Tractinsky, N., Katz, A.S., Ikar, S.: What is beautiful is usable. Interacting with Computers 13(2), 127–145 (2000)
29. Birkhoff, D.G.: Aesthetic Measure. Harvard University press, Cambridge (1933)
30. Holzinger, A., Kickmeier-Rust, M.D., Wassertheurer, S., Hessinger, M.: Learning performance with interactive simulations in medical education: Lessons learned from results of learning complex physiological models with the HAEMOdynamics SIMulator. Computers & Education 52(2), 292–301 (2009)
31. Holzinger, A., Kickmeier-Rust, M., Albert, D.: Dynamic Media in Computer Science Education; Content Complexity and Learning Performance: Is Less More? Educational Technology & Society 11(1), 279–290 (2008)

Context Information in Guiding Visual Search: The Role of Color and Orientation

Sonja Stork[1], Laura Voss[1], Andrea Schankin[2], and Anna Schubö[1]

[1] Ludwig Maximilian University Munich, Department Psychology, Leopoldstrasse 13,
D-80802 Munich, Germany
sonja.stork@lmu.de
[2] Ruprecht Karls University Heidelberg, Institute of Psychology, Hauptstrasse 47-51,
D-69117 Heidelberg, Germany

Abstract. At work and at leisure people perform various visual search tasks, e.g. they search for a particular icon in software tools, on Web sites or on mobile phones. With an increasing number of items, visual search becomes difficult. Recently, it has been suggested that the so-called contextual cueing effect, which is known from psychological experiments, can be applied to improve visual search performance. Contextual cueing leads to decreased search times for target objects within familiar context configurations. It is assumed that associations between context configurations and target locations are learned implicitly and then used to guide the allocation of attention to the relevant object. In accordance with demands for interface consistency, this mechanism could be interesting for the development of user interfaces. The present study investigated which object features (e.g. color or orientation) can establish the learning process. The results show that implicit learning of color and orientation arrangements are possible, but the transfer to configuration with changed features depends on the recent learning history. Implications of these results are discussed with respect to the design of user interfaces.

Keywords: Interface Consistency, Contextual Cueing, Visual Attention, Learning.

1 Introduction

At work and at leisure people often have to search for certain visual objects in various contexts like software applications and Web sites. In general, humans are doing quite well in finding a task-relevant object (target) among other task-irrelevant objects (distractors), for example, a relevant menu button among a variety of irrelevant buttons within the taskbar.

However, with increasing numbers of icons on the desktop or of "apps" (applications) on the mobile phone, the difficulty to find a certain icon increases. Especially, if the icons are very similar to one another or very small, they are difficult to distinguish. The similarity of icons depends on their features, e.g. color, shape, and size. Depending on these features and their combinations, the icons are more or less easily to distinguish and the relevant icon can be found easily

G. Leitner, M. Hitz, and A. Holzinger (Eds.): USAB 2010, LNCS 6389, pp. 291–304, 2010.

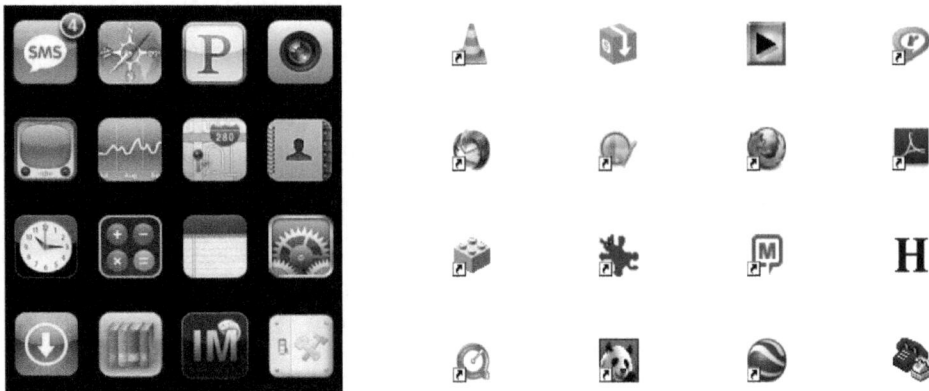

Fig. 1. Example for icon list on a mobile phone (left: Apple® iphone icons) and on the computer screen (right: Microsoft Windows® desktop icons)

or not. Fig. 1 shows examples of typical icon lists. The left icons are very similar because they share the rectangle shape. The right icons have different shapes but they are often rather small on laptop displays. Accordingly, the task to find a particular icon within these lists might be hindered. Users may facilitate their search of relevant icons by classifying and sorting them according to different purposes. However, this method can become rather time consuming depending on the number of icons. Here, another method is suggested that might facilitate user's search by applying a mechanism found in psychological research.

It is well-known that the human visual system is limited with respect to the number of objects which can be processed simultaneously. Therefore, objects have to be selected for further processing – a mechanism known as selective visual attention. Two mechanisms are supposed to allocate attention appropriately and efficiently to areas of interest. Bottom-up or stimulus-based mechanisms guide visual attention to objects with certain physical properties [1, 2]. For example, salient features, dissimilarities to other surrounding objects or abrupt onsets [3] can enhance target selection.

Moreover, also top-down or knowledge-based factors like familiarity [4] and novelty [5] can guide visual attention. Knowledge-based allocation of attention can be introduced by instructions or acquired without intention over time. The latter mechanism is known as implicit learning. Implicit learning occurs within a variety of daily life activities, for example in motor learning, in the control of complex situations, in language acquisition, or in sequence learning. The advantage of such an implicit mechanism is that it does not need additional processing capacities or any additional instruction of the user.

Accordingly, implicit learning is expected to be of relevance also for user interface design. As stated by Steve Krug in his book "Don't make me think" [6], Web sites and applications for human computer interaction (HCI) should be designed in an intuitive way. An implicit learning mechanism can help to facilitate HCI, because this mechanism works completely effortlessly, i.e. without thinking about it.

One mechanism which makes use of implicitly learned information is known as contextual cueing. If people are asked to search for a target object and to identify it as fast as possible based on a certain object features like color or orientation, they are faster in a familiar environment, also called the visual context. In a typical experiment, the effect of the visual context is investigated by manipulating the spatial arrangement of task-irrelevant distractor objects, within which a task-relevant object has to be found. If these arrangements are presented repeatedly, the participants become faster in finding the target object compared to novel arrangements never seen before. It is proposed that this effect is based on learned associations between the target location and the surrounding context elements [7], which can be used to guide visuo-spatial attention more efficiently to the target location.

Applying this mechanism to the design of user interfaces touches the topic of interface consistency. The three-dimensional model of interface consistency [8, 9] distinguishes conceptual consistency, communicational consistency and physical consistency. The physical consistency includes visual features like color, size, shape, and location. These features typically describe properties of the target itself. Another possibility to enable interface consistency could be the consistency of context elements. In this sense, contextual cueing is expected to enhance search performance of certain interface elements which are embedded in a familiar context. So far, there are inconsistent results whether consistency really enhances performance [10, 11], but the investigation of the contextual cueing effect could shed more light to this question.

2   Contextual Cueing Based on Color and Orientation

A precondition to transfer this kind of learning mechanism to real world applications is the ecological validity of contextual cueing. So far, it has been shown that implicit learning occurs not only with artificial stimuli but also with pictures of real objects like LEGO® bricks [12]. However, in all previous contextual cueing experiments, the visual context was defined by the spatial arrangement of distractor objects, that is, all objects were arranged in a kind of matrix but not all possible positions were filled. Thus, it is impossible to decide whether object positions (i.e., the spatial arrangement of the objects) or other object properties (features, such as color, size, and shape) were learned. Although it has been shown that contextual cueing occurs if only the spatial arrangement and not the object features were informative for the target location [13], it is unclear so far whether visual contexts defined by object features can also establish the learning process. However, for the implementation of contextual cueing to HCI applications, it is essential to know which target properties can be used to enhance the search performance.

Because the object identity can be specified as the combination of different features, for example color and shape, it is important to know whether single features of context stimuli can be learned as well as feature combinations. For example, certain icons could be distinguished by either their color, their form, or both. One interesting question is whether certain object features support the implicit learning process better than others.

Another important question is whether learned context information can be transferred if one additional feature is added to the context objects. So far, it has been shown that transfer is possible if one feature is missing and matches are incomplete, for example if object shapes remain but if color information is deleted [14]. Therefore, it seems as if object shapes can be learned separately, which can lead to an improvement of search performance.

One general problem in interpretations of contextual cueing effects is the assumed allocation of attention because other explanations are also possible. For example, it has been proposed that contextual cueing might also enhance response selection [15, 16]. If it is intended to improve visual search in HCI applications via contextual cueing it is important that the mechanism modulates attention allocation rather than the selection of button presses. One method to demonstrate the involvement of attentional selection is the recording of eye movements. Because saccades are typically preceded by attention shifts [17], eye movements can be used as indicator of attention allocation.

To summarize, the goal of the present experiment was to clarify whether contextual cueing occurs also without gaps or pattern in the context configuration. It was investigated whether the features color and orientation can be learned separately to form visual contexts and whether the implicit knowledge about these contexts can be transferred to a test phase, in which feature combinations are presented. Moreover, the involvement of attentional processes in the contextual cueing effect was tested by eye movement recordings.

3   Methods

3.1   Participants

Eight subjects (age 20-33 years, mean age 24.4 years) participated in this experiment. Six of them were right-handed and all had normal or corrected-to-normal vision according to self-report. All participants were naive as to the purpose of the study and received 8 Euro per hour for their participation. Most of the participants were students of the Ludwig Maximilian University.

3.2   Stimuli and Apparatus

The experiment was conducted in a dimly lit room to control for interferences from the outside. The experimental setup consisted of a table equipped with a LCD projector, which was mounted on top above the search area, a mirror system, and a remote eye tracker [18].

The participants sat on a (non-rotating) stool in front of the table. The height of the stool was adjusted individually, so that the unrestrained viewing distance from participant's eye to the centre of the search area was approx. 60 cm. If necessary, participants were provided with a foot rest in order to maintain a comfortable position.

The stimulus displays were generated and displayed with MATLAB R2006b (The MathWorks Inc.) on a Dell Latitude D830 laptop running Microsoft Windows XP Professional. They were projected on the table (size: 100 x 80 cm) via the mirror and appeared in an area of approx. 20° x 20° of visual angle in the centre of the display.

The eye tracker was placed in an opening at the bottom part of the table. The lower edge of the display area projected on the table was adjusted to the same level as the upper edge of the opening for the eye tracker. During the experiment the left eye's gaze position and eye movement duration during the search was recorded via an Eyelink 1000 system (2007 SR Research Ldt.; sample rate 500 Hz, pacing interval 1000 Hz, 100% illuminator power) in remote mode. Eye movement data were recorded by a portable Host PC under DOS mode.

Two response buttons were located left and right of the eye tracker, and the participants were instructed to press the buttons with their left or right index finger, respectively.

All search displays consisted of 4 x 4 pictures of six different LEGO® bricks, which were created with LeoCAD (cf. Fig. 2). Lego bricks offer a good possibility to control item features in contrast to more complex items. The size of the bricks varied from approx. 1.6° x 0.9° to 3.2° x 1.7° of visual angle. Visual angles were adjusted to a natural view based on the real size of LEGO® bricks. The bricks were colored in either red or green, and they were oriented either horizontally or vertically. The participants were instructed to search for the brick with 1 x 3 units (target stimulus). All other bricks were task-irrelevant distractors. In the test phase, the stimuli were basically the same, but there was an additional either light grey (75% grey value) or dark grey (25% grey value) dot on one of the knobs.

3.3   Design

The goal of the present experiment was to examine whether a visual context defined by object features can guide spatial attention. Similar to previous experiments, the visual context was defined as the arrangement of distractor objects. The advantage of a learned visual context is reflected by faster responses to repeated search arrays relative to novel ones. In the present experiment, the repeated set of stimuli consisted of 16 search displays, randomly generated at the beginning of the experiment and then repeated throughout the entire experimental session. It is important to note that the target (i.e. the 3 unit brick) always appeared at the same location within a particular repeated search array, but at different locations across different displays. The response-relevant target dimension (color or orientation) was selected randomly also in repeated trials, in order to ensure that the whole display is not associated with a specific response. The novel stimulus displays consisted of configurations that are shown only once in the entire experiment. These trials measured baseline search speed as a control because search times may decrease in the time course of the experiment. To rule out location probability effects, the target appeared equally often at each of 16 possible locations throughout the experiment. Each location was used twice during one block, once in a repeated configuration and the second time in a novel configuration. All configurations were generated separately for each participant and presented intermixed.

As we were interested in whether specific object features can guide attention more efficiently, we varied the object feature defining the context. In one condition, only the color was task-relevant whereas the orientation was held constant (color condition, cf. Figure 2, left panel), in another condition the orientation was task-relevant whereas the color was held constant (orientation condition, cf. Figure 2, middle panel). In the color condition, displays consisted of red and green LEGO® bricks that were always oriented horizontally. In the orientation condition, displays consisted of bricks that were oriented horizontally and vertically and always colored in red. In both conditions, the objects used as distractors were the bricks consisting of 2, 4, 6, or 8 units, and the target stimulus was always the 3 unit brick. The participants were instructed to find the target brick as fast as possible and to press one of two buttons, corresponding to the targets color (in the color condition) or orientation (in the orientation condition), respectively. More precisely, the right button had to be pressed if the target was green and the left button if it was red in the color condition. In the orientation condition, the participants were asked to press the right button if the target had a horizontal orientation and the left button if it had a vertical orientation.

The effect of object features was assessed in two separate experimental sessions to exclude transfer effects. Furthermore, to control for sequence effects, half of the participants started with the color condition, the other half with the orientation condition. This part of the experiment – the learning phase – consisted of 20 blocks for each condition. Within each block, each of the 16 repeated displays

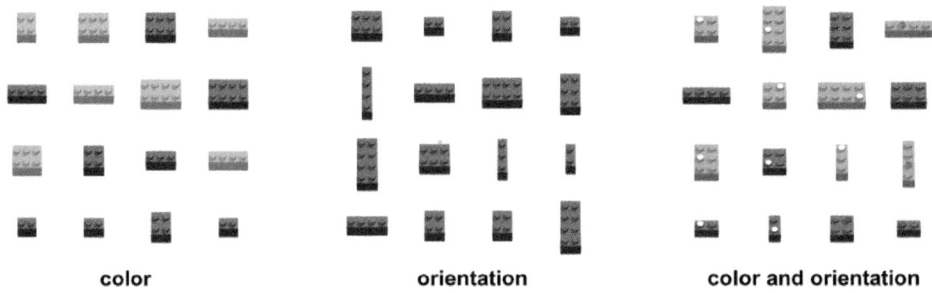

Fig. 2. Examples of search arrays. Each array consisted of 16 LEGO® bricks, arranged in a 4 x 4 matrix. The target was always a brick with 3 units, the distractors were bricks with 2, 6, or 8 units. Color condition (left): stimuli were always horizontal, red or green bricks, Orientation condition (middle): stimuli were always red, horizontal or vertical bricks, Test condition (right): stimuli were horizontal or vertical, red or green with a dark or narrow dot as response-relevant target feature.

was presented once, intermixed with 16 novel search displays for a total of 32 trials per block. The data of 4 subsequent blocks were grouped into an epoch, resulting in 5 epochs. Thereby, variations in response times and eye movements could be assessed depending on the time course of the experiment.

In a second phase of the experiment, we wanted to assess whether the context formed by one critical feature can be transferred to novel contexts that are defined by two features. Therefore, each of the previously described condition was followed by a test phase. In this test phase, search displays were presented that consisted of red and green LEGO® bricks that were oriented horizontally and vertically, each with one light or dark grey dot on one of the knobs. For the distractors, the dot appeared with equal probability on each of the knobs. Participants had to press one of two buttons, corresponding to the dot's color on the target (left button for a light grey dot, right button for a dark grey dot). Novel trials were again randomly generated. For the repeated trials, however, one feature was exactly as in the previous 20 blocks, one was randomly assigned to each stimulus: In the color condition (red and green horizontal bricks in the first 20 blocks), color patterns were taken from the 16 repeated trials from the first 20 blocks, but the orientation level was randomly assigned to each brick. In the orientation condition (vertical and horizontal red bricks in the first 20 blocks), orientation patterns were taken from the first 20 blocks, but the color was randomly chosen for each brick.

The whole experiment consisted of two sessions, conducted on two different days. Each session consisted of a learning and a test phase (cf. Table 1). In the learning phase only one object feature (color or orientation) was varied to establish the context configuration, and in the test phase also the previously absent object feature was added to the context stimuli in order to assess transfer of learning to novel contexts. In the learning phase, three main variables were manipulated: the visual context (repeated vs. novel search displays), the object feature (color vs. orientation), and the epoch (1-5). In the testing phase, the visual context (repeated vs. novel) was manipulated and analyzed depending on the condition of the learning phase.

3.4 Procedure

Each participant attended two sessions of the experiment, one for each condition. Half of the participants started with the color condition and the other half with

Table 1. Task design for the two experimental groups, who performed the color and orientation condition in balanced order

group	session 1		ca. 1 week later	session 2	
	learning	test		learning	test
1	color	color & orientation		orientation	color & orientation
2	orientation	color & orientation		color	color & orientation

the orientation condition. The two sessions were on average 7 days apart (min. 4, max. 9 days).

After being positioned at the workbench, the participants were given a written instruction projected on the display area. They were asked to search for the three-unit LEGO® brick among 15 other LEGO® bricks and to press one of the buttons, depending on the identity of the target. Importantly, participants were not informed about the repetition manipulation of trials.

For eye movement recordings, a 13-dot calibration and validation, and a drift check was conducted before the first trial. Then participants performed 20 blocks of the learning phase followed by 3 blocks of the test phase. After each block participants could take a short break to rest their eyes, but were instructed not to move too much.

They then could start the next block by pressing one of the buttons. A block consisted of 32 trials. Each trial started with the presentation of a black fixation cross in the center of the display area which remained for 1000 ms. After an interval of variable length (300-1000 ms), the stimulus array was presented on the search area. The variable interval prevents the prediction of the stimulus onset and the occurrence of rhythmic pressing of the response buttons. The participant searched for the target and pressed one of the buttons as fast and as accurately as possible, depending on the target's feature identity. The stimulus display remained visible for 500 ms after the button press, and participants were instructed to fixate the target until the display disappeared. The duration of one session of the experiment was about 100 minutes.

3.5   Data Analysis

Reaction times (RTs) were measured as the time from the onset of the search display until the participant's response. Eye movement data were analyzed with the Eyelink data viewer and the fixation counts were computed for each trial. Trials with wrong button presses were defined as errors and excluded from the further analysis. Outliers were defined as values of more than 2 standard deviations below or above the mean value within a subject and block and excluded. The 23 blocks were grouped in sets of 4 blocks each into 5 epochs for the learning phase and into the test epoch consisting of 3 blocks. For the learning phase, mean reaction times and fixation counts were entered into separate repeated-measures ANOVAs with the factors context (repeated vs. novel configurations), object feature (color vs. orientation) and epoch (1 to 5). An effect of epoch reflects changing RTs in the time course of the experiment (i.e. general learning or practice). More interestingly, if the context defined by object features is learned and affects the visual search for a target (i.e. contextual learning), this effect would be reflected by a statistical effect of context. An interaction between the factors feature and context would indicate different learning processes for the features color and orientation. To analyze transfer effects statistically, reaction times in the last epoch of the learning phase and reaction times in the test phase were compared.

4   Experimental Results

Reaction times and fixation counts of the color and orientation condition are shown in Fig. 3.

During the learning phase (epoch 1 to 5), reaction times decreased over time $(F(4, 28) = 10.46, p < 0.001)$. A significant contextual cueing effect occured for the reaction times, that is, shorter search times in the repeated condition across all object features $(F(1, 7) = 14.017, p < 0.01)$. There was no significant difference in RT between color and orientation condition in the learning phase $(F(1, 7) < 1)$ and no interaction between context and feature $(F(1, 7) < 1)$. Regarding the transfer, the comparison of the last epoch of the learning phase and the test phase revealed a significant interaction between phase and object feature $(F(1, 7) = 20.51, p < 0.01)$. That is, in the color condition reaction times increased after adding orientation information to the distractors, whereas in the orientation condition reaction times decreased after adding the color to the distractor configuration. A further analysis of reaction times, which compared the first and last block of the test phase separately for the two feature conditions, showed no reliable effect of context in the color condition $(F(1, 7) < 1)$, but a significant benefit for the repeated trials in the orientation condition $(F(1, 7) = 8.98, p < 0.05)$.

The eye movement analysis in the learning phase revealed a decreasing number of fixations for both object features, which was only marginally significant $(F(4, 28) = 2.146, p = 0.68)$. A contextual cueing effect occurred during the learning phase across color and orientation, that is the fixation count was lower with repeated contexts $(F(1, 7) = 8.35, p < 0.05)$. Similar to the reaction times, no significant difference between the color and the orientation condition was obvious in the learning phase $(F(1, 7) < 1)$ and no interaction between context and feature $(F(1, 7) < 1)$. The last epoch of the learning phase and the test phase showed a significant interaction between object feature and phase $(F(1, 7) = 11.53, p < 0.05)$. That is, in the color condition the number of eye fixations necessary to find the target increased after adding orientation information. In contrast, adding color information led to an decrease of the number of fixations in the orientation condition.

5   Discussion of the Results

The aim of the present experiment was to clarify whether the object features color and orientation are learned differently in a contextual cueing paradigm with complex pictures of real-world objects. Moreover, the interesting question was whether implicit knowledge about context configurations based on color or orientation information could be transferred if an additional feature is added to the context configuration during the test phase. For evaluation of ecological validity it was tested, whether the contextual cueing effect occurs also without gaps in the contextual matrix.

First of all, a contextual cueing effect was present also with the use of a completely filled contextual matrix. This result demonstrates that object features and not only locations are learned. In general, the results show that context configurations based on the features color and orientation can be learned equally well. In both feature conditions a contextual cueing effect could be demonstrated during the learning phase. The benefit did not differ between both feature conditions. Moreover, also the use of more complex real-world objects enabled the development of a benefit for repeated displays over time. Overall, reaction times were longer than in previous experiments with artificial stimuli. Probably, the use of a greater number of distinct context elements together with the presentation of a completely filled matrix lead to longer search times. Interestingly, when the previously absent feature (color or orientation) was added to the context configuration in the test phase, impressive differences occurred in the two feature conditions. Reaction times decreased below the level of the previous learning phase and a benefit for repeated displays (that is displays with the same orientation configuration) was present, if color was added in the test phase. If, however, orientation information was added, reaction times increased in comparison to the learning phase and the contextual cueing effect disappeared. In other words, changing the orientation of context elements after having learned configurations based on pure color information seems to disturb the implicit learning effect. This result is unexpected from a real-world perspective: We have often experienced familiar objects to occur in

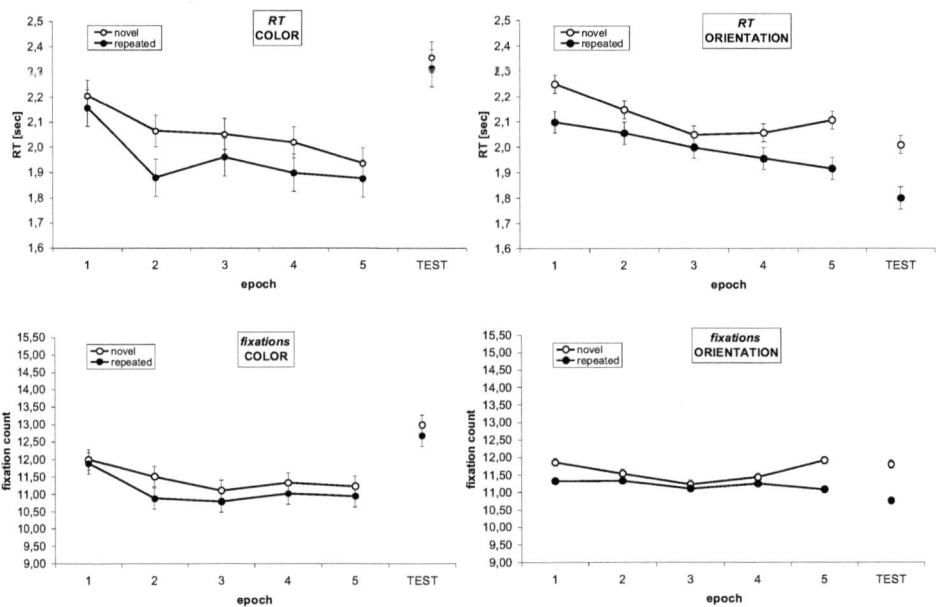

Fig. 3. Reaction times (top; mean and standar error) and fixation counts (bottom; mean and standard errors) for the two condition color (left) and orientation (right) as a function of epoch (x-axis) and context (filled vs. unfilled symbols)

different orientations, however, we would not expect them to suddenly change their color.

In contrast, adding the grey dot to the bricks seemed not to disturb the performance, at least not in the orientation condition. A possible explanation for performance differences can be found in the experimental setting. During the learning phase of the color condition the action-relevant dimension was color and the subjects had to decide whether the target object was colored in red or green. In the subsequent test phase subjects had to decide whether the grey dot was bright or dark. Again, the decision is based on some kind of color dimension, a fact that might lead to interferences in response selection processes because the previously learned color-response association has to be inhibited. However, this assumption can not be evaluated with the present data.

The eye movement pattern, that is the fixation count across epochs in the learning phase and the test phase, resembles nicely the pattern of reaction times. These similarities can be interpreted in favor of an involvement of attentional processes. In accordance to the reaction times, also the fixation counts in the test phase differed between the color and orientation condition.

It might be discussed whether contextual cueing is based on an implicit or explicit learning mechanisms. Although we did not perform an explicit memory test in the current experiment, previous experiments (e.g. [7]) have shown that participants are usually unable to distinguish repeated from novel displays in a memory test after the experiment. In a prestudy with identical stimuli and similar search displays compared to the current experiment, most participants reported that they did not have noticed the repetition of displays. In that experiment, an explicit memory test demonstrated no significant difference between the detection of repeated displays and false identification of new displays. This could be interpreted in favor of an implicit learning mechanism also in the present experiment.

The present experiment nicely shows that contextual cueing is due to a more efficient guidance of attention in repeated displays. However, some questions remain open. For example, the fixation counts show that also with repeated displays several fixations are necessary to find the target, that is, with repeated displays the necessary fixations are only reduced. In contrast to visual search of targets with homogenous distractors [19] the present task seems to be too difficult to be solved with peripheral vision. The stimuli resemble each other too much and focal vision is necessary in order to identify the relevant target as well as to discriminate the relevant target feature (color, orientation or dot color). Because of the similarities between target and distractors several stimuli must be scanned in succession before the target is found and several search strategies can be used [20]. Nevertheless, the benefit of repeated displays might have different reasons. If the familiarity of the context configuration has an immediate effect, the first saccade could already land at a position close to the target. Another possibility is that the context configuration turns to be familiar during the scanning process and therefore saccadic eye movements are directed to the target region after some saccades. Further experiments and more detailed analyses of eye scanpaths will shed light to the mechanism of contextual cueing. Moreover, also the observed asymmetry of the transfer effect for color and orientation stimuli could be better understand if, for example, different eye scanpaths would be found.

In sum, the present study shows that implicit learning can occur in visual contexts based on simple features, such as color and orientation. However, the transfer to configuration with additional features depends on the recent learning history with respect to the order of context features to be learned.

6   Conclusions and Application

An important result for the application of the described implicit learning mechanism is the fact that it does not depend on gaps in spatial configurations. This is relevant for ecological validity and for possible fields of application. For example, the icons for "apps" on mobile phones often form a completely filled matrix without any gaps between the icons, if the maximal amount of icons per page is used (see Fig. 1).

Moreover, the results show that it is possible to use more complex pictures of real-world objects in the described paradigm. Objects in the environment, on Web sites, and in software applications differ in a variety of feature aspects. The generality of the contextual cueing mechanism is necessary, if it should serve for the enhancement of user interfaces.

It should be noted that although the participants of the present experiment were students with a relative low mean age, the result are expected to be generalizable. It has been shown that the contextual cueing effect is present also with older people, that is, it seems to be stable over age [21].

As stated at the beginning, it is essential to understand the underlying mechanism for deciding which features of the context elements can improve visual search performance. With the present study, it has been shown that separate features can be learned. However, how this knowledge is transferred to contexts with additional objects features depends on the feature type learned before. For physical interface consistency, this means that search performance could benefit from constant context elements, which are implicitly learned. The fact, that color and orientation of context elements can be learned equally well suggests that these features should be used for user interface design. Moreover, it seems that certain features can be added (i.e. color) without disturbing the representation of the previously learned context. This could enable a more flexible realization of interface consistency, depending on the task or environment. For example, one could imagine that, depending on a chosen menu, the color of an icon changes. But by keeping the form or orientation of the other icons constant, the target icon is still found more easily. In sum, the present results demonstrate, in contrast to other studies [11], a performance benefit for a specific kind of consistency, namely the consistency of the context. In the future, the implementation of a contextual cueing mechanism into user interface design may help to enhance performance and satisfaction of end users.

Acknowledgments

This project is partially supported within the Cluster of Excellence CoTeSys (Cognition for Technical Systems), funded by the German Research Foundation (DFG). We also want to thank Shanshan Cui who has designed the stimuli and contributed to the setup.

References

[1] Treisman, A., Gormican, S.: Feature analysis in early vision: evidence from search asymmetries. Psychological Review 95, 15–48 (1988)

[2] Bravo, M.J., Nakayama, K.: The role of attention in different visual-search tasks. Perception & Psychophysics 51, 465–472 (1992)

[3] Yantis, S., Jonides, J.: Abrupt visual onsets and selective attention: Evidence from visual search. Journal of Experimental Psychology: Human Perception & Performance 10, 601–621 (1984)

[4] Wang, Q., Cavanagh, P., Green, M.: Familiarity and pop-out in visual search. Perception & Psychophysics 56, 495–500 (1994)

[5] Johnston, W.A., et al.: Attention capture by novel stimuli. Journal of Experimental Psychology: General 119, 397–411 (1990)

[6] Krug, S.: Don't Make Me Think! A Common Sense Approach to Web Usability. New Ryders, Indianapolis (2000)

[7] Chun, M.M., Jiang, Y.H.: Top-down attentional guidance based on implicit learning of visual covariation. Psychological Science 10, 360–365 (1999)

[8] Ozok, A.A., Salvendy, G.: Measuring consistency of Web page design and its effects on performance and satisfaction. Ergonomics 43(4), 443–460 (2000)

[9] Holzinger, A., Stickel, C., Fassold, M., Ebner, M.: Seeing the System through the End Users Eyes: Shadow Expert Technique for Evaluating the Consistency of a Learning Management System. In: Holzinger, A., Miesenberger, K. (eds.) USAB 2009. LNCS, vol. 5889, pp. 178–192. Springer, Heidelberg (2009)

[10] Schneider, W., Shiffrin, R.M.: Controlled and automatic human information processing: detection, search and attention. Psychological Review 84, 1–66 (1977)

[11] AlTaboli, A., Abou-Zeid, R.: Effect of Physical Consistency of Web Interface Design on Users Performance and Satisfaction. In: Jacko, J.A. (ed.) HCI 2007. LNCS, vol. 4553, pp. 849–859. Springer, Heidelberg (2007)

[12] Schankin, A., Stursberg, O., Schubö, A.: The role of implicit context information in guiding visual-spatial attention. In: Caputo, B., Vincze, M. (eds.) ICVW 2008. LNCS, vol. 5329, pp. 93–106. Springer, Heidelberg (2008)

[13] Endo, N., Takeda, Y.: Selective learning of spatial configuration and object identity in visual search. Perception & Psychophysics 66(2), 293–302 (2004)

[14] Song, J.-H., Jiang, Y.: Connecting the past with the present: How do humans match an incoming visual display with visual memory? Journal of Vision 5, 322–330 (2005)

[15] Kunar, M.A., Flusberg, S., Horowitz, T.S., Wolfe, J.M.: Does Contextual cueing Guide the Deployment of Attention? Journal of Experimental Psychology: Human Perception and Performance 33(4), 816–828 (2007)

[16] Schankin, A., Schubö, A.: Cognitive processes facilitated by contextual cueing. Evidence from event-related brain potentials. Psychophysiology 46, 668–679 (2009)

[17] Godijn, R., Pratt, J.: Endogenous saccades are preceded by shifts of visual attention. Evidence from cross-saccadic priming effects 110(1), 83–102 (2002)

[18] Stößel, C., Wiesbeck, M., Stork, S., Zäh, M.F., Schubö, A.: Towards Optimal Worker Assistance: Investigating Cognitive Processes in Manual Assembly. In: Proc. of the 41st CIRP Conference on Manufacturing Systems, pp. 245–250 (2008)

[19] Findlay, J.M.: Saccade Target Selection During Visual Search. Vision Research 37(5), 617–631 (1997)

[20] Findlay, J.M., Brown, V.: Eye scanning of multi-element displays: I. Scanpath planning, Vision Research 46, 179–195 (2006)

[21] Howard, J.H., Howard, D.V., Dennis, N.A., Yankovich, H., Vaidyab, C.J.: Implicit Spatial Contextual Learning in Healthy Aging. Neuropsychology 18(1), 124–134 (2004)

Exploring the Possibilities of Body Motion Data for Human Computer Interaction Research

Johann Schrammel[1], Lucas Paletta[2], and Manfred Tscheligi[1,3]

[1] CURE - Center for Usability Research & Engineering
Modecenterstrasse 17, 1110 Wien, Austria
`{schrammel,tscheligi}@cure.at`
[2] Joanneum Research
Wastiangasse 6, 8010 Graz, Austria
`lucas.paletta@joanneum.at`
[3] HCI-Unit, ICT&S, Universität Salzburg
Sigmund-Haffner-Gasse 18, 5020 Salzburg, Austria

Abstract. The ability to move is an important characteristic of the human condition and an important aspect for interactive settings. The role of body movement however was not addressed with priority in human computer interaction until now. In this paper we explore the possibilities and issues for usability and user experience research utilizing body motion data. We provide an overview of relevant related work and report the setup and initial results of two studies utilizing body motion capture. We discuss the experiences made in using motion capture approaches for human computer interaction research and provide an outlook on future directions of research.

1 Introduction

The possibility to move is an important aspect of the human condition, and body motion is a natural and essential element of interactive settings and scenarios. Until now the role of body movement however was not addressed with priority in human computer interaction and user experience research. This relative lack of interest probably can be explained by the limitations of available technologies capable of collecting motion data reliably and economically. Recently these technological restrictions have become less and less severe, and in future we expect an almost complete removal of restrictions stemming from technical limitations. More and more tools become available that allow to easily access and utilize body movements for interaction purposes. Until recently game controllers for example only used the tiny movements of the fingers to control the action, and current office applications rely almost exclusively on mouse and keyboard input. This is about to change, as the example of the huge success of the Nintendo Wii indicates.

The main goal of this paper is to explore the resulting possibilities and issues for usability and user experience research. We firstly want to outline the theoretical background and present related research focusing on existing work on capturing motion data, the role of movement in human computer interaction. Secondly we present two

G. Leitner, M. Hitz, and A. Holzinger (Eds.): USAB 2010, LNCS 6389, pp. 305–317, 2010.

examples using different technological approaches in addressing these issues and provide information on how we used these approaches in human computer interaction research. We discuss the possibilities, advantages, shortcomings and research implications of these approaches. Finally we provide thoughts on future direction of research using body motion detection and open issues to be solved.

2 Capturing Motion Data

Eadweard Muybridge introduced motion capture 1887 in his now famous experiments entitled Animal Locomotion, in which he studied the way in which animals and birds moved by taking series of photographs. Driven by similar interests in 1973 psychologist Johansson conducted his Moving Light Display (MLD) experiments. Johansson attached reflective markers to the joints of test subjects and recorded their motions [1]. He then asked subjects to identify known movements after being shown only the trajectories of the markers. Since then numerous different approaches to capture and analyze human motion have been suggested, developed and commercially used. This high interest is driven by numerous promising application domains for motion capture e.g. advanced user interfaces, motion analysis for clinical and sports training purposes, surveillance systems or virtual reality applications. Motion capture systems have been developed using very different types of technologies.

Vision based techniques capture body movement by use of cameras, either using markers or working markerless. Vision-based human motion estimation and analysis has been a thriving area of research within the past years. In an overview article Moeslund [2] for example identified over three-hundred related publications over the period of 2000–06 in major conferences and journals dealing with this topic. In a recent special issue of the Int. Journal of Computer Vision on the topic of human motion tracking Sigal and Black [3] characterized it as a "mostly solved problem in constrained situations". However, in unconstrained contexts and for real-time applications there are still important issues to be adressed.

Another approach uses feedback from *angle sensors attached to the human body joints*. Such systems are commercially available, provide reliable data and have been used successfully in HCI-studies [e.g. 4, 5]. However, they are rather cumbersome and obtrusive for the user. The latest model of the GYPSY-6 exoskeleton by Animazoo for example still weights over 6 kg and takes about 10 minutes to setup.

A third approach uses data from *position, orientation and accelerometer sensors* attached to the human body. Knight et al. [6] report various uses of accelerometers ranging from physics teaching, science education, posture measurement and ambulatory monitoring. Examplary applications within the field of HCI are Shoogle [7], DJogger [8] or ubifit [9]. The advantage of this tracking approach is that the used sensors are rather cheap, easy to track and relatively unobtrusive for the user. However, the information these sensors provide on body motion is typically either not very accurate (position) or provides only relative data (accelerometers), and therefore is more difficult to use and interpret than complete motion information. A popular implementation variant due to its ease of implementation for this approach is to utilize the controllers of the Nintendo Wii as accelerometer sensors [e.g. 10, 11, 12, 13].

Next we also want to briefly mention approaches that focus only on *capturing single elements of body motions*. For example big size touch screens such as used in tabletop computing could be considered as type of motion capture devices as they have the capability of tracking the position of the body part in contact with the screen (typically the fingers) [e.g. 14, 15, 7].

Summarizing we can say that cheap controllers and sensors that allow to recognize and track the movement of users have become available, and that they are more and more used in dedicated interaction devices. Examples include accelerometer based (e.g. Nintendos Wii) or computer vision based (Microsofts' project Natal) game controllers. Also, more and more mobile devices such as handheld phones or tablet computers are equipped with build-in accelerometer and tilt sensors, and therefore allow to be used as motion controllers and enable new interactive experiences. Another driver fostering increased importance of movement in interaction is the continuing success of touch-based interaction combined with decreasing costs of big-size screens. This two effects lead to the inclusion of semi-natural and intuitive body and movement-gestures in the interaction. Furthermore progress in gesture recognition and mobile augmented reality applications fosters the application possibilities of whole body interaction.

We think that these developments drive interaction towards more and more involvement of movement resulting in interaction styles that could be summarized as *whole body interaction*.

3 Analyzing Motion Data

In many cases the available motion data can be directly used for interaction purposes e.g. if the movement and position of the users lower arm is tracked correctly it can be used as input device e.g. as a pointer. However, human motion data contains more information than the position and orientation of body parts alone. Analyzing movement patterns across time researchers have identified several possibilities to interpret the data in a semantically meaningful way.

A first popular direction of analysis is the automated detection and recognition of user behavior and activity. Research has shown that state-of-the-art systems are able to successfully detect different types of user behavior and activities such as walking, running, standing, and sitting based on their specific movement patterns [e.g. 16, 17, 9]. Also everyday activities such as brushing ones teethes or vacuuming the floor could be learned and detected successfully by these systems [18].

However, it is not only possible to detect physical activities of the user or his context, motion data also allows to derive data about the cognitive and emotional state of users. [19] showed that humans are capable of judging the emotional state of a human body from motion information alone. Similarly [20] showed that it is possible to recognize emotions better than chance based solely on gait information. Since then efforts have been made to automatically detect and estimate the emotional state of users based on motion data (more details on the relationship between motion and emotion are discussed in the next chapter). It has also been shown that personality traits correlate with characteristics of music-induced movement [21], suggesting that motion data can bee used to estimate personality traits.

Another possible application that has been addressed in research is the usage of the uniqueness of movement patterns of a user for authentication purposes. Applications in the context of security and disambiguation between users in multi-user contexts have been proposed. For example gait recognition has been successfully demonstrated [e.g. 22].

4 Motion, Emotion, Interaction and Experience

The previous paragraphs showed that from a viewpoint of analysis and application scenarios several relevant directions exist. To fully utilize the potential of these analyses it is helpful to also take a phenomenological view on the different functions of body movements. For the context of interactive scenarios in general and gaming in specific Berthouze [23] distinguishes between five different types or functions of body movements:

Table 1. Categorization of body movement types as proposed by Berthouze [23]

Body movement	Description
Task-control	necessary to control the game
Task-facilitating	facilitating the control
Task(role)-related	typical of the role defined by the game scenario
Enjoyment and emotional expressions	expressing affective states related to or induced by the game experience
Social behavior (attention seeking, synchronized movement, etc.)	supporting social interaction

Taken a closer look, Table 1 above shows that important aspects of the functionality of body motions are related to the expression of emotional experiences. Motion and Emotion are even very similar literally, and researchers suspect that there are causal relations between these two concepts. The direction of this causality and the details of the involved mechanisms are not clear yet and subject to ongoing research.

A study by Riskind and Gotay [24], for example, revealed how "subjects who had been temporarily placed in a slumped, depressed physical posture later appeared to develop helplessness more readily, as assessed by their lack of persistence in a standard learned helplessness task, than did subjects who had been placed in an expansive, upright posture."

With regard to the relationship between movement and user experience common sense and results from UX research suggests that the interaction with products, tools, and artifacts can be enriched by allowing people to move naturally and unrestrictedly [4, 25]. If people can express themselves using their whole body, they immerse into another world more naturally and easily. Results show that even engagement and social interaction are encouraged by controllers that afford movement [26]. Izard et al. [27] describes neural, sensorimotor, motivational and cognitive processes that can influence emotions. Body posture and movement can activate emotions by afferent processes.

These examples of the important role of motion for experience in interactive settings highlight the need to include data on this aspect in user experience research and to further research the involved processes in more detail.

5 Example Studies Utilizing Body Motions

In the previous chapters we analyzed that utilization of motion data and embodied interaction from a technological and theoretical viewpoint. We conclude that there seems to be a high potential to enhance interactive experiences by including motion data in interaction design and user experience. In the next sections we want to present two different approaches we have used in praxis for studying user experience and human computer interaction aspects considering motion. We briefly report selected results of this studies to show the possibilities of the chosen approaches. However, the full analysis of data and the discussion of the individual results are not within the scope of this paper and are subject of (future) dedicated publications.

Study 1: Using accelerometer data to track users' movement during gameplay

A first setting we want to describe to be able to discuss and analyze the possibilities of motion capture for user experience research is in the context of game research.

Research Questions. In detail we were interested in answering the question whether a more embodied way of controlling the interaction is amplifying experience in a gaming context as expected?

Study Design. To control weather our hypothesis of enhanced experiences is correct we conducted a simple comparison of self-reported experiences in two different gaming conditions either controlling a game by Wii-controllers designed to be used with body gestures and traditional joystick-like controllers using only the thumbs to control the game.

Six female and six male subjects participated in the study. Participants were between 20 and 36 years old and had extensive experience in computer game playing. Each participant brought a friend of the same sex along, against whom they were playing in the gaming session of the study.

Participants were playing two different tasks (food tracing and cow tossing) from the game "Rayman Raving Rabbids" on the Sony Playstation 2 (seated condition) and on the Nintendo Wii (motion condition). Play time to finish the tasks on either type of console typically was between 10 and 15 minutes. Amount of movements of the player was tracked by use of a second Wii Remote attached to the dominant arm (see below for detailed description of setup). Participants played against the friend they brought with them. "Rayman Raving Rabbids" has very similar graphics on the two consoles and gaming sites give them the same rating. Half of the participants started with the Wii, and half with the Ps2.

After each condition participants were asked to rate their average experience during playing by use of Emocards [28]. Additionally, participants were asked to describe the emotionally most outstanding situation during play. They were also asked to fill out a questionnaire using Likert-scale items regarding perceived agitation and emotions.

Additionally facial muscle activity of the zygomaticus major muscle (the "smile" muscle) and the currogator supercilii muscle (the "frown" muscle) was measured by use of electromyography to gather continous uindicators for user experience.

Motion capture setup: For Capturing the motion of the users we used Wiimotes from Nintendo. Wiimotes are equipped with three-axis accelerometer sensors, and they are ideal for rapid deployment since they are equipped with wireless connection functionality to a host computer using Bluetooth, and free open source code for accessing the sensor data exists. In detail we used the DarwiinRemote (Version 0.3.1) Software (available at http://sourceforge.net/projects/darwin-remote/). As the Wiimotes communicate using Bluetooth it is unfortunately not possible to read out the movement data of a Wiimote and to use it at the same time as a controller in the standard Wii configuration. The Wiimotes are also equipped with an infrared camera, a vibration sensor, and a loudspeaker. These are not used for the experiments reported here, but present interesting possibilities for usage in future projects. Figure 1 below shows the readings of the accelerometer-sensors provided by DarwiinRemote-Software. In the pictured sequence the Wiimote was first moved back and forth along all three main dimensions resulting in the dominance of the data from the regarding accelerometer, and then wiggled without specific direction. To use the data in analysis the readings from all sensors can be recorded in a time-stamped logfile.

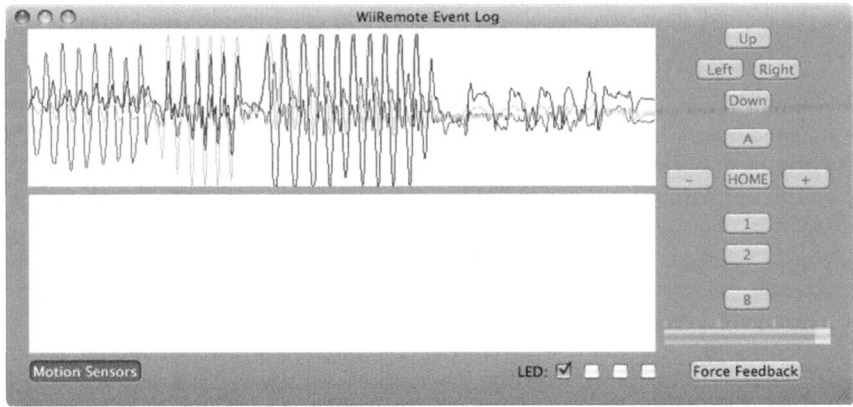

Fig. 1. Screenshot from DarwiinRemote-Software Showing Readings from Accelerometers

Comparing Gaming Conditions: Users reported more positive experience when using the Wii compared to the Ps2. Two-way repeated measures ANOVA with sex and game condition as independent variables showed a significant main effect for self-reported experience.

Correlation of Motion and EMG: Situational motion data (as provided by the Wii) and experience indicators (EMG data) was correlated to further analyze the relationship of these two data sources. The motions of gamers show a highly significant correlation with both, the EMG-values of the zygomaticus (r=0.139, p<0.01) and the currogator (r=0.256, p<0.01). One might suspect that this correlation is caused by a slight activation of the tracked muscles related to an overall increased tension during movements. However, several arguments point against this interpretation. First, in this analysis only a binary representation of EMG data was used and threshold values were manually assigned to the data taking care they are set high enough to only detect meaningful activation. Second, several random samples of video data from different study participants were analyzed regarding the plausibility of the binary EMG-outputs. No indication for erroneous data was found.

Qualitative results support this interpretation, as the following example statements from participants show:

"Playing on the Wii is more fun, the whole body is in movement and not only fingers and thumbs."

"I preferred playing on the Wii better. You have to do more with the arm and move more. If you are allowed to do this, you can better feel the game play"

Study 2: Using position data to study the relationship of users' attention and motion in public outdoor scenarios

Research Questions. The main question of the second study was to better understand, which areas and objects receive attention by pedestrians in a shopping street, and whether there is a significant influence of the users movement on the direction of attention.

Study Design. 16 study participants where equipped with mobile eye-tracking systems and various sensors (detailed description below) which were used to track the users motion. Participants were asked to perform a realistic task within the inner city of Graz, which was to stroll through the Grazer Herrengasse and inform themselves about shopping possibilities in the street. Overall time of data capture per test person was about 15 minutes.

Motion capture setup. In this study a different motion capture setup was chosen. For capturing the users body and head movements two low-cost Inertial Measurement Units (IMUs) of manufacturer XSens (http://www.xsens.com) were used. Xsens MTi-G was used to capture head data (the sensor was mounted to the helmet of the eye-tracking equipment), and Xsens MTx was used to capture body movement (the sensor was attached to the participants' waist using a customary belt pouch). Both sensors were connected via USB to a Laptop-Computer the test participant carried in a rucksack. "MT Manager"-Software provided by the manufacturer of the sensors was used to record the data.

We also used the build-in sensors of the Google Nexus One smartphone to capture GPS-position data. The position fixing component of the device is a GPS receiver, which is integrated directly within the chipset. Unfortunately, the manufacturer does not provide publicly available specifications. The device is also equipped with integrated accelerometers and a tilt compensated magnetic sensor. Only the GPS-data was used as the x-sensors provide more accurate data. However, using the build-in sensors would be a very attractive option for application scenarios that require only tracking the body position and do not call for very high accuracy.

Additionally a mobile eye-tracking system was used during the study. This analysis of this data is still underway, and results with regard to gaze fixations are not yet available and will be the subject of future publications. Figure 2 below shows a photograph of a participant equipped with the full set of sensors.

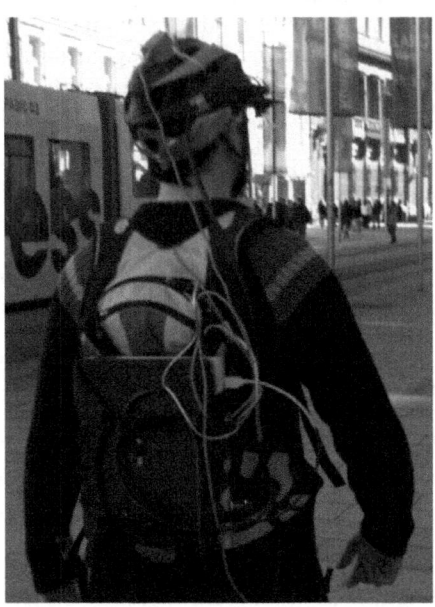

Fig. 2. Participant equipped with tracking technology in the Grazer Herrengasse

Body and Head Orientation of Pedestrians: A first focus of analysis of the data was to analyze the area of the attention of the pedestrians in the urban setting. Our basic reference system for the field of attention is the human body itself. Regarding horizontal direction of attention the reference is the body orientation of the user (measured by the sensor at the waist), and the relative orientation of the head (measured by the sensor mounted on the helmet). For vertical orientation we chose to use the perpendicular axis as main reference. Figure 3 provides an overview of the average horizontal orientation of the users head relative to the body orientation. The graphic shows a distribution of orientation as might be expected: In the majority of cases the head orientation is aligned with the body orientation, with decreasing numbers for relative orientations to the sides. There are almost no cases with a relative angle of more than 60 degrees in either direction.

Figure 4 shows the results for the vertical alignment of the head of pedestrian users on the move. The image clearly shows that the most attention is directed towards a slightly lowered position, and that there is much more attention towards the lower sphere than the upper sphere. This can easily be explained by the needs of pedestrians to navigate between other pedestrians, the usage and consultation of personal devices (e.g. looking on the watch, consulting written materials, using electronic devices, etc.) and watching objects of interest in shopping windows.

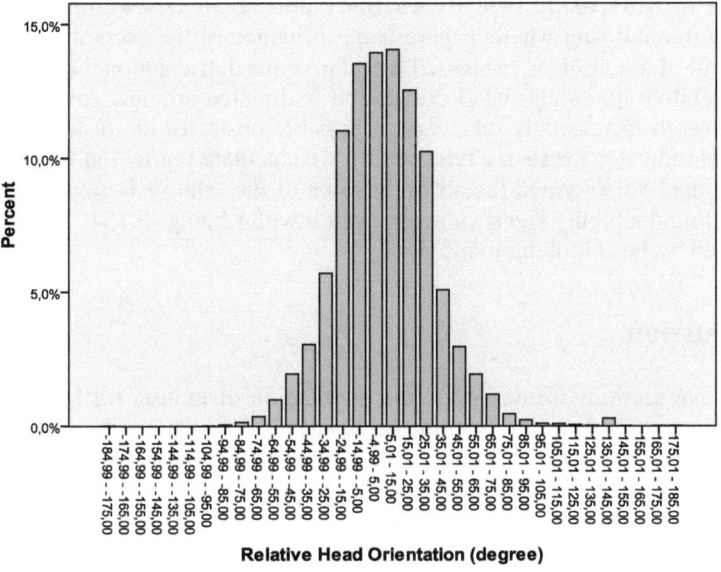

Fig. 3. Relative horizontal head orientation expressed in degrees across all test participants

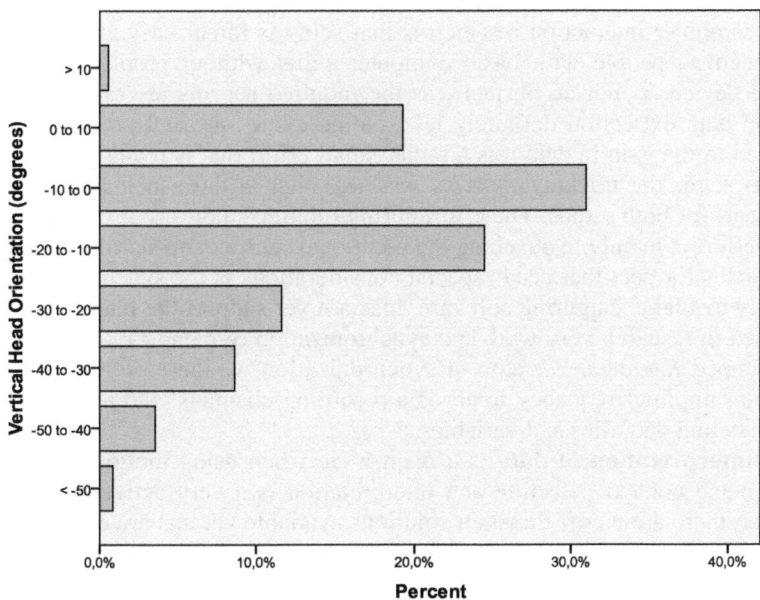

Fig. 4. Relative vertical head orientation expressed in degrees across all test participants

Influence of Movement Velocity on Body and Head Orientation: We next were interested in analyzing whether there is an influence of the users movement velocity on the field of attention as expressed by relative head orientation. Our hypothesis was that the relative horizontal head orientation is directed stronger towards the front as the user has to increasingly take care of possible obstacles the faster he moves. As a first initial indicator for such a relationship we calculate regression (Pearson) between the movement velocity and the absolute value of the relative horizontal head orientation. We found a highly significant correlation with r being -0.154. The faster the user moves the less he is looking to his sides.

6 Discussion

In the above sections we described the application of motion tracking technology in two different studies. In this section we want to discuss the individual results of the studies in much detail but focus on the experiences made with the different approaches and discuss the possibilities of tracking technologies for HCI research.

Both study setups show that the utilization of motion capture provides valuable data for the research. The finding of study 1 directly support our hypothesis that increased involvement of motion provides positive chances for enhanced user experiences, and study 2 showed that tracking that can provide helpful information of the users attention, that would not be available otherwise.

Practical issues. A first experience from applying motion tracking technology for human computer interaction research is that setup is rather easy and can be done by non-specialists people with basic computer skills without problems. Also, cost of tracking devices is not an obstacle, as the required sensors are rather cheap. Setup-time and data extraction definitely takes some extra time and precautions, however compared to the gain in data it is a rather small effort that is required. In detail initial effort to setup the tracking systems was less than a day (including testing of the equipment) for both setups. The effort during running studies is also very small, as the needed effort is mainly in attaching the additional sensors and starting data recording.

A practical aspect that needs special considerations is the synchronization of data. Currently available capturing software does not yet support the integration with other tools used in research very well, and synchronization of data has to be done based on time-stamped raw data. For ease of synchronization we therefore recommend to use the same sampling frequency in all data recording channels, and to follow god practice of labeling data files and variables.

The interpretation of data is a main issue when using motion data. Automated behavior and context detection and interpretation is a very active field of research. However, there are no off-the-shelf solutions available yet that are easy to use by non-experts and provide reliable data. Typically, the available approaches and algorithms need to be specifically targeted to the used context of the study, and extensive calibration and fine-tuning of parameters by experts is needed to achieve good results. However, there are several aspects of body motion that can be easily interpreted, do not need extensive setup and anyhow provide valuable data. In Study 1 we showed that accelerometer data and the conveyed information about the amount of movement can be helpful for a better understanding of gaming experience, and study 2 showed that basic movement data such as velocity and orientation allow to better understand patterns of attention of pedestrians in urban outdoor settings.

On very big advantage of using motion data is the availability of **continuous and unobtrusively captured user data**. This allows to study user behavior and experience related to the sensed variables across time, without the need to interrupt the user with frequent questions and thereby artificially altering the interactive process. Also such setups allow the study facilitator to observe data online, and to take targeted interventions if required by the study goals or to asked focused questions in follow-up interviews referring to the specifics of a situation brought to attention of the researcher by the online data. This aspect will be especially interesting once reliable detection mechanisms become available, however already now with very unreliable data or only human interpretation this capturing mechanisms could form a good basis for analysis. Another interesting possibility for research is to use the recorded data to identify sequences of special interest and to discuss these situations with participants after the test.

A further advantage of utilizing body motion data in HCI-research is the possibility to easily **compare the behavior of different study participants** with regard to their interaction styles. The availability of recorded data fosters the comparative analysis either by use of statistical procedures or by the visual analysis of movement patterns.

Another relevant application context for body motion data is the **facilitation of Wizard-of-Oz studies**. In the section on related work numerous possibilities for the application of body motion data in different types of interfaces has been shown, and research is needed on how to optimally design these interfaces. Wizard-of-Oz studies with a human operator simulating the targeted behavior of different algorithms could help to identify the most valuable directions of research early in the research process. Visually displaying the readings of motion sensors could very much ease the task of the wizard, which is known to be a very challenging responsibility.

To even more broaden the possibilities of motion data in **future research** we want to especially focus on the following areas:

- Include eye tracking data and integrate with motion data to generate unified method for studying users' attention in outdoor scenarios. We also work on integrating this model with a virtual model of the environment.
- Expand classification of body movement types to more general scenarios and framework for understanding the meaning and function of body movements.
- Develop set of methods that allows recognizing relevant behavior for HCI automatically. We do not expect to achieve 100% accuracy, but preprocessing of data will enormously speed up the annotation of observation data.

7 Conclusions

In this paper we showed the relevance and potential of body motion data for human computer interaction research and provided examples from real studies in the field of HCI. The approaches we described and discussed can and easily be used by other researchers, and valuable inputs for HCI can be generated.

References

1. Johansson, G.: Visual Perception of Biological Motion and a Model for Its Analysis. Perception Psychophysics 14(2), 201–211 (1973)
2. Moeslund, T.B., Hilton, A., Krüger, V.: A survey of advances in vision-based human motion capture and analysis Comput. Image Underst. 104(2), 90–126 (2006)
3. Sigal, L., Black, M.J.: Guest Editorial: State of the Art in Image- and Video-Based Human Pose and Motion Estimation. Int. J. Comput. Vision 87(1-2), 1–3 (2010)
4. Bianchi-Berthouze, N., Kim, W.W., Patel, D.: Does Body Movement Engage You More in Digital Game Play? and Why? In: Paiva, A.C.R., Prada, R., Picard, R.W. (eds.) ACII 2007. LNCS, vol. 4738, pp. 102–113. Springer, Heidelberg (2007)
5. Pasch, M., Berthouze, N., van Dijk, E., Nijholt, A.: Motivations, Strategies, and Movement Patterns of Video Gamers Playing Nintendo Wii Boxing. In: ECAG 2008 (2008)
6. Knight, J.F., Bristow, H.W., Anastopoulou, S., Baber, C., Schwirtz, A., Arvanitis, T.N.: Uses of accelerometer data collected from a wearable system Personal Ubiquitous Comput., vol. 11(2), pp. 117–132. Springer, Heidelberg (2007)
7. Williamson, J., Murray-Smith, R., Hughes, S.: Shoogle: excitatory multimodal interaction on mobile devices. In: Proceedings of the SIGCHI conference on Human factors in computing systems, CHI 2007, pp. 121–124. ACM, New York (2007)
8. Biehl, J.T., Adamczyk, P.D., Bailey, B.P.: DJogger: a mobile dynamic music device. In: CHI 2006 extended abstracts on Human factors in computing systems, CHI 2006. ACM, New York (2006)
9. Consolvo, S., McDonald, D.W., Toscos, T., Chen, M.Y., Froehlich, J., Harrison, B., Klasnja, P., LaMarca, A., LeGrand, L., Libby, R., Smith, I., Landay, J.A.: Activity sensing in the wild: a field trial of ubifit garden. In: Proceeding of the twenty-sixth annual SIGCHI conference on Human factors in computing systems, CHI 2008, pp. 1797–1806. ACM, New York (2008)
10. Hafner, V.V., Bachmann, F.: Human-Humanoid Walking Gait Recognition Humanoids 2008. In: 8th IEEE-RAS International Conference on Humanoid Robots (2008)
11. Schou, T., Gardner, H.J.: A Wii remote, a game engine, five sensor bars and a virtual reality theatre. In: Proceedings of the 19th Australasian conference on Computer-Human Interaction, OZCHI 2007, pp. 231–234. ACM, New York (2007)
12. Schlömer, T., Poppinga, B., Henze, N., Boll, S.: Gesture recognition with a Wii controller. In: Proceedings of the 2nd international conference on Tangible and embedded interaction, TEI 2008, pp. 11–14. ACM, New York (2008)
13. Schreiber, M., Wilamowitz-Moellendorff, M., Bruder, R.: New Interaction Concepts by Using the Wii Remote. In: Proceedings of the 13th International Conference on Human-Computer Interaction. Part II, pp. 261–270. Springer, Heidelberg (2009)
14. Patten, J., Recht, B., Ishii, H.: Interaction techniques for musical performance with tabletop tangible interfaces. In: Proceedings of the 2006 ACM SIGCHI International Conference on Advances in Computer Entertainment Technology, ACE 2006, p. 27. ACM, New York (2006)
15. Collins, A.E.: Exploring tabletop file system interaction. In: CHI 2007 Extended Abstracts on Human Factors in Computing Systems, CHI 2007, pp. 2171–2176. ACM, New York (2007)
16. Ravi, N., Dandekar, N., Mysore, P., Littman, M.L.: Activity recognition from accceleration data American Association for Artificial Intelligence (2005)
17. Györbiro, N., Fabian, A., Homanyi, G.: An activity recognition system for mobile phones Mob. Netw. Appl. 14(1), 82–91 (2009)

18. Yang, J.-Y., Wang, J.-S., Chen, Y.-P.: Using acceleration measurements for activity recognition: An effective learning algorithm for constructing neural classifiers. Pattern Recognition Letters 29(16), 2213–2220 (2008)
19. Dittrich, W.H., Troscianko, T., Lea, S.E., Morgan, D.: Perception of emotion from dynamic point-light displays represented in dance. Perception 25 (1996)
20. Montepare, J.M., Goldstein, S.B., Clausen, A.: The identification of emotions from gait information. Journal of Nonverbal Behavior 11 (1987)
21. Geoff, L., Saarikallio, S., Toiviainen, P.: Personality traits correlate with characteristics of music-induced movement. In: 7th Triennial Conference of European Society for the Cognitive Sciences of Music, ESCOM 2009 (2009)
22. Gafurov, D., Snekkenes, E.: Gait recognition using wearable motion recording sensors. EURASIP J. Adv. Signal Process, Hindawi Publishing Corp. 2009, 1–16 (2009)
23. Berthouze, N.: Body movement as a means to modulate engagement in computer games. In: Workshop on Whole body Interaction II: The future of the human body, HCI 2008 (2008)
24. Riskind, J.H., Gotay, C.C.: Physical posture: Could it have regulatory or feedback effects on motivation and emotion? Motivation and Emotion 6 (1982)
25. Moen, J.: From hand-held to body-worn: embodied experiences of the design and use of a wearable movement-based interaction concept. In: Proceedings of the 1st International Conference on Tangible and Embedded Interaction, TEI 2007, pp. 251–258. ACM, New York (2007)
26. Lindley, S.E., Le Couteur, J., Berthouze, N.L.: Stirring up experience through movement in game play: effects on engagement and social behavior. In: Proceeding of the CHI 2008 SIGCHI Conference on Human Factors in Computing Systems. ACM, New York (2008)
27. Izard, C.: Four Systems for Emotion Activation: Cognitive and Noncognitive Processes. Psychological Review 100 (1993)
28. Desmet, P., Overbeeke, C., Tax, S.: Designing products with added emotional value: development and application of an approach for research through design. The Design Journal 4(1) (2001)

International Workshop on Enabling User Experience with Future Interactive Learning Systems (UXFUL 2010)

Sabine Graf[1], Kinshuk[2], and Andreas Holzinger[3]

[1,2] Athabasca University, School of Computing and Information Systems
1100, 10011-109 Street, Edmonton, AB T5J-3S8, Canada
sabineg@athabscau.ca,
kinshuk@athabscau.ca
[3] Medical University Graz, A-8036 Graz, Austria
Institute for Medical Informatics, Statistics & Documentation (IMI)
Research Unit HCI4MED
andreas.holzinger@medunigraz.at

Abstract. Nowadays most educational institutions use learning systems in order to provide blended or fully online courses in a formal setting with high similarity to learning in a classroom. However, new technologies such as mobile, pervasive and ubiquitous technologies can enable learners to have richer learning experiences through learning that can take place whenever learners are interested in learning, at anytime and anywhere. Multimodal, smart and intelligent devices make the interaction between the learners and the system more natural and intuitive and considering the learners' current situation and characteristics allows the personalization and adaptation of learning material and activities, leading to more effective learning by providing learners with information that is relevant for them. This workshop brings together researchers from Psychology and Computer Science, aiming at discussing research on using and incorporating such new technologies in learning systems and therefore, providing learners with rich learning experiences at anytime and anywhere, in a more intuitive and personalized way.

Keywords: User experience, multimodal devices, mobile/pervasive/ubiquitous learning, adaptivity & personalization, smart & intelligent technologies, learning environments/systems.

1 Introduction and Motivation

Standard information systems for learning purposes have matured, technology is stable and masses of information can be made available to the learner. However, Data is not Information, Information is not Knowledge. The increasing amount of information and the shorter time for learning processes with respect to higher quality forces us to think about possibilities of finding new ways to optimize learning management systems (e.g. [1, 2, 3, 4]).

G. Leitner, M. Hitz, and A. Holzinger (Eds.): USAB 2010, LNCS 6389, pp. 318–321, 2010.

Most educational institutions are already using such learning systems either in a blended or purely online way for delivering parts of courses or fully online courses to their students. These systems allow the management and presentation of online courses, which include different types of resources and activities such as learning material, quizzes, forums, etc. Most of these systems are desktop-based, supporting a formal way of learning, which is in many matters similar to learning in traditional classrooms. However, new technologies provide us with much more opportunities, supporting learning in a more informal way, whenever a learner wants to learn, in the real world, from real learning objects and in a personalized way considering the learners' current situation, previous knowledge and experiences as well as their individual characteristics [5].

We are surrounded by multimodal interfaces which enable the inclusion of all human senses, and mobile, ubiquitous and pervasive technology is available everywhere and at all time [6]. Current research deals with using such new technologies for the purpose of learning, integrating them in current learning systems, and building learning environments where students are provided with more authentic learning experiences both inside and outside of the classroom. Through using mobile devices as well as sensors that communicate with those mobile devices, learners can learn from real-life objects, having learning experiences in real life situations at the time learners are interested in learning. Furthermore, new technologies allow students to interact with the learning environment in more natural and intuitive ways, using multimodal and smart interfaces from various types of devices ranging from mobile phones to smart boards/tables and ubiquitous computing [7] and to interactive simulations [8]. By using all these devices and sensors, a huge amount of information about learners as well as their environment can be detected and stored. Such rich information can be used to make learning more personalized and adaptive to learners' needs by considering data available about a learner's current context/situation (e.g., location, environment, surrounding people, surrounding real-life learning objects etc.) as well as data about a learner's characteristics (e.g., interests, experiences, prior knowledge, cognitive abilities, learning styles, etc.), enabling provision of adaptive and personalized learning resources and activities. While there are masses of learning resources, activities and information available, concrete data about learners' situation and characteristics enables new technologies to filter and decide on how to present relevant information, resources and/or activities to learners, avoiding the provision of irrelevant materials.

The focus of this workshop is on the provision of enhanced user experience (UX), including making information, resources and activities more useful, usable and enjoyable. This is a challenge for interdisciplinary research on the intersection of Psychology and Computer Science, aiming at using technology in the way it is most effective for supporting the learning process of learners.

2   The Workshop Papers at a Glance

In this section, we briefly introduce the papers of this workshop. The first paper, by Giovannella, Spadavecchia and Camusi, deals with ubiquitous learning environments, liquid places and the "organic" era, discussing the design in education and educational experiences in such environments. Furthermore, the paper presents a set of tools and methodologies that can help monitoring the social level of the interactions and the quality of social emotions in such environments.

The second paper by Granić and Nakić focuses on user modelling and identifying individual differences of learners in order to provide adaptivity and personalization. Based on a comprehensive literature review, individual characteristics of learners, which are used in adaptive systems, are discussed and a framework for their classification is proposed.

The next two papers are in the area of technology enhanced language learning. The paper by Eimler, von der Pütten, Schächtle, Carstens and Krämer deals with using a robot for supporting children in starting to learn English as second language. The paper introduces the robot rabbit Nabaztag and presents an evaluation of the robot with respect to hedonic aspects, motivating function, as well as the general usability and overall impression evoked by the robot. On the other hand, the paper by Romero, Zarraonandia, Aedo and Díaz, discusses design and usability aspects for courses delivered through mobile learning. The paper describes the design process for creating courses to develop English grammar, reading and listening skills through mobile learning scenarios and presents respective guidelines.

The paper by Tomberg, Laanpere and Lamas deals with enhancing blog-based learning environments with functionality that brings such environments closer to traditional learning management systems and therefore proposes the incorporation of learning flow management and semantic data exchange in blog-based learning environments.

3   Program Committee

We are most grateful for the support of this workshop to

Reinhold Behringer, Leeds Metropolitan University, UK
Maiga Chang, Athabasca University, Canada
Nian-Shing Chen, National Sun Yat-sen University, Taiwan
Matjaz Debevc, University of Maribor, Slovenia
Carlo Giovannella, ScuolaIaD University di Roma Tor Vergata, Italy
Vlado Glavinic, University of Zagreb, Croatia
Ray Yueh-Min Huang, National Cheng-Kung University, Taiwan
Gwo-Jen Hwang, National University of Taiwan, Taiwan
Jiyou Jia, Peking University, China
Charalambos Karagiannidis, University of Thessaly, Greece
Vive Kumar, Athabasca University, Canada
Chung Hsien Lan, Nanya Institute of Technology, Taiwan
Chien-Sing Lee, Georgia Institute of Technology, USA
Jimmy Lee, The Chinese University of Hong Kong, Hong Kong
Gerd Mietzel, University Duisburg-Essen, Germany
Toshio Okamoto, University of Electro-Communications, Japan
Elvira Popescu, University of Craiova, Romania
Carsten Roecker, RWTH Aachen, Germany

Demetrios Sampson, University of Piraeus & CERTH, Greece
Jean Underwood, Nottingham Trent University, UK
Geoff Underwood, Nottingham University, UK
Stephen J.H. Yang, National Central University, Taiwan
Martina Ziefle, RWTH Aachen, Germany.

References

1. Stickel, C., Ebner, M., Holzinger, A.: Useful Oblivion Versus Information Overload in e-Learning Examples in the Context of Wiki Systems. Journal of Computing and Information Technology (CIT) 16(4), 271–277 (2008)
2. Graf, S.: Adaptivity in learning management systems focussing on learning styles. Ph.D. thesis, Vienna University of Technology (2007)
3. Graf, S., Kinshuk, I.C.: A Flexible Mechanism for Providing Adaptivity Based on Learning Styles in Learning Management Systems. In: Proceedings of the IEEE International Conference on Advanced Learning Technologies (ICALT 2010), pp. 30–34. IEEE Computer Society, Sousse (2010)
4. Graf, S., MacCallum, K., Liu, T.-C., Chang, M., Wen, D., Tan, Q., Dron, J., Lin, F., McGreal, R.: Kinshuk: An Infrastructure for Developing Pervasive Learning Environments. In: Proceedings of the IEEE International Workshop on Pervasive Learning (PerEL 2008), pp. 389–394. IEEE Press, Hong Kong (2008)
5. Graf, S., Kinshuk: Adaptivity and personalization in ubiquitous learning systems. In: Holzinger, A. (ed.) USAB 2008. LNCS, vol. 5298, pp. 331–338. Springer, Heidelberg (2008)
6. Holzinger, A., Nischelwitzer, A.K., Kickmeier-Rust, M.D.: Pervasive E-Education supports Life Long Learning: Some Examples of X-Media Learning Objects. Paper presented at the World Conference on Continuing Engineering Education, Vienna (2006), http://www.wccee2006.org/papers/445.pdf
7. Holzinger, A., Softic, S., Stickel, C., Ebner, M., Debevc, M., Hu, B.: Nintendo Wii Remote Controller in Higher Education: Development and Evaluation of a Demonstrator Kit for e-Teaching. Computing & Informatics 29(3), 1001–1015 (2010)
8. Holzinger, A., Kickmeier-Rust, M.D., Wassertheurer, S., Hessinger, M.: Learning performance with interactive simulations in medical education: Lessons learned from results of learning complex physiological models with the HAEMOdynamics SIMulator. Computers & Education 52(2), 292–301 (2009)

Following the White Rabbit – A Robot Rabbit as Vocabulary Trainer for Beginners of English

Sabrina Eimler, Astrid von der Pütten, Ulrich Schächtle,
Lucas Carstens, and Nicole Krämer

University of Duisburg-Essen, Department of Social Psychology: Media and Communication,
Forsthausweg 2, 47048 Duisburg, Germany
{Sabrina.Eimler,Astrid.von-der-Puetten,
Nicole.Kraemer}@uni-due.de,
{Ulrich.Schächtle,Lucas.Carstens}@stud.uni-due.de

Abstract. The current paper presents a case study conducted to evaluate the robot rabbit Nabaztag functioning as a vocabulary trainer for beginners of English. Hedonic aspects and motivating function, as well as the general usability and overall impression evoked by rabbit, were tested. A group of 18 5th grade students of an English class at a German junior high school were instructed to practice 20 pairs of vocabulary. Ten students were assisted by the speaking robot rabbit, while eight learned by applying an ordinary paper-and-pencil method. Results show that after one week, students who had learned with the Nabaztag had, on average, a higher recall than the control group. Moreover, the evaluation of the hedonic and pragmatic quality of interacting with the rabbit was high, as was the evaluation of both ease of use and perceived usefulness. Students learning with the rabbit were in a better mood afterwards than those who learned by means of the traditional method.

Keywords: Robots, robot-assisted learning, hedonic quality, motivation, vocabulary training, human-robot interaction, e-learning, intelligent tutoring systems.

1 Introduction

In Germany, learning English as a second language is an integral part of public education. Only recently, learning English has been established as part of the curriculum of many elementary schools and is sometimes even part of kindergarten education. In contrast to neighboring countries like the Netherlands, there has traditionally generally been only mediocre knowledge of English among the German population, which might be explained not simply by a lack of motivation but by the absence of opportunities to speak English. Children do not need to speak English during class, and the average German child only rarely encounters English-speaking foreigners in their daily life or watches English-language TV programs (see also [1]). However, second language acquisition is promoted and encouraged as an important prerequisite for intercultural communication not only across Europe but worldwide.

G. Leitner, M. Hitz, and A. Holzinger (Eds.): USAB 2010, LNCS 6389, pp. 322–339, 2010.
© Springer-Verlag Berlin Heidelberg 2010

Among other factors that positively influence second language acquisition, such as personality or experience, researchers stress the importance of motivation [2], [3], [4], [5]. However, many children and school students are not motivated to study English [1]. Children often do not see the importance of speaking another language and often cannot be motivated to practice vocabulary.

As an answer to these problems, the number of computer-supported vocabulary trainers available on the German market has increased in the last years. Ranging from mere storing lists of vocabulary for repeated interrogations to complex interactive language learning games with animated virtual characters, they have become increasingly popular. In parallel, academic research from computer science, psychology and education has presented Intelligent Tutoring Systems, e.g. [6], and pedagogical agents [7], [8], [9], [10], [11], [12]. Results of evaluations regarding learning outcomes, however, are mixed [13].

A solution that probably leads to even more positive results might be provided by toy robots, which have become available (and affordable) on the consumer market outside research laboratories and have found their way into children's bedrooms. As robots have always been equally fascinating for children and adults alike, they might especially impress the learner through their emotionally appealing qualities. In line with research from the field of human-centered design, they are likely to provide a high degree of fun and enjoyment and exert an inherent motivating function in children's language learning training - combining tangibility and playfulness.

With the aim of making use of these qualities, we present an application for the robot rabbit Nabaztag, introduced by the French company Violet, acting as a vocabulary trainer for beginners of English. We developed a vocabulary training application for beginners of English that works with a computer and the Nabaztag. The rabbit has an integrated speech synthesis module, LED lights and movable ears. These features were combined with an integrated adaptive feedback mechanism for the individual performance of the user, with the aim of designing an application that is simultaneously easy to use and motivating, appealing and pleasurable to young language learners.

The article begins with an overview of relevant aspects of user-centered design, drawing attention to the expected appeal of the little white rabbit. Furthermore, a review of effects of the related development of pedagogical agents and work on robot-assisted learning is provided. These sections are followed by a description of the Nabaztag and the training application, in particular the feedback mechanism as an integral part of an Intelligent Tutoring System adding to a positive user experience. Subsequently, details on the evaluation and its results are described before a conclusion is drawn and an outlook given in the last section.

2   Background and Related Work

2.1   User-Centered Design - More Than Just Usable

As pointed out in the introduction, emotional and motivational aspects are essential when it comes to a successful learning application. In recent years, a shift can be observed from a mere concentration on the pragmatic or functional qualities of a product or the prevention of usability problems, respectively, to the consideration of the emotional role and importance of positive experiences associated with the objects or systems [14], [15], [16], [17], [18]. According to Overbeeke et al. [15], humans look for products that are not necessarily easy to use, but rather "challenging, seductive, playful, surprising, memorable or even moody, resulting in enjoyment of the experience" ([15], p.9). Against the background of calls by the HCI researcher community for a more holistic view on human-computer interaction (e.g. [19], [20], [21], [22], [23], [24], [25], [26], [14]), the presented application is designed to combine both the consideration of cognitive, predominantly rational aspects of the experience, and its emotional and sensual values. While the cognitive parts are mainly realized by the implementation of a rudimentary user model and adaptive feedback (see sections 2.2 and 2.3), attention is drawn in this section to the emotional and sensual qualities. However, it should be mentioned that both aspects go hand in hand and contribute to the overall experience.

What makes the Nabaztag different from other vocabulary training solutions is first and foremost its tangibility. It has a surface, a texture and a certain weight. By combining the tangible rabbit and an on-screen application, the presented solution even goes beyond mere tangibility, as it bridges the abstractedness of computer screen solutions for vocabulary training, and taps into the emotional and physical pleasure provided by tangible objects [14]. Added to this is the rabbit's capability to move its ears, flash its LED lights and to speak, meaning that it provides a multi-sensual experience: audio, visual and haptic.

Moreover, it is conceivable that people like the novelty of the Nabaztag's appearance and its cuteness. The fact that the beauty of an object matters for its evaluation is shown, for instance, by Tranctinsky et al. [27]. Furthermore, against the background of Jordan's [20] suggestions to conceive products as "living objects with which people have relationships" (p.7), the rabbit might have a certain appeal because of its reference to a real rabbit. Besides tangibility, novelty and aesthetic appeal, owning and interacting with the rabbit might help people to communicate and express a specific image of themselves to others [24], [25]; it might in the long run become an emotionally meaningful object to its user.

In sum, the Nabaztag has a high potential to exert a specific appeal to children and make the interaction pleasurable. Moreover, the chances of succeeding in getting learners to engage in and be motivated for vocabulary training with the Nabaztag are good.

2.2 Pedagogical Agents and Robot-Assisted Learning

A different perspective is taken by researchers in the field of pedagogical agents. The following section adds to the aspects outlined above insofar as agent systems add to the establishment of a positive user experience. How this is achieved is explained in the following. Since extensive research about the effects of robot-assisted learning is still lacking, it is useful to look at research on pedagogical agents in order to deduce some guidelines and expectations. For some time now, virtual teachers and tutors have been introduced not only within computer science and educational psychology, but also in commercial applications (e.g. the Wii Fit agent by Nintendo). While commercial agents are often simple graphical characters not capable of interaction, scientific implementations provide largely autonomous computer agents enhancing students' learning and motivation [13]. This shows that the benefits in learning and motivation resulting from a positive user experience have also been recognized in this area. As a major advantage of pedagogical agents, it has been claimed that because of their ability to communicate verbally and nonverbally, they will allow for personalized interactions which will motivate the learner (e.g. [7], [13]). However, as can be read in several reviews on the effects of pedagogical agents (e.g. [10], [13], [28], [29], [30]), the large amount of studies that have investigated their effect on the learning outcome do not reach a consistent conclusion advocating the positive effect of these applications for the learner. Additionally, positive effects of pedagogical agents have largely been attributed to the voice of the agent rather than the visual presence [31].

It has recently been argued that the social, emotional and motivational effects of pedagogical agents have been largely neglected, even though they are an integral aspect of the agents´ presumed effectiveness [32], [13]. In fact, social and motivational aspects have rarely been measured. One exception is the study by Domagk [29], who demonstrated that likeability appears to be a crucial point for motivation (see also section 2.1). She did not find a positive effect of pedagogical agents on motivation or learning on the general level, but demonstrated that likeable agents lead to a higher motivation and increased transfer performance. All of these findings, which add to and support assumptions from the field of user-centered design, are important for the design of learning applications that motivate and encourage the user. They motivate the learner to engage in vocabulary training not only in the short term, but also ensure that vocabulary is regularly practiced in the long term.

Often, results gained from research with agents and the effects they evoke are assumed to be valid for robots as well. This is a simplification that results from a lack of research into pedagogical robots and may not apply in every case. Also in this area, it has been argued that with regard to motivation, a tangible object might have an even stronger effect than an embodied agent or a software application (see for example [33], [34]).

The spread of robot-assisted learning and the benefit of these tangible learning robots, which is combined with the idea of playfulness, has also been put forward and tested by Han and colleagues [35]. They present a study in which they compared the effects of traditional media-assisted learning and web-based instruction with the effects of home robot-assisted learning. Results show that children felt a home robot to be friendlier than other media-assisted learning applications. Compared to other learning programs, the home robot was superior in promoting and improving students' concentration, interest, and academic achievement.

Furthermore, Kanda, Hirano, Eaton and Ishiguro [1] endeavored to develop the humanoid robot "Robovie", which encourages children to engage in conversations in the English language. They placed it in an elementary school for two weeks and compared the interaction frequency with the students' achievement in an English test score. They concluded that: "[T]he robot did encourage some children to improve their English, and [...] was more successful in engaging children who already knew at least a little English." (p. 78). While this does not necessarily allow for conclusions about the cognitive effects, i.e. students' learning success, it does draw attention to the motivating function that this tangible tutor has with regard to engaging students in language learning.

In summary, findings outlined from the field of pedagogical agents emphasize the importance of the agent's appearance, i.e. nonverbal and verbal expressiveness as well as voice, for learner motivation. The few results available suggest that robots are not only capable of engaging students but are superior in eliciting concentration and interest. It remains open whether a robot other than a humanoid is able to not only cause positive (cognitive) learning outcomes but to provoke learner's motivation in a one-to-one teaching situation with a structured vocabulary training application.

2.3 The Robot Rabbit as an Intelligent Tutor

While the aspects outlined above primarily focus on the emotional qualities of the robot for the user, this section introduces Intelligent Tutoring Systems (ITS) and sheds light on the implementation of rational qualities, i.e. didactic strategies that foster motivation and interest. However, as stated above, both rational and emotional aspects of a product's design have to be considered to enable a positive user experience.

In a review article, Chih-Yueh Chou, Tak-Wai Chan and Chi-Jen Lin [36] provide an overview of the development and components of ITS and conclude that the vision of using a computer as an agent, a so-called intelligent tutor, to assist students to learn has not been abandoned since Carbonell's simulation of a Socratic tutor in the 1970s. A great deal of effort has since been made in terms of developing computers that simulate tutors, Intelligent Tutoring Systems [37], [38]. The underlying assumption is that a one-to-one teaching situation with direct and adaptive feedback is the ideal learning scenario in which the computer is tutoring interaction [36]. In line with this, Chou, Chan and Lin [36] refer to results achieved by Bloom [39] who demonstrated that one-to-one tutoring is far more effective than classroom teaching.

According to Wenger [38], Intelligent Tutoring Systems consist of a domain expert module, a student model, a pedagogical module and an interface. The expert domain knowledge can usually be presented to the student and is used to evaluate the learner's performance. This is often represented as facts (e.g. correct matches between translations) or rules. As a precondition to provide adaptive feedback, the learner model usually detects or infers learner's beliefs and misconceptions from the received answers, for example by tracing the student's actions. Various approaches for modeling students have been proposed (e.g. [40], [41], [42]), some of which collect a number of mistakes and misconceptions to gain a picture of the learner [43]. A third essential part of Intelligent Tutoring Systems is the pedagogical module, which includes pedagogical strategies and instructions to tutor the student and determines when and how to instruct the student. Finally, the ITS is completed by the interface, e.g. text, voice, animation, virtual reality etc., through which ITS and learner communicate and exchange information [36].

Since mentoring has also shown to be relevant for learner motivation in the context of pedagogical agents [44], we consider the implementation of an adaptive feedback mechanism working on the basis of a user model to be an essential characteristic for the newly developed application. In the following section, we will describe in detail the features of the vocabulary training application that has been developed under consideration of findings from human-centered design, pedagogical agents research and features of an ITS in order to achieve not only a positive learning outcome but first and foremost a positive user experience going along with a high level of motivation.

3   System Design and Functionality

3.1   The Robot Rabbit Nabaztag and Its Technical Features

The Nabaztag is a robot in the shape of a rabbit (see Fig. 2) offered by the French company Violet. It is a Wi-Fi enabled ambient electronic device which can connect to the internet to process specific services via a server located at http://www.nabaztag.com. It is 23 cm high and weighs 1 kg. It is equipped with 5 LED lights (rgb, in total 15 LEDs), one at its "nose", three on its "belly" and one at the bottom, a microphone ("belly button"), two interchangeable magnetic ears with output/input motors, an RFID reader (ISO14443 Type-B), a Wi-Fi card (SoftMAC 802.11) and a built-in speaker. The rabbit is controlled by a microprocessor and features a text-to-speech synthesizer. The Nabaztag receives all of its information from a server, with which it exchanges information in 30-second intervals. The rabbit is capable of reading out loud written texts in 32 languages via text-to-speech synthesizer or mp3. It can also react to specific predefined spoken commands. The developers provide an open API to customize existing or a program's own applications. The user controls the Nabaztag fully via the company's website.

3.2   Drawing on the Idea of Intelligent Tutoring

As outlined above, research results prove that ITSs as well as pedagogical agents positively influence learning motivation and success. In our application, we try to combine conceptual aspects of both. This section describes in detail the process students go through when interacting with the rabbit.

In a first step, students confirm a start-up dialog appearing on the screen of the laptop. Once the student presses the start button, the introduction sequence is initialized. Since the establishment of a personal relationship by introducing oneself is also a characteristic feature of a student-teacher relationship in human-human communication, we considered it important to give the rabbit a name and have it introduce itself to the student. Consequently, the Nabaztag introduces itself in German as a teaching rabbit that wants to help the student and repeats the same in English: "Hallo. Mein Name ist Clara und ich komme aus einer Kiste. Ich bin ein Lern Hase. Ich lerne gerne Vokabeln und will dir helfen, besser in der Schule zu werden. Du kannst mit mir gemeinsam lernen, Spiele spielen und viele andere Dinge machen. Ich kann sprechen, meine Ohren bewegen und in vielen verschiedenen Farben leuchten. I can speak English, too, and this is why I can teach you so many things." - "Hello. My name is Clara and I live in a box. I am a teaching rabbit. I like to learn vocabulary and want to help you to improve in school. If you like you can learn and play with me. I can speak, rotate my ears and glow in a lot of different colors." Following the personal introduction, the Nabaztag gives instructions on how the course of action is going to be from that point on. It instructs the student to type a list of vocabulary in the GUI that is shown next. To prevent typing errors from affecting the learning outcome at this point, the words are double-checked with a list stored previously in the computer.

As an integral part, we implemented an adaptive feedback mechanism that would provide variable feedback depending on the student's performance. Following a set of three translated words, the student receives feedback about his errors and is presented with the correct spelling of the incorrectly recalled words. The GUIs present the student with one piece of German vocabulary at a time, with a text field in which the student is to type in the proper English translation. After three pieces of vocabulary, the student is given feedback if he/she has typed in one or more faulty translations. The whole questioning process, as well as the correction feedback, is accompanied vocally by the Nabaztag. In addition to the correction feedback, the Nabaztag utters a motivational feedback after nine pieces of vocabulary, i.e. after three sets of three translated words, the student receives motivational feedback adjusted accordingly depending on the student's performance in this sequence. Feedback consists of short, one-sentenced, motivational statements. For example, when the student is performing poorly, the Nabaztag utters something like "You can only improve from here on" or when the student performs outstandingly, the Nabaztag says "Great, I am impressed". Moreover, the feedback given also depends on the feedback provided in the previous sequence: if a student performed well in one sequence and is performing badly in the next, he is given different feedback from a student who, for example, performed badly in two consecutive sequences (see Table 1).

Table 1. The Adaptive Feedback Mechanism (Examples)

Sequence of right (1) and wrong (0) answers			Feedback	Translation
{1,0,0}	{1,0,0}	{0,0,1}	Du kannst Dich nur	You can only get better.
0	0	0	noch steigern	
{1,1,1}	{1,1,1}	{1,1,1}	Toll - ich bin	Wow - I am impressed.
1	1	1	beeindruckt	
{0,0,1}	{1,0,1}	{1,0,1}	Du wirst immer	You are getting better and
0	1	1	besser	better.

The adaptive feedback is accomplished through generating strings that contain ones for correct translations and zeros for faulty translations. An increased count of wrong answers in the generated string indicates a low performance of the student, thus changing the motivational feedback to a tone that differs from the feedback a student performing well would receive. Providing motivational feedback every ninth piece of vocabulary made it necessary to simplify the generated strings of right and wrong answers before matching them with appropriate feedback. Since matching every single combination of right and wrong answers would have made it necessary to take into account 512 different possible outcomes of performance, three digits were compressed into one, thus shortening the strings to three digits. If wrong answers outnumbered right ones, the result was compressed to "wrong"; if right answers outnumbered wrong ones, the result was "right" (see Table 1). In this way, a manageable number of possible combinations was considered for the matching between performance and feedback.

In order to enhance the training effect and to retain the idea of playfulness, we integrated a memory game. Thus, when the student reaches the next stage, the Nabaztag instructs him on the upcoming game. The student is presented with a game board with 16 overturned stylized memory cards (see Fig. 1), each containing either a German or an English word. These pairs of words are a random selection from the previously learned vocabulary. When the student clicks on one of these cards, it turns over and reveals the English or German word. Through performing the described task, the student is told to match the English words with their German counterpart and vice versa. Whenever the student finds two pairs, the Nabaztag utters positive feedback, saying that the student is doing a good job. This feedback switches between German and English. It is invariable, but differs with increased headway. For example, "Zwei Paare. Weiter gehts!"("Two pairs. Keep it up!) or "You are really good! Three pairs!"

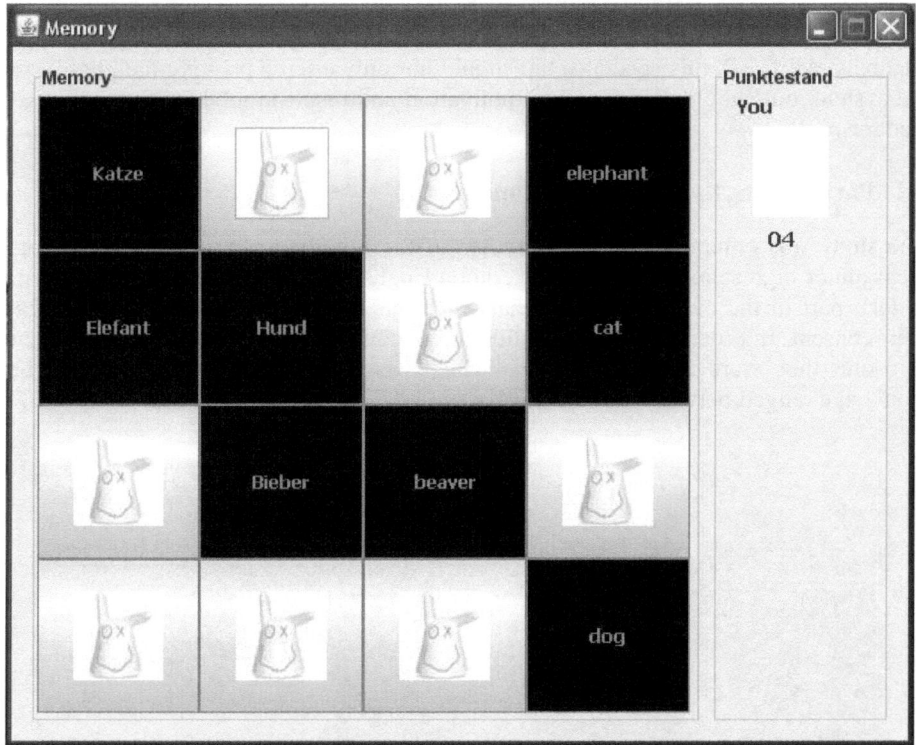

Fig. 1. Screenshot of the Memory Game

4   The Case Study

4.1   Aim and Expectations

The findings outlined in chapter 2 lead us to ask whether a verbally and non-verbally expressive robot like the Nabaztag might have positive effects on learners' motivation. If we assume that the robot rabbit's appearance and tangibility are capable of triggering a certain degree of motivation and interest, its verbal and nonverbal expressiveness would, according to the findings outlined above, even add to that. By explicitly addressing the user and the adaptive feedback mechanism, there is at least the illusion of a personalized interaction. This is even supported by the rabbit, who introduces itself as Clara. Instructions appear not only on the screen but are additionally uttered by the

Nabaztag, which in line with Atkinson's [31] results, should increase positivity of the user's experience. The outward appearance of the small, white rabbit might evoke feelings of sympathy or liking in the user.

Moreover, considered here are not only the emotional/social and relational aspects discussed above, but also the cognitive ones.

Our application requires not just the typing of the English word and its German translations, but also represents multimodal interaction. The application includes verbal and nonverbal aspects and the rabbit expresses itself both by means of hearable input of vocabulary and by simultaneously providing the written word, which can be read on the screen to ensure that the vocabulary is "grasped" in a variety of sensual channels. All in all, this special setup should not only elicit a positive feeling towards the system, but should also increase motivation and result in a better performance of students.

4.2 Participants, Spatial and Personnel Setup

The study was conducted with 5th graders of the Steinbart Gymnasium Duisburg, a local junior high school, during an afternoon English class. Students had been invited to take part in the evaluation beforehand. Parents were informed in detail and gave their consent. In order to make the children feel comfortable, the study was conducted in rooms they were familiar with and which were provided by the school. Participants' age ranged between 9 and 11 years, with the mean age being 10.28 ($SD = .57$).

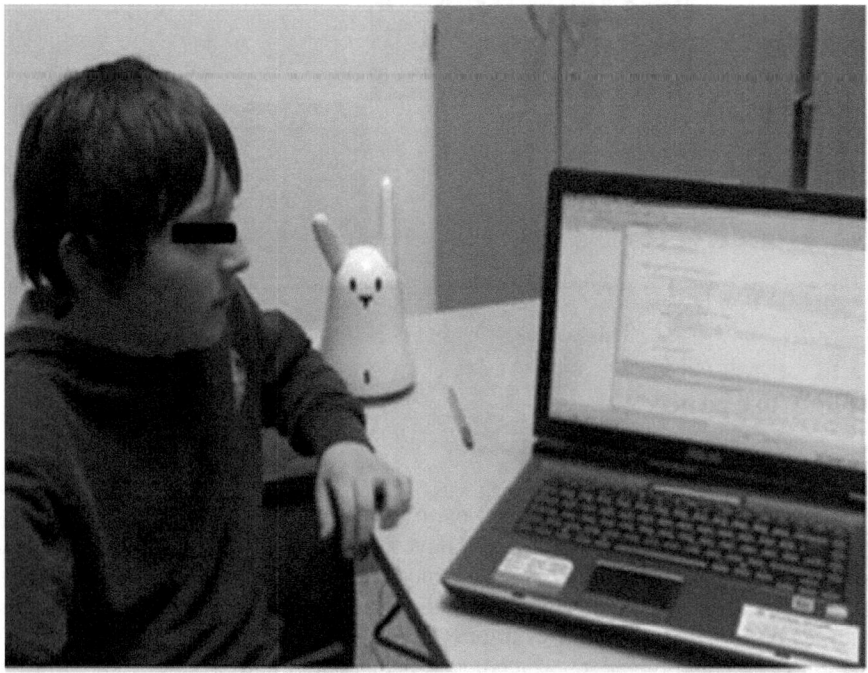

Fig. 2. Setup with the Nabaztag, a notebook and a student

Eighteen participants were randomly assigned to one of the two conditions (with rabbit vs. without rabbit) by drawing lots that would identify them as a member of one or the other condition. The experimental group was comprised of ten students and the control group contained the remaining eight students. The students in the experimental group went through the experimental setting with the Nabaztag and were seated in separate rooms equipped with a robot rabbit, a notebook with mouse and a wireless network in order to enable a server connection for the rabbit (see Fig. 2), with one supervisor for each participant. The control group studied vocabulary in a separate room with one supervisor present. They were given a list with the designated German-English vocabulary and an additional piece of paper which they had to hand in after the training.

4.3 Procedure

The group that learned in the traditional way was given the material. After 20 minutes, students had to hand in all the material (vocabulary list and additional pieces of paper) that had been given to them in order to ensure that recall results were not distorted by children practicing at home. Subsequently, they were given a questionnaire that asked for information on their gender and age as well as their mood measured by the PANAS items (refer to section 4.4 for details).

In the rabbit condition, two runs were conducted with five children each. The instruction was limited to showing the students the setup they were to work with, namely the laptop with mouse and the Nabaztag. They were also told that the Nabaztag would guide them through the whole process but should any problems occur they were to ask the supervisor for help. Then, students were left alone up until the end of the studying tasks, when the questionnaire had to be filled out.

Once the student had pressed the start button, the introduction sequence was initialized and the Nabaztag introduced itself as described in section 3.2. Following the personal introduction, the rabbit instructed the student to type in the list of 20 German words with their English equivalent, which had been selected from their official school text book in the GUI, and to confirm each piece of vocabulary by pressing "Save vocabulary" and the "I am ready" button at the end. The students' list was validated with a previously stored list to ensure that students would not learn wrong spellings or translations. All students were confronted with the same words. Once the student had typed in all of the words, the system initialized the vocabulary learning sequence in which the rabbit started asking the student for the translation of the vocabulary in random order.

The learning sequence made use of simple GUIs and variable feedback depending on the student's performance uttered by the Nabaztag as outlined in section 3.2.

This phase was terminated either when the student reached 80% correct words or after 20 minutes. On the PC desktop, a memory game started, choosing a number of eight pairs of words in random order from the vocabulary list. Once the student had finished the memory game task, the Nabaztag uttered a final positive feedback and instructed the student to let the supervisor know that he/she had finished the studying exercise.

After this, the students completed a questionnaire containing the same items as the control group (mood and demographics) as well as several scales for the evaluation of the Nabaztag and the overall impression it evoked. Students were thanked for their participation and returned to their afternoon activities.

4.4 Questionnaire

In order to design the questionnaire in a way that was appropriate for children of a young age, it was written in a personal and easily readable manner. The questionnaire contained six parts and was four pages long. Each section of the questionnaire was preceded by instructions informing the students on how to fill in the different parts. All instructions and questions were written in German. In order to assess not only the students' mood but also their general impression of the interaction with the robot rabbit, a number of different scales were included in the questionnaire: the Positive Affect Negative Affect Schedule (PANAS) scale [45], the AttrakDiff 2 scale [46], the Perceived Usefulness Scale and the Perceived Ease of Use Scale [47], [48], as well as several ad-hoc items.

The PANAS scale [45] is a psychometric scale that measures the constructs of positive and negative affect in the participant and was used to obtain participants' mood after the learning exercise and to enable a comparison of the average mood of the group that had learned with the rabbit with that of the group that had pursued the paper-and-pencil vocabulary practice. The PANAS scale contains 20 items (e.g. enthusiastic, interested, confused, nervous) to effectively describe the affective state of the person on a 5-point Likert scale ranging from "not at all or very little" to "extremely". While the PANAS scale was used for both groups, the group learning with the rabbit and the group learning without it, the following scales were only included in the questionnaire given to the students in the rabbit condition.

Besides participants' mood, we were interested in the user experience in learning with the Nabaztag. In order to assess this, the AttrakDiff 2 scale [46] was included in the questionnaire. It consists of a 21-item semantic differential containing, for example, the opposing pairs complicated vs. simple or unimaginative vs. creative, and measures the pragmatic quality as well as the hedonic quality of the Nabaztag application. According to Hassenzahl [46], "pragmatic attributes are connected to the users' need to achieve behavioral goals" (p. 322). Since utility and usability are important prerequisites for the achievement of specific goals, an object that ensures effective and efficient goal achievement is perceived as having pragmatic quality. Hedonic attributes are, in contrast, related to the user's self. They can be distinguished into stimulation (e.g. novelty, challenge etc., see also [49, 50]) and identification (e.g. self-presentational function, communicating personal values, see also [51]).

The Perceived Usefulness Scale and the Perceived Ease of Use Scale, taken from the Technology Acceptance Model [47] [48], were used to assess students' acceptance of the Nabaztag and the complementary desktop application. While the Perceived Usefulness Scale contains seven statements on how useful or useless the student considers the Nabaztag to be (e.g. "All in all, I consider the rabbit useful for school" or "I think the rabbit could help me to perform better at school"), the Perceived Ease of Use scale consists of six items for the evaluation of how easy or complicated the use of the Nabaztag is perceived to be (e.g. "The rabbit is easy to use and behaves as expected" or "Learning with the rabbit is exhausting"). Both scales are measured on a 7-point Likert scale ranging from "I don't agree at all" to "I fully agree".

The ad-hoc items assessed the personal opinion of the students. There were four questions, each measured on a 5-point Likert scale ranging from "I fully disagree" to "I fully agree". The first question asked whether or not the student wanted to use the Nabaztag again in the future. The second question asked whether the student would recommend the Nabaztag to a friend, the third question asked whether the student preferred the Nabaztag over traditional learning techniques, and the final question asked whether or not the student had already used a learning tool in the past. In the final section of the questionnaire, age and sex of the participant were recorded.

4.5   Results

The following description of the results follows the order in which the items were arranged in the questionnaire.

4.5.1   Students' Mood

Items from the PANAS scale were grouped into positive (e.g. enthusiastic, interested etc.) and negative (e.g. distressed, hostile etc.) items as suggested by Watson, Clark, and Tellegen [31]. Values were subsumed for the experimental group as well as for the group learning without the Nabaztag. The average value for the group interacting with the robot rabbit was $M = 3.52$ ($SD = .91$) for the positive items and $M = 1.28$ ($SD = 1.81$) for the negative items. In contrast, the average values for the other group were $M = 2.78$ ($SD = .60$) for the positive items and $M = 1.40$ ($SD = .48$) for the negative items.

Albeit only at the 10% level, differences between the groups were significant with regard to the positive affect factor (F (1, 16) = 3,935; $p = .065$; p$art. \eta^2 = .197$). Since this low significance level might be explained by the small sample size, the effect size d was additionally calculated and resulted in a very high effect size of $d = .97$, showing that the difference is relevant.

4.5.2   AttrakDiff2: Hedonic Identification /Stimulation and Pragmatic Quality

Hedonic stimulation reached the highest average value, with a mean value of $M = 6.04$ ($SD = .69$). Items adding up to the hedonic identification of the Nabaztag and its application were slightly lower, resulting in a mean value of $M = 5.53$ ($SD = .99$). Finally, the pragmatic quality of the application reached an average value of $M = 5.47$ ($SD = .926$). This shows that with regard to the evaluation of the rabbit, the attribution of, for instance, novelty and challenge was most prominent, while aspects of personal values and self-presentation as well as usability were attributed to a smaller extent.

Correlations were calculated between the AttrakDiff2 constructs and participants' mood. The hedonic identification value of the AttrakDiff 2 questionnaire correlated with the positive mood value of the PANAS questionnaire ($r = .78$, $p < .05$). Correlations between hedonic identification or pragmatic quality and the participants' mood were not found.

4.5.3 Technology Acceptance: Perceived Ease of Use and Perceived Usefulness

The constructs of Perceived Usefulness (PU) and Perceived Ease of Use (PEU) from the Technology Acceptance Model (TAM) were tested in terms of predicting user acceptance. Since Davis [47; 48] does not state reliability measures for the scales, Cronbach's alpha values were calculated for both sets of items. Cronbach's alpha was shown to be very high ($\alpha = .931$) for the items constructing the Perceived Usefulness Scale, in contrast to the alpha value of the Ease of Use Scale ($\alpha = .611$). Items of both scales were summed together to obtain an average value for the perceived usefulness ($M = 6.49$, $SD = .79$) and the system's ease of use ($M = 6.23$, $SD = .69$). Both emerged as very high.

Correlations between PU and PEU and the AttrakDiff 2 constructs, as well as participants' mood, were calculated. Results show that the hedonic identification ($r = .71$, $p < .05$) as well as the hedonic stimulation ($r = .85$, $p < .05$) correlated with the perceived usefulness. The pragmatic quality of the AttrakDiff 2 questionnaire correlated with the perceived ease of use ($r = .67$, $p < .05$). Calculations for the other dependant variables did not show any significant effects.

4.5.4 Ad-Hoc Items

With regard to the ad-hoc items the following results emerged: Measured on a 5-point Likert scale the average answer to the question if the participant wanted to learn with the rabbit again was $M = 4.90$ ($SD = .32$). With regard to recommending it to a friend, a mean value of $M = 4.5$ ($SD = .97$) was assessed. And finally, the average answer to the question of whether learning with the rabbit was better than traditional learning methods was $M = 4.9$ ($SD = .97$). Thus, all in all, the rabbit was evaluated positively.

A t-test comparing the group of students that had indicated using a computer-based vocabulary trainer at home ($N = 2$) showed that students who do not have a vocabulary trainer at home ($N = 8$) perceived the vocabulary training as more comfortable ($M1 = 4.5$, $SD = .7$, $M2 = 5.0$, $SD = 0$, $t(8) = -2.53$, $p < .05$). In addition, t-tests were conducted with regard to the PANAS scale and the AttraktDiff 2 in order to discern differences between the evaluations of students used to computer based vocabulary training and those who are not. However, these analyses failed to reach significance level.

4.5.5 Recall

The group that had learned with the Nabaztag performed slightly better in the vocabulary test that was conducted. The maximum number of right answers that could be achieved was 20 pairs. The group that had learned with the rabbit (1) recalled on average more than one word more than the group that had learned the traditional way (2) ($M1 = 13.7$, $SD = 3.83$, $M2 = 12.13$, $SD = 4.22$). However, the comparison between the two groups failed to reach significance level. The additional calculation of the effect size d resulted in $d = .389$, which is a medium size effect.

5 Discussion and Outlook

In the previous text, we presented ideas of changing an off-the-shelf consumer robot in the shape of a rabbit into a vocabulary trainer that children like to interact with. We described a case study of a robot-assisted learning setting that includes the robot rabbit Nabaztag as well as an additional on-screen application that complements it. This setup involves not only the use of speech synthesis technology in order to be able to interact verbally with the user (at least one-sided) but is also nonverbally expressive – both aspects being identified as relevant to learner motivation and success. It also combines the idea of tangible objects dedicated to learning assistance with playfulness realized by means of the memory game that completes the actual training phase.

As a positive user experience is an important precondition for initial and long-term motivation, one of the primary goals of the study presented was to evaluate whether the user's experience is a positive one. We were interested in finding out whether students would assign not only pragmatic qualities but also beneficial emotional, hedonic qualities to the rabbit. In addition to the characteristics of the rabbit itself, such as tangibility, cuteness, verbal and nonverbal expressiveness, the adaptive feedback mechanism (as an essential part of an ITS) was implemented to ensure that the learner is individually motivated and informed about his performance. Although it is a rather rudimentary approach in our case, there is a user model which is generated "on the fly" on the basis of the user's performance, i.e. the number of the right and wrong answers given. In contrast to the general idea of a user model, our model is not persistent over time and not yet refined over a number of sessions. Although the implemented learner model could be more elaborate, it is questionable whether a vocabulary trainer needs an elaborated user model at all. One might as well argue that in the sense of adaptive learning, it is primarily important to react to the learner's actual state or performance, respectively, which the current implementation does.

The results of our evaluation show that the 5th graders we tested generally liked interacting with the rabbit. All our results indicate that although some differences do not reach significance level and have to be interpreted with caution, there is an indication of differences between the group learning with the rabbit to the control group as indicated by the effect size d: Students in the rabbit condition were in a more positive mood and recalled more words in the vocabulary test conducted one week after the interaction. A positive feeling evoked by learning with the rabbit is a necessary precondition not only for motivation but also for factors that influence a generally positive evaluation of the learning experience and interaction with the application. Hedonic stimulation and identification as well as the pragmatic quality were rated relatively highly. Furthermore, the ease of use and the perceived usefulness were rated to be very high on average. The fact that participants were not only willing to learn with the rabbit again but would even recommend learning with it to a friend does show that the application fulfills a decisive precondition for the establishment of motivation: People feel positive about it and would like to return to practicing vocabulary with the rabbit again. Interestingly, the students who are used to a vocabulary trainer were less excited. Although results are based on a small number of students only, this might be an indication of decreasing motivation and interest over time – an aspect that has also been observed by Karapons et al. [16] but which needs to be explored in more detail and in further long-term research.

With regard to the evaluation, there are some points that have to be mentioned as critical. The small sample of 10 and 8 only allows for tentative conclusions and should not be generalized. Despite the fact that students were distributed randomly to the conditions, it cannot be ruled out that one or the other sample might have consisted of especially skilled or unskilled learners. Furthermore, the exact mechanism of the effects was not addressed by the study. Since we compared a complex learning system with a control group, we cannot conclude whether it is actually the embodied rabbit, the feedback function or the gaming elements that contribute to the positive mood and better performance of our sample. Besides this, there are a number of further limitations to our results. For example, we did not test whether the children really did not know the vocabulary before but proceeded on the information given by the teacher that the vocabulary selection had not been part of the curriculum. Moreover, it would have been helpful to additionally assess the recall of vocabulary directly after the interaction instead of merely after one week.

For further uses of the application, especially in long-term settings, it will certainly be beneficial to establish a user model that might function like methods working with index cards that are sorted according to the learner's performance and relate back to previous learning sessions. As progress in speech recognition is made, it will become possible to interact via natural speech rather than via predefined sets of words, with a robot that not only speaks, but also generically "understands" what is being said. Vocabulary could not only be checked for the right spelling but also with regard to pronunciation. Systems available today may be able to produce utterances; however, difficulties remain in recognizing human utterances without being trained to recognize a specific voice or domain-specific sets of words and distinguish them from background noise. Other aspects that might be considered refer to the rabbit´s nonverbal expressions. First results show that people associate certain feelings of the rabbit with its ear position [52].

From this first evaluation, it can be concluded that it provided us with many useful insights that will be used to refine the application. As our results show, not only was the quality of the application in terms of ease of use and usefulness rated highly but, more importantly, the children indicated a highly positive experience with regard to particularly hedonic aspects of the setup. Besides this, our study draws attention to the fact that it is easy to get people to engage with the robot and cause an initial motivation.

However, as also observed by Kanda et al. [1] in their field trial with the "Robovie" English trainer, students reduced the number of interactions with the robot considerably after one week. This shows that keeping the students engaged with the vocabulary trainer over time probably still remains a challenge for future research.

Acknowledgments. The authors would like to thank the following persons and institutions that contributed to the successful completion of this project: Steinbart Gymnasium Duisburg, Michael Euteneuer, Peter Michael Minnema, Sebastian Feltgen, Clarissa Salisbury and Florian Hardt, Sabrina Sobieraj, Tina Ganster and Lars Bollen. Special thanks go to Anja Thieme. The research leading to these results has received funding from the European Community's Seventh Framework Program [FP7/2007-2013] under grant agreement no. 231868.

References

1. Kanda, T., Hirano, T., Eaton, D., Ishiguro, H.: Interactive Robots as Social Partners and peer Tutors for Children: A Field Trial. Human Computer Interaction 19, 61–84 (2004)
2. Bialystok, E., Hakuta, K.: In other words. Basic Books, New York (1994)

3. McLaughlin, B.: Second language acquisition in childhood. In: Preschool children, 2nd edn. Erlbaum, Hillsdale, NJ (1984)
4. Wong Fillmore, L.: When learning a second language means losing the first. Early Childhood Research Quarterly 6, 323–346 (1991)
5. Tabors, P.: One child, two languages. Paul H. Brookes, Baltimore (1997)
6. Koedinger, K.R., Anderson, J.R.: Intelligent tutoring goes to school in the big city. International Journal of Artificial Intelligence in Education 8, 30–43 (1997)
7. Lester, J.C., Towns, S.G., Callaway, C.B., Voerman, J.L., FitzGerald, P.J.: Deictic and emotive communication in animated pedagogical agents. In: Cassell, J., Sullivan, J., Prevost, S., Churchill, E. (eds.) Embodied Conversational Agents, pp. 123–154. MIT Press, Boston (2000)
8. Baylor, A., Kim, S.: The effects of agents' nonverbal communication on procedural and attitudinal learning outcomes. In: Prendinger, H., Lester, J.C., Ishizuka, M. (eds.) IVA 2008. LNCS (LNAI), vol. 5208, pp. 208–214. Springer, Heidelberg (2008)
9. Baylor, A.L., Ryu, J.: Does the presence of image and animation enhance pedagogical agent persona? Journal of Educational Computing Research 28, 373–395 (2003)
10. Baylor, A.L.: Permutations of control: Cognitive considerations for agent-based learning environments. Journal of Interactive Learning Research 12, 403–425 (2001)
11. Graesser, A.C., D'Mello, S.K., Craig, S.D., Witherspoon, A., Sullins, J., McDaniel, B., Gholson, B.: The relationship between affect states and dialogue patterns during interactions with AutoTutor. Journal of Interactive Learning Research 19, 293–312 (2008)
12. Graesser, A.C., Jackson, G.T., McDaniel, B.: AutoTutor holds conversations with learners that are responsive to their cognitive and emotional states. Educational Technology 47, 19–22 (2007)
13. Krämer, N.C., Bente, G.: Personalizing e-learning. The social effects of pedagogical agents. Educational Psychology Review 22, 71–87 (2010)
14. Norman, D.A.: Three levels of design: Visceral, behavioral, and reflective. In: Norman, D.A. (ed.) Emotional Design, pp. 63–98. Basic Books, New York (2004)
15. Overbeeke, K., Djajadiningrat, T., Hummels, C., Wensveen, S., Frens, J.: Let's make things engaging. In: Blythe, M.A., Overbeeke, K., Monk, A.F., Wright, P.C. (eds.) Funology. From Usability to Enjoyment, pp. 7–17. Kluwer Academic Press, Netherlands (2003)
16. Karapanos, E., Zimmerman, J., Forlizzi, J., Martens, J.-B.: User experience over time: An initial framework. In: Proceedings of the International Conference on Human Factors in Computing Systems, pp. 729–738 (2009)
17. Seligman, M.E.P., Csikszentmihalyi, M.: Positive psychology: An introduction. American Psychologist 55(1), 5–14 (2000)
18. Jordan, P.W.: Human factors for pleasure in product use. Applied Ergonomics 29(1), 25–33 (1998)
19. Gaver, B., Martin, H.: Alternatives: Exploring information appliances through conceptual design proposals. In: Proceedings of the SIGCHI Conference on Human Factors in Computing Systems, pp. 209–216 (2000)
20. Jordan, P.W.: Designing pleasurable products: An introduction to the new human factors, pp. 1–57. Taylor & Francis, London (2000)
21. Wright, P., Wallace, J., McCarthy, J.: Aesthetics and experience-centered design. Transactions on Computer-Human Interaction 15(4), 1–21 (2008)
22. Olivier, P., Wallace, J.: Digital technologies and the emotional family. International Journal of Human-Computer Studies 67(2), 204–214 (2008)
23. Hassenzahl, M.: The effect of perceived hedonic quality on product appealingness. International Journal of Human-Computer Interaction 13(4), 481–499 (2001)

338   S. Eimler et al.

24. Hassenzahl, M.: The thing and I: Understanding the relationship between user and product. In: Blythe, M.A., Mink, A.F., Overbeeke, K., Wright, P.C. (eds.) Funology: From usability to enjoyment, pp. 31–42. Kluwer Academic Press, Netherlands (2003)
25. Burmester, M., Hassenzahl, M., Koller, F.: Usability ist nicht alles - Wege zu attraktiven Produkten [Beyond usability: Appeal of interactive products]. I-com 1, 32–40 (2002)
26. Kaptelinin, V., Nardi, B.A.: Acting with technology: Activity theory and interaction design, pp. 1–116. MIT Press, Cambridge (2006)
27. Tractinsky, N., Katz, A.S., Ikar, D.: What is beautiful is usable. Interacting with Computers 13, 127 (2000)
28. Clarebout, G., Elen, J., Johnson, W.L., Shaw, E.: Animated pedagogical agents. An opportunity to be grasped? Journal of Educational Multimedia and Hypermedia 11, 267–286 (2002)
29. Domagk, S.: Pädagogische Agenten in multimedialen Lernumgebungen. Empirische Studien zum Einfluss der Sympathie auf Motivation und Lernerfolg [Pedagogical agents in multimedia learning environments. Empirical studies on the influence of likability on motivation and learning]. Logos, Berlin (2008)
30. Moreno, R.: Animated pedagogical agents in educational technology. Educational Technology 44, 23–30 (2004)
31. Atkinson, R.K.: Optimizing learning from examples using animated pedagogical agents. Journal of Educational Psychology 94, 416–427 (2002)
32. Kim, Y., Baylor, A.L.: A social-cognitive framework for pedagogical agents as learning companions. Educational Technology Research & Development 54, 569–590 (2006)
33. Powers, A., Kiesler, S., Fussell, S., Torrey, C.: Comparing a Computer Agent with a Humoid Robot. In: Proceedings of the ACM/IEEE international conference on Human-robot interaction table of contents Arlington, Virginia, USA, pp. 145–152 (2007)
34. Yamato, J., Shinozawa, K., Naya, F., Kogure, K.: Evaluation of Communication with Robot and Agent: Are robots better social actors than agents? IEIC Technical Report 100, 15–19 (2001)
35. Han, J., Jo, M., Park, S., Kim, S.: The Educational Use of Home Robots for Children. In: IEEE International Workshop on Robots and Human Interactive Communication (2005)
36. Chou, C.Y., Chan, T.-W., Lin, C.-J.: Redefining the learning companion: the past, present and future of educational agents. Computer and Education 40, 255–269 (2003)
37. Sleeman, D., Brown, J.: Intelligent Tutoring Systems. Academic Press, London (1982)
38. Wenger, E.: Artificial Intelligence and Tutoring Systems. Morgan Kaufmann, Los Altos (1987)
39. Bloom, B.S.: The 2 Sigma Problem: the search for methods of group instruction as effective as one-to-one tutoring. Educational Researcher 13, 4–16 (1984)
40. Greer, J.E., McCalla, G.I.: Student Modelling: The Key to Individualized Knowledge-Based Instruction. Springer, Heidelberg (1994)
41. Mizoguchi, R.: Student Modeling in ITS. In: Chan, T.W., Self, J. (eds.) Emerging Technologies in Education, pp. 35–48. AACE (1995)
42. Carr, B., Goldstein, I.P.: Overlays. A theory of modeling for computer-aided instruction. AI Lab Meno 406, MIT, Cambridge, Massachusetts (1977)
43. Brown, J.S., Burton, R.R.: Diagnostic models for procedural bugs in basic mathematical skills. Cognitive Science 2, 155–191 (1978)
44. Bente, G., Breuer, J.: Making the Implicit Explicit: Embedded Measurement in Serious Games. In: Ritterfeld, U., Cody, M.J., Vorderer, P. (eds.) The social science of serious games: Theories and applications, Routledge/LEA, Philadelphia, PA (2009)

45. Watson, D., Clark, L.A., Tellegen, A.: Development and validation of brief measures of positive and negative affect: The PANAS scale. Journal of Personality and Social Psychology 54, 1063–1070 (1988)
46. Hassenzahl, M., Burmester, M., Koller, F.: AttrakDiff: Ein Fragebogen zur Messung wahrgenommener hedonischer und pragmatischer Qualität. In: Ziegler, J., Szwillus, G. (eds.) Mensch & Computer 2003. Interaktion in Bewegung, pp. 187–196. B.G. Teubner, Stuttgart (2003)
47. Davis, F.D.: Perceived Usefulness, Perceived Ease of Use, and User Acceptance of Information Technology: A Comparison of Two Theoretical Models. MIS Quarterly 13, 319–340 (1989)
48. Davis, F.D., Bagozzi, R.P., Warshaw, P.R.: User Acceptance of Computer Technology: A Comparison of Two Theoretical Models. Management Science 35, 982–1003 (1989)
49. Hassenzahl, M.: The Interplay of Beauty, Goodness, and Usability in Interactive Products. Human Computer Interaction 19, 319–349 (2004)
50. Csikszentmihalyi, M.: Beyond boredom and anxiety. Jossey-Bass, San Francisco (1975)
51. Wicklund, R.A., Gollwitzer, P.M.: Symbolic self-completion. Lawrence Erlbaum Associates, Inc., Hillsdale (1982)
52. Eimler, S., von der Pütten, A., Ganster, T., Krämer, N.: Lass die Ohren nicht hängen - Eine explorative Studie zum Eindruck des nonverbalen Verhaltens eines Kommunikationsroboters in Form eines Hasen. In: Kongress der deutschen Gesellschaft für Psychologie (2010) (accepted as poster)

Learning Flow Management and Semantic Data Exchange between Blog-Based Personal Learning Environments

Vladimir Tomberg, Mart Laanpere, and David Lamas

Tallinn University, Narva mnt 25, 10120 Tallinn, Estonia
vtomberg@tlu.ee, mart.laanpere@tlu.ee, david.lamas@acm.org

Abstract. The use of blogs as Personal Learning Environment is an emerging trend in higher education. While many teaching and learning tasks are easy to implement in a blog-based PLE, this type of tools still lacks some of the important features that made traditional Learning Management Systems efficient for both teachers and learners.

This paper addresses the challenges of enhancing blog-based learning environments with two new functionalities: learning workflow management and semantic data exchange.

Keywords: Blogs, assessments, learning flow, WordPress, plug-ins, development, LePress, semantic metadata, microformats.

1 Introduction

The use of personal blogs in teaching and learning has increased significantly during the last five years, becoming one of the major trends in the domain of technology-enhanced learning. Whereas this trend is clearly related with the simplicity of publishing, reading and discussing through blogs, these still miss relevant functionality, which hinders their systematic adoption in educational settings. For instance, it is quite difficult to manage assignment related workflows and to promote semantic data exchange between multiple blog instances.

This paper reports on an approach to bring assignment related workflow management and context specific semantic data exchange to WordPress.

We start with a review of the background on blog-based Personal Learning Environments, followed by a conceptualization of learning flow management between multiple blog instances. Finally, we describe a usage scenario and the prototype of LePress – a learning flow management extension for WordPress blog engine – and discuss its implementation and potential applications.

2 Personal Learning Environments

Nowadays universities generally use some kind of Learning Management Systems (LMS). Such popularity is the result of the maturity of the inherent concepts as well

G. Leitner, M. Hitz, and A. Holzinger (Eds.): USAB 2010, LNCS 6389, pp. 340–352, 2010.

as of the fact that LMS are now stable environments featuring high availability, scalability, usability, interoperability, stability, security performance [1].

However, technology enhanced learning researchers argue that the adoption of Personal Learning Environments might result in a quantum leap over LMS based approaches. As envisioned, PLE facilitate learner-based constructivist learning processes and promote the usage of open resources, and Web 2.0 tools by opposition to the teacher-centric tactics enabled by typical, Web 1.0 associated LMS [2].

Nevertheless, even in the most progressive universities, the adoption of PLE is still incipient both due to its novelty [3] and to the fact that the concept is unknown still to most faculty. Integrating PLE in the learning process is further deterred by the lack of knowledge on how to used the emerging tools to facilitate the achievement of learning goals – on one hand, people wait with great enthusiasm the announcement of new communication tools quickly declaring them as very suitable add-ons for the PLE concept, on the other hand, there is no common understanding of how to integrate such new tools into the learning processes as there is also insufficient understanding of how to methodologically benefit from such an integration.

Additionally and although the number of tools potentially useful in a PLE is growing everyday, there still is no common understanding on how to sustainably articulate them in order to scaffold learning workflows. In part, these results from the implicit untidy nature of PLE, as there are no strict rules and ordered sequences of actions such as found on LMS – from this point of view, the usage of PLEs is harder to analyse, describe and manage when compared to that of a typical LMS. This downside also results from the lack of shared knowledge those using these artefacts – the educators – and those developing them.

Finally it should also be mentioned that there is a probability that the acceptance PLE will not overcome that of LMS in the near future. As Anderson argues, the impact of using Web 2.0 tools on results and cost of learning is not enough studied yet: "It is also unclear how energetically formal education institutions should build in social spaces that were originally designed for informal socialization and networking" [4]. We believe that this process will likely take place little by little, simultaneously with the growing understanding role of PLE in education and with the understanding of ways for supporting traditional learning activities with PLE. For a start it is necessary to learn how to implement such functionalities in PLE and only after that take it away from LMS.

In the research work herein reported we explore the idea of implementing typical learning workflow activities on PLE based on a popular open-source blog tool.

3   Blogs as Learning Tools

Blogs and other so-called Web 2.0 tools are proving to be suitable building blocks of more learner-centred learning environments. Initially blogs were just personal diaries that were being used mainly for publishing author's texts over the Internet together with the possibility of eliciting comments from their readers for readers. The nature of these digital diaries has been changing progressively as bloggers discovered and understood the newly enabled possibilities. Eventually blogs became much more than digital diaries and we can now find entire websites and services built on top of the initial weblog concept. Further, blogging functionality is nowadays supported by most social network – micro blogging is a core service for the majority of mainstream social services such as Facebook and Twitter [5].

Using blogs in education and especially in learning processes has active supporters as not less active opponents. There is significant body of research confirming the advantages of blogs as replacements of other computer-mediated communication tools in learning processes. For example, the usage of Really Simple Syndication (RSS) motivates students to participate in discussions [6] by continually supporting "pull" synchronization rather than requiring "push" actions on the teacher's or students' side, which makes users feel less intrusive [7]. Another foremost feature of almost any blog engine is the simplicity of the publication process, which easily relates better to any young student profile than centrally administrated LMS [8]. The same feature contributes towards the students' feeling of confidence that he/she has some level of control over the learning process.

The first attempts of using blogs in education started in the early 2000-s. For example Betts and Glogoff proposed such variants of using blog in class, as assignments, reflections, and journal entries. Analysis of several courses conducted using blogs demonstrated that students showed high level of interest towards this new tool. Indeed students began to propose additional variants for the course activities, such as literacy inventories, purposive reading, observation notes and linguistic analysis [9].

Later, Du and Wagner examined the use of blogs in constructivist education approaches and classified the basic advantages of blog use highlighting three of them: support for active learning, support for collaborative learning and reinforced individual accountability [10].

Collaborative learning, according to Du and Wagner 'results in better learning outcomes, compared with individual-oriented learning' Because of the web nature of blogs, they promote the facilitation of the power of linking, of providing feedback, and of enabling different forms of connections between participants in the learning process.

An important advantage of using blogs in education, still according to Du and Wagner, is the ability fostered by blogs to reinforce individual accountability. This is accomplished in three ways: non-anonymity — personal responsibility of students to progress; individualized feedback — embedded in blog capabilities for receiving feedback from teacher and students; benchmarking and self-assessment — possibility for student to compare own work with works of other students.

The blogosphere is a collection of interconnected blogs. As any open and decentralized environment and any free community, it is difficult to be controlled. Therefore the use of blogs is usually not as widespread in universities and schools as institutional LMS. On the contrary, shifted locus of control in blogs presupposes their smooth integration into the PLE concept space as it builds on minimizing top-down administration and maximizing the self-directedness of the students.

By analysing typical uses of blogs in learning, Laine had classified many different uses for blogs, such as: problem solving tool, discussion tool, reporting tool, learning diary, preparation tool, link dump, collaboration tool, bonding tool, fun factory, and shield against shyness [11]. It should be noted that highlighted uses contain many activities that can be found in traditional learning courses. This allows us to establish the theoretical possibility of implementation online, blog based, courses.

4   Beyond Blogging

In order to accomplish our goals, we started by identifying which blogging workflows were already used in learning processes. Specifically, our interest lied on studying how assignments could be posted and assessed using blogs. We assumed that teachers had previous experience in using blogs, for instance in the delivering of learning materials. We also assumed that the posting of assignments and their assessment would be desirable.

Further, we also assume that each student would use its own blog as an e-portfolio publishing accomplished assignments and getting feedback from teachers and fellow students in the form of comments or grades. Using their blogs in any other ways should never be a problem for either teachers or students.

Current blog platforms usually provide both categories and tags as semantic annotation tools, which are suitable aggregation mechanism within each blog but not across blogs. Tramullas and Garrido [12] stated that the semantic Web been integrated into blogs is yet to happen, although this can be done through the development of new functionalities.

Again, current blog platforms provide the ability to comment, which on top of its basic purpose, can also be used to link different messages on distinct blogs. Other possibilities for linking messages are mechanisms such as pingback and trackback. Unfortunately, all fail to provide suitable semantic annotation.

As we believe that a blog platform should remain a blog platform, we attempted to address our problem extending the basic blog feature set with a blog extension prototype, which adds an extended feature set without disabling any of a blog system's central characteristics.

For implementing described above task we developed a blog extension prototype LePress. LePress is a WordPress plug-in; this name is a combination of the words Learning and WordPress.

5   Usage Scenario

Let's consider the following usage scenario: A teacher is about to begin a new course. She has most of her learning materials already hosted in her teaching blog but she would like to reorganize them for this new course. With the LePress plug-in installed, the teacher gets to create courses and easily aggregate the available learning materials in logical units. Further, she can even use some of the learning materials as assignments upon which student assessment is planned.

The teacher's next step is the registration of the students. If a multiuser version of WordPress is being used then, setting LePress powered blogs for the students is straightforward. Otherwise, students have the option of either using their own existing blogs or creating new blogs and install the LePress Student plug-in by themselves. The teacher may then ask students to register by automatically sending them email invitations.

Once the registration of the students is completed, a special relationship between the blogs of the teacher and the students is established and the learning process may start. From this moment the teacher now has access to the roll of students, their blogs and e-mail addresses and vice-versa, all from their blog's extended interface. This virtual integration allows participants to coexist in a common information space and to follow the process of the course concurrently. This also fosters the creation of some classroom awareness and the communication among classmates.

Further, the teacher can now assign tasks for students to carry out using her blog. Students are automatically notified about the assigned tasks in their blogs and may publish the assignment's outcomes directly in their own blogs. Later, the teacher is also automatically notified about students' completion of tasks and may assess, comment and grade the students' work in their blogs.

Of course, one can argue that some of what was described in the previous paragraphs could also be accomplished with a blog's basic feature set. Whereas this might be true for some tasks such as the publication of task assignments, the posting of assignments outcomes, and the sharing of comments, it surely doesn't hold for the case of logical aggregation of course materials, course enrolment, assignment setting, tracking and assessing.

Hence, we can now identify two types of activities when delivering a course using a blog: Activities that can be achieved using the blog's basic functionalities and activities that require additional functionalities and it is the latter type of activities that is addressed by the LePress blog extension prototype.

6   Blogs and Courses

The conceptual design of LePress was based on three main guidelines: ensuring that both teacher's and learners' usual learning flows are supported in an usable, natural and simple way; aiming for minimal or absent blog architecture interference ensuring all basic feature set while leaving extended functionality transparent and ready to be used when needed; and achieving maximum or total blog architecture reuse ensuring that no feature is implement it doesn't carry substantial s added value.

With these guidelines in mind, the first challenge was to help the teacher deploy she's course. This was addressed interpreting a course as a collection of learning activities, which happened on and during predetermined moments in time (figure 1). Activities are themselves blog postings, which may relate to such elements as learning materials, discussions, assignments, and assessments. A course would also count with one teacher and a number of students.

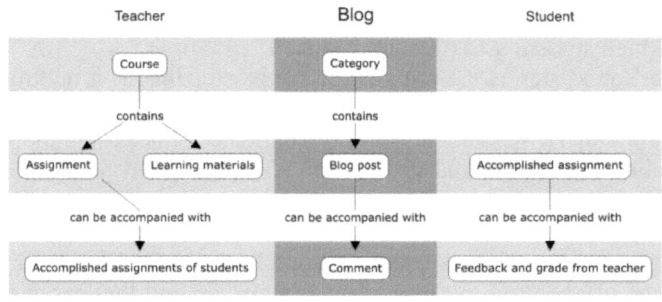

Fig. 1. Mapping the entities of blogs to concepts of LePress courses

Blog postings are organized in categories and the same happens with postings of learning activities. The difference is that the latter are assigned to special LePress course categories. These LePress categories enable additional functionalities such as binding of users and specific category to tie enrolled students to a specific course. Course categories are standard WordPress categories labelled by a 'new course' attribute.

Both teacher and students are also parts of a given course in LePress. The teacher is the author and owner of course, which she deploys on her blog using a course category. Course categories store metadata on course designation, teacher details and institution. The form with mentioned above filled data is shown on figure 2.

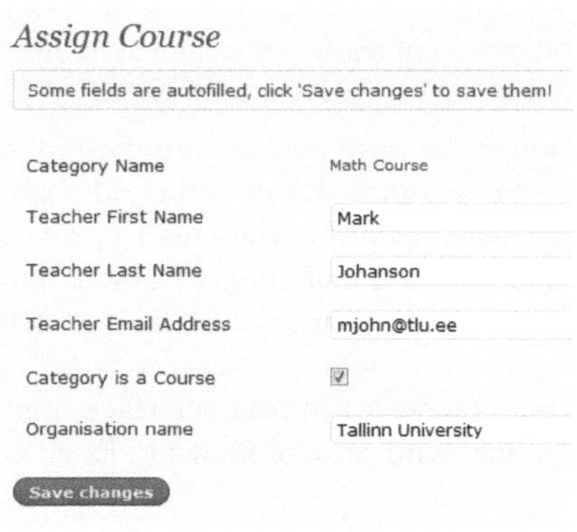

Fig. 2. Course category description in LePress' user interface

Another one advantage of this approach is the possibility of using RSS feeds to track the course's evolution with tools other than the teacher or students' blogs. This broadens the boundary of the course to all RSS enabled devices.

The second challenge was to bind the teacher and her students to a course. As the owner of the blog within which the course is deployed, the teacher is naturally bound to her course.

As for binding the students to a course, this was addressed by allowing the definition of communities of users based on specific blog categories. With this feature, the teacher can track all of her courses' students and related performance indicators; the students can get to know who their classmates are thus fostering the creation of the classroom awareness and facilitating communication among classmates.

The third challenge was an implementing of a mechanism of assignment and assessment. As noted before, all the course activities are published as regular blog posts. Assignments, however, are published using a special assignment post, which stores some additional metadata – for the time being only start and end dates are stored – and which is automatically announced to all students' blogs in their LePress interfaces (figure 3).

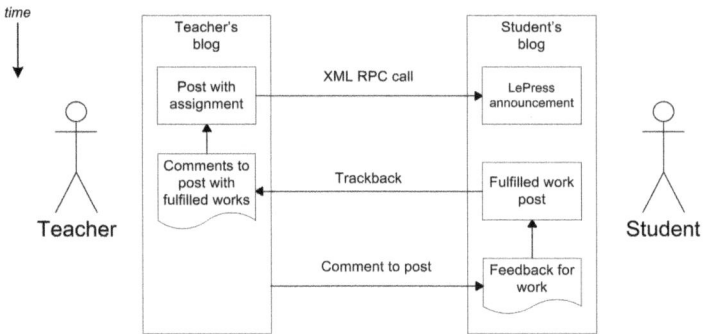

Fig. 3. Interaction of teacher and student during a course

Students should accomplish the assigned task in theirs blog and may refer to their own LePress interfaces for the assignment's content and deadline.

Finally, the teacher may use standard comments to provide the user with the feedback that she sees fit or she may use her blog's LePress interface to write her comments, grade the assignments and keep track of students' activities and accomplished assignments.

Comments written on the teacher's LePress interface appear in the students' blogs as standard comments together with an eventual grade given by the teacher. Grades are free form.

7   Supported Learning Workflow

The general architecture of a blog-based PLE involving the LePress module is depicted in Figure 4. We propose to conceptualise the use of PLE into three layers: the User, the Learning Flow, and the Learning Content layers.

The Learning Flow layer is in the middle, consisting of multiple blog instances, each of them with either the LePress Teacher or LePress Student plug-in installed. It is the LePress plug-in that supports the envisioned learning workflow.

In following we are describing the main parts of LePress learning workflow.

Course creation: the courses are deployed by creating a new course category in the teacher's blog and by assigning it all the relevant metadata (see figure 3).

Announcement and enrolment: the teacher can announce each course by filling in an invitation form with the students e-mail addresses from within LePress' interface or she can use LePress to import a text file containing the students' email address to automatically generate the invitations. In context of LePress environment the enrolment is the subscription to the 'course' blog category. It may only results in true enrolment if achieved within a student's blog LePress interface. Subscribing to the course using a standard RSS reader will not enable any of LePress' features; it can be used by students as additional way for receiving information.

To complete the enrolment process the teacher must accept the subscription requests.

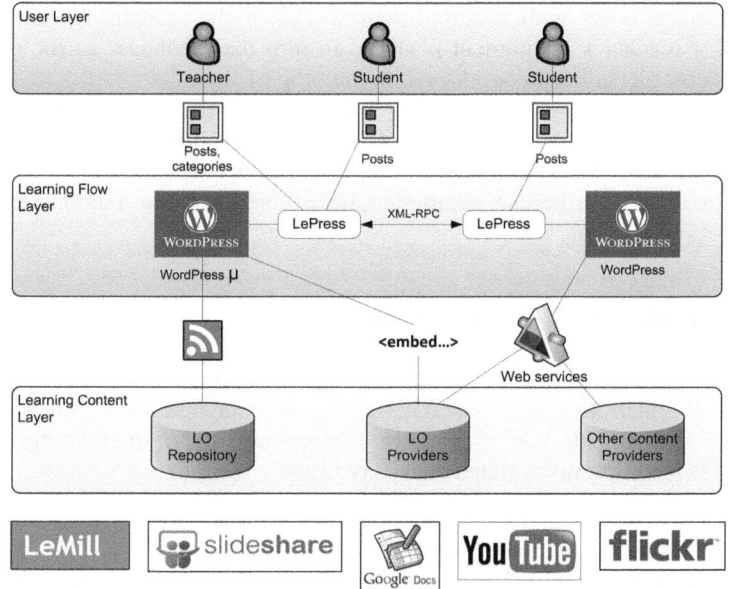

Fig. 4. LePress provides assessment workflow in layered architecture of modern PLE

Publishing course materials: the teacher publishes course materials as standard blog posts assigned to the course category.

Announcing assignments: assignments are announced within the teacher's blog using the LePress interface. As said before, assignments are special metadata-enabled posts, which have a start and finish date. These posts are automatically tracked by LePress using an XML-RPC call (see figure 3) and listed in all blogs belonging to enrolled students. The assignment is also announced to each enrolled student via an e-mail message.

Submitting assignments by the students: a submitted post will only be identified as an assignment submission if published from LePress Results page. Such the posts will appear as standard posts in the student's blog and as trackbacked comments associated with the original assignment post in the teacher's blog. This way, a permanent link is maintained between the assignment and the assignment's results.

Assessment: all assignment-related posts submitted by students appeared as comments in the blog of teacher and also tracked at the LePress results page of teacher as a list of links to originals. The teacher can view works of students in their blogs by following the link from LePress results page. When the teacher wants to evaluate a work of the student, he/she can do it from the same LePress Results page also. By clicking to link he gets a special form where it is possible to write text notes and to grade the work. LePress maintains a record by automatically placing its content into the blog of student as comment under accomplished work (figure 3).

This way LePress supports efficiently three most typical learning flow scenarios for the blogs of the teacher and students: assignment announcement, assignment submission, and assessment.

The published posts with accomplished works of the student are duplicated as comments for teacher's assignment-post and in turn the feedbacks of the teacher are appeared as comments for the work-post in the blog of students.

All these comments look very natural for blogs, but they can be implemented as described above only with the support of LePress. Any other standard functionality directly provided by WordPress can be used, for example if teacher or student gets a comment for blog post, he can automatically receive an email announcement about this.

8 LePress' Backend and Frontend

To enable course management an additional LePress menu was added to the teacher's WordPress administrative interface. This menu has four options: Courses, Subscriptions, Write assignments and Manage assignments. Each of these options enables some of the teacher's course related everyday tasks:

- In the Courses screen the teacher can manage his/her blog's categories assigning them course status as well as other metadata elements;
- The Subscriptions screen facilitates the management of the students. It provides tools to invite, track and delete students from any of the teacher's courses;
- The Write assignment screen allows for the publication of assignments within each of the teacher's courses;
- The Manage assignments screen offers the teacher a class-book like interface which lists students name, blog links and assignment status. Assignments can be accomplished or not accomplished. Accomplished assignments are graded and commented upon by the teacher and are automatically linked to the relevant post in the student's blog.

Students have a similar backend menu in their blog's administrative interface, but this has only two options, Subscriptions and Assignments:

- The Subscriptions option allows students to manage their enrolments to courses;
- The Assignments screen lists all published assignments together with the links to forms that enable the fulfillment of each assigned task.

To enable higher levels of usability and productivity, teachers and students have also access to 'frontend' LePress interface. We developed a separate user interface that caters for the control and management of almost all course-related tasks. In contrast to the form of implementation of the LePress 'backend' this 'frontend' is implemented as a WordPress widget. Widget is a small portion of an HTML code that can be embedded into a web page. LePress widget contains of data related to course management, e.g. course calendar, deadlines of assessments, names and emails of participants and so on (Figure 5).

This data can be accessed at any time straight from the blog's user interface, without the necessity to move into WordPress dashboard. These widgets can be switched on/off in the teacher's or students' blog using standard WordPress widgets management interface.

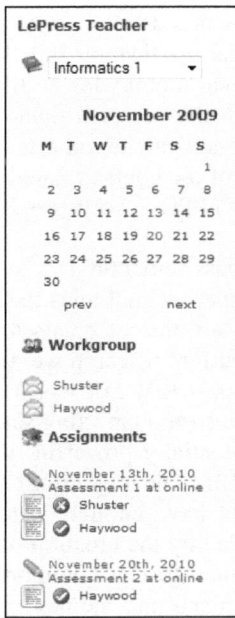

Fig. 5. LePress widget

Figure 5 depicts the teacher's widget; the student's widget has the same functionality but without possibility to manage the assignments. On the top, there is a dropdown box for choosing a course, which causes all related content to be displayed.

Assignments related to the selected course can be accessed either using the calendar or the list of assignments displayed at the bottom of the widget.

Within the calendar, assignments are available as links established over their respective end dates.

Within the list of assignments, for each assignment the widget lists the students who already completed the assignment and providing direct access to each student's work and facilitates the grading and feedback functionality. Icons differentiate the assessment status as accessed and not accessed.

LePress widget also fosters within course communication by listing all course members together with their e-mail addresses and blog links.

One of interesting opportunities that can be integrated into existing software by help of widgets is a semantic data exchange. This will be explained in next chapter.

9   Semantic Data Exchange

As with most social services, data exchanged within LePress might not be easily reusable unless some meaning is attached to it. LePress uses data that can be reused by instructors and students, typical examples of such data is the deadline of an assessment or names and e-mail addresses of the course participants. The question is: how to allow the users to reuse such data outside of a blog in other various tools? For example, the date for an assessment's deadline can be exported from the browser and imported into a personal calendar application in a local computer, Internet services like Google Calendar or a personal mobile device like phone or iPod. The same procedure can be implemented with the personal data of the students and teachers, for example names and e-mail addresses can be imported to the personal address book.

In order to facilitate the flow of the course related data between course participants and improve usability of using LePress software, we developed the semantic data exchange in LePress.

There are not many ways to pass semantic data to the end user in the web environment. The most known and popular technologies that allow the embedding of semantic markup into web documents are microformats for HTML, RDFa for XHTML 2, and microdata for HTML 5. In current research we do not consider microdata because of its novelty and the lack of tools that can work with it. RDFa and microformats seem like more suitable candidates for supporting semantic data exchange in LePress. However, although RDFa is potentially powerful, it lacks the browser side support microformats currently have [13]. The biggest disadvantage of microformats is a limited vocabulary that does not have enough means for describing course related data. This limitation can be settled by the creation of new microformats that must be proposed and accepted by the microformat community. Also, the existing elemental microformats can be easily combined into the new compound microformats if such a combination will give new meaning to the data. Microformats are very wide-spread and supported by global services like search engines, such as Google and Bing. Because of this, and in spite of its semantic shortcomings, microformats were chosen to provide the context for the LePress data.

The course-related microformat data is embedded into the code of the LePress widget. When a page with the LePress widget is loaded into the browser, the microformat data can be read and interpreted. Popular browsers enable the interpretation of microformats either natively or by means of third-party extension. Figure 6 depicts an example of accessing the microformat data using the Tails Export extension for Firefox.

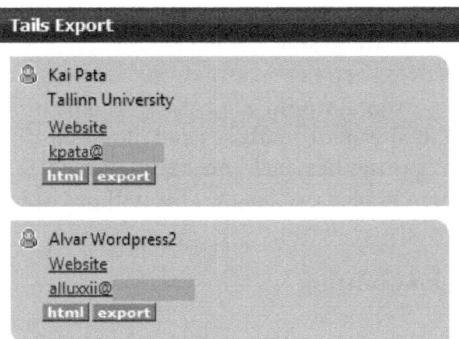

Fig. 6. Tails Export add-on for Firefox with ready to export microformat data from LePress widget

At the present time, LePress supports two of the most popular microformats: hCard and hCalendar. The hCard format is perfectly suited to convey a course participant's personal data. When using the microformat-enabled browsers or browser plug-ins, the LePress hCard data can be exported to a vCard file or directly to a contact manager application such as Microsoft Outlook.

With the hCalendar format, LePress enables a similar functionality for the course related events such as the assignments. They can be exported into the iCalendar file or directly into the calendar application or service, providing a seamless integration of LePress with the day-to-day tools of the course participants.

As illustrated by these two simple examples, the use of microformats can provide countless potential cases of using data mash-ups from different sources, which can be especially interesting in the context of educational settings. With the two above presented microformat data exchange implementations, we only demonstrated a small part of the foreseen possibilities for the use of semantic data. Today, microformats can represent many commonly published things like people, events, blog posts, reviews and tags, and these possibilities can be implemented in LePress in the future. We believe that this facet of LePress can and should be further investigated in order to enable richer LePress interactions among users and integration within its own components and with the surrounding functionalities and applications.

10   Current Implementation and Future Developments

WordPress was the blog platform chosen to test our ideas and to implement the current blog extension prototype. One of the reasons was the size of its userbase, but the main motive for choosing WordPress was its easy plug-in extensibility. WordPress is, however, not a final solution for implementing and testing the concepts outlined in this paper, but rather as a first draft that might be ported to other blog platforms should our approach prove successful. In fact, interoperability among distinct blog platforms would be an inherent goal from a PLE perspective.

The latest release of LePress is a stable version 1.02; the user manual is being developed so that the plug-in can be made available to the entire WordPress community. The plug-in is distributed in two editions – LePress Teacher and LePress Student. Both are required for enabling the simple learning flow management in LePress.

We see some interesting perspectives that open the current research. At first, it is possible to mash up assignment-related data. On the given example we have shown how a blog category that is interpreted as a course can be subscribed to with a standard RSS reader. This way is already widely used by educators. In our case we propose not only RSS data, but data that is semantically rich by means of microformats. This opens up new ways to make mash-ups of courses.

Widgets can further foster the PLE concept. The example illustrated in this paper is but a small step compared to what else can possibly be achieved. The mainstream blog platforms are becoming more open towards accommodation of diverse widgets.

The weakest point of LePress is that it works only on these WordPress instances where user is able to install our plug-in. However, many bloggers use different blogging platforms (Blogspot, Movable Type etc). This is why we plan to explore the possibilities for implementing learning flow management across different blog engines.

11 Conclusion

The simplest learning flow taking place in a Web-based environment contains announcement of assignment by the teacher, assignment submission by students, review and assessment of submitted assignments by the teacher and receipt of feedback/grade by students. By developing the LePress plug-in for WordPress we demonstrated how this learning flow can be automated using the typical features of blog engines: trackback, categories and sidebar widgets. We also explored how course- and assignment-related semantic data could be distributed using Microformats. Within our laboratory tests, potential users (teachers and students) were satisfied with the user experience. However, in order to prove the applicability of LePress on the wider scale, pilot tests should be conducted in a real-life context with large groups of users.

References

1. Hall, J.L.: Assessing Learning Management Systems. In: Chief Learning Officer, `http://pttmedia.com/newmedia_knowhow/KnowHow_Deploy/LMS/Docs/Assessing_LMS.doc` (accessed January 2010)
2. Dron, J., Anderson, T.: Lost in social space: Information retrieval issues in Web 1.5. Journal of Digital Information 10 (2009)
3. Attwell, G.: The Social Impact of Personal Learning Environments. In: Connected Minds, Emerging Cultures: Cybercultures in Online Learning. Information Age Publishing, Incorporated (2008)
4. Anderson, T.: Open Educational Resources Plus Social Software: Threat or opportunity for Canadian Higher Education? In : Congress at UBC (2008)
5. Baker, S., Green, H.: Social Media Will Change Your Business. Business Week Online (2008)
6. Brooks, C., Montanez, N.: Improved annotation of the blogosphere via autotagging and hierarchical clustering. In: 15th International Conference on World Wide Web, Edinburgh, Scotland, pp.625–632 (2006)
7. Nardi, B., Schiano, D., Gumbrecht, M., Swartz, L.: Why we blog. ACM Commun. 47, 41–46 (2004)
8. Maag, M.: The potential use of "Blogs" in nursing education. CIN: Computers, Informatics, Nursing 23, 16–24 (2005)
9. Betts, D., Glogoff, S.: Instructional models for using weblogs in elearning: A case study from a virtual and hybrid course. Syllabus (2004)
10. Du, H., Wagner, C.: Learning with Weblogs: An Empirical Investigation. In: 38th Hawaii International Conference on System Sciences (HICSS), p. 7b (2005)
11. Laine, T.: Mobile Blogs in Education: Case of ViSCoS Mobile. University of Joensuu, Department of Computer Science and Statistics, Joensuu (2007)
12. Tramullas, J., Garrido, P.: Weblogs Content Classification Tools: performance evaluation. In : I International Conference on Multidisciplinary Information Sciences & Technologies, Mérida (2006)
13. Tomberg, V., Laanpere, M.: RDFa versus Microformats: Exploring the Potential for Semantic Interoperability of Mash-up Personal Learning Environments. In: 2nd workshop on Mash-Up Personal Learning Environments (MUPPLE 2009) at EC-TEL (2009)

Educational Complexity: Centrality of Design and Monitoring of the Experience

Carlo Giovannella[1,2], Chiara Spadavecchia[1], and Andrea Camusi[1]

[1] ISIM Garage-ScuolaIaD
[2] Phys. Dept. - University of Rome Tor Vergata
via della ricerca scientifica 1, 00133 Rome, Italy
giovannella@scuolaiad.it, info@mifav.uniroma2.it

Abstract. In the first part of the paper we discuss why the characteristics of the "organic" era of interaction, we are living, make us claim the centrality of the "Design" as an element of possible innovation for the whole educational scene of this new century and more so for educational processes that have strong relationships with design domains and practices (HCI, IxD, Design for experience, TEL, etc.). The dissemination and the acquisition of the "design literacy" require, however, the adoption of complex educational processes, like the "organic process", that, in turn, requires the development of an equally complex monitoring system, able to assist teachers/tutors in the evaluation of qualities of the educational Experience and individual Experience styles, to customize, contextualize and, more in general, improve the experiences. In the second part of the paper, thus, we present, as a first step toward the realization of such monitoring system, the development of tools and methodologies that allow to monitor in quasi-real time the social level of the interaction and the quality of the social emotions, i.e. individuals' emotional feelings and emotional nuances of their relationships.

Keywords: Design centrality in education, Design literacy, Design for the experience, Liquid learning places, Person in place centered design, Organic era of interaction, Organic process, Learning styles, Experience styles, SNA, Automatic Text Analysis, Emotional interaction, Evaluation of design process.

1 Introduction: Liquid Places and Organic Era

As well known the development of the knowledge society has marked the transition into the post-industrial era where the primary good is the immaterial knowledge that, thanks to the complexity and robustness of the net of distribution and to the simplicity to reproduce intangible assets, overrides the boundaries of law, becomes liquid, magma, "open", "in progress".

At the same time we are currently witnessing the reshaping of the physical environment: the pervasive "machine", more and more hidden in spaces and artifacts [1,2], "dissolves" itself in the everyday life leaving over as unique trace the "computability"; in parallel the development of infrastructures and of wireless communication is completely reshaping the approach to the nets, so that people are increasingly transforming into active net terminals with which they will be constantly connected,

G. Leitner, M. Hitz, and A. Holzinger (Eds.): USAB 2010, LNCS 6389, pp. 353–372, 2010.
© Springer-Verlag Berlin Heidelberg 2010

independently from the physical place in which they operate during their nomadic traveling, with the consequent emergence of new lifestyles.

The integration of the above phenomena brings to inevitably foresee scenarios in which people will nomadically populate more and more sensitive and responsive physical spaces through which they will interact with socially dense virtual environments. The disappearance of machine within the everyday life's objects and spaces will enable individuals to interact with the latter ones in an extremely natural way using gestures, words and emotions. A more natural interaction will then bring individuals to give less importance to functional aspects and more to the so called "use qualities" [3] that will contribute to define the one's personal EXPERIENCE. Environments will become able to perceive individual's conditions and to co-evolve in order to respond to each one's personal needs. They will be populated by social relations, increasingly simple to start up and, at the same time, increasingly complex to be managed: they will become what we defined LIQUID PLACES. Their configuration is regularly redefined by each active entity's action according to more and more unpredictable "open" [4] and "baroque" [5] trajectories.

The range of the design is not any longer "local" and one has to consider also long range consequences in space and time, as for instance social acceptability and eco-sustainability [6]. In such a new frame, one has to put more and more attention to the way in which individuals – being both cornerstone and target of the mediated interaction and experience – communicate and learn.

All the above features - diffused intelligence and complexity, places' liquidity and co-evolution, more natural interactions and higher unpredictability of the interaction's trajectories, attention to the experience's qualities, design expanding over time and space - concur to draw the features of a new era that we may define: "organic era" [7].

2   Centrality of the Design in Education

In this framework, the practices of design and meta-design, although readapted to the new situation, may become the cornerstone of all educational processes (in particular of those dealing with subjects like: Instructional Design, Design for the Experience, Interaction Design, HCI, TEL, etc.). Indeed the Design, as compared to the fluctuations that have characterized the history of education [8] - nature/culture, utopia/pragmatism, humanities/sciences, theoretical/practical activities - places itself in a central position that can integrate the various opposites. Due to the limitations in space, this is certainly not the most appropriate forum to retrace the history of education, however it may be worthwhile to list a set of key issues that emerged recently, that are driving our present educational practices and that may help the reader to understand better our claim about the "Centrality of Design":

a) the "machine" and the mediated communication are complex, although they may have been designed and produced to appear simple; they may appear simple but as simple as they appear more complex is the design process that they are hiding, especially in the presence of a large number of interacting entities; therefore it is not correct to persuade the students that design complexity is simple and even easier to hide the complexity to the end-users;

b) environments and situations in which the artifacts/services are used, and processes put in practice, are complex and the trajectories of use are not always predictable; this means that there can no longer entrust to fully deterministic design (especially if we are dealing with Design for Experience); we must embrace "open design" and be able to provide experiential re-configurability (not just the physical one);

c) processes, besides being complex, must possess a high degree of flexibility and re-adaptability, which implies, for their management, the acquisition of meta-design capacity;

d) design practices cannot neglect to consider the "time", from different points of view: the maintenance in time, the sustainability in time (not only of scale) also in terms of environmental compatibility (physical and virtual), the timing of experience (before , during, post), the perception of time;

e) users' experiences have qualities that, even in the complexity of their identification, one should be able to monitor, in order to derive quantitative indicators and thus references.

Considering all above, we believe that the centrality of Design for educational experiences can be claimed on several levels:

i) pedagogical, for what concerns the purpose of training processes; the ultimate aim, indeed, should be to enable learners to acquire reflective and meta-design skills in order to be able to continuously readjust design processes and, even, their own project of life; in other words learners should be able to put into practice the critical method [9] that makes the so-called reflective practitioner [10] a sort of a reference model in the complexity of contemporary society – renewing a tradition that from Socrates comes to date [8];

ii) process level, because the Design enable to respond to complexity by structuring flexible processes that can, from one side acquire the organicity of the natural systems and on the other include the iterativity typical of the scientific method; to this latter, the design adds the pragmatic aimed at finalizing a modification of the world (not only its understanding); therefore the design processes are not only problem-based, but also project and process based, i.e. P^3BL [11, 12];

iii) methodological, for the ability to absorb the best of what is expressed by various disciplines and to integrate it within the processes mentioned above; consider, for example, the methodologies derived from cultural anthropology, that suitably readjusted, are used in the process of problem setting; those derived from cognitive science and used in the design and implementation of the tests; those derived from the engineering reused in the medium- and high-fidelity rapid prototyping, etc ... [13, 14]

iv) didactic, as demonstrated by the continuing tension in readapting the methods outlined above and in developing tools and procedures that allow their practical implementation in different contexts and situations, in other words by the effort to be at the same time general and flexible [15, 16].

We wish to emphasize that the recognition of the pedagogical centrality of Design automatically leads to the need of an effort to spread among the new generations a sufficient level of "design literacy".

3 Education as an Experience

At this point we may understand that learning is becoming an increasingly complex activity, as complex as the interactions and relationships that the actors participating in it give rise and as the places where such activity is being conducted, that – does not matter if real or virtual - day after day, are becoming more and more stratified, sensitive and co-evolutive.

Regardless of whether the educational process will be conducted face-to-face, in blended or fully on-line configurations, the framework described above requires the development of complex PB^{3}L (Problem- Project- and Process-Based Learning) [11] educational processes, as 'organic' [7] as the era we are living in, able to accommodate the parallel developments of functional layers, characterized by an high level of flexibility. These processes, which have their cultural background in the activism, can be regarded as "experiences", characterized by their own experience's qualities.

Table 1. Summary of the Experience Styles and of their correlation with the functional layers of the Organic Process

Organic Process		Experience Styles					
			Interaction				
	Explore / Learning	motivational	perceptive (exploring)	physical cognitive	creative, innovative	subjective time	ludic (alea, ilinx, mimicry, agon)
	Elaborate / Design		info processing, working, design	cognitive emotional, social			
	Actuate / Communicate		extroversion introversion	social, emotional, cognitive			

Although the identification of all the dimensions of an experience is still a very open issue, in a general manner, one can say that every experience, including the learning ones, is based on interactions, or communicative acts, performed by the individuals simultaneously on multiple levels, see Tab. 1, the main fuels being the personal motivation. It is not possible, therefore, to describe an experience separately from the personal characteristics of each individual, because this latter is, at the same time, focus and active element of the experience. Because of this, recently we have introduces a set of "Experience styles" [16] that operate a integration among characteristic of the educational process (organic one, see next paragraph), personal characteristics (e.g. learning styles [17, 18] the specific dimensions of the human interaction

(Tab. 1) and any further significant dimension that can help to describe as completely as possible an EXPERIENCE (e.g. use qualities [3]).

4   The "Organic Process"

Over the last twenty years the structure and characteristics of the most popular "processes" changed a lot: as examples we moved from a prevalent push character to a prevalent pull one and the activities underwent a clear segmentation and organization into phases. Still in the current days the design process more widely diffused and applied is a cyclical process based on the four phases - observation/analysis, design, prototyping/implementation, evaluation/validation – which is a transposition of the classical scientific method based on the repetition of the following phases: observation, correlation (problem setting), development of models and theories (problem solving), design of new experiments and experimental assessment of predictions. Such process, despite the passage from a circular iteration to a spiral one (aimed to a better representation of the constructive effect of iterations), always tends to partially hide the linearity associated to the time dimension that necessarily characterize any productive process.

Nowadays some industrial processes became inter-iterative, others intra-iterative, and with the increase of their complexity tend to resemble more and more to the parallel flow of turbulent streams, characterized by local vortices (iterations), linear drift and unavoidable convergence in a mainstream - the river – which, in turn, cannot avoid to flow into the sea (deployment) in a well defined time.

In the past - in order to get students to understand and operate within such complex dimension in a short time - we developed and applied an educative process, called ISIM process, composed by a well defined series of phases (an exploratory-competitive phase, three collaborative design sub-phases - devoted respectively to static, dynamics, interfaces -, a development phase - soft & hard prototyping - and a deployment phase) characterized by interactive activities, milestones and deliverables [19]. The f2f ISIM process was augmented by parallel online activities that took place within a homemade on-line learning platform, called Life (former Home-University) [20]. Such on-line activities, moreover, were essential to favor students' approach to constructivism, as well as to expand the operative time-window that, in turn, resulted in a larger amount of time devoted to experiment creative and ethnographic methodologies. Even though such strategy and the related process were rather successful, the complexity of the challenges presented by the "organic era" and the differences among the various educative contexts brought us to further reflect upon the process we designed, upon on-line environment's potentialities and organization and also upon the evaluation methodologies.

Indeed we realized that - in order to improve the responsiveness to the complex challenges posed by real world and DULP vision [11,12] - we needed a more flexible process within which the activities could be represented and organized in meaningful layers rather than exclusively in phases.

Our vision and our alternative proposal is inspired by the "living organisms" that, at any level, fulfil three basic functionalities:

- investigate: the environment to collect information & learn;
- elaborate: the information to design/produce;
- communicate: the "products" by means of "actions" that, in the case of very complex organisms, can make use of highly structured and conventional languages.

The above vital functions, can be carried on as collective activities and are always active during the whole development of what we may consider our inspirational process: "life". In fact, we believe that we can organize and describe productive and/or educative processes (see the case studies presented in par. 5) in a way that appears quite alike to the one in which the "life" of an organism living in a co-evolving environment is organized. That is why we called it "*organic process*" [7].

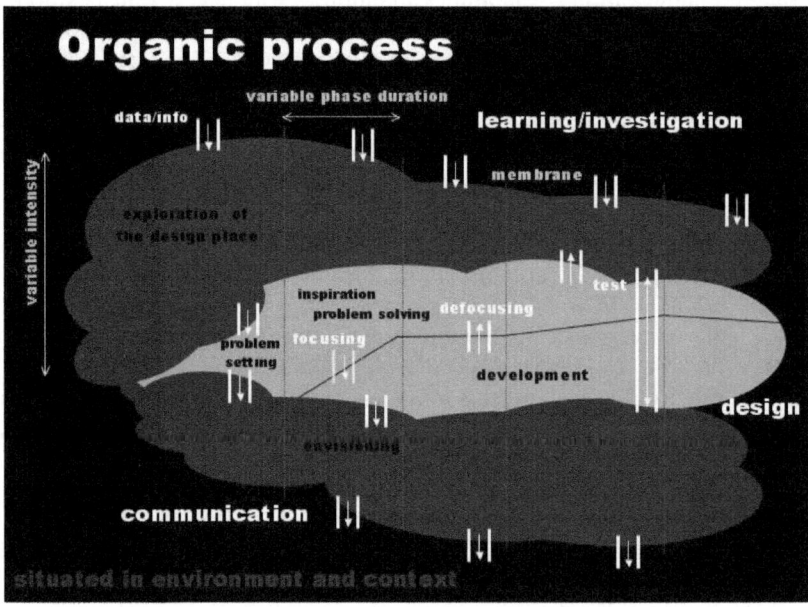

Fig. 1. Blob representation of the "organic process"

An "organic process", see fig. 1, can be represented in the plane "time vs. intensity (of the functionalities)" as an "organic blob" within which the three main functionalities (layers) are active and fulfilled during the whole time-window of the process (apart from an initial transient). The organic process/blob, much the same as a living cell, is supplied with many different channels enabling it to communicate with the external world: inlet channels set on the top of the membrane of the learning/investigation-layer and outlet channels set along the membrane of the communication layer. Moreover there are internal channels acting as gates and enabling to exchange information between the different layers. For instance: information crosses a gate while going from the "exploration of the design place" to the "problem setting" activities, from the "inspiration and problem solving" to the "development" during the fulfilment of sub-functionalities (see the black border line) and vice-versa, from the "development" to the "envisioning" and "communication", toward the learning/investigation layer when tests are needed, etc.. Obviously, just like a river must flow into the sea, also the "organisms" are compelled to concretely act so as to fulfil their vital activities in a given time. Due to this, each "phase" internal to the layers (schematically represented by the red dotted vertical lines) should be accomplished according to a precise time schedule.

It is notorious that a wider flexibility of the process also implies more difficulties in its application especially if it is necessary to achieve given results in a given time window, regardless of the specific peculiarities of the context. This is an apparently easy result to achieve in a deterministic process where "knowledge" transfer is carried out through behaviouristic methodologies. The situation is completely different when one is dealing with project-based learning processes in which the students are left free to proceed along their own path, according to constructivist modalities implying collaborative-cooperative behaviours. In such situations the tutor has to operate a constant supervision on the on going process to avoid turning aside the proper way and to reach the expected goals within the timing forecasted, despite the huge number of possible paths. To help those people who may wish to apply the "organic-process" we have defined a set of general guidelines:

- consider the learning space & process as parts of a unique "design place" that can be continuously redefined as function of the specific context and process's evolution;
- keep the three functional layers active during the whole educative process;
- expose students to an as larger number of methodologies (and/or to a mixture of them) as possible, compliant with the process's time-window;
- stimulate scaffolding, collaborative work and also the development of social awareness according to the constructivism's guide-principles; balance all this by encouraging a sane competition based on creativity and innovation ability;
- adapt the on-line environment to host a creative and enjoyable process to be considered as a valuable "experience";
- put the strongest attention possible to timings and recovering of the weakest students;

Although the organic process's principles and the above mentioned guidelines, don't enable us to provide receipts that are mechanically applicable, nevertheless, we may supply some methodological indications derived from our experience that hopefully may help:

- "learning" can be kept always active because of the continuous need of inputs to understand the design place, to decide how to develop the project (for instance tech benchmarking), to test and improve solutions, etc.; in our case, therefore, "learning" is continuously stimulated by the tutor's request to enlarge the basis of the data or to verify the data collected;
- "design" should be switched on as soon as the first data enter the organic process; indeed, also the analysis can be considered a design and creative activity whenever people are asked to give original representations, to imagine the strategy enabling them to get further data, to define personas, scenarios, etc ...
- "communication" is always an active layer since our process makes a large use of the on-line environment designed to favor the application of constructivism and of socializing practices; this implies that students learn to communicate with the external world far before the "reporting activities", by learning to expose themselves to their community of practice.

5   Monitoring the Experience

The logical consequence of increasingly complex educational processes, like the "organic" one, is that assessment and evaluation should converge and integrate the monitoring of the educational experience's quality. It is not an easy task, which, usually one tries to accomplish by defining grids and rating scales containing both qualitative and quantitative criteria derived upon her/his own personal idea of training experience.

Being well aware of the objective difficulty in defining the relevant qualities of an experience and what may be their weight in the learning processes (see par. 2), we may wonder whether it would be possible to equip the teachers/tutors with tools able to help them in the quantitative and qualitative monitoring of the activities that are carried on during the processes. A request that becomes even more stringent in online processes which lack multimodal face-to-face interaction.

Fortunately, the educational processes mediated by the machine, like those taking place on-line or in blended configuration, generate copious amounts of electronic *traces* that, when properly channeled and analyzed, can come to our aid.

Whatever the tools and methodologies used, a shrewdness of those who design educational processes should be to pay attention that each activity leave at least some traces in a given place. Ideal from this point of view is the forum because it is particularly suited to collect analysis, brainstorming, storytelling, design diaries, etc. .

Texts, in fact, are still the traces that are left more likely by the learners in their training and the text analysis is still the most ecological way to obtain information on individuals, their socio-relational skills, the learning process.

Of course, once that traces have been collected we must ask ourselves what aspects of the educational experience we intend to monitor and which indicators are the most appropriate to use. This is a very wide and quite new field of investigation!

In the past we have already shown how it is possible to monitor the cognitive evolution by mean of a quantitative evaluation of concept maps; here, in the following, we shall focus ourselves on how, starting from an analysis of the interaction occurred in a forum, it would be possible to monitor the social and emotional characteristics of educative design processes, by integrating social network analysis (SNA) [21] and automatic text analysis (ATA) [22].

5.1   Description of Case Studies

As case studies we took the traces produced during three editions, 2007-2009, of the blended course in "Interfaces and multimodal systems" (ISM) of the bachelor degree in Media Science and Technologies of the University of Rome Tor Vergata and those produced during the project work phase of the Scuola IaD's Master on process' design for the Technology Enhanced Learning (TEL). This latter is attended mainly by high and secondary schools' teachers and is carried on fully on-line.

All learning processes mentioned above have been carried on according to the "organic process" described in the previous paragraph. It is important to stress that: a) the layer of "learning" has been kept constantly active at first by means of a critical exploration of students' design places and of various research activities carry on the web, thereafter with the launch of periodic discussions on subjects intended to usefully complement the other activities that gradually were developing within the other functional layers; b) the "design" layer was kept constantly active first by applying various methods of analysis to the data collected and by the design of concept maps, then through the elaboration of a project work; c) the "communication" layer, although has been kept constantly active by the need to present and discuss the results of the various activities through the forum (using text, image and, in some cases, movies), was also constantly stimulated by storytelling activities, the request to develop the student's personal blog and e-portfolio, and to reorganize the design diary in a form useful for a written report and an oral presentation. Although the organic process is composed by parallel layers of activities, nevertheless, for sake of clarity and convenience of analysis, we offer to the reader, here below, its macro-phases representations: 8 for the master and 5/6 for the bachelor course.

Master. I) opening phase of acclimatization (8 days long); II) preliminary exploration activities; III) critical analysis of one's own working place (after 21 days); IV) data processing and problem setting (after 50 days); V) preliminary discussion on project works (after 66 days); VI) project work development (after 84 days); VII) debriefing and preparation for the final examination (after 130 days); VIII) "take leave" and plans for the future session (ten days long, after 140 days).

Bachelor. I) opening phase of acclimatization (5-15 days long); II) preliminary exploration activities; III) critical analysis and problem setting (after 40 days); IV) preliminary discussions on project works and tests (after 80-90 days, Easter holidays included); V) project work design and development, opening of the on-line design diary (after 95-105 days); this phase goes on till the final examination and includes also the debriefing (after 160-170 days); VI) recovering phase (starts the last week of July), only for the groups that are lagging behind on the delivery date. Students have to give two presentations after Easter holidays and at the end of the course.

5.2 Activity Tracking and Its "Social Quality"

In fig.2 we show the results of monitoring the modalities adopted by the participants to interact during the design process through the forum. The recordings concern the opening of new thread, the post replies and the comments (indeed the forum of the on-line learning environment we adopted, LIFE [20], allows to comment single words or phrases). Two sets of broken curves show respectively the intensity of exchanges produced exclusively by students and by students plus the tutors (3 for the master and 1 for ISM courses); the latter are identified by the T. Fig. 1a) shows how students participating in the ISM 2009 process use comments much less than master students and, more in general, produce a lower volume of activity (despite the eventual data normalization for the lower number of participants in the ISM process).

To understand the meaning of these observations is necessary to go further into data analysis. After the integration in LIFE of a module devoted to Social Network Analysis, we were able to study the characteristics of the network that developed during the design processes. Figure 2 shows, as an example, a series of snapshots on the network status as it appears during the various phases of the process for the case of ISM 2009. Even at a quick glance, the graphs show that the collaborative network developed progressively over the first three phases - although the net remains still heavily centralized on the tutor - and then suffer a setback during the phase devoted to the discussion of design proposals, before to acquire new vigor during the phase of collaborative design and development; during this latter the strongest relationships appear to be the intra-group ones and those with the tutor.

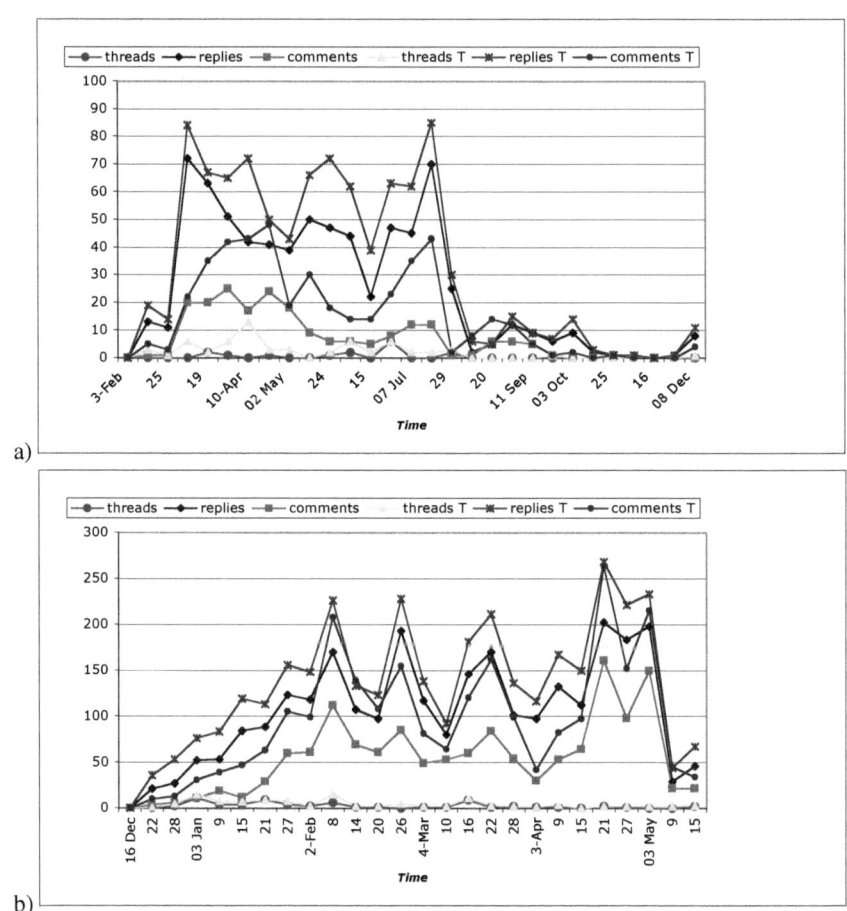

Fig. 2. Forum exchanges as function of time. a): ISM 2009; b): Master.

This set of observations are confirmed more quantitatively by the data reported in fig. 4. In fact they tell us that:

a) despite the noticeable difference from process to process the average density of the ISM processes, conducted in blended configuration, is on average quite low compared to that observed in the Master, which was conducted entirely on-line;

b) the analysis of the network centralization and of the tutor centrality shows that in the case of ISM processes the values of these two quantities are practically equivalent; this demonstrate that the networks form around the leading figure of the tutor and the on-line activities does not help in inducing a denser collaborative interaction among learners, except for the intra-group interaction already mentioned above.

Further supports to this analysis comes from measuring the average number of nodes (ANIN) with which each learner interacts during the design process: in the case of ISM 2009 ANIN take the value of 4.7, just slightly higher than the sum of the two group companions and the tutor. Not unlike is the situation for ISM 2007 in which ANIN is even lower: 3.4. In 2007, however, the localized comment functionality of the forum was not available. Such functionality, indeed, helps in increasing the level of the interaction as demonstrated by ISM 2008; for this cohort, indeed, ANIN was 6.4 considering only post replies and 8.3 if comments are also included. The largest number of contacts found in 2008, compared to that of 2009, however, must not mislead as it has to be normalized to the number of students participating in the cohort: 23 in 2008 and 15 in 2009. From the foregoing it follows that in the blended design processes the online activities are mainly used to develop a denser interaction with the tutor and to maintain the design diary design of the group;

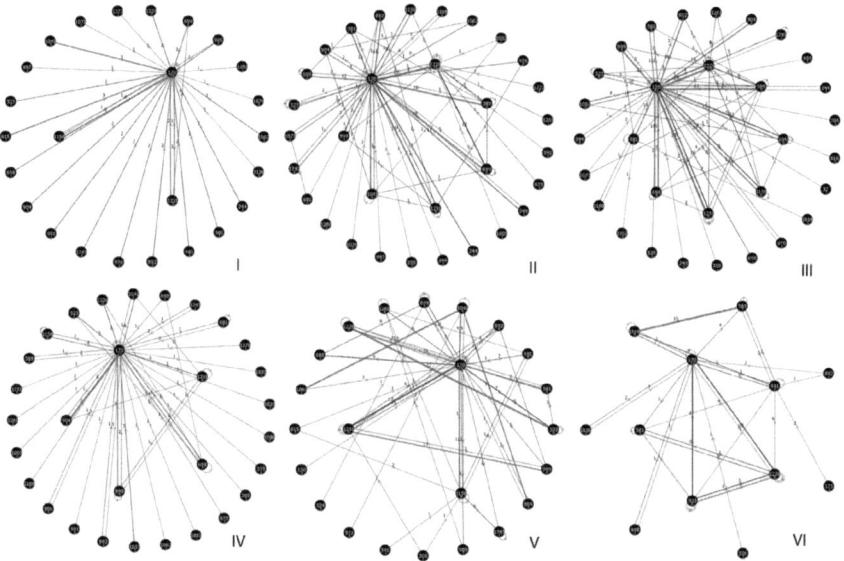

Fig. 3. Snapshots of the relationships developed during the six phases of the design process ISM 2009. Red links refer to post replies, blue links to comments.

c) in case of the master, conducted completely on-line, the density of the interaction is much higher, despite the high average number of participants in the design process: 30 units; during the phase of "concept design and development" the net density came up to 0,32%, correspondingly the value of input network centralization decreased and also the output network centralization greatly increases by touching the tip of 0.6. It is no by chance, then, that ANIN took the value of 15.1, i.e. half of the participants in the design process. Such data, in our opinion, demonstrate the effectiveness of the online activities in the realization of valuable collaborative processes, when these latter are developed fully on-line.

The question that comes next is, of course, the following: is the intensity of social interaction correlated with the overall performance of the students?

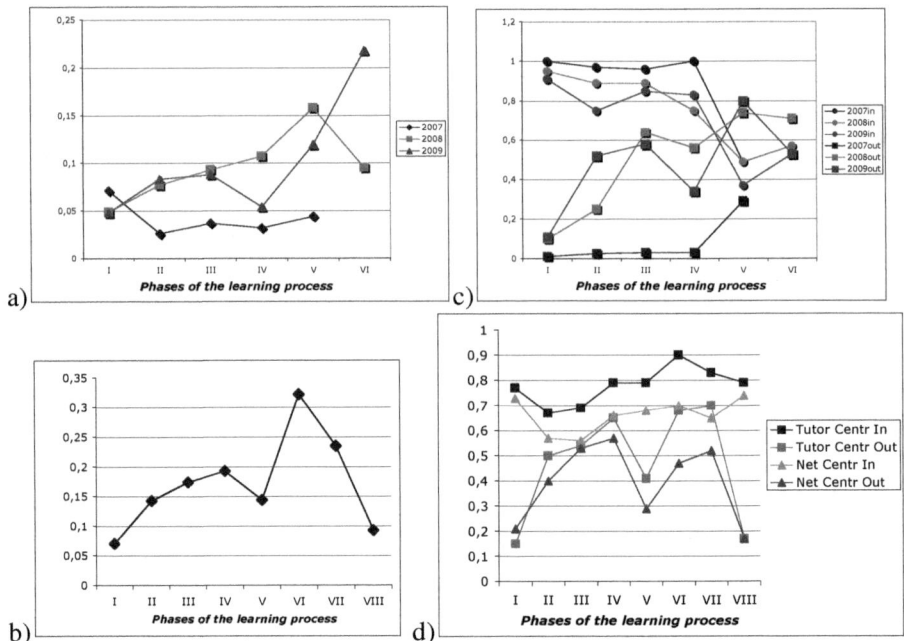

Fig. 4. Variation of the net density with the phases of the design process: a) ISM processes; b): Master. c) variation of the network centralization during the ISM processes; d) variation of the network centralization and of the tutor centrality during the master process.

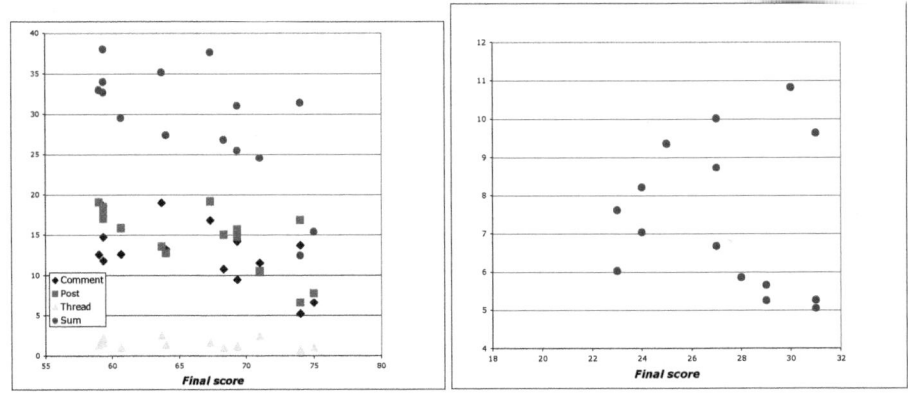

Fig. 5. Standard deviation of the student activities with respect to the average activity of the whole group integrated over the whole duration of the process vs. the score reported during the final examination. Left: Master; right: ISM 2009.

To try to answer this further question we calculated, for each student, the standard deviation of the intensity of the various forms of interaction - threads, replies, comments - with respect to the average activities recorded for the design process as a whole. In Fig. 5, these values are shown vs. the mark obtained by the students during the final examination. It is clear that there is no conclusive answer. In the case of the Master, i.e. a process carried on completely on-line, the correlation seems to exist and the weight of such correlation appears to be distributed equally on post replies and comments.

In the case of ISM 2009 (the data analysis of other cohorts is ongoing), instead, we are faced with possibly a double trend: on the one hand there seems to be a group of students who benefits from on-line social interaction, on the other seems to be another group that shows an opposite trend to indicate a predisposition for working in a more confidential manner. This is the first clue indicating the possible existence of measurable design styles.

The data analysis performed to date could be developed further to obtain detailed information about each single student, but the study of the characteristics of the individuals goes well beyond the scope of this article and is left for the future.

5.3 The "Emotional Quality" of the Learning Experience

It is well-known fact that emotion is a quality of the learning experience that can affect memory, attention, decision making and performance of a learner who participates in educational processes and social interactions mediated by the machine [23]. Unfortunately, at present is not a quality that is monitored systematically and in an ecological manner. The main difficulties are: a) the development of tools able to obtain information in "quasi-real time" without disturbing the on-going process; b) the integration of such tools in the workflow, i.e. within the on-line environment where, usually, the learning processes are carried on.

Currently, research on the subject have been conducted using techniques typical of sociology and ethnography that allowed pre-and post-surveys on the learning experience [24] or through the detection of physiological parameters that can be hardly defined "ecological". Recently some research groups start to work, with good results, on the collection and real-time analysis of para-verbal elements such as facial expression [25] or the emotional nuances of the voice. Although of great interest at the stage of laboratory demonstrations and experiments, such methods are still quite far from being used in real learning contexts.

Another possible approach is under investigation by groups working on text analysis, but not specifically on education, through the adaptation of the Latent Semantic Analysis to detect affective semantic similarities among words contained in a corpus and an affective hierarchy based on the WORDNET-AFFECT lexical database [26]. The method is promising but is based on an affective hierarchy derived arbitrarily with a top-down procedure, while it is important that relations among words and emotions emerge from the thought of the users through a bottom-up procedure.

Therefore the identification of methods and tools able to monitor the emotional state during a learning process and that have also a high probability of penetration is still an open issue. Our proposal is to use as input the texts produced by members of a learning community and to evaluate them in quasi-real time, in situ, to extract their emotional content thanks: a) to the integration in LIFE of a module to perform automatic text analysis (ATA); b) to the building up of a reference corpus of words whose affective weight is determined with a bottom-up procedure. Preliminary results have been published in reference 27.

Compared to the analysis of facial expressions and voice one loses in immediacy but gains in portability and integrability within the flow of real educational experiences. Respect to the method proposed in ref. 26 our starting point – the weighted affective corpus - is probably much closer to the common feeling. Of course, it is not impossible that in the future one may find a convergence between the two approaches.

As discussed above the extraction of the emotional content of a text requires, necessarily, the existence of a benchmarking reference: i.e. a weighted affective corpus in the same language of the text to be analyzed. Unfortunately, such affective corpus for the Italian language was not available and we had to create it through a complex testing procedure that entailed: a) selecting a first group of words potentially significant (direct and indirect affective words); b) their presentation to a quite relevant number of subjects to obtain a distribution of their affective weights.

In this early phase of the implementation, to speed the comparison procedure, we decided to create an affective dictionary based on graphic forms, rather than lemmas. Moreover, we postponed to future developments also the identification of the dependence of the weights on the context of use.

We first selected a large number of graphic forms candidate to transmit emotions and then, after a random extraction, we presented a subset of 30 of them to volunteers who had to indicate which emotion they were able to convey.

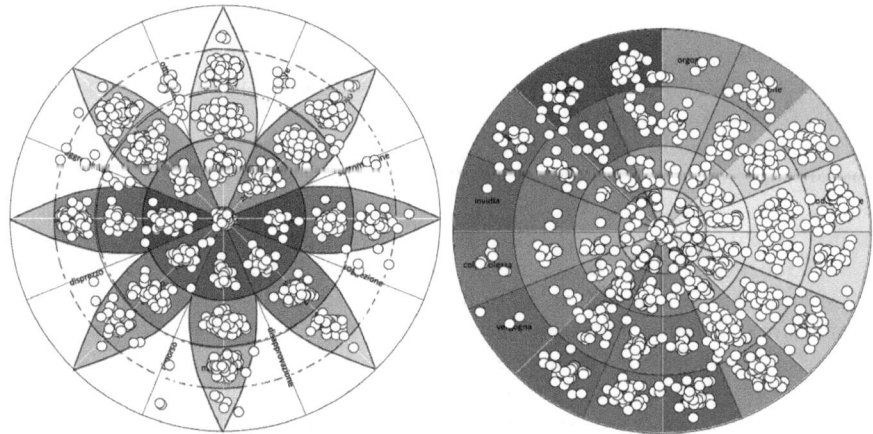

Fig. 6. Coverage of the emotional palettes representing the Plutchik model (left) and the GEW (right)

To put the subjects in as much as possible "ecological" situation we ask them to read the word and, then, to indicate the emotion by clicking on the colored representation of one among the most popular models of emotions. In particular, we concentrated on two models whose representations, by including a large variety of emotions, offer to the subjects a wide choice, very similar to what happens in real life when one tries to determine, in a more or less conscious way, the emotional content of a text: the model of Plutchik [28] and the model described by GEW (Emotional Geneve Wheel) [29] see fig. 6. The first was chosen as representative of the family of the so called finite-state models of emotions in which every emotion - sometime defined force - represents a state that is supposed to be culturally invariant, although expressible with different intensity. The second, on the other hand, is inspired to the so called multidimensional models, which have their precursor in the 2 dimensional model based on valence and intensity. The test was executed by 98 subjects (44 used its on-line version), 18-35 years old, half male and half female. Apart from the first 24 tests, used for text calibration, in all the remainders we included 8 control items that have been used to determine the reliability of results, a procedure that maybe particularly necessary in the case of texts performed on-line. Fig. 6 shows the coverage of emotional palettes we obtained. It is immediate to see that the coverage obtained for the Plutchik model is currently quite satisfactory; the same cannot be stated for GEW. This result suggests that before to use the GEW in the phase of analysis one should increase the number of tests and extend, as well, the selection of the emotionally meaningful words. For this reason the discussion of the case studies, presented in the following sections, have been based solely on the Plutchik model.

Fig. 7 a) shows examples of emotional distributions associated to affective words: as might be expected, after having integrated the results of the tests, all the words can be associated to a more or less broad distribution of emotional states (and/or their nuances), i.e. affective weights. These distributions have been stored in the database and used to extract the emotions carried by the textual corpora.

Fig. 7 b) shows one of the most critical point of the extraction of the emotional content from texts: the models of emotion do not fully overlap, even when one considers only the six fundamental emotions defined by Ekman [30] and included in both the models considered here. The same graphical forms used in different model context generate different results. A reasonable overlapping (around 70%) is obtaneid by joy, anger, fear and sadness. Only around 40% the overlapping for surprice and disgust. This results raises even more doubts about the use of top-down approaches in the classification of the affective words. A closer study on the equivalence between the models of emotion used, and between these and other models of emotion, such as bi and tridimensional model or WORDNET-AFFECT (for which there is a valid emotional vocabulary in English) is left to the next future.

After the extraction of the corpora of texts produced during the development of educational processes described in Sec. 4.1, we calculated the average distributions of emotion conveyed by all the texts written by students and tutors. The first strip of histograms in fig. 8.1) refers to the Master in e-learning and shows how after an initial transient, the emotional state of the group is stabilized and remains unchanged over time, reflecting a process that has been kept under control and that was carried on without major problems. The situation of ISM has been somewhat different. The average emotional state of the group was much less stable and shows peaks of negative "mood" in the proximity of the deadlines for deliveries or oral presentations. Among the three processes of the ISM the more problematic one was that held in 2007.

As far as individuals are concerned, the strip b of fig. 8.2) shows how the emotional pattern of the main tutor (ID 1404) was dominated by the 'anticipation' (central emotion of one of the petals of the Plutchik flower that integrate also 'vigilance' and 'interest') which can be translated into a constant presence and encouragement to the needs of the learners and to the schedule of the process. Strip c of the same figure shows, on the other hand, that other tutors (e.g. ID 1433) may play a different and complementary role, namely to foster in the learners a positive attitude (represented by the 'joy' - that include also 'serenity' and 'ecstasy') and, as well, a continued

368   C. Giovannella, C. Spadavecchia, and A. Camusi

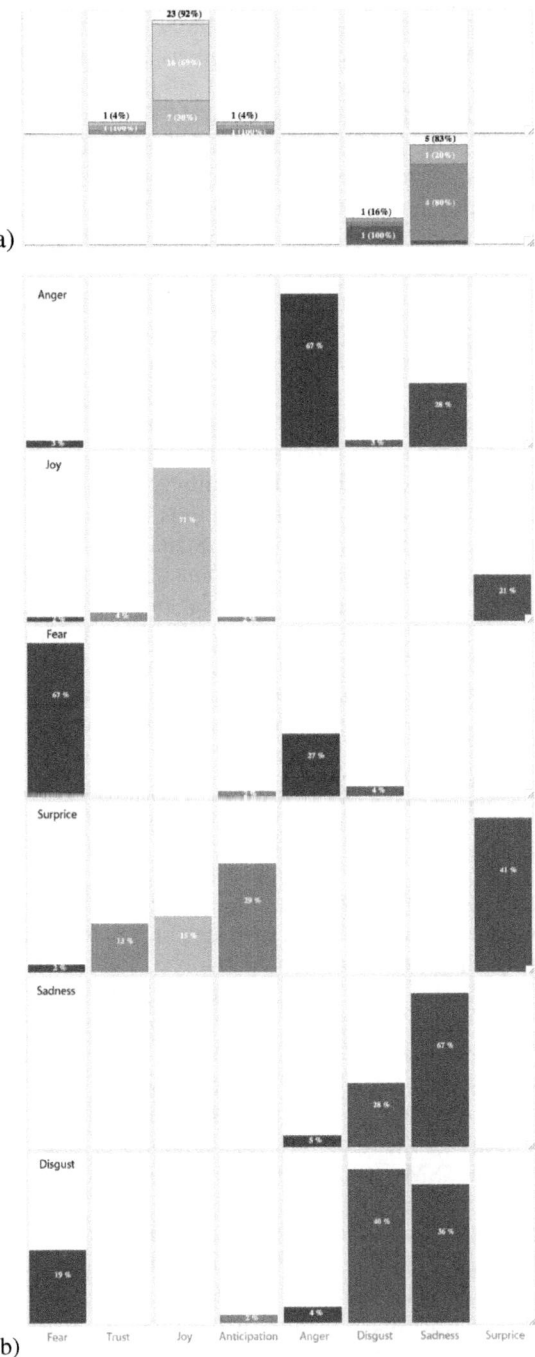

a)

b)

Fig. 7. a): Examples of emotional distributions associated with the graphical form; cheers (above), abandoned (below); b): overlapping between results obtained GEW (rows) and Plutchik model (columns)

confidence in the process and in themselves. Strip d shows the case of learner ID 1799 that after a cautious approach, stabilizes her emotional profile, aligns with the process and get a very good final score. The learner to which refers strip e, while in tune with the process, shows also large doses of fear and sadness and close to the examination (April), boredom and anger, to indicate an increasing state of fatigue that did not allow to perform at the best of her possibility. Strip f shows the case of learner ID 1910, emotionally not very stable and not easy to deal with; in the last month, however she got in harmony with the process and was able to pass the exam. Finally, in strip g is shown the case of learner ID 1899, that deserved very little interest in the process at the beginning (hence the emotional instability of the distribution) and that did not pass the examination; it is not by chance that toward the end sadness, fear and anger reach a significant proportions before to fall down again during the "take leave" phase where reappeared a higher level of confidence for the future.

The system allows also for a more detailed, day by day, analysis, but its description is beyond the scope of this article.

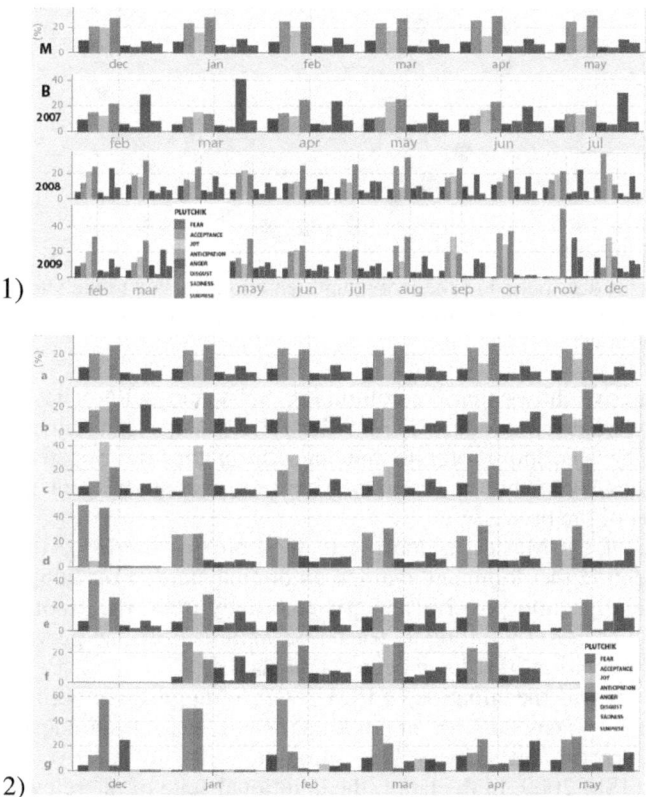

Fig. 8. 1): Time evolution of the distributions of the average emotions, as detected by means of automatic text analysis, for the four educational processes described in sec. 3; 2): comparison among the dynamics of the average distributions of emotions of the group (a) and that of some individuals (b and c: tutors; d-f: students) for the case of the Master in e-learning

Lastly we want to show how the average emotional state of the individuals can be disaggregated and distributed over the relationships that each one has with other members of the community. Focusing on the IV phase of the process, fig. 9 shows a visualizations of how the individual emotions distribute on the various relationships identified by means of another tool integrated in LIFE that allows to perform SNA. The representation is centered on the ID 1404. The colored halo around the ID of the individuals represents the dominant average emotional state, while the flags (stacked histograms) show the distribution of the emotional content of the relationship (whether post or comment) from both sides.

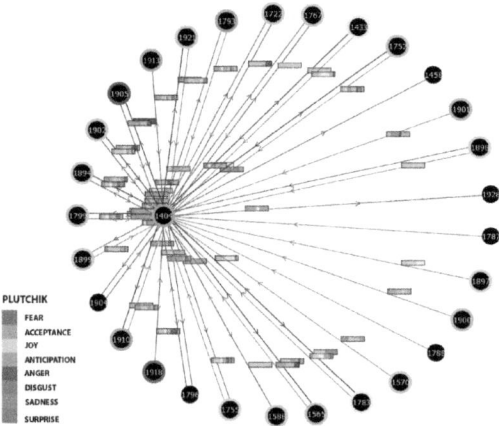

Fig. 9. Example of distribution of the individual's emotions related to the interactions that have characterized her/his work in the forum. Red link: replies to post comments; blue link: comment to portions of text.

Fig. 10, finally, shows that by combining SNA and ATA it is possible also to monitor the average emotional state of the relationships entertained by the whole community. The snapshots refer to the interaction that developed during the four design processes taken into consideration here as case studies, integrated along the whole duration of the processes.

In the case of the Master, according to the color of the halos that surround the nodes (representing the dominant average emotional state of the subject), the climate has been generally quite positive and permeated by trust; the emotions spans from 'joy', expressed at most by tutors, to 'trust' and 'anticipation' that pervades most of the learners and the relations that have been established.

Very different was the situation of ISM 2007: to the positive vigilance of the tutor the group seems to respond with an emotional status that, if not negative, seem to be pervaded by surprise and sadness. The situation seems to improve progressively in ISM 2008 and ISM 2009. In the latter, the emotional state of the relevant actors of the process - i.e. those with a higher degree of centrality, and thus placed in the inner circle - seem to be reasonably positive.

One point that remains unclear is how much the emotion of the individual can be influenced by the emotional state of the group and / or by that of the group leaders, i.e. by what we may call, respectively, the social emotionality and leadership.

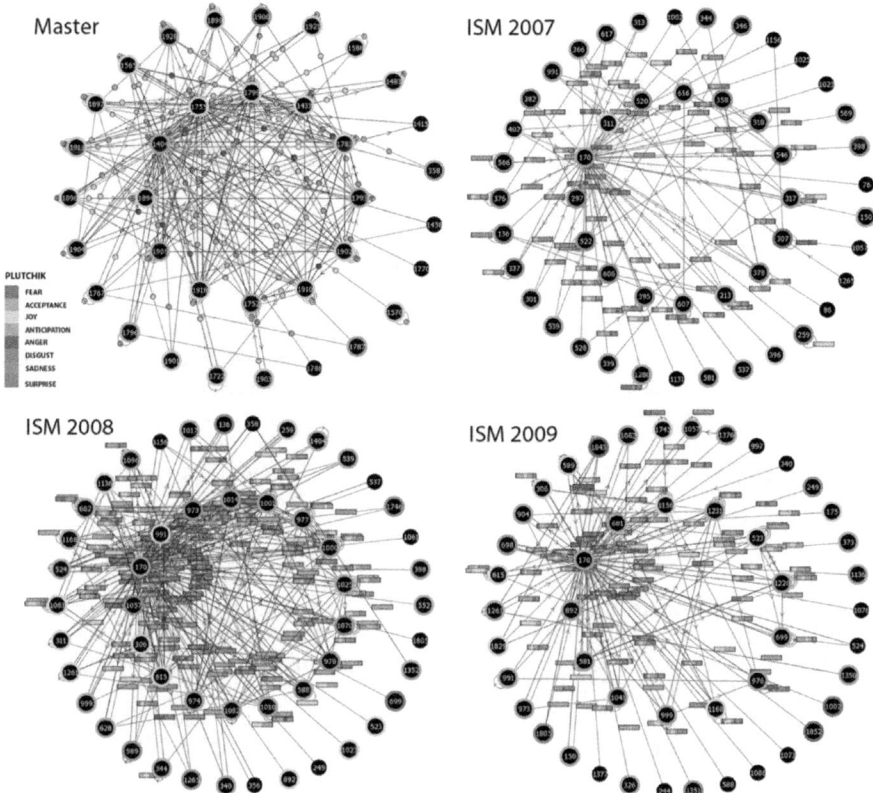

Fig. 10. Integrated view of the interaction developed during the design process enriched by emotional halos. Color of the halos according to the Plutchik model and to legend.

The study of this, like many other aspects that we mentioned, is left for the close future.

In conclusion we think that the results presented here above, although refer to an experimental use of new methodologies and tools - worthy of further study – are still sufficient to demonstrate the feasibility of an "experience's monitoring system" and, more in general, the enormous potential of the automated and selective analysis of the traces left by the members of a learning community during on-line and blended educative processes.

References

1. Weiser, M.: Some Computer Science Problems in Ubiquitous Computing. Communications of the ACM (1993)
2. Greenfield, A.: Everyware. In: The Dawning Age of Ubiquitous Computing, AIGA & New Riders, Berkley (2006)
3. Löwgren, J.: Articulating the use qualities of digital designs. In: Aesthetic Computing, pp. 383–403. MIT Press, Cambridge (2006)
4. Eco, U.: The Open Work. Harvard U.P., Cambridge (1989)

5. N.B. the term "baroque" is used in the acceptation of "baroque ensembliste", see Moretti L., Tapié M.: Le Baroque Généralisé. Manifeste du Baroque Ensembliste. Centro Internazionale di Ricerche Estetiche, Dioscuro (1965)
6. Thackara, J.: In the bubble. In: Designing in a complex world, MIT Press, Cambridge (2005)
7. Giovannella, C.: An Organic Process for the Organic Era of the Interaction in HCI. In: Educators 2007: Creativity3 - Experiencing to Educate and Design, pp. 129–133. Univ. of Aviero press (2007)
8. Cambi, F.: Manuale di storia della pedagogia. Editori Laterza, Roma-Bari (2003)
9. Adorno, T.: Cultural Industry. Routledge, New York (2001)
10. Schön, D.A.: The Reflective Practitioner. How Professionals think in action. Ashgate, Aldershot (1983)
11. Giovannella, C.: DULP: Complexity, organicity, liquidity. IxD&A (7-8), 11–15 (2009)
12. Giovannella, C., Graf, S.: Challenging Technology, Rethinking Pedagogy, Being Design Inspired. eLearn Magazine (2010), http://www.elearnmag.org/subpage.cfm?section=articles&article=114-1 (retrieved August 15 2010)
13. Moggridge, B.: Designing Interactions. The MIT Press, Cambridge (2007)
14. Benyon, D., Turner, P., Turner, S.: Design Interactive Systems. Pearson Education, Harlow (2005)
15. Jones, J.C.: Design Methods. Wiley, New York (1980)
16. Lidwell, W., Holden, K., Butler, J.: Universal Principles of Design. Rockport, Beverly (2003)
17. Giovannella, C., Camusi, A., Spadavecchia, C.: From Learning Styles to Experience styles. In: ICALT 2010, pp. 732–733. IEEE Press, New York (2010)
18. Coffield, C., Mosely, D., Hall, E., Ecclestone, K.: Learning styles and Pedagogy in Post-16 Learning. LSRC, Univ. of Newcastle upon Tyne, London (2004)
19. Graf, S., Viola, S.R., Leo, T.: Kinshuk: In-Depth Analysis of the Felder-Silverman Learning Style Dimension. J. of Res. on Tech. in Education, 79–93 (2007); and references therein
20. Learning in an Interactive Framework to Experience, http://life.mifav.uniroma2.it
21. Wasserman, S., Faust, K.: Social network analysis: methods and applications. Cambridge University Press, Cambridge (1994)
22. Bolasco, S.: Analisi Multidimensionale dei dati. Carocci, Roma (1999)
23. Picard, R.W., et al.: BT Technology Journal 22, 253–269 (2004)
24. Pekrun, R.: Progress and open problems in educational emotion research. Learning and Instruction 15, 497–506 (2005)
25. El Kaliouby, R., Robinson, P.: Real-Time Vision for Human-Computer Interaction, pp. 181–200. Springer, Heidelberg (2005)
26. Strapparava, C., Valitutti, A., Stock, O.: The affective Weight of Lexicon. In: Proceedings of the Fifth International Conference on Language Re- sources and Evaluation, LREC, Genoa, Italy (2006)
27. Spadavecchia, C., Giovannella, C.: Monitoring learning experiences and styles: the socio-emotional level. In: ICALT 2010, pp. 445–449. IEEE Press, New York (2010)
28. Plutchik, R.: Emotion: A Psychoevolutionary Synthesis. Harper & Row, New York (1980)
29. Scherer, K.R.: What are emotions? And how can they be measured? Social Science Information 44, 695–729 (2005)
30. Ekman, P.: An Argument for Basic Emotions. Cognition and Emotion 6(3/4), 169–200 (1992)

Designing Usable Educational Material for English Courses Supported by Mobile Devices

Rosa Romero, Telmo Zarraonandia, Ignacio Aedo, and Paloma Díaz

Universidad Carlos III de Madrid
Departamento de Informática
Escuela Politécnica Superior
Av. Universidad 30 Leganes, Madrid, España 28911
{rosa.romero,tzarraon,pdp}@inf.uc3m.es, aedo@ia.uc3m.es

Abstract. Mobile Learning (M-Learning) may offer many advantages when designing educational processes as it can help to overcome restrictions of time and place. However, it is necessary to consider the special features of the type of devices used to follow these type of courses in order to guarantee the usability of the learning objects produced for this eLearning modality. In this document we describe the process of designing a set of courses which aim to support learners when developing English grammar, reading and listening skills, explaining the guidelines we have followed to ensure the usability of the final product.

Keywords: Language learning, Usability, M-learning, learning material design.

1 Introduction

The application of information and communication technology to the area of education has changed the learning processes from the perspective of the student, the instructor and the instructional designer. The growth and rapid evolution of wireless technology have created new opportunities for an anytime and anywhere learning paradigm, commonly know as Mobile Learning (M-Learning) [1].

Among the many benefits that the m-learning modality can provide, what most stands out is the ability to access and follow the learning material simply and without undue effort. M-learning offers a new way to integrate learning into daily life. In this way, students can follow the course material making use of their spare time whilst travelling on public transport. This has been perceived by many educationalists as offering flexibility in learning and presents a multitude of unique educational advantages [2]. Additionally, a constant exposure to digital technologies, gadgets, games, and mobile devices has led to a new breed of student; learners who can rapidly adopt and adapt new technologies because the interaction with these tools is innate for them. Moreover, mobile technologies offer students the possibility of constructing their interpretations of a subject and to communicate those understandings to others. Those technologies, if employed effectively, expand discussion beyond the classroom and

G. Leitner, M. Hitz, and A. Holzinger (Eds.): USAB 2010, LNCS 6389, pp. 373–383, 2010.

provide new ways for students to collaborate and communicate their knowledge in class and in the outside world [3]. However, together with its many benefits, the implementation of m-learning processes also poses considerable design challenges, many of which are related to the restrictions that its portability impose on the devices normally used in this learning modality.

In this position paper we describe the process of designing a set of courses to support the learning of English which can be followed using mobile devices. In order to guarantee the usability and increase the effectiveness of the produced material, the design process has been carried out taking into account different guidelines found in the literature. In this paper we describe how these guidelines have been adapted for implementing activities from training three different language learning skills: *reading, listening and grammar*. The set of learning objects produced could be followed using domestic PCs, PDAs or mobile devices which support Flash technology, and have been grouped making a total of 41 courses. The work has been carried out as part of the MW-TELL project (Mobile and Wireless Technologies for Technology-Enhanced Language Learning) [4], funded by European Commission under the Leonardo da Vinci (LdV) Sectoral Programme of the Lifelong Learning Programme. The MW-TELL project addresses the urgent need for building a new generation of vocational training services for the provision of on-demand lifelong learning competence and skills development, not subject to time and place restrictions. Following this objective different software has been produced for facilitating the authoring (MW-TELL Courses Authoring Toolkit), annotation (MW-TELL Learning Objects Metadata Authoring Toolkit) and delivering (MW-TELL Course Player) of educational material to handheld devices. A free access repository has also been set up with the aim of storing and sharing educational resources, which may adopt several forms such as presentations, exercises, graphs or self-assessments. The educational resources can also be retrieved grouped under the form of a course in a specific subject, and in this case the student will require the use of the MW-TELL Player software to follow the different activities proposed.

The rest of the paper is organized as follows. In section 2, we outline the need of our approach by presenting some related research on Mobile Learning English systems that have proved the suitability of these for type of devices for this specific area of education. Following on from that, the design process of the learning objects is explained, detailing the guidelines followed to ensure the usability and efficiency of the material produced. Finally some conclusions and future work lines are presented.

2 Related Works

Foreign language learning is a critical issue in the field of education, and the effectiveness of this type of learning could be greatly enhanced by the application of m-learning techniques. These learning processes normally take place in a traditional classroom and students may not be provided with many opportunities to practice what they have learned outside that context. Therefore the use of m-learning in this domain seems particularly appropriate, as it can tackle different skills and activities related to this type of learning.

For instance, to enhance the learning of vocabulary, the personalized system described in [5] recommends appropriate English vocabulary to learners according to individual learner vocabulary ability and memory cycles. To promote reading ability the PIMS (Personalized Intelligent Mobile System) system proposed in [6] can be adapted to automatically retrieve unknown or unfamiliar vocabulary from English news articles according to the English vocabulary ability of the individual learner. Following a similar purpose, the mobile-device-supported peer-assisted learning system (MPAL) described in [7] supports collaborative EFL (English as a Foreign Language) reading activities. Moreover, several studies have been conducted on the use of M-Learning to improve English listening and speaking abilities. For example, the Mobile Adaptive CALL (MAC) [8] is aimed at helping Japanese-English speakers in perceptually distinguishing the non-native /r/ versus /l/ English phonetic contrast. In [9] the development of a system for one-on-one English oral practice and assessment in classroom supported by handheld devices is described.

The findings of these studies have demonstrated that students increased their performance in the above mentioned abilities, and readily accepted the use of handheld devices for English learning. The analysis of the related systems evidenced the necessity of providing different sets of learning objects, depending on the basic skill in which development is sought. Furthermore, in this way the learner is offered the possibility of practising the skill in which he/she needs more training. However, the analyzed systems mentioned above did not pay sufficient attention to providing a system interface which responds to the very specific requirements of this learning modality. As the evaluation of the last system depicted, this could lead to some interaction drawbacks, which in turn could decrease the effectiveness of the system as a learning tool.

This way, in order to fully enjoy the benefits offered by the devices used in this learning modality, the designers of both software and content have to consider the special restrictions associated to their use. The screen size and resolution limitations of these devices and their special input mechanisms are clearly two restrictive factors, but attention should also be paid to the bandwidth limits, network reach or the expenses associated with data usage when designing how to access the content. The wide range of hardware and operative systems available, and the different rendering obtained from different browsers should also be taken into account as they may seriously limit the compatibility and usability of the software. The rapid changes in the context of use of mobile devices should also be considered, as changes in noise level, brightness or other environmental conditions may also change the usability or appropriateness of an application [10].

In order to improve the usability of their applications, designers can follow different recommendations and guidelines found in the literature. For instance, the World Wide Web Consortium (W3C) proposes a series of best practices for delivering Web content to mobile devices [11]. Gong and Tarasewich, in turn, [12] propose extending the general HCI recommendations of Shneiderman [13] and to adapt them to the case of handheld computers. For the specific area of learning object design for mobile applications the recommendations described by Churchill and Hedberg in [14] can help to avoid common mistakes.

3 Educational Material Design Process

In order to ensure the usability and, more generally, the quality of the final training material, the design process has taken into consideration several design guidelines proposed by different authors. This section describes the main guidelines followed, and the way they have been implemented in our material.

3.1 Learning Content Design

There are many different definitions of the concept of learning object in the literature. In our case, the definition chosen is based on two fundamental predicates of the learning objects, learning and reusability [15]: "A Learning Object is an independent and self-standing unit of learning content that is predisposed to reuse in multiple instructional contexts". The key to a successful object is, naturally, whether it actually does facilitate learning [16]. Part of the answer, of course, is that it is not possible to ensure that learning always occurs. However, in the design of our training material some of the steps proposed by Rachel S. Smith [16] have been considered in order to make it more likely. Next, we will describe how these steps have been conducted along the learning objects design process.

Step 1: Keep Your Educational Goal in Focus. Every choice taken during the design and development of the learning material must refer to the learning objective we seek the learner to attain. The question to be raised is: What educational problem are you trying to solve?

The aim of our material is to support university students who are trying to obtain the Europass skills level B1 certificate whilst generally improving their English reading, listening and grammar skills. At this stage of the project the development of writing skills has not been considered as only the implementation of basic interactions such like drag and drop or click have been taken into account. Hence, dividing the courses content into grammar, reading and listening blocks is the most logical option. Only assets which support the development of each specific skill have been considered in each block of courses.

Step 2: Choose Meaningful Content that Directly Supports your Educational Goal. This second step recommends that each part in a learning object should relate to and support the others. Learners can become confused, distracted, or even lost in a maze of too much information. This guideline also encourages us to follow some specific design strategies like choosing content and examples that are concrete rather than abstract.

Our course contents are adapted to English students of the Europass skills level B1 certificate. The material used to create the learning objects has been provided by English teachers from the University Carlos III of Madrid. Accordingly, these contents have been built on learner´s existing knowledge. In listening courses, examples have been drawn from real-world data to keep the content focused on everyday functional language, and to demonstrate how the learner may use the new knowledge in his/her own life. Those examples have also served as a base for the ones used in the grammar theory. With regard to the reading courses, the comprehension of the student has been trained and evaluated by using English riddles.

Step 3: Select Appropriate Activity Structures. The basic structure of the activities in a learning object will have a direct effect on whether learning occurs easily, with difficulty, or rarely. Students who are solving problems, drawing conclusions, comparing options and thinking about what they are doing are likely to be actively engaged in the learning process. Besides, these types of activities make use of the higher-order thinking skills of synthesis, analysis, and evaluation.

The MW-Tell project proposes six generic Mobile Training Scenarios Templates for constructing courses: Competence Based Learning, Problem Based Learning, Project Based Learning, Experiential Learning and Tutorial Based Learning. The development of our courses is based on two of these pre-defined templates: Tutorial Based Learning and Experiential Learning. When following courses based on the former scenario, students analyze information related to a concept, search for data, identify the best solution and apply their knowledge in practice. When following courses based on the latter scenario, the learner trains a particular English skill by direct practice. In order to increase student engagement both types of courses make extensive use of multimodal information, and both include several short exercises to provide the learner with continuous and immediate feedback about his/her learning.

Step 4: Consider Assessment Issues. Assessments are used to determine how much learning actually takes place. This fourth step advises that choosing a method of assessment should be considered as part of the design problem: should comprehension indicators, like multiple-choice quizzes, be used? Or should we ask the leaner to produce a written document like an essay or research paper?

Each of the courses developed following the Tutorial-based Learning template includes a specific module of assessment. Two basics methods of assessment have been used in these modules: single or multiple-choice quizzes and drag and drop exercises (Fig 1). On the other hand, the exercises included in the courses developed according to the Experiential Learning template, try to replicate normal teaching methods on a

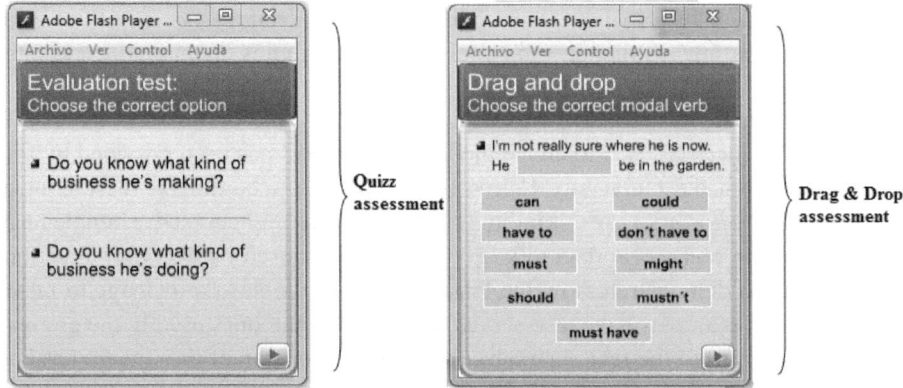

Fig. 1. Examples of assessment modules produced

traditional English course. This way, for instance, during a listening exercise the student can only listen twice to the recording.

3.2 Usability Guidelines

The term usability is defined by the ISO 9241-11 as *'the extent to which a product can be used by specified users to achieve specified goals with effectiveness, efficiency and satisfaction in a specified context of use'* [17].

The ultimate goal of usability is meeting the needs of the user's satisfaction [18]. In order to produce training material as usable as possible, the designers should take into account the special characteristics and limitations of the devices which are going to be used to follow the course. Following this idea and before properly starting with the process of designing the learning objects we reviewed different recommendations and guidelines for designing mobile learning portals and learning, and chose the most well-known ones. Next, we will describe the main guidelines which were finally followed, as well as the way they were implemented in the particular case of our training material.

User Analysis: The User/Learner. This guideline advised paying special attention in examining the user´s characteristics, such as age, nationality, user´s degree of familiarity with mobile devices and special needs or physical disabilities.

The content of these courses is targeted to learners of Europass Skill Level B1 (User Independent). It is expected that the courses will be used in the university context, by students who make use of mobile technology as part of their daily life and do not have special needs. The courses material will all be in English in order to allow its use by students from different nationalities.

Interface Design: The Small Screen Display / Overuse of the Screen. Two different usability guidelines have been followed in order to facilitate the visualization of the educational material and not to hamper its comprehension.

The first one recommends that the height and width of the display area should not exceed the screen size. Long pages should be segmented into smaller chunks and an effective mechanism to view and navigate to the desired page should be provided. Extensive scrolling and the number of clicks should be well thought out. The second guideline recommends paying close attention to the amount of relevant information included in each page.

In order not to exceed the screen size of a PDA, the size of the learning objects has been set at 240 x 268 pixels, and the minimum font size used was 13 pt. These choices have been taken after analyzing opinions about the clarity and legibility of the material gathered from the students targeted by the courses. In the same way, in order to keep the learner attention, the use of paging is prefered over the use of scrolling. Long scrolling pages may cause students to abandon and not fully complete the task. Setting criteria to determine the amount of relevant information on each page has been especially important in the case of the learning objects of the grammar block. In this way, no more than two examples have been included on each page of the learning objects which include grammar theory (Fig 2).

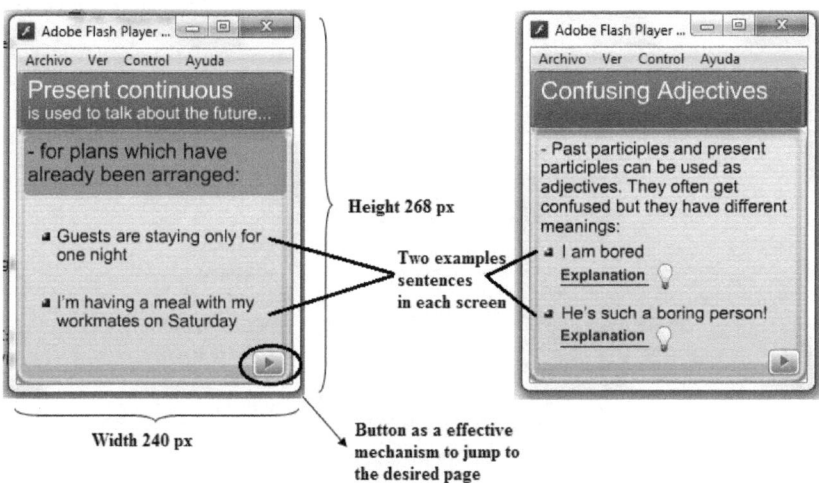

Fig. 2. Example of implementation of the usability guideline "The small screen display"

Interface Design: Navigation and Consistency. This guideline points out that the selection of appropriate navigation structures may be of a great importance in the usability and presentation clarity of the learning material in small screen displays. The consistency of the implemented mechanism for navigating from one screen to another is also of major importance as it maintains the learners' pace and stimulates learning interest.

All the screens of the learning objects produced have a consistent layout, colour scheme and overall look (Fig 3 and 4). The same icons are allays used to denote the same types of information or actions (tips, sounds, correct, incorrect,..).

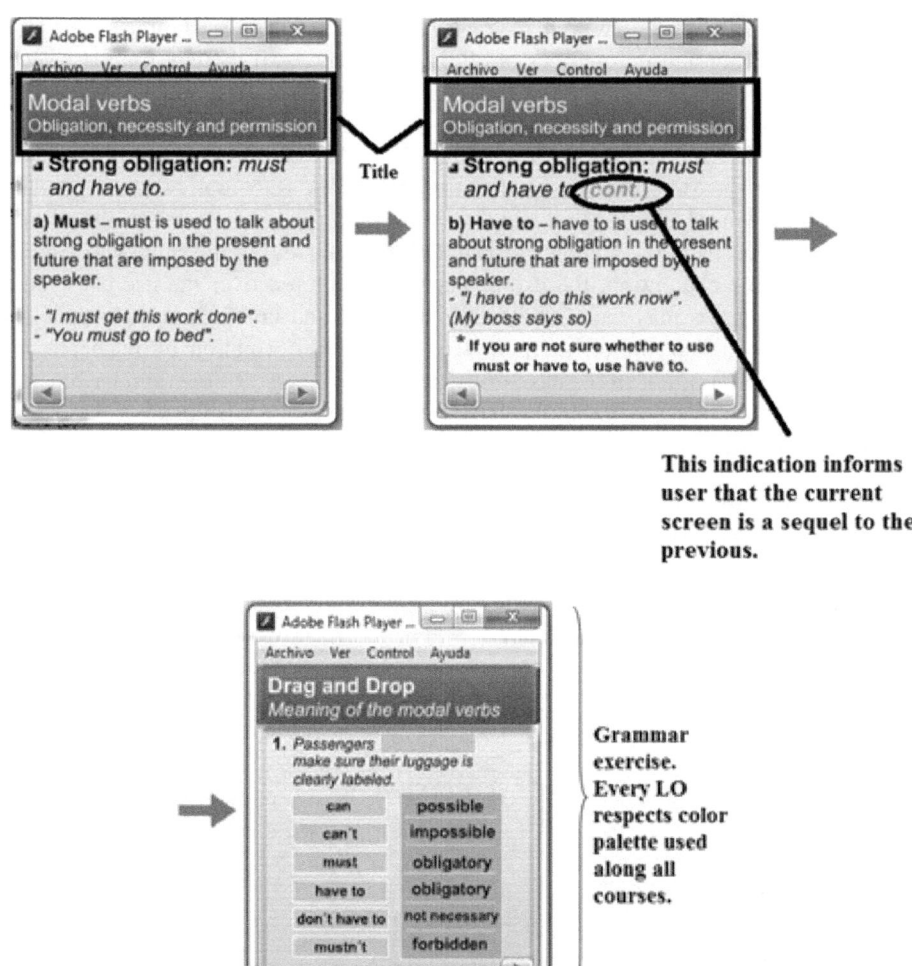

Fig. 3. First example of implementation of the usability guideline *"Navigation and Consistency"*

In all courses the same typeface in the text content is used. Navigation design follows established standards and uses conventions to ensure that, for instance, link colours contrast sufficiently with text, visited and unvisited links.

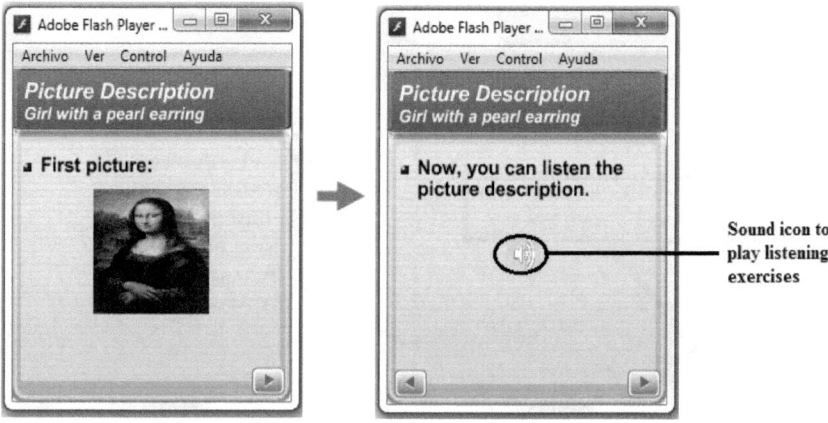

Fig. 4. Second example of implementation of the usability guideline "Navigation and Consistency"

Interface Design: Allow Learners to Control their Interactions. There is some common agreement about the convenience of giving the users the freedom to choose how to complete the proposed tasks. Learners may be more likely to explore a topic if they are confident that they can return to previously visited pages, and can find their way around easily.

Fig 5 and 6 depict examples of how this guideline has been implemented in different learning objects. For instance, as shown in the pictures, every learning object include *Back* buttons to allow learners to find their way back to previously visited pages easily.

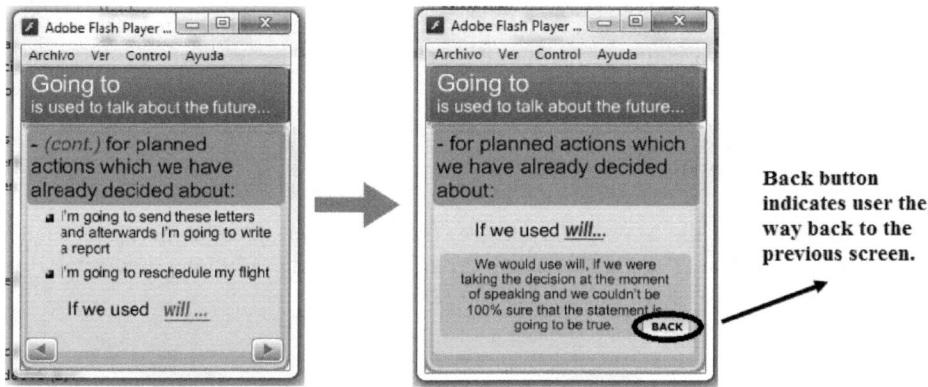

Fig. 5. First application example of the usability guideline "Allow learners to control their interactions"

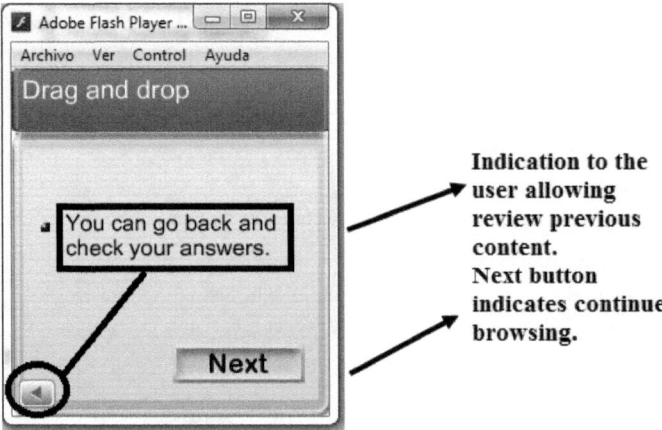

Fig. 6. Second application example of the usability guideline "Allow learners to control their interactions"

4 Conclusions

In the same way as learners of many other areas, the students of foreign languages may benefit greatly from the use of m-learning technology. M-learning provides new opportunities to follow the educational material, overcoming many restrictions about the time and place in which the learners can access them. However, due to the special characteristics of the devices used in this learning modality, it is necessary to follow different design recommendations for guaranteeing the usability of the material, and for increasing the effectiveness of the provided resources. In this document we have described the most important guidelines that have been followed in order to produce a set of courses whose aim is to assists English language students when developing their reading, listening and grammar skills. The next step will be to carry out an evaluation in order to estimate the users' satisfaction on the usability of the system and on the effectiveness of the final product.

Acknowledgement

This work is part of the MW-TELL project funded by European Commission under the Leonardo da Vinci (LdV) Sectoral Programme of the Lifelong Learning Programme. Contract No: 2008-1-GR1-LEO05-00693.

References

1. Chen, Y.S., Kao, T.C., Sheu, J.P.: A mobile learning system, for scaffolding bird watching learning. Journal of Computer Assisted Learning 19, 347–359 (2003)
2. Goodison, T.A.: The implementation of m-learning in UK higher education. In: Proceedings of ED-MEDIA 2001, pp. 613–618. AACE Press, Tampere (25-30, 2001)

3. Gay, G., Stefanone, M., Grace-Martin, M., Hembrooke, H.: The effects of wireless computing in collaborative learning environments. International Journal of Human-Computer Interaction 13(2), 257–276 (2001)
4. Mobile and Wireless Technologies for Technology-Enhanced Language Learning, http://www.mobile2learn.eu/index.php
5. Chen, C.-M., Chung, C.J.: Personalized mobile English vocabulary learning system based on item response theory and learning memory cycle. Computers & Education 51, 624–645 (2008)
6. Chen, C.-M., Hsu, S.-H.: Personalized Intelligent Mobile Learning System for Supporting Effective English Learning. Educational Technology & Society 11(3), 153–180 (2008)
7. Lan, Y.-J., Sung, Y.-T., Chang, K.-E.: Mobile-device-supported peer-assisted learning system for collaborative early EFL reading. Language Learning & Technology 11(3), 130–151 (2007)
8. Uther, M., Zipitria, I., Singh, P., Uther, J.: Mobile Adaptive CALL (MAC): a case-study in developing a mobile learning application for speech/audio language training. In: Proceedings of the Third International Workshop on Wireless and Mobile & Technologies in Education (WMTE 2005), pp. 187–191. IEEE Computer Society, Los Alamitos (2005)
9. Yang, J.C., Lai, C.H., Chu, Y.M.: Integrating speech technologies into a one-on-one digital English classroom. In: Proceedings of the 2005 IEEE International Workshop on Wireless and Mobile Technologies in Education (WMTE 2005), pp. 159–163. IEEE Computer Society, Los Alamitos (2005)
10. Kim, H., Kim, J., Lee, Y., Chae, M., Choi, Y.: An Empirical Study of the Use Contexts and Usability Problems in Mobile Internet. In: Proceedings of the 35th Hawaii International Conference on System Sciences (2002)
11. Mobile Web Best Practices 1.0, http://www.w3.org/TR/2006/WD-mobile-bp-20060412/#bpgroupnavlinks
12. Gong, J., Tarasewich, P.: Guidelines for Handheld Mobile Device Interface Design. In: Proc. of Decision Sciences Institute Annual Meeting (2004)
13. Shneiderman, B.: Designing the User Interface: Strategies for Effective Human-Computer Interaction. Addison-Wesley Longman Publishing Co., Inc., Amsterdam (1997)
14. Churchill, D., Hedberg, J.: Learning object design considerations for small-screen handheld devices. Computers & Education 50, 881–893 (2008)
15. Polsani, P.R.: Use and abuse of reusable learning objects. Journal of Digital Information 3(4), Article No. 164 (2003)
16. Smith, R.S.: Guidelines for Authors of Learning Objects. NMC: The New Media Consortium, http://www.nmc.org/publications/learning-object-guidelines (retrieved May 1, 2010)
17. ISO/IEC, 9241-11: Ergonomic Requirements for OfficeWork with Visual Display Terminals (VDT)s – Part 11 Guidance on Usability. 1998: ISO/IEC 9241-11: 1998 (E)
18. Nielsen, J.: Usability Engineering. Morgan Kaufman Publishers, Academic Press (1993)

Enhancing the Learning Experience: Preliminary Framework for User Individual Differences

Andrina Granić and Jelena Nakić

Faculty of Science, University of Split, Nikole Tesle 12, 21000 Split, Croatia
{andrina.granic,jelena.nakic}@pmfst.hr

Abstract. A system able to adapt to different user characteristics may increase user's learning outcome and advance her/his personal learning experience. This paper reports on research identifying and appraising user personal differences employed in user modelling for adaptive educational systems. A preliminary set of individual characteristics relevant for adaptation is proposed, along with a framework for their categorization. The framework is derived on the basis of empirical studies and survey papers reviewing the usage of these variables in adaptive and adaptable systems. Each variable is addressed from the perspective of its definition, implementation in existing systems and relevance for adaptation. Methods for variable detection and quantification are discussed as well. Suggested framework represents authors' perspective of the state-of-the-art in analyzing user individual differences and adds to the body of knowledge related to the user analysis as an essential part of an adaptive system development process.

Keywords: User experience; user individual differences, user modelling, web-based learning.

1 Introduction

Current research acknowledges that understanding users and diversity in their backgrounds, skills, goals and needs is at the core of successful design of information society technologies (IST) products and services. Furthermore, the need for accessible and usable learning in knowledge society for all promotes e-learning that engages users effectively. From this perspective, the role of transparent system interface and intuitive interaction tailored to unique personal requirements is crucial. Regarding the design of effective e-learning systems, the interface adjusted to individual differences of each particular user/learner should be able to advance users' personal learning experience and consequently increase their learning achievements. In such a context, it is crucial to conduct research that embraces and relies on innovations in user sensitive design. The influence of user goals, knowledge, preferences, styles and experience on her/his interaction with a system is unquestionable and studies have already empirically proved that system intelligent behaviour relies on individual differences e.g. [4, 6, 14, 36]. However, adaptive systems development is the process that includes comprehensive research, in relation to the application domain of a particular

G. Leitner, M. Hitz, and A. Holzinger (Eds.): USAB 2010, LNCS 6389, pp. 384–399, 2010.
© Springer-Verlag Berlin Heidelberg 2010

system. Designing intelligent interaction needs to take into account several research questions: how to identify user characteristics relevant for the application domain, how to model the user, what parts of the adaptive system shall change and in what way and finally how to employ user model to implement adaptivity, cf. [4, 40]. Research presented in the following addresses the first issue in the context of the web-based learning design.

The goal of this paper is to summarize and report on a survey on user individual differences that aid in the development of successful e-learning applications able to increase users' learning outcomes and advance their personal learning experience. Based on empirical studies and surveys on existing adaptive systems we have constructed a preliminary framework for categorization of user individual characteristics employed as sources for adaptation in adaptive educational systems (AESs).

Each adaptive application has certain specific features and specific target user groups, so there is no unique "set" of user model variables appropriate for all AES's. Having that in mind, the recommended framework could be considered as an authors' perspective of the state-of-the-art in analyzing user individual characteristics and intends to serve as a basis for user analysis as a starting point of any adaptive system design. User analysis in a learning context encompasses identification and acquisition of relevant user's information. Specifically, it enables the recognition of the individual user features that are the most important for the enhancement of user experience, the increase of learning achievements (as an objective measurable effect), along with the improvement of satisfaction in system usage.

The paper is structured as follows. Section 2 offers a brief review of studies of individual differences from a historical perspective. Section 3 describes related work and presents a framework for user individual characteristics as sources for adaptation. Section 4 summarizes and discusses the suggested framework, while the final section concludes the paper.

2   Brief Historical Background on User Individual Differences

The initial comprehensive overview of individual differences in the HCI field is Egan's [15] report on diversities between users in completing common computing tasks such as programming, text editing and information search. He pointed out that the ambition of adaptivity is that not only "everyone should be computer literate" but also that "computers should be user literate", suggesting that user differences could be understood and predicted as well as being modified through the system design. Since then, the diffusion of technology brought computers to the wide user population with extensive variety of knowledge, experience and skill dimensions in different areas. Accordingly, identification of individual differences relevant for a system adaptation became a critical issue. In their early consideration of adaptivity, Browne, Norman and Riches [3] provided one of the first classifications of candidate dimensions of user differences that may impact computer usage. They included diversities in cognitive styles (field dependence/independence, impulsivity/reflectivity, operation learning/comprehension learning), personality factors, psycho-motor skills, experience, goals and requirements, expectations, preferences, cognitive strategies and a number of cognitive abilities. Later on, Dillon and Watson [14] reviewed a century of individual differences work in psychology stressing the role of differential psychology in the HCI field. They have identified a number of basic cognitive abilities that have reliably influenced the performance of specific tasks in predictable ways. Based on their own analyses, they concluded that measures of ability can account for approximately 25% of variance in performance, thus being suitable for usage in decision making for most systems, especially in addition to other sources of information (previous work experience, education, domain knowledge, etc.). According to their recommendations, psychological measures of individual differences should be used to increase possibilities for a generalization of HCI findings. There is a number of studies confirming these pioneer work suggestions, showing for example that cognitive abilities, such as spatial and verbal ability, do affect the interaction, particularly the navigation performance of the user [2, 10, 33, 49, 61].

The influence of user goals, knowledge, preferences and experience on her/his interaction with an intelligent system is unquestionable [4]. Moreover, these characteristics have been successfully employed in many adaptive systems, for example AHA! [12], InterBook [5], KBS Hyperbook [29], INSPIRE [41], AVANTI [51], PALIO [52].

On the other hand, the matter of adaptation to cognitive styles and learning styles has been mainly ignored or marginally addressed until a last decade. Nevertheless, latest research confirms that navigation preferences of users reflect their cognitive styles in several dimensions: field dependent vs. independent, as defined by Witkin, Moore, Gooddenough and Cox [60], holist vs. serialist [42], verbalizer vs. imaginer [46]. In a related study, Chen and Macredie [9] found that field dependent learners prefer guided navigation, while field independent favour navigation freedom. Graff [26] also showed that individuals identified as having verbaliser and imager cognitive styles apply different browsing strategies.

In the educational area, many authors have concluded that adaptation to learning styles, as defined, for example, by Kolb [35] or Honey and Mumford [30], could bring potential benefits to students' learning activities. This is evident from an increasing number of AES's having implemented some kind of adaptation (adaptability or adaptivity) to learning styles, see for example CS388 [8] or INSPIRE [41].

Evidently, the effect of user individual differences on her/his performance has been the topic of a very fruitful research for the last few decades. However, the obtained results are not quite consistent, partially because the user performance while using a particular system depends greatly on the system itself [3]. In addition, the research on cognitive styles and learning styles in the HCI field is emerging. There is yet no strong evidence of their relevance concerning user's interaction with an intelligent system, as also discussed in [50]. Furthermore, even if these user styles were proved to be relevant, the question of potential benefits from personalized interaction still remains. System adaptation, even when well designed, does not necessarily imply user's performance improvement *cf.* [9]. Moreover, it can be disadvantageous to some classes of users [11]. From this rationale, it is worthwhile to consider possible alternatives before deciding to include adaptation into a system. An enlargement of learner's experience to overcome her/his low spatial ability [1] or an appropriate redesign of a non-adaptive interface [31] could be considered as alternatives.

Based on these reflections, we have conducted an empirical user analysis regarding a web-based learning application [38]. User individual characteristics concerned as predictor variables included age, personality factors, cognitive abilities, experience, background knowledge, motivation and expectations from e-learning. The study revealed that the students' intelligence, in terms of the Spearmans' "g" factor [53], hyperspace experience and motivation has a statistically significant correlation with learning outcomes acquired in e-learning environment. Obtained results are in line with general expectations, but now have been empirically proven, adding to the body of knowledge on user individual differences.

3   Preliminary Framework for User Individual Differences

There is a large amount of related work summarizing the influence of user individual differences on user's interaction with an adaptive system. A majority of such papers have listed adaptive systems with their user model variables, detection mechanisms and adaptation techniques applied, e.g. [47]. However, there is a significantly lower number of papers attempting to summarize all the variables employed as user model attributes in existing systems. One can easily find reviews of adaptive systems accommodating one user individual characteristic, for example cognitive styles [9] or learning styles [41, 23], but there is a lack of papers offering a systematization of variables used as sources for adaptation in existing adaptive systems.

Focusing on variables instead on systems, Triantafillou and Georgiadou [55] examined variables that can initiate adaptation and discussed their potential use in a hypothetical student model for computerized adaptive testing. Their list of "adaptive variables" emerged from five survey articles. On the contrary, Thalmann [54] concluded his own list of "adaptation criteria" based on structured content analysis of 30 existing adaptive hypermedia systems. His review provided suggestions for the preparation of a learning material with respect to the identified adaptation criteria, even though it did not consider any cognitive abilities or cognitive styles. Grimley and Riding [28] concluded that cognitive style, gender, working memory, prior knowledge and anxiety have significant impact on web-based learning. They have described those concepts, placed them within the context of learning and proposed the ways of adapting the learning environment to each individual user. Still more applicable suggestions for user model construction and maintenance could be found in [7]. This review represents user models of adaptive web-based systems from three aspects: what is being modelled, how it is modelled, and how the models are maintained.

Regarding user models of existing adaptive systems, in this paper a preliminary framework is established for user individual characteristics that are, or could be employed as sources for adaptation in e-learning systems. The classification is derived from the review of empirical studies and survey papers on existing AES's, acknowledging the relevance of those variables for system adaptation. Identified characteristics are classified in three broad categories:

ii)   *personal user characteristics*: age, gender, cognitive abilities, personality, cognitive style and learning style;

iii)   *previously acquired knowledge and skills*: experience, psycho-motor skills and background knowledge;

iiii)   *system related user characteristics*: goals, requirements, preferences, interaction styles, motivation and expectations.

Following subsections describe each one of the identified characteristics in detail. For each recognized variable three significant aspects are addressed – its definition, implementation in existing systems and evaluation of its relevance for adaptation. Additionally, methods used for detection and quantification of described characteristics are also reported. The framework is briefly summarized in Table 1, subsequent to the descriptions of the identified variables.

3.1 Personal User Characteristics

This category comprises general user information, such as age and gender, along with user individual traits. Concerning diversities in *age*, the more heterogeneous the user population is, the influence of age on user performance is greater. Age, experience and background knowledge are certainly not independent variables. Their influence on success of user interaction is naturally overlapping to some extent. Still, age is often a good predictor of user performance for individuals who are novices in using complex systems [15]. In addition to that, Ford and Chen [20] found differences in navigation behaviour of students using a hypermedia learning system, related to their age. In the same study they have obtained a statistically significant correlation of *gender* with the number of requests for guidance. Female students asked for less guidance, they have displayed a relatively extrinsic motivation for attending the learning session and have successfully completed a greater number of tasks compared to males. *Individual traits* are user features that define a user as an individual: cognitive abilities, personality, cognitive styles and learning styles. These features are very steady over time and they are usually assessed by reliable psychometric tests, under the supervision of a psychologist conducting the tests and interpreting the results. The research on individual traits and their use for adaptation is emerging, especially on the use of cognitive and learning styles. Progress is also evident in examining new methods for detection and quantification of individual traits during the interaction.

Cognitive abilities. Among many classifications of cognitive abilities [14], there are several characteristics which seem to be relevant for HCI: general intelligence, spatial, verbal and visual ability, reasoning aptitudes, perceptual speed, working memory capacity and others. The impact of these characteristics on users' interaction was confirmed in numerous studies, both early and recent [2, 15, 25, 39].

Spatial ability is the ability to perceive spatial patterns, or to maintain orientation with respect to objects in space [16]. HCI research often uses this term to annotate the ability of mental manipulation of 2-dimensional and 3-dimensional figures, and sometimes to annotate the ability of memorizing spatial arrangement of objects, e.g. [3]. However, among all cognitive abilities, spatial ability is the most cited as a good predictor of user performance, especially considering navigation [2, 10, 33, 49, 61]. Spatial ability is traditionally assessed by psychometric tests; yet another approach to dynamic detection of spatial aptitudes could be found in AKBB [27].

Compared to spatial ability, a significantly smaller part of literature deals with other cognitive abilities. Norcio and Stanley [39] reported few studies that have found the influence of *reasoning aptitudes* and *verbal ability* on computer usage. Dillon and

Watson [14] quoted several studies that examined the influence of user's *perceptual speed*, logical reasoning and *visual ability*. They reported differences in user performance related to logical reasoning and visual ability and confirmed that these user differences could be reduced by appropriate training and/or interface design. More recent work acknowledges the effect of *working memory capacity* on educational achievement in terms of problem solving, reasoning and reading comprehension [28], but possibilities for adaptation of e-learning systems to models of learning concerning working memory are still in an exploratory phase.

Personality. According to Eysenck [17] two main personality factors are *extraversion vs. introversion* and *neuroticism vs. emotional stability*. The extraverts tend to be more physically and verbally active whereas the introverts are independent, reserved and steady. The person in the middle of the dimension likes a mix between social situations and solitude. Neuroticism is the tendency to experience negative emotions or nervousness. On the other hand, emotional stability is related to calm, stable and relaxed persons. Personality concerns characteristics which remain stable over time and across situations, often considered as part of user individual traits that generally reflects on the way she/he uses a computer system [3, 4, 47]. In particular, Richter and Salvendy [45] compared the performance of extraverts and introverts using system interfaces with personality attributes added. Their results showed that the interface designed with introverts' personality attributes generally results in the fastest performance for both extraverts and introverts.

Cognitive styles. This is a relatively stable category of user individual differences related to information processing patterns in general context. Among various dimensions of cognitive styles, *field dependence/independence* (FD/FI) is probably the most exploited in adaptive systems, especially in the educational domain. According to Witkin, Moore, Gooddenough and Cox [60], FI individuals follow an analytical approach and study one topic in detail before reading the other. Conversely, FD users see the global picture first and concentrate on the details afterwards. FI users tend to develop self-defined goals and reinforcements, while FD individuals require externally defined goals and reinforcements.

   In related research, Pask [42] studied global/analytic differences concerning learning of complex academic subject matters and identified *holist vs. serialist* approach to learning. Holist individuals process information in relatively global ways, similar to FD users, whereas serialist individuals use relatively analytic approach, similar to FI users. Moreover, Ford and Chen [20] found statistically significant correlations between these cognitive style dimensions. According to the scores of psychological tests, Pask's holistic cognitive style is connected with FD style, while serialist cognitive style is connected with FI style. This result suggests that the holist and FD learner use similar learning strategies, as do the serialist and FI learner.

   User differences in cognitive styles result in different learning strategies in virtual learning environments. Chen and Macredie [9] found that FD learners use guidance through instructional content, while FI learners prefer to create their own path of learning topics. In the same study, they have empirically confirmed that FI learners explore each topic in depth before reading another topic. On the other hand, FD learners first run through the whole content of the course and then concentrate on a single topic. User differences in cognitive styles have been successfully applied in implementation of different strategies for instructional design in several AESs, e.g. [20, 50]. On the basis of different learning behaviour displayed by FI and FD learners [9], De Bra, Smits and Stash [13] speculate that at least field dependent learners should benefit from providing an introductory page on each major topic that would be offered before presenting the whole material on the topic. They also recommend two different ways of designing such introductory pages.

Another commonly exploited dimension of cognitive styles is *verbaliser/imager* [46]. Verbalisers usually prefer textual modes of presentation while imagers prefer non-textual modes (for example pictorial and diagrammatic information), especially while illustrating, or elaborating on initial textual information. This dimension of cognitive styles has been shown to affect browsing strategies [26] and learning preferences [48]. It is implemented, e.g. in AHA! [50] using the conditional inclusion of objects, but without enforcing the use of certain media types.

Graff [26] showed that imagers tend to see their environment as a whole in a complex hypermedia architecture. However, measurement of the depth of browsing did not show differences between verbalisers and imagers. Comparing this result with findings of Ford and Chen [20], it appears that imagers do not display exactly the same strategies as holists and field dependent learners in their tendency to see the overall structure of the learning content. This is just another empirical confirmation for the rationale that various dimensions of learner cognitive styles produce different learning strategies and that they should be considered as different variables in development of AES's.

Learning styles. In HCI literature, newer research emerged on a variety of learning style models and categorizations, e.g. [23, 40]. Here, we consider learning styles strictly as user preferred strategies of learning, contrary to some authors who consider cognitive styles displayed in the learning process as learning styles.

On the basis of Kolb's theory of experiential learning [35], Honey and Mumford [30] classify learners into four types: *activists, pragmatists, reflectors* and *theorists*. This learning style model is commonly implemented in existing AES's, for example INSPIRE [41]. Implementations of Felder–Silverman learning style model [18] can also be frequently found in adaptive systems, e.g. CS388 [8] and SAVER [22]. This model characterizes each learner according to four dimensions: *active/reflective, sensing/intuitive, visual/verbal* and *sequential/global* learner.

A number of researchers have reported improved learning performance of students whose learning styles matched the presentation mode. Ford and Chen [21] have found a significant difference in performance on conceptual knowledge for students learning in matched and mismatched conditions. Learning performance in matched conditions was significantly higher than the one in mismatched conditions.

The common method for obtaining learning styles from the user is using some kind of questionnaire. There are specific questionnaires for each one of the learning style models, for example, Kolb's Learning Style Inventory [34]. Although this method enables a very reliable diagnosis of learning styles, filling out a questionnaire is usually boring and time-consuming for students. Researchers continuously seek for methods to infer student's learning style from her/his interaction with a system. One approach is using Bayesian networks, as implemented in SAVER [22] for detection of the Felder–Silverman learning style model. Graf and Kinshuk [24] proposed another approach, applicable to learning management systems in general instead to a single e-learning system. They have designed general patterns indicating user preferences for a learning style dimension and calculated the level of those dimensions on the basis of the patterns values.

Explicit detection of user learning styles is a quite difficult process, either for user to fill out the questionnaire, or for AES developers to design and implement dynamic detection of learning styles from user interaction. In order to simplify the learning styles identification process and to develop a more reliable user model, Graf, Lin and Kinshuk [25] investigated relationships between learning styles and cognitive abilities. They have identified connections between learning styles in the Felder-Silverman learning style model and the working memory capacity as an example of cognitive abilities. The learners with a low working memory capacity display an active, sensing, visual and global learning style, while the learners with a high working memory capacity tend to be reflective, intuitive and sequential. These results show that the identification process of both learning styles and cognitive abilities can be supported by each other, thus contributing to the user modelling process.

3.2 Previously Acquired Knowledge and Skills

The second broad category of user characteristics encompasses prior experience in using computers and Internet, previously acquired psycho-motor skills and background knowledge.

Experience. It is generally understood that prior experience in using computers is a good predictor of user performance [2, 3, 39]. Since the diffusion of Internet and growing number of systems delivered as web-based applications, the same claim stands for the experience in using hyperspace, as confirmed in [4, 20]. The experience in the usage of a concrete system is not included since it cannot be perceived as a previously acquired skill.

Psycho-motor skills. Early research suggested the importance of certain psycho-motor abilities, e.g. using the keyboard when using complex computer systems [3]. This is not so evident in recent research, probably due to the fact that the participants of most empirical studies are recruited from student population already familiar with computers. However, considering general population as potential target users of e-learning systems, this user characteristic becomes again an important variable that could influence the interaction. In addition to that, HCI research specifically considers users with limited psycho-motor skills such as disabled and elderly people. An example of information retrieval system adapted to these groups of users is AVANTI [19].

Background knowledge. This category is considered as two-sided. First, it refers to the user's knowledge related to the subject matter that is acquired prior to AES usage. Previously acquired knowledge is often functionally different from the knowledge to be attained in interaction with the system. Second, background knowledge encompasses prior experience in fundamental skills related to the subject, but acquired in a different context. For example, if user objective is a creation of a HTML page, then her/his HTML experience is considered as background knowledge. The relevance of background knowledge for adaptation is very well recognized in the HCI research and this variable is often implemented in AES's, *cf.* [7].

3.3 System Related User Characteristics

Goals and requirements. User goals and requirements (considered as short-term goals) are one of the main variables directing the adaptation in many adaptive and adaptable systems. In instructional systems, user goals usually depend on teaching strategies (and sometimes are even set by the system), so the techniques for adaptation to learning goals are various, see for example ELM-ART [56] for problem solving support, KBS Hyperbook [29] for project-based learning and INSPIRE [41] for a goal-driven approach.

Preferences. In general, every user has individual preferences related to the style of displaying information on screen. A user may prefer larger fonts, link annotation in different colours, coloured background, less information on the page, etc. However, user preferred styles of presentation modes are limited by the facilities of the system interface, so they can be considered as system dependent variables to some extent. User preferences are extremely hard to deduce by the system, so in most cases the user provides that information to the system, directly or indirectly. The preferences provided by the user are often a very reliable part of the user model [31]. Still, this is a changeable variable, which complicates the process of user modelling. Probably the most successful way of modelling preferences is enabling user customization of her/his user model, the way it is done in AHA! [12] or ELM-ART [56].

Interaction styles. Interaction styles in existing systems include menus, command entries, questions and answers dialogues, form-fills and spreadsheets, natural language dialogue and direct manipulation [44]. Each user may individually prefer a certain interaction style, but it is a general opinion that menus are more useful for novices than commands, because users do not have to remember much information. Conversely, commands are usually quicker and are preferred by experienced users [*ibid*]. Adaptation to user interaction styles is implemented for example in AKBB [27].

Motivation. The role of motivation in the learning process is generally acknowledged in educational psychology. Students with higher levels of intrinsic motivation and self-efficacy achieve better learning outcomes [43]. In a traditional classroom the teacher knows how to perceive the level of students' motivation, how to adapt his teaching strategies to the students' current motivational state and sometimes even how to increase their motivation for learning. However, in computer-assisted learning, the possibilities of exploiting motivation to improve learning performance are mainly neglected [58]. Recent studies make certain progress in this area. Specifically, Hurley and Weibelzahl [32] have developed a recommender tool, named MotSaRT, which suggests intervention strategies for teachers to increase student's motivation.

Intrinsic motivation is a rather personal user feature, mostly reflecting the user's desire and willingness to make an effort towards a specified goal. Still, it is very natural to consider motivation as a system dependent feature, for two reasons. First, to some extent the level of user motivation is dependent on the goal, and the goal is commonly defined by the system. Second, the means and manners of presenting the learning material can greatly affect user motivation. Thus, regarding the features of the system that form motivation (e.g. making the system visually attractive, well structured, highly usable and effective) designers can make significant progress in increasing the level of user motivation.

Expectations. User's previous interactions with the same or similar system often create expectations of system usage. If a user was satisfied in previous interactions, she/he will probably have positive attitude towards the system and expect a pleasant and beneficial session. A recent study showed that learners with greater expectations of e-learning have experienced higher levels of fulfilment in using e-learning systems, although they did not achieve higher learning outcomes [38]. Older reports confirming the influence of users' expectations on usage of interactive systems could be found in [3].

4 Framework Summary and Discussion

Summarizing the previous section, Table 1 gives a brief overview on the user individual characteristics exploited as user model variables of various adaptive and adaptable systems. The table is derived from eight survey papers and provides a comparison of researchers' acknowledgments of each particular variable as a source for adaptation.

The framework proposed in this paper and synthesized in the table has certain limitations regarding the first intention of this study, which was to consider only evaluated AES's, that is, precisely the studies that have confirmed adaptation success. However, studies on the evaluation of adaptive and adaptable systems are rarely conducted, unfortunately keeping track with the lack of empirical studies in the HCI field in general, cf. [11, 57]. Additionally, methods and approaches for evaluation of adaptive systems are still explored and not yet strongly established [59]. Consequently, the table also quotes a number of survey papers where an empirical confirmation of the influence of identified variables on learning process in non-adaptive learning systems is offered. It can be assumed that adaptation of the system to those user characteristics that significantly correlate with learning outcomes acquired in non-adaptive learning systems could bring substantial benefits to students' learning performance. Such variables could be then considered as relevant for adaptation.

A number of user individual characteristics seem to have been validly and reliably identified in the HCI literature, but the terminology used (the features names) and their precise relationships to each other is not always clear. That was the most significant practical difficulty that we faced in the attempt to suggest a set of relevant user characteristics. For example, identification of cognitive and learning styles from case studies was challenging due to interchangeable usage of these terms. Accordingly, in this paper cognitive styles are considered as information processing strategies in general, while term learning styles refer only to the user preferred learning strategies, as described in the previous section. Similar reasoning is applied when considering spatial ability. We have chosen to explain various dimensions of spatial ability instead of using different terms for different dimensions.

Table 1. User individual characteristics potentially relevant for adaptation

		Egan, 1988	Norcio & Stanley, 1989	Browne et al., 1990.	Dillon & Watson, 1996	Brusilovsky, 2001	Rothrock et al., 2002	Brusilovsky & Milan, 2007	Grimley & Riding, 2009
Personal characteristics and preferences	Age			•					
	Gender	•							•
	Cognitive abilities	•	•	•	•				•
	Personality			•			•		
	Cognitive style		•	•			•	•	•
	Learning style					•		•	
Previously acquired knowledge and abilities	Experience	•	•	•			•	•	
	Psycho-motor skills			•	•		•		
	Background knowledge	•	•				•		•	•
System related user characteristics	Goals and requirements			•		•	•	•	
	Preferences		•	•			•		
	Interaction styles		•						
	Motivation			•					
	Expectations			•					

It is important to take into account that some variables, although clearly identified, do not affect user interaction independently (e.g. age, experience and background knowledge) and they should be considered regarding their natural overlap with each other. Recent research suggests that relationships among variables in some cases could be exploited for simplifying user modelling process, e.g. the relationship between learning and styles and cognitive abilities [25, 28].

Relevant user individual characteristics, even when clearly identified and properly evaluated, certainly do not represent the sufficient set of variables to guarantee adaptation success. Some research emphasizes that user environment plays an important role in user interaction e.g. [4]. *Environment data* comprise all aspects of the user environment that do not directly translate to user characteristics, but may have an impact on user's goals and resources. A number of systems (for various purposes) are able to adapt to environment data (*ibid.*). It is also recognized that the adaptation to *groups of users* and to *user situation specificity* [47] is important. More recently, growing research on mobile and ubiquitous computing has expanded the notions of user environment and user situation specificity and has recognized the need of adapting to a broader *context of user's work*, including user platform, location, environment and a number of human dimensions [7].

Concerning all variables suggested in the framework, in addition to the ones mentioned above, the most often used trigger for adaptation is the user progress in system usage. In adaptive educational systems, *knowledge* is the best indicator of user status and commonly used variable to initiate adaptation, e.g. in ELM-ART [56], KBS Hyperbook [29], Interbook [5] and AHA! [50].

Many researchers disagree on the importance of modelling of some of user individual characteristics and about their usage for adaptation purposes, as shown in Table 1. Sometimes even the same authors over the years have recommended different set of user model attributes (compare [4] with [7]). Although Brusilovsky's six-category classification [*ibid*] is clear and applicable, the framework offered in this paper reflects human features which are classified into three broad "user-related" categories and then fine-grained into particular features which are appropriate as attributes for user model. Nevertheless, the framework is just a preliminary result of a comprehensive ongoing research. The field is emerging, thus it may be possible to include new user features over time. That is, research concerning affective state of the learner and its influence on interaction is innovative and promising (several approaches can be found in [37]).

The proposed framework represents the authors' perspective of the state-of-the-art in analyzing individual differences, and intends to serve as a staring point for AES's design/research teams. Respecting the fact that user performance considerably depends on a particular system, designers are encouraged to conduct their own user analysis concerning the system being developed, searching for the appropriate set of user model variables that will lead to the adaptation success. It is important to have an open mind in searching for user characteristics relevant for a particular system *cf.* [31], also taking into account the target users group. A subset of variables hypothetically relevant for a particular system and target user group could be selected and implemented. However, evaluation of system adaptation to these variables should follow the implementation to ensure that the adaptive system advances users' interactions. Initially selected set of hypothetical sources for adaptation can be refined through formative evaluation in any stage of the developing process. In addition, it is important not to consider each variable separately, but to find a combination of characteristics that would ensure a major benefit. The cost ratio issues of the adaptation should not be ignored. In that context, a preliminary assessment of the potentially relevant variables enabled by this survey can contribute in disregarding unnecessary variables and consequently decrease efforts and expenses of the developed system.

5   Conclusion and Future Work

This paper presents a survey on user individual differences employed in user modelling of adaptive learning systems. The set of user individual characteristics employed as sources for adaptation of e-learning systems was established and the framework for their categorisation is suggested. The identified characteristics are classified into three broad categories: personal user characteristics, previously acquired knowledge and skills as well as system related user characteristics. For each recognized variable, three significant aspects are addressed – its definition, implementation in existing systems and evaluation of its relevance for adaptation – whether in adaptive (where available), or non-adaptive learning systems. In addition, methods used for detection of described characteristics are reported and discussed.

Depending on the nature of the system being developed and the target user groups, this categorisation may be considered as an initial set of possible variables that can be embraced as candidate sources for adaptation. Careful evaluation of system's adaptive behaviour should reveal the combination of characteristics that will cause the biggest impact on both learning performance and satisfaction in system usage.

This framework represents an initial attempt to construct a set of user individual characteristics significant for system adaptation. Further research is needed to investigate successful methods and approaches for implementation of adaptive or adaptable behaviour to the identified characteristics, following the motto "do not diagnose what you cannot treat" [31]. The future research will include an in-depth analysis of existing adaptive systems, focusing on evaluated systems that provide effective and efficient adaptations.

Acknowledgments. This work has been carried out within project 177-0361994-1998 Usability and Adaptivity of Interfaces for Intelligent Authoring Shells funded by the Ministry of Science and Technology of the Republic of Croatia.

References

1. Benyon, D., Höök, K.: Navigation in Information Spaces: Supporting the Individual. In: INTERACT 1997, pp. 39–46 (1997)
2. Benyon, D., Murray, D.: Developing Adaptive Systems to Fit Individual Aptitudes. In: Proceedings of the 1st International Conference on Intelligent User Interfaces, Orlando, Florida, USA, pp. 115–121 (1993)
3. Browne, D., Norman, M., Rithes, D.: Why Build Adaptive Systems? In: Browne, D., Totterdell, P., Norman, M. (eds.) Adaptive User Interfaces, pp. 15–59. Academic Press Inc., London (1990)
4. Brusilovsky, P.: Adaptive Hypermedia. User Modeling and User-Adapted Interaction 11, 87–110 (2001)
5. Brusilovsky, P., Eklund, J.: InterBook: an Adaptive Tutoring System. UniServe Science News 12 (1999)
6. Brusilovsky, P., Kobsa, A., Nejdl, W. (eds.): Adaptive Web 2007. LNCS, vol. 4321. Springer, Heidelberg (2007)
7. Brusilovsky, P., Milan, E.: User Models for Adaptive Hypermedia and Adaptive Educational Systems. In: Brusilovsky, P., Kobsa, A., Nejdl, W. (eds.) Adaptive Web 2007. LNCS, vol. 4321, pp. 3–53. Springer, Heidelberg (2007)
8. Carver, C.A., Howard, R.A., Lavelle, E.: Enhancing student learning by incorporating learning styles into adaptive hypermedia. In: Proc. of 1996 ED-MEDIA World Conf. on Educational Multimedia and Hypermedia, Boston, USA, pp. 118–123 (1996)

9. Chen, S., Macredie, R.: Cognitive styles and hypermedia navigation: development of a learning model. Journal of the American Society for Information Science and Technology 53(1), 3–15 (2002)
10. Chen, C., Czerwinski, M., Macredie, R.: Individual Differences in Virtual Enviroments – Introduction and overview. Journal of the American Society for Information Science 51(6), 499–507 (2000)
11. Chin, D.N.: Empirical Evaluation of User Models and User-Adapted Systems. User Modeling and User Adapted Interaction 11, 181–194 (2001)
12. De Bra, P., Calvi, L.: AHA! An open Adaptive Hypermedia Architecture. The New Review of Hypermedia and Multimedia 4, 115–139 (1998)
13. De Bra, P., Smits, D., Stash, N.: Creating and Delivering Adaptive Courses with AHA! In: Nejdl, W., Tochtermann, K. (eds.) EC-TEL 2006. LNCS, vol. 4227, pp. 21–33. Springer, Heidelberg (2006)
14. Dillon, A., Watson, C.: User Analysis in HCI – The Historical Lessons From Individual Differences Research. Int. Journal on Human-Computer Studies 45, 619–637 (1996)
15. Egan, D.: Individual Differences in Human-Computer Interaction. In: Helander, M. (ed.) Handbook of Human-Computer Interaction, pp. 543–568. Elsevier Science B.V. Publishers, North-Holland (1988)
16. Ekstrom, R., French, J., Harman, H., Dermen, D.: Manual for kit of factor referenced cognitive tests (1976)
17. Eysenck, H.J.: Four ways five factors are not basic. Personality and Individual Differences 13, 667–673 (1992)
18. Felder, R.M., Silverman, L.K.: Learning and Teaching Styles in Engineering Education. Engineering Education 78(7), 674–681 (1988)
19. Fink, J., Kobsa, A., Nill, A.: Adaptable and adaptive information provision for all users, including disabled and elderly people. The New Review of Hypermedia and Multimedia 4, 163–188 (1998)
20. Ford, N., Chen, S.Y.: Individual Differences, Hypermedia Navigation and Learning: An Empirical Study. Journal of Educational Multimedia and Hypermedia 9(4), 281–311 (2000)
21. Ford, N., Chen, S.Y.: Matching/mismatching revisited: an empirical study of learning and teaching styles. British Journal of Educational Technology 32(1) (2001)
22. Garcia, P., Amandi, A., Schiaffino, S., Campo, M.: Evaluating Bayesian Networks' Precision for Detecting Students' Learning Styles. Computers & Education 49, 794–808 (2006)
23. Graf, S.: Adaptivity in Learning Management Systems Focussing on Learning Styles. Ph.D. Thesis. Faculty of Informatics, Vienna University of Technology (2007)
24. Graf, S.: Kinshuk: An approach for detecting learning styles in learning management systems. In: Proceedings of the International Conference on Advanced Learning Technologies, Kerkrade, Netherlands, pp. 161–163 (2006)
25. Graf, S., Lin, T.: Kinshuk: The relationship between learning styles and cognitive traits – Getting additional information for improving student modelling. Computers in Human Behavior 24, 122–137 (2008)
26. Graff, M.G.: Individual differences in hypertext browsing strategies. Behaviour and Information Technology 24(2), 93–100 (2005)
27. Granić, A.: Foundation of Adaptive Interfaces for Computerized Educational Systems. Ph.D. Diss (in Croatian) University of Zagreb, Faculty of Electrical Engineering and Computing. Zagreb, Croatia (2002)

28. Grimley, M., Riding, R.: Individual Differences and Web-Based Learning. In: Mourlas, C., Tsianos, N., Germanakos, P. (eds.) Cognitive and Emotional Processes in Web-Based Education: Integrating Human Factors and Personalization, pp. 209–228. IGI Global, Hershey (2009)

29. Henze, N., Nejdl, W.: Adaptivity in the KBS Hyperbook System. In: 2nd Workshop on Adaptive Systems and User Modeling on the WWW, Toronto, Banff, Held in Conjunction with the World Wide Web (WWW8) and the International Conference on User Modeling (1999)

30. Honey, P., Mumford, A.: The Manual of Learning Styles, 3rd edn. Peter Honey, Maidenhead (1992)

31. Hook, K.: Steps to Take Before Intelligent User Interfaces Become Real. Journal of Interaction with Computers 12(4), 409–426 (2000)

32. Hurley, T., Weibelzahl, S.: Using MotSaRT to Support On-line Teachers in Student Motivation. In: Duval, E., Klamma, R., Wolpers, M. (eds.) EC-TEL 2007. LNCS, vol. 4753, pp. 101–111. Springer, Heidelberg (2007)

33. Juvina, I., van Oostendorp, H.: Individual Differences and Behavioral Metrics Involved in Modeling web Navigation. Universal Access in the Information Society 4(3), 258–269 (2006)

34. Kolb, D.: Learning Style Inventory, Self-Scoring Test and Interpretation booklet. McBer and Company, Boston (1976)

35. Kolb, D. A.: Experiential Learning: Experience as the Source of Learning and Development. Prentice-Hall, Englewood Cliffs (1984)

36. Magoulas, G.D., Chen, S.Y., Papanikolaou, K.A.: Integrating Layered and Heuristic Evaluation for Adaptive Learning Environments. In: Weibelzahl, S., Paramythis, A. (eds.) Proceedings of the Second Workshop on Empirical Evaluation of Adaptive Systems, held at the 9th International Conference on User Modeling UM 2003, Pittsburgh, pp. 5–14 (2003)

37. Mourlas, C., Tsianos, N., Germanakos, P.: Cognitive and Emotional Processes in Web-based Education: Integrating Human Factors and Personalization. Advances in Web-Based Learning Book Series. IGI Global (2009)

38. Nakić, J., Granić, A.: User Individual Differences in Intelligent Interaction: Do They Matter? LNCS, vol. 5615, pp. 694–703. Springer, Heidelberg (2009)

39. Norcio, A., Stanley, J.: Adaptive Human-Computer Interfaces: A Literature Survey and Perspective. IEEE Transactions on System, Man and Cybernetics 19(2), 399–408 (1989)

40. Papanikolaou, K.A., Grigoriadou, M.: Accommodating learning style characteristics in adaptive educational hypermedia systems. In: Individual Differences in Adaptive Hypermedia Workshop at the Third International Conference on Adaptive Hypermedia and Adaptive Web-based systems, AH 2004, Eindhoven, Netherlands (2004)

41. Papanikolaou, K.A., Grigoriadou, M., Kornilakis, H., Magoulas, G.D.: Personalising the Interaction in a Web-based Educational Hypermedia System: the case of INSPIRE. User-Modeling and User-Adapted Interaction 13(3), 213–267 (2003)

42. Pask, G.: Styles and Strategies of Learning. British Journal of Educational Psychology 46, 128–148 (1976)

43. Pintrich, P.R., De Groot, E.V.: Motivational and self-regulated learning components of classroom academic performance. Journal of Educational Psychology 82(1), 33–40 (1990)

44. Preece, J., Rogers, Y., Sharp, H., Benyon, D., Holland, S., Carey, T.: Human-Computer Interaction. Addison-Wesley, Harlow (1994)

45. Richter, L.A., Salvendy, G.: Effects of personality and task strength on performance in computerized tasks. Ergonomics 38(2), 281–291 (1995)

46. Riding, R.J., Buckle, C.F.: Learning styles and training performance. Training Agency, Sheffield (1990)
47. Rothrock, L., Koubek, R., Fuchs, F., Haas, M., Salvendy, G.: Review and reappraisal of adaptive interfaces: Toward biologically-inspired paradigms. Theoretical Issues in Ergonomic Science 3(1), 47–84 (2002)
48. Sadler-Smith, E., Riding, R.: Cognitive style and instructional preferences. Instructional Science 27, 355–371 (1999)
49. Stanney, K., Salvendy, G.: Information visualization: Assisting low spatial individuals with information access tasks through the use of visual mediators. Ergonomics 38(6), 1184–1198 (1995)
50. Stash, N., De Bra, P.: Incorporating Cognitive Styles in AHA! (The Adaptive Hypermedia Architecture). In: Proceedings of the IASTED International Conference Web-Based Education, pp. 378–383 (2004)
51. Stephanidis, C., Paramythis, A., Karagiannidis, C., Savidis, A.: Supporting Interface Adaptation: the AVANTI Web-Browser. In: 3rd ERCIM Workshop on User Interfaces for All (UI4ALL 1997), Strasbourg, France (1997)
52. Stephanidis, C., Paramythis, A., Zarikas, V., Savidis, A.: The PALIO Framework for Adaptive Information Services. In: Seffah, A., Javahery, H. (eds.) Multiple User Interfaces: Cross-Platform Applications and Context-Aware Interfaces, pp. 69–92. John Wiley & Sons, Ltd., Chichester (2004)
53. Sternberg, R.J.: Cognitive Psychology, Wadsworth, a division, 3rd edn. Thompson Learning, Inc. (2003)
54. Thalmann, S.: Adaptation Criteria for Preparing Learning Material for Adaptive Usage: Structured Content Analysis of Existing Systems. In: Holzinger, A. (ed.) USAB 2008. LNCS, vol. 5298, pp. 411–418. Springer, Heidelberg (2008)
55. Triantafillou, E., Georgiadou, E.: Applying adaptive variables in computerised adaptive testing. Australasian Journal of Educational Technology 23(3), 350–370 (2007)
56. Weber, G., Brusilovsky, P.: ELM-ART: An Adaptive Versatile System for Web-based Instruction. International Journal of Artificial Intelligence in Education 12, 351–384 (2001)
57. Weibelzahl, S.: Problems and pitfalls in the evaluation of adaptive systems. In: Chen, S., Magoulas, G. (eds.) Adaptable and Adaptive Hypermedia Systems, pp. 285–299. IRM Press, Hershey (2005)
58. Weibelzahl, S., Kelly, D.: Adaptation to Motivational States in Educational Systems. In: Proceedings of the Workshop Week Lernen - Wissensentdeckung - Adaptivität (LWA 2005), pp. 80–84. Saarland University, Saarbrücken (2005)
59. Weibelzahl, S., Masthoff, J., Paramythis, A., van Velsen, L. (eds.): Proceedings of the Sixth Workshop on User-Centred Design and Evaluation of Adaptive Systems, Held in Conjunction with the International Conference on User Modeling, Adaptation, and Personalization (UMAP 2009), Trento, Italy (2009)
60. Witkin, H., Moore, C., Gooddenough, D., Cox, P.: Field-dependent and field-independent cognitive styles and their educational implications. Review of Educational Research 47, 1–64 (1977)
61. Zhang, H., Salvendy, G.: The implication of visualization ability and structure preview design for web information search tasks. Int. J. of Human–Computer Interaction 13(1), 75–95 (2001)

Scene Segmentation in Artistic Archive Documentaries

Dalibor Mitrović, Stefan Hartlieb, Matthias Zeppelzauer, and Maia Zaharieva

Interactive Media Systems Group
Vienna University of Technology
Favoritenstrasse 9-11, Vienna, Austria
{mitrovic,hartlieb,zeppelzauer,zaharieva}@ims.tuwien.ac.at

Abstract. Scene segmentation is a crucial task in the structural analysis of film. State-of-the-art scene segmentation algorithms usually target fiction films (e.g. Hollywood films). Documentaries (especially artistic archive documentaries) follow different montage rules than fiction films and consequently require specialized approaches for scene segmentation. We propose a scene segmentation algorithm targeted at artistic archive documentaries. We evaluate the performance of our technique with archive documentaries and contemporary movies and obtain satisfactory results in both domains.

Keywords: Archive film material, documentaries, scene boundary detection.

1 Introduction

Films have a hierarchical structure that is the result of the editing process. On the lowest structural level there is the single *frame*. A number of continuously recorded frames form a *shot* and a sequence of shots belonging together a *scene*. The set of all scenes is the *film*. In modern fiction films, such as Hollywood films, scenes usually depict activities with the same dramatic incident or location [1]. This definition is not applicable to documentaries and especially not for artistic archive documentaries. In artistic archive documentaries, shots constituting a scene are related on a higher abstraction level. For example, in a fiction film, a scene may show two people driving in the car and talking to each other. All the shots depicting this conversation form the scene. In an artistic archive documentary, a scene consists of shots that e.g. show how electricity is brought to a village. These shots show someone installing a power line, peasants using an electrical thresher and several houses of the village with electrical lighting. All these shots are recorded at different locations and at differing times. Their cohesion is much lower than for the shots in the fiction film example. Due to the low cohesion of shots there is only little a priori knowledge (e.g. about composition

G. Leitner, M. Hitz, and A. Holzinger (Eds.): USAB 2010, LNCS 6389, pp. 400–410, 2010.

rules) that can be incorporated into the segmentation process. The most important clue for scene segmentation in documentaries is the repeated appearance of visually similar shots and motives. We aim at exploiting this clue by applying several *orthogonal* features for the detection of visual similarities in parallel and by merging their individual results. By this approach we attempt to compensate for the lack of a priori knowledge.

Existing techniques for scene segmentation are usually tailored to modern films. The techniques can be divided into three categories: graph-based approaches [5,9], model-based approaches [2,11], and merge-(and-split)-based approaches [4,8]. Yeung et al. propose a graph representation for video content where nodes represent the shots and edges represent the temporal flow of the story [9]. The graph is split into sub-graphs representing scenes based on temporal (time windows) and visual constraints (color and luminance similarity). In general, graph-based approaches are not applicable to scene detection in artistic archive documentaries since these films are mostly shot in an open and highly dynamic environment. Zhai et al. present a statistical method for the detection of video scenes. The method is based on the Markov Chain Monte Carlo technique and relies on model priors, visual constraints (color similarity), and temporal consistency [11]. Such model-based approaches work well for scenes where scene content can be represented by a parametric probabilistic model. The experimental nature of artistic archive documentaries does not allow for the definition of such generic models. Rasheed et al. propose a two-pass approach for scene boundary detection in Hollywood films and TV shows [4]. In the first stage, the authors perform shot clustering based on color similarity. In the next stage, over-segmented scenes are merged again based on shot lengths and motion content analysis in the scenes. Recently, Wang et al. proposed a method based on overlapping links for the detection of video scenes [8]. The authors perform an iterative backward and forward search for similar shots in a video. Shot similarity is defined as the combination of visual (color) similarity and consistent motion characteristics. Since artistic archive documentaries frequently have no color information and exhibit a large amount of shaking and flicker that reduces the reliability of motion features, scene segmentation in this context requires more robust content-based features. In this paper, we adapt the overlapping links method (which is independent of content-based features) for the segmentation of scenes in artistic archive documentaries.

2 Material

The material employed in this investigation are artistic documentaries produced in the Soviet Union in the 1920s and 1930s. In contrast to news- and sports broadcasts and fiction films, these documentaries do not contain any narrative structure. In fact the director Dziga Vertov strongly opposed any narration in the Hollywood sense. Consequently, the films share a collage-like style. Vertov relied on the viewer's mind to connect the depicted activities and locations. Scenes in the context of Vertov's films represent topics on an abstract level. For example one scene shows people and machines building a hydro-electric dam. The next scene shows the flooding of different villages to symbolize that villages are flooded with energy. Eventually, it is shown how the villages are electrified.

The original material is 35mm black-and-white silent film. We employ frame-by-frame digitized backup copies of the films, because the original films do not exist anymore. The films are digitized at PAL resolution. Unfortunately, the state of the material has degraded significantly, during storage, copying, and playback over the last decades. Numerous artifacts were introduced into the material (see Figure 1). The most common artifacts we have to deal with include scratches, introduced by dirt in the projectors during playback, dust, liquids, etc. copied into the images, visible framelines, and frame displacements introduced by shrinking[1] and copying under suboptimal conditions.

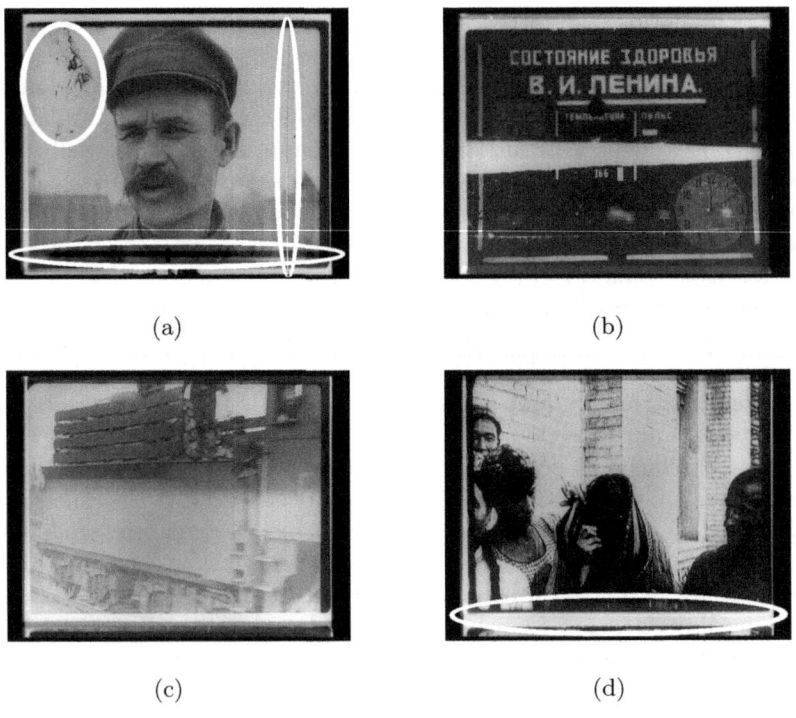

(a)   (b)

(c)   (d)

Fig. 1. Artifacts often found in archive film. Figure 1(a) shows a frame with several artifacts: dirt (top left), vertical scratch (right), frameline copied into the image (bottom). The frame in Figure 1(a) has a tear in the middle. Errors introduced during copying include unwanted changes in intensity and contrast as well as visible framelines depicted in Figures 1(c) and 1(d), respectively.

---

[1] Shrinking refers to the process of physical (horizontal and vertical) contraction of the filmstrip over time.

3 Method

We propose a merge-based approach which is optimized for artistic archive documentaries. Firstly, we employ local features to identify shots. Secondly, we extract different orthogonal features for the detection of visual similarities. Thirdly, we extend the *overlapping links method* of Wang et al. [8] (for the grouping of visually similar shots into scenes) to multiple features by adding a merging step. Finally, we introduce a postprocessing step that assigns shots that were not assigned to scenes in the previous steps.

3.1 Shot Boundary Detection

The employed shot boundary detection (SBD) technique consists of two stages. The first stage utilizes scale-invariant feature transform (SIFT) keypoints [3] to measure the similarity between two consecutive frames. We take the number of matched keypoints in two frames as an indicator for similarity. If the number of matching keypoints drops below a fixed threshold the technique recognizes a shot boundary. The results of this simple approach deteriorate in two cases, namely dissolves and sequences with fast motion. During dissolves (frames of the preceding shot are blended with frames of the following shot) the number of matching keypoints does not drop below the threshold and the shot boundary is missed. We observe that missed dissolves do not impede scene segmentation because dissolves usually do not coincide with scene boundaries in the material under consideration.

Fast motion causes difficulties for the SBD technique because fast motion introduces significant differences in consecutive frames. The number of matching SIFT keypoints drops to zero and a shot boundary is detected. The false differences lead to over-segmentation and motivate a second stage of our SBD technique. The second stage heuristically corrects over-segmentation by combining shots that are below a reasonable length. Note that over-segmentation is not critical, because similar but falsely split shots are later merged during scene segmentation.

3.2 Scene Segmentation

Our scene segmentation technique relies on the results of the SBD to extract keyframes which are used for the similarity measurements. Each shot is represented by the first frame of the shot. After these keyframes have been selected, additional preprocessing is necessary. This preprocessing consists of image cropping in order to remove the frame borders that do not carry any important information, see Figure 2. For the selected film material the crop masks were determined manually for each film.

The next computational step is the extraction of visual content-based features. We employ three content-based features: block-based intensity histograms (BBH), the edge change ratio (ECR) and SIFT keypoints. For the BBH we divide the image into blocks and compute the intensity histogram for each block.

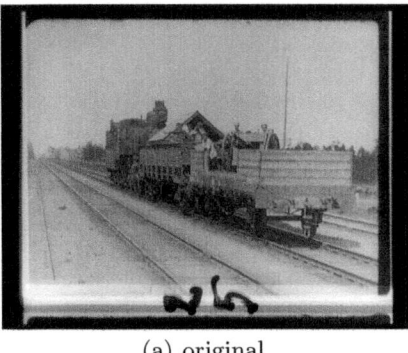
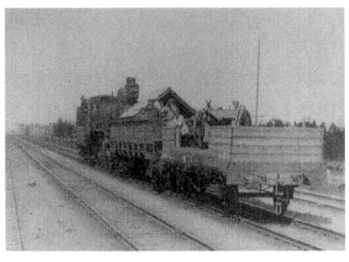

(a) original   (b) pre-processed

Fig. 2. A frame prior to (Figure 2(a)) and after (Figure 2(b)) preprocessing. Entirely black areas are cropped to facilitate similarity matching. Cropping further removes potentially misleading information like the horizontally handwritten numerics *2* and *5* at the bottom of Figure 2(a).

The edge change ratio (ECR) is an edge-based measure for the dissimilarity of images [10]. ECR is the ratio of appearing and disappearing edges in two (consecutive) frames. SIFT provides descriptions of salient points in the image. These three features represent orthogonal information, namely intensity, edges, and salient keypoints. Consequently, by combining the features we are able to capture a larger spectrum of visual similarities. Furthermore, the features have the potential to mutually compensate for weaknesses. For example in situations where keypoints can hardly be detected (e.g. in a shot that mainly shows homogeneous areas like sky), the intensity histograms may provide a more accurate description).

We compute the similarities between the shots using appropriate distance measures for the features. We can limit the similarity computation to a time window of several preceding and following shots without losing too much information. The similarity for the SIFT feature is expressed by the number of matching keypoints. If the number of matching keypoints of two frames exceeds the threshold T_{SIFT} we consider the frames as similar. We compare BBHs using the absolute sum of bin-wise differences and the number of matching blocks. We employ two thresholds $T_{BBH_{Bin}}$ for the bin-wise differences and $T_{BBH_{Block}}$ for the number of matching blocks. $T_{BBH_{Bin}}$ is used to decide whether two image blocks are similar and $T_{BBH_{Block}}$ is used to decide whether two frames are similar. The ECR is a feature which is always computed for two frames and therefore it is used directly as a measure for dissimilarity. If the ECR is lower than the threshold T_{ECR} the frames are considered to be similar.

These similarity computations yield three different similarity scores for each pair of shots. We use these scores separately for scene segmentation. The scene segmentation algorithm groups all shots that are similar and inside a specified time window into scenes. Additionally, shots that are between two similar shots

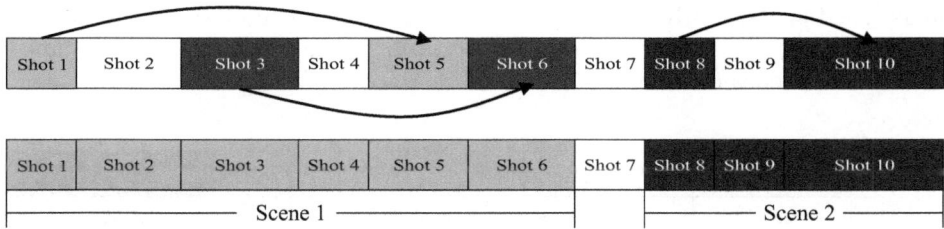

Fig. 3. The similarity computations show which shots belong together (indicated by the arrows and shading). Shots that have no similarities (Shot 9) but exist between matching shots are assigned to the scene defined by the surrounding matching shots (Shot 8 and Shot 10).

are assigned to the group of the surrounding similar shots. Figure 3 illustrates this process. At the end of the shot grouping we obtain three different scene segmentations (one for each content-based feature).

We merge these three segmentations using the set operation *union*. For an illustration see Figure 4. For example consider Shot 2-4 in the first and second row of Figure 4. Shot 3 and Shot 4 are part of one scene according to BBH (first row in Figure 4). Shots 2 and 3 are part of one scene according to SIFT (second row in Figure 4). The union operation combines these overlapping sets of shots into one scene with the shots 2, 3, and 4. The output of this procedure are the so called *core scenes* (last row in Figure 4).

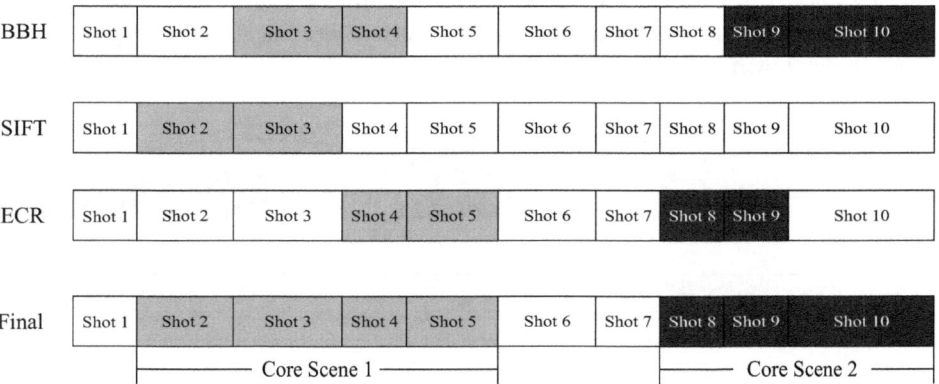

Fig. 4. The three scene segmentations obtained by the content-based features, BBH, SIFT, and ECR are combined. The result of this combination are the core scenes.

3.3   Post-processing

Usually, there are still unassigned shots between the core scenes. These shots are assigned to scenes by iteratively repeating the scene segmentation for the unassigned shots. With each iteration we decrease the similarity requirements (manipulating the similarity thresholds accordingly) until the shots are assigned to adjacent scenes (see Figure 5).

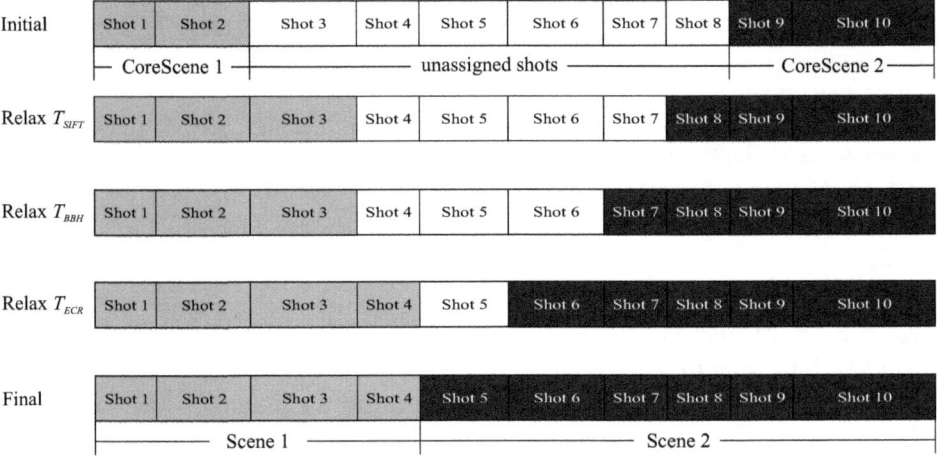

Fig. 5. Iterative repetition of the scene segmentation in order to assign the unassigned shots. The similarity requirements are decreased until all shots are assigned.

The *iterative* reduction of the similarity thresholds avoids the unwanted merging of scenes. If we set the thresholds too low from the beginning, scene segmentation would be too tolerant yielding an under-segmentation of the film. An example is shown in Figure 6.

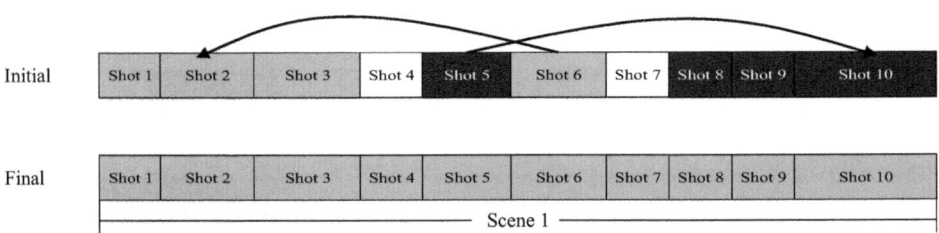

Fig. 6. Unwanted scene merging occurs, when the initial similarity requirements are too low. Arrows indicate similar shots, shading indicates assignment to scenes. The iterative reduction of similarity thresholds prevents this situation.

4   Experiments and Results

The investigated artistic archive documentaries have an experimental style and a complex temporal structure. We perform experiments with two films from the soviet filmmaker Dziga Vertov: "The Eleventh" and "Man with a Movie Camera". The films were selected because there is a common agreement among film scientists about the scene segmentation of these films. This is not the case for all films originating in this time where the segmentation into scenes usually is highly interpretative. The characteristics of the two films are summarized in Table 1.

Table 1. Characteristics of the investigated films

Title	Length	Frames	Shots	Scene boundaries
The Eleventh	58'	63123	660	21
Man with a Movie Camera	1h28'	95768	1782	38

We perform a detailed analysis of the approach (as a whole) and the different components (features, processing steps, etc.). The experiments are structured as follows:

1. Performance of single features: which of the employed features are most beneficial for scene segmentation.
2. Evaluation of the overall system' performance (based on the selected features from the first step).
3. Analysis of postprocessing: what is the benefit of the proposed postprocessing step (assignment of unassigned shots to core scenes)?
4. Performance on contemporary material: we perform scene segmentation on contemporary movies enabling a comparison with the performance of other state-of-the-art methods.

In a preliminary study, we analyze the performance of single features. Therefore, we select a subset of the video material (the first 200 shots of "The Eleventh") and analyze how many similar shots are detected by the individual features. A manual annotation reveals that 98 shots show significant similarities. For each feature we empirically optimize the decision thresholds. Similarity comparison by single features focuses on the optimization of precision while the next step (scene scegmentation) targets the improvement of recall. The results for all three features are summarized in Table 2.

The three features show an equally good performance (recall of approximately 0.50 at a precision of 1.00). This does not mean that the features represent the same information. An evaluation of the results reveals that each feature finds a different subset of similar shots. That means that they capture different types of similarities and complement each other. Consequently, we select all three features for the final system to retain as much information about similarities as possible.

For the SIFT feature the optimal decision threshold T_{SIFT} is 40, which means that two frames are considered similar if more than 40 feature points are similar. The decision threshold for ECR, T_{ECR} is 23% which means that two keyframes are similar if less than 23% of their edges are different. The two thresholds for BBH are: $T_{BBH_{Bin}} = 0.5$ and $T_{BBH_{Block}} = 55\%$. That means that two keyframes

Table 2. Performance of the single features

Feature	Correct	Missed	False Positives	Recall	Precision
Block-based histogram (BBH)	50	48	0	0.51	1.00
Edge Change Ratio (ECR)	46	52	0	0.47	1.00
SIFT	48	50	0	0.49	1.00

are considered similar if the difference between their histogram is lower than 0.5 in more than 55% of the blocks. Experiments with block-size (5x5, 10x10, 20x20) showed that this parameter has only little influence on the results. A block-size of 10x10 is chosen for the final system. The thresholds are set rather strict to avoid false positives at this stage of processing.

The performance measures for the entire system for the investigated films are summarized in Table 3. Recall is the ratio of correctly detected shot boundaries (SBs) and the total number of SBs according to the ground truth. Precision is the ratio of correctly detected SBs and the total number of retrieved SBs. For both films recall is above 90%. In "The Eleventh" only one scene boundary is not detected. For "Man with am Movie Camera" three scene boundaries cannot be detected. The (compared to recall) lower precicion values indicate that the approach performs an over-segmentation of the films.

Table 3. The performance of scene segmentation for the historic documentaries

Title	Correct	Missed	False Positives	Recall	Precision
The Eleventh	20	1	11	0.95	0.65
Man with a Movie Camera	35	3	50	0.92	0.41

Next, we investigate the performance of the proposed postprocessing step (iterative assignment of unassigned shots to core scenes). An analysis of the core scenes obtained by the scene segmentation (without postprocessing) reveals that a significant amount of shots are not assigned to any core scene, see Table 4. These results show that the postprocessing is crucial for robust scene segmentation.

The postprocessing iteratively makes the decision thresholds more tolerant to assign the unassigned shots to core scenes. Our experiments show that the largest benefit in this postprocessing is provided by the SIFT feature followed by BBH and ECR. From this observation we conclude that the SIFT feature is the most expressive feature in our study. Additionally, we observe that only a few iterations are necessary to assign all unassigned shots (3 iterations for "Man with a Movie Camera" and 5 iterations for "The Eleventh").

Finally, we evaluate the performance of our method for contemporary film material which enables the comparison with other state-of-the-art shot segmentation approaches. We apply the proposed approach to two films that are often used for scene segmentation in literature: "Forest Gump" and "Blade Runner". The results for "Blade Runner" are summarized in Table 5. This film is also

Table 4. Assignment of shots to core scenes results in a significant portion of shots that are not assigned to any core scene

Title	# Shots	# Unass. Shots	Percentage unassig. shots
The Eleventh	660	203	31%
Man with a Movie Camera	1787	460	26%

Table 5. The performance of scene segmentation for the film "Blade Runner" compared to the approach of [6]

Approach	SBs	Found	Correct	Missed	False Positives	Recall	Precision
"naive case" [6]	24	n/a	20	4	n/a	0.83	n/a
"using refinement" [6]	24	n/a	18	6	n/a	0.75	n/a
proposed approach	24	40	18	6	22	0.75	0.45

analyzed in [6] where Sundaram and Chang apply two versions of their algorithm ("naive case" and "using refinement"), see Table 5.

From Table 5 we observe that our method performs comparably well to the approach in [6] although our method is not optimized for (high-quality) color video (for example we do not make use of color information). Furthermore, we do not use audio information as in [6]. Note that the comparison is limited in expressiveness since the authors of [6] do not provide information about the precision of their approach.

We further analyze the movie "Forest Gump". Since no ground truth segmentation is available, we manually analyze the film and identify 52 scene boundaries. The proposed method finds 68 scene boundaries, where 44 are correct and 8 are missed. The number of false positives is 24 which yields a recall of 0.85 and a precision of 0.65. This is a satisfactory result for state-of-the-art scene segmentation algorithms. We compare our method with that proposed by Vendrig and Worring [7]. The authors segment the movie into 152 "'logical story units". If we apply the same rules and preconditions for segmentation as in [7] we obtain 143 segments. A more precise comparison is not possible since the authors in [7] employ different evaluation criteria.

5   Summary

The specific characteristics of artistic archive documentaries require adapted analysis techniques. We have presented a novel scene segmentation technique that has been designed specifically for this type of film. The technique employs orthogonal features to group similar shots into scenes in a two-step process. In the first step, we identify core-scenes based on visual similarity. In the second step, we assign the remaining unassigned shots to the core scenes, by iterative adaptation of thresholds. We evaluate the technique using archive documentaries and contemporary fiction films. The results for fiction films are satisfactory with an average recall of 0.80 and an average precision of 0.55. We achieve significantly higher recall for archive documentaries. An average recall of 0.94 and a precision of 0.53 prove the suitability of our technique to archive documentaries. We will direct future work toward reducing over-segmentation and thus increase the precision of the presented scene segmentation technique.

Acknowledgments

This work has received financial support from the Vienna Science and Technology Fund (WWTF) under grant no. CI06 024.

References

1. Beaver, F.E.: Dictionary of film terms: the aesthetic companion to film art. Peter Lang Publishing (2009)
2. Gu, Z., Mei, T., Hua, Z.S., Wu, Z., Li, S.: EMS: Energy minimization based video scene segmentation. In: IEEE International Conference on Multimedia and Expo., pp. 520–523 (2007)
3. Lowe, D.: Distinctive image features from scale-invariant keypoints. International Journal of Computer Vision 60(2), 91–110 (2004)
4. Rasheed, Z., Shah, M.: Scene detection in Hollywood movies and TV shows. In: IEEE Conference on Computer Vision and Pattern Recognition (CVPR 2003), vol. 2, pp. II- 343–II- 348 (2003)
5. Rasheed, Z., Shah, M.: Detection and representation of scenes in videos. IEEE Transactions on Multimedia 7(6), 1097–1105 (2005)
6. Sundaram, H., Chang, S.F.: scene segmentation using video and audio features. In: IEEE International Conference on Multimedia and Expo., pp. 1145–1148. IEEE, Piscataway (2000)
7. Vendrig, J., Worring, M.: Systematic evaluation of logical story unit segmentation. IEEE Transactions on Multimedia 4(4), 492–499 (2002)
8. Wang, X., Wang, S., Chen, H., Gabbouj, M.: A Shot Clustering Based Algorithm for Scene Segmentation. In: Proceedings of the 2007 International Conference on Computational Intelligence and Security Workshops, pp. 252–259. IEEE Computer Society, Washington (2007)
9. Yeung, M., Yeo, B.L., Liu, B.: Segmentation of video by clustering and graph analysis. Computer Vision and Image Understanding 71(1), 94–109 (1998)
10. Zabih, R., Miller, J., Mai, K.: A feature-based algorithm for detecting and classifying scene breaks. In: Proceedings of the 3rd ACM International Conference on Multimedia, pp. 189–200. ACM, New York (1995)
11. Zhai, Y., Shah, M.: Video scene segmentation using markov chain monte carlo. IEEE Transactions on Multimedia 8(4), 686–697 (2006)

Issues in Designing Novel Applications for Emerging Multimedia Technologies

Hyowon Lee

CLARITY: Centre for Sensor Web Technologies
School of Computing
Dublin City University, Ireland
hlee@computing.dcu.ie

Abstract. Emerging computational multimedia tools and techniques promise powerful ways to organise, search and browse our ever-increasing multimedia contents by automating annotation and indexing, augmenting meta-data, understanding media contents, linking related pieces of information amongst them, and providing intriguing visualisation and exploration front-ends. Identifying real-world scenarios and designing interactive applications that leverage these developing multimedia technology is certainly an important research topic in itself but poses a number of challenges: the currently practiced methodologies and tools in the field of Human-Computer Interaction and Interaction Design seem to work better when the target users and usage requirements have been clearly identified and understood in advance whereas much of what emerging multimedia technology could offer is expected to create completely new user activities and usage that we are not aware of; immature multimedia tools currently being researched are not good enough to be the core engines of real-world applications today, making realistic user studies through deployment difficult; our future interaction platforms will be more than just desktop PC, Web, or mobile devices but many other forms of tangible, embedded, physical appliances which we expect the currently developing multimedia technology would be coupled with. In this paper, these challenges and the insights into how we could get over them are explored based on the author's decade-long experience in designing novel interactive applications for multimedia technology.

Keywords: Human-Computer Interaction, Multimedia, Interaction Design, Innovation, Design Methodology, Novel Technology.

1 Introduction

With so much R&D in multimedia research in developing various novel techniques and algorithms promising effective and efficient access to our growing media archives and collections, thinking about how to channel those developments into usable and feasible usage scenarios and actual, practical, innovative and high-impacting real-world applications is certainly a significant issue today.

G. Leitner, M. Hitz, and A. Holzinger (Eds.): USAB 2010, LNCS 6389, pp. 411–426, 2010.
© Springer-Verlag Berlin Heidelberg 2010

The "demonstration systems" often featured in many multimedia research papers are in a sense such an effort to bring the developing computational tools in multimedia into real-world applications, even though they tend to be short-sighted, technically-oriented, poorly-designed and usually lack an understanding of end-users and contexts in which such a system is to be used.

On the one hand, most multimedia research groups' lack of expertise in Inter-action Design and Human-Computer Interaction (HCI) knowledge and perhaps their lack of collaboration with neighbouring HCI groups within their departments may be to blame. But on the other hand, the HCI community itself does not seem to offer more prescriptive methods or procedures to help develop novel scenarios and applications in such a way as to leverage the technologies developed by these multimedia researchers. Monitoring and interviewing end-users and coming up with requirements to develop a better version of an existing application is one thing, but trying to come up with a usable application not based on end-user data but based on emerging technology itself is another.

While acknowledging the power of User-Centred Design and how the strong emphasis on end-users and establishing comprehensive user requirements promotes a product that satisfies existing user needs and thus fitting the system well to their work context, an attempt to develop a completely novel application that does not have existing user base or current practice of use tends to face a lack of methodological support due to the HCI tools and procedures that seem to be focused on supporting today's tools and activities rather than tomorrow's.

The culprit of the plethora of complex technology demos with poor usability in multimedia witnessed today is not only the lack of inter-disciplinarity or lack of collaboration between multimedia and HCI, but the lack of general understanding of how a novel application could and should be developed where the starting point is technological possibility instead of an identified, unmet user needs in a specific domain.

The focus of this paper is on "emerging" or "novel" multimedia techniques rather than well-studied or already-robust techniques since the latter group of tools, once matured enough, become the realm of "conventional" technologies that any software house or companies can readily adopt in developing a highly usable multimedia application with the well-established software development and usability assessment processes available today. With this in mind, this paper will describe three interweaving issues that make it challenging in developing future interactive applications that incorporate emerging multimedia tools and techniques, and in doing so draw on the author's hands-on experience of designing a variety of novel multimedia applications in a large multimedia research group over the past ten years.

To name but a few of these novel applications, a Web-based video retrieval system where a user can search a video collection by semantic features such as the existence of faces/people, indoor/outdoor, and cityscape/landscape [3]; an object-based photo archive where a user can search for objects in photos (e.g. a vase, a car or a ship) in terms of the object characteristics rather than whole photos [25]; a security video search system where CCTV video footage in a

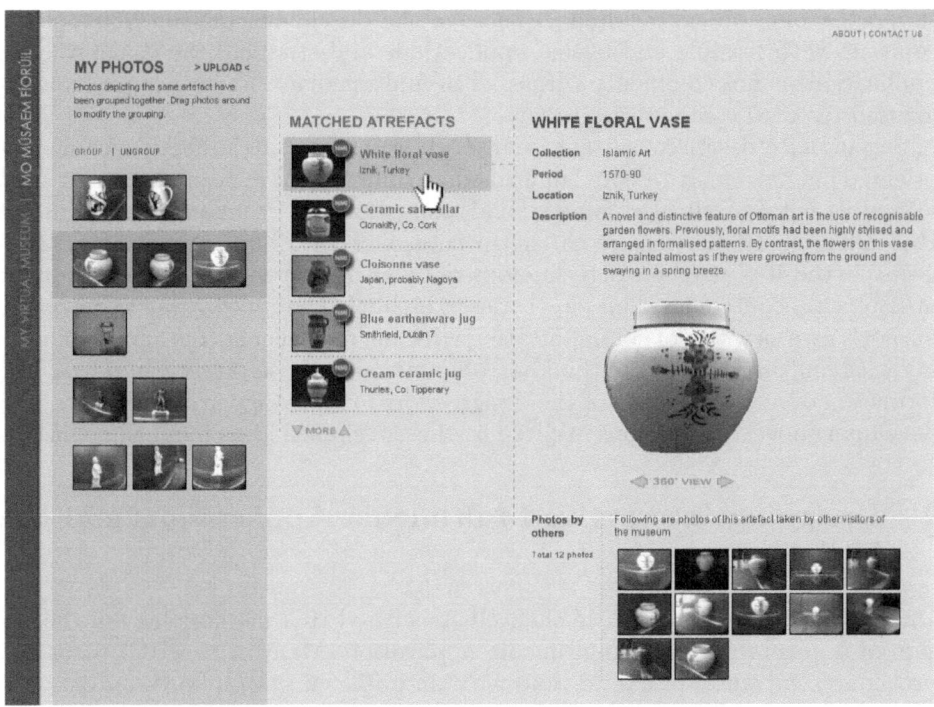

Fig. 1. Photos taken from a museum are automatically grouped by individual arte-facts (left panel), and matched to the museum's authoritative photo collection (middle panel), then linked to detailed information about that artefact (right panel)

university campus is captured and indexed by people's contours and later a se-curity staff can trace whereabouts of a suspicious person appearing in multiple camera locations [14]; a museum artefact explorer where a user can upload the photos taken at the museum to match and group the same artefacts even if the photos show different angles or sides, and display information on them (see Figure 1 for a screen shot) [2]; an online photo organiser where the uploaded per-sonal photos are automatically annotated by the people appearing in the photos [23]; a Lifelogging browser where a large number of passively captured photos from a wearable camera are automatically structured by individual events, their relative importance identified and presented in an intriguing comic-book style montage as to help the user review their day [15]; a route finder where a collection of in-vehicle video footage is automatically indexed and seamlessly interweaved with the vehicle routes on a geographic map [19], and many more. All of these applications incorporated one or more combinations of multimedia techniques that were on-going research topics at the time (and many of them still are), and were more than just "technology demos" in the sense that an extensive Inter-action Design effort was expended in developing them and specially designed to support some form of novel activities that conventional applications do not support. Going one extra mile to package the developing multimedia tools to come up with feasible and usable applications and studying the usage of such applications is not commonly witnessed in multimedia or any other technology-focused research communities today.

Serving as a "design consultant" and "usability expert" in the highly technically-oriented but extremely talented multimedia group that have been generating such a great variety of exciting computational tools, the author's unique position as the HCI and Interaction Design researcher-practitioner contributing to "all things end-users" in the 40+ members of technology researchers over the past decade brought many exciting outcomes. This paper tries to highlight the issues by reflecting on the author's own practice of communicating with his multimedia colleagues, of dealing with multimedia ways of thinking, of monitoring the aggressive and dynamic formation of new ideas, and of the design effort in applying various HCI tools to developing novel applications inspired by these technical ideas in multimedia.

2   Designing Interactive Multimedia Applications and the HCI Stance

One might attempt bringing in the well-structured HCI methodology in the design of a novel interactive multimedia application. Many of the HCI tools and procedures currently practiced (and with desirable effects), however, are geared towards those applications that we currently use, with relatively well-understood domains and with an existing user base. Involving the target end-users at various stages of the development process in order to reflect the users' wishes and needs into the design is the central premise of the User-Centred Design (UCD) approach. Currently popular ethnographic methods such as Cultural Probes [7] and Contextual Inquiry [9] as well as other traditional interviews, questionnaire, interaction logging and eye-tracking, are the examples of these methods where the purpose is to obtain the information about people's current practice of certain activities in order to incorporate them into the design.

Some of the multimedia technologies do promise an enhancement of existing tools in existing practices. For example, *face detection and recognition* technique could be plugged in to an existing personal photo or video management service such as Flickr and YouTube, to help reduce the user's manual annotation burden by automatically tagging the photos or video clips by the appearance of individual persons' names. *Advertisement detection* in a video stream could be plugged in to our VCR/DVD recorders at home to help save the storage and skip the annoying ad breaks in the middle of a movie, by automatically identifying them and removing or at least tagging them at the time of recording. These scenarios are certainly a useful target for the computational multimedia tools to be applied to and be made useful in the real-world, in the way that makes people's life easier and more convenient by automating those elements that so far had assumed human labour and intervention.

There are, however, ways in which technologies could support very new activities, or rather, *create* new activities that people have not done before: online chatting was not a known activity that anybody did until the infrastructure of the Internet and the software that supported it appeared; the activity of blogging did not exist only 5 years ago until web blogging services appeared and people started using them; video sharing/voting and twitting are also the examples of recently invented activities whereby those technological applications appeared first then the uptake of the usage happened afterwards. Designing for these novel applications (albeit the lack of any technological innovations in some of the above examples) that will support new activities is fundamentally different from designing, for example, a next generation of a word processor or a better version of a library management system.

We expect the tools and techniques researched in many multimedia R&D groups today will in time create many such new activities in the form of "novel interactive applications." Because the design for the new activities expected to be invented cannot rely solely on existing user data or precedent design examples, the starting point of designing such an application is on shaky grounds (Section 3.1). While the novel multimedia tools themselves might not provide robust and accurate performance today thus making any decent user-experiment or deployment effort difficult (Section 3.2), we expect by the time these tools become better understood and more mature in terms of their performance, the kinds of interaction platforms that we will be interacting with on a day-to-day basis will be much more diverse (Section 3.3). The next section will address these issues in more detail.

3   The Issues

3.1   Shaky Starting Point

An interaction designer typically gets input from (1) engineers, who provide technologies; (2) anthropologists, who provide field data; (3) behavioural scientists, who provide models and theories to support the design of artefacts [31]. While the modern HCI practice strongly advocates the User-Centred Design approach where the emphasis is on establishing requirements by understanding the users and the environment where the system in concern is to be located and used, designing novel multimedia applications often do not have the "field data" or the information on the existing users' practice of the application area, as that application scenario itself is something new. Also, many successful designers rely on their past experiences of designing similar artefacts [11], and many aspects of design activity itself are based on building on successful precedences. Designing novel applications, as there is no such initial exemplar or successful products, has a very shaky starting point.

Some inspirations do come from observing people's current lives and their activities. Trying to use ethnographic studies to explore new possible scenarios and innovations [22] and studying a particular practice to learn about the underlying motivation for a more grounded innovation [17] have been suggested.

These approaches try to start by studying end-users in developing technological innovations. Also, we could first study the usage of existing applications of a similar nature (probably a manually-intensive equivalent that the new application is to supersede) and hope that they could help inform the design of the new. For example, in order to design a novel application that uses a *video summarisation* technique, we could study how people browse their DVD collections using a chapter selection feature provided in most DVD movies, or use an Electronic Program Guide to quickly get the gist of the contents, and identify how the current experiences in these activities could be enhanced with the automatic video summarisation. Collecting usage data from the "proxy users" in this way is one of the ways to ground the new technological development to the real-world. In a recent article in interactions [18], Norman warns against the tendency to rely on ethnography in technological inventions by explaining how major breakthroughs and innovations in history came from technologists who had very little understanding of users, and how most often "technology will come first, the products second, and then the needs will slowly appear."

Because it is often impossible to predict whether a newly-supported activity is something that people will want to do, or rather, impossible to predict how people will accommodate and assimilate a novel activity afforded by the new application into their lives, it is more important to quickly develop a robust application first then get people to start using it. In this sense, the design decisions for novel multimedia applications should be made as to come up with an artefact that is open-ended in terms of its eventual usage or purpose (because we don't know what they would be at the time of design) but that strictly adheres to usability principles [26]. Thus, quickly prototyping an application and conducting a usage study with it is one sure way to go about developing a novel multimedia application, without spending too much resources on trying to establish initial requirements or understanding the usage context at the beginning. As more and more people have the access to the Web, developing a Web-based application has the great benefit of being able to easily deploy it for a number of users to use although this can be a problem in limiting the usage scenarios for near future (see Interaction Platform Issues Section below).

The shaky starting point tends to result in longer design time to produce an initial application scenario and the user-interface, as having no previous examples to follow and having no good understanding of usage makes it difficult to structure and streamline the design process in any way. For example, it took the author well over full-time 4 months to design a video clip searching application where a clip-to-clip content similarity measure is used to support a "find more like this" type of query and interactive refinement of the query and retrieval results in a highly efficient way [20]. Having a query panel on the left where example video clips and their associated transcripts are added and retrieval results on the right showing matched shots' keyframes as well as a few preceding and following shot keyframes in different sizes, had no such precedences and everything had to be designed from scratch. For this, a series of iterative sketches and brainstorming sessions with the technical members were undertaken as the main process over a 4-month period. After the system was fully implemented and a user experiment conducted, we had much better understanding of the application in terms of people's opinions about such a tool and how it might be further refined or re-branded into a product. It has been noticed that a number of other multimedia groups designed similar user-interfaces in the subsequent years, and now designing a similar interface can be a matter of days (precedences and practical know-how/experience makes such a big difference in design).

The design of a lifelogging photo browser where a large number of a person's lifelog photos from a SenseCam can be reviewed [15] took more than a year during which the strategies to connect between the supporting back-end techniques and their possible front-end manifestation and interaction schemes gradually developed - there was no precedence of such an application and there still is no usage of such an application as it will take many more years for the passive capture device such as SenseCam to be used by the general public. Many of the novel applications incorporating multimedia techniques developed in our group took months for each of them to form any concrete user-interface, because of the lack of understanding in the application areas and the lack of examples to narrow down the design space.

While in engineering fields the lack of initial understanding or requirements generally poses challenges in formulating the questions and problems to work on, design studies show that the inherent quality of designers is the ability to work on an ill-defined problem space and quickly reach an initial design solution by framing the problem space in a creative way, then going back and forth between the problem and solution space over time [5]. When it comes to designing novel multimedia applications, such quality will be very much needed and it may be an important clue in any attempt to make explicit the procedure for innovative design that lacks user/usage information.

3.2 Imperfect Back-End Performance and Implications

Developing effective video *shot-boundary detection* and *keyframe extraction* techniques have been a very active sub-topic in the multimedia field since the late 90s and early 2000s and their accuracy level is said to have reached above 95-98% today (for straightforward hard-cut transitions anyway) [29]. We call this a "solved problem" and these well-understood techniques are today featured in many video editing tools to help quickly browse the video contents. *Face detection* has been, as its potential value for such a technique is huge, an another active research topic in computer vision and now many digital cameras feature real-time face detection and highlighting in the camera viewfinder to help the user focus the camera to those face areas. Some of these older topics in the field are having fruition today by being featured in these commercial products. There are a variety of different techniques in multimedia that are currently being studied and sooner or later to come out of the laboratories into real-world applications.

One of the problems of making a working prototype of a novel multimedia application is that the multimedia technique that the system is to demonstrate

418   H. Lee

is, almost by definition, an imperfect technology that multimedia researchers are working very hard today to improve in their laboratories. As the technology research community, it is important to design novel applications *now* even though their back-end multimedia techniques themselves may not yet be good enough to be used in the real-world, in order to envision and shape the near-future when such techniques will have become sufficiently matured.

Having an immature technology as a back-end of a system not accurate or robust enough to be used un-supervised in a real-world application is a big handicap as an interactive application: users will notice the inaccurate results on the front-end and this lowers the perceived value and attraction of the application enormously, even if all other usability aspects are crafted to high standards. It can be compared to, say, an online shopping mall site where product information is occasionally incorrect or some times wrong photos are displayed for a product - whatever the reason, it is simply unacceptable. This means the precious comments, feedback and usage of the test users that otherwise could have shown valuable information about possible new usage or wishes will be clouded by the obvious functionality flaws.

In order to remove such complaints on the performance of the system (and to get useful comments on all other aspects), we need to manually correct the results of the imperfect algorithms and show the perfect outcome to the users.

For example, we had an online video retrieval system we called Físchlár ("Fís" means *video*, and "chlar" means *programme* in the Irish language) which was deployed within the university campus for over 6 years (1999-2006) during which more than 2,000 students and staff users registered and actively used the system. The system ingested video streams from broadcast TV signal on our users' requests and processed, indexed, and structured the incoming video stream for browsing, searching and playback. One of its latest variations incorporated an automatic *news story segmentation* technique and processed daily 9pm news from the national TV channel RTÉ, and presented a news story-based searching and browsing interface to the users. A lot of effort was put into capturing the real usage of this system with interaction logging, diaries and questionnaire [16]. While the system had to be made robust and accessible at all times (our users used the system in the morning before they start working, at lunch breaks, between lab sessions and in late evenings), the most problematic aspect was that the story segmentation engine itself did not produce 100% accurate results, thus our users would frequently see incorrect story units in their browsing. In order to prevent this, the newly added news videos were manually checked every morning to correct wrong segmentation with a simple editing tool before our users started accessing the site in the morning. This early-morning manual intervention continued every day for more than 5 months during which this particular study was conducted. Costs associated with deploying an application, especially when its back-end uses an experimental multimedia techniques that is not mature, can be so high that it may seem almost a luxury to be able to conduct this kind of long-term deployment study with such an application.

In this particular study, our users thought the system fully-automatically indexed the news stories without any human intervention, but the more illuminating fact for us was that they did not really *care* whether it was automatically done or otherwise: all they wanted was to be able to locate the news stories they were interested in and watch them to kill some time, as if it were a regular online news service such as Irish Times Online or BBC News Online. They instead complained about the system not presenting the news stories by overall categories such as "International", "Politics", "Entertainment" and "Sports", which did provide us with future desired features of the application.

An alternative strategy is to design the user-interface in such a way that whenever a user notices such imperfect output of the back-end processing, he/she could very easily fix or correct it while doing the task. The corrected facts can then be fed back to the back-end processing and propagate to the rest of the data, overall improving the accuracy of the system. Encouraging or motivating the user to provide annotation during the use [27] is probably a good strategy for providing a service with imperfect performance as long as the task of annotation is not lengthy or laborious. For example, in a personal photo management system we developed in 2007 [21], uploaded photos were automatically annotated with the name of the people present in each of the photos using face recognition augmented with a body-patch algorithm. As the accuracy of these algorithms was not 100% accurate, sometimes the users noticed incorrect names being labeled for some faces in the photos. Using a simple mouse-over action over the photo and the selection of a predicted alternative names pushed to the user by the system, he/she corrected the annotation with a minimal effort whenever such error was noticed and the system re-calculated remaining photo collection with the revised certainty based on that manual correction, just as is done in current systems like Apple iPhoto.

Another stream of strategy is that when the back-end performance is imperfect, we could develop usage scenarios and the user interaction in such a way that such imperfection would not be so blatantly noticeable or crucial in the user's task. For example, our online Movie Browser application [1] used movie *scene segmentation and classification* techniques to present movie content by chunks of Exciting, Dialogue, or Montage scenes (see Figure 2 for a screen shot). While the state-of-the-art scene segmentation tools are still not mature enough to ensure reliable results, our user-interface arranged the browsing mechanism with a large timeline where the segmented scene blocks are highlighted in different colours depending on its identified scene types. When a user clicks any of the highlighted blocks on this timeline, the series of scenes around that time region is presented and the user can browse movie events around that time region. In our deployment study of this system with over 260 students in a Media Study course for a full semester, the students used the system freely to help write their movie analysis assignments. Interviews, focus group and questionnaire were used to obtain their usage and opinions, and the inaccurate scene boundaries and classification appearing on the interface was not an issue partly because the interface

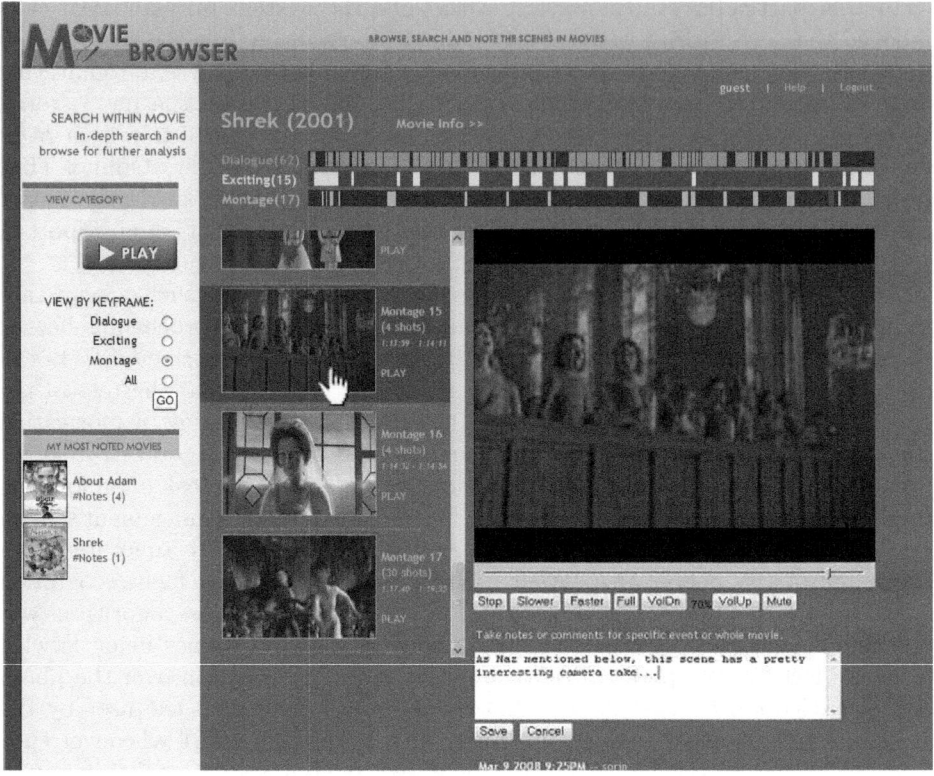

Fig. 2. Three-band timeline shows where dialogue, exciting, and montage scenes are in the movie, and clicking any area on the timeline will show the scene keyframes around that area below

naturally reduced any negative effects by showing neighbouring scenes but also partly because the concept of scene boundary itself cannot be objectively defined or agreed upon by everybody: as long as the users were able to roughly reach a point of their interest quickly and navigate around, they were happy and did not complain about the segmentation inaccuracy.

The choice of these strategies will depend on the domain and the way the usage scenario is drawn for that application. Thus, it will probably be more difficult to design the above-mentioned news story browsing interface in such a way that the incorrect story segmentation results will not be too obvious or matter, because news stories are generally more well-defined and are often the isolated unit of contents that news consumers will want. Even so, there might be some novel scenarios that we could develop where the blending of adjacent news stories is the main feature, perhaps a visualisation of an aggregation of daily news stories over a long period.

3.3   Interaction Platform Issue

Consider some of the multimedia tools and techniques we are currently developing are packaged into an intriguing application running on an Apple iPad, with which a user can use a simple finger touch to easily command the functions, search and browse with the powerful automatic indexing and visualisation techniques in a way that conventional applications cannot. Are there particular multimedia tools that might be better suited for this "Multimedia iPad" scenario than others?

So far, whenever somebody showed a "demo" of a multimedia research project, it was shown on a desktop PC or a laptop displaying a stand-alone or Web-based user-interface in some way. Large databases of complex and colourful multimedia information in image, video and text may be nicely visualised on a large monitor with a mouse and keyboard, and help explore the data, adjust sophisticated parameters, pinpoint the area of interest, draw a region, and navigate a deep hierarchy of menus relatively efficiently. More recently some demos were shown on mobile devices, with academic events specifically dealing with mobile multimedia appearing such as the International Workshop on Mobile Multimedia Processing (ICPR 2010), the International Conference on Mobile and Ubiquitous Multimedia (MUM 2010) and the ACM Multimedia Workshop on Mobile Video Delivery (MoViD 2010).

The great thing about Web-based and mobile multimedia applications is that they can be packaged to be more or less readily accessible for anybody who has access to the Internet or has an appropriate mobile device. Deploying a Web-based prototype application or an iPhone app is methodologically very effective in terms of getting people to use it to get feedback and monitor the emerging usage of such applications.

However, *by the time* many of the emerging multimedia tools studied today become mature enough to be used outside the lab and into real-world applications (say in 5-10 years as a ballpark figure for a cycle in which a newly proposed computational tool becomes a commercialisable piece of technology), we will be interacting in our daily lives with more variety of devices and platforms, most likely far *more frequently* than with desktop PCs or mobile platforms: interactive tabletops, with such a ubiquity of physical tables at home, restaurants, cafes, airplanes and schools, will probably become one of the most commonly encountered interaction platforms in the near future; interactive TV, augmenting conventional TV boxes with social connectivity, storage and processing power, will become the future way of watching TV; large multi-touch walls will dominate our streets, at bus stops and shopping malls providing novel public spaces with multi-user interactivity; other embedded appliances will be around us such as electronic magazines, sophisticated digital picture frames, touch-screen in-home displays (perhaps a variation of the next generation of iPad), door panels with media alerts and weather forecasts, etc.

Thus we envisage that it will be more constructive and forward-thinking to try to couple the emerging multimedia techniques that we are developing today with these more novel interaction platforms, than just demoing on a desktop PC or a laptop. As different interaction platforms assume different physical and contextual characteristics and consequently different appropriate modes and styles of interaction, we should consider that some types of multimedia tools currently being developed might be more suitable to manifest on particular types of platforms than others in order to maximise or best leverage their potential power and benefits.

For example, an earlier project involved developing an automatic news story segmentation tool from daily TV broadcast news videos and recommended individual news stories to mobile users based on user preference, viewing history and collaborative filtering [8] - the mobile platform with small screen and awkward input mechanism makes the content analysis and structuring techniques coupled with automatic recommendation of meaningful units of information quite ideal for providing the kind of user interaction where the interaction effort is minimised by the system intelligently digesting the information, structuring it, summarising it, then selectively presenting the most useful piece of information to the user on the mobile screen. Thus, multimedia techniques that result in elaborate visualisation or explorative interaction is less of a value to mobile platforms but summarising, structuring, and selective pushing types of techniques seem more promising for mobile applications. For example, the sports summarisation technique we have developed [24] analyses any field-sports video content and identifies those segments that contain high probability of important events happening in the game. Stitching up those identified segments can result in a 3-minute video summary of important events from a 90-minute football match. Such a summarised form of a playable video could very well support a mobile entertainment service where the user's interaction with the device is to simply watch a 3-minute summary video rather than typing in text, selecting options, dragging panels, and exploring a sophisticated visualisation scheme which all cause interaction burden to the mobile user.

Down the road, we can imagine an ideal mobile device where its back-end mechanism is so advanced that as soon as the user turns on the device he/she will see only those information and interface that the user wanted to use without any menu navigation selection of options requiring visual attention, as a result of the combination of accurate information processing, intelligent inference and adaptive interface.

Exploring the suitability of various interaction platforms for emerging multimedia techniques should be one very important part of the interactive multimedia application design. The obvious challenge in trying to develop such applications is that the developed system (whether it being on a tabletop, iTV, Multitouch Wall, or any other platforms) is difficult to deploy due to the current unavailability of such platforms to the test users, unlike Web-based systems or iPhone apps that could relatively easily be deployed as many users have access to these platforms anyway.

In 2005, our group developed an interactive tabletop application that incorporates a number of video retrieval techniques to allow multiple users sitting around the table to collaboratively search for video clips [28]. While the back-end multimedia tools were used to segment video streams to manageable chunks and to allow similarity-based searching amongst the chunked clips, the front-end table interface tested how the interaction can be arranged in such a way that the collaboration amongst the users could be encouraged and conducted smoothly. The tabletop is still an on-going field of study in the HCI community, and coupling multimedia techniques on an interactive table gives very interesting research opportunities to this line of study. Because regular users do not have an interactive tabletop and in most cases have not even used such a platform, studying people's use of the application required for us to arrange appointments with the test users in the room where we showed it and got them to do training tasks, in a typical laboratory user testing style.

In 2008, we developed a "Multimedia TV" application which featured a number of multimedia techniques (including shot/scene/story boundary detection, sports highlight detection, face detection, clip similarity calculation, etc.) in a TV set and a viewer with a conventional remote control can use a small number of buttons to use these capabilities [12]. *Lean-back interaction* that characterises a TV interaction requires extremely simplistic screen element design and the mechanism to invoke the functions while watching the TV. During the design stage of the TV widgets and screen elements, we brought in test users to our TV set and informally observed their behaviour and discussed with them. Even though realistic usage can only be tested in people's own homes, deploying such a TV to a home is currently impossible as nobody has such a TV.

It is not easy to see any effort in experimenting the emerging multimedia techniques on novel interaction platforms, as most multimedia researchers are busy with their algorithms and techniques to seriously think about applying them to these platforms and the HCI researchers often have little understanding of what emerging multimedia tools offer.

While quite a lot of interaction design knowledge, experience and skill set are today available for the desktop PC/Web platform, relatively little is understood or practiced for the mobile platform, and far less for other more novel platforms. The design knowledge for each of these platforms are, however, slowly growing today as more and more experimental applications appear in the labs and the trial-and-error process starts identifying what makes good interaction strategies for each of these platforms. Growing design knowledge for each of these platforms is highlighted and summarised in [13]. Leveraging the increasing amount of design knowledge for various novel platforms will be one of the keys to successfully deploying usable interactive multimedia applications of the future.

4   Conclusion

The way we can interact with multimedia data depends on how the data is organised, indexed and presented, so there is certainly a very important link between multimedia technology and interaction design [10]. A competent interaction designer for multimedia applications will be someone who is equipped with HCI tools, design thinking and skills while at the same time understands the nature of multimedia technologies and the trend of their progress over time.

In highlighting the issues, this paper did not emphasise the lack of design thinking by the multimedia researchers although this is most likely one of the factors slowing down the development of highly usable and attractive multimedia applications. Multimedia researchers without practical design skills usually like to argue a multimedia application's user-interface with such HCI terms and concepts as "click distance", "screen real-estate", "consistency" as it seems they find these concepts most comfortable to understand in their scientific and engineering frame of mind. The fact of the matter is that a competent interaction designer usually does not constrain himself to such terms in designing or assessing the interface. For designers these terms are largely a hindsight, post-design analysis or post-design rationale. He tries to find a wholesome solution that can elegantly solve a range of issues in a single, coherent and unifying theme (sometimes called "primary generator" [11] or "first principle" [4]), even at the cost of a sub-optimal level of, say, click distance or screen real-estate, more drawn from his/her experiences and intuition, frequently ignoring an elaborate requirements analysis that multimedia researchers in the science and engineering tradition prefer to start with. Certainly design decisions are based on a series of good judgements of the designer [30] who can juggle with many unknowns and known factors, and the success of a design is at the designed outcome, not the way design choices were argued and rationalised [6]. It is understandable how multimedia researchers struggle to understand and often become frustrated when their interaction design colleagues immediately start working on the final solution in a sketch when given a description of the technologies to be incorporated.

The way forward would be on the one hand for the multimedia community to embrace these "designerly ways of knowing" [5] and leverage their ability in developing the new generation of interactive applications that incorporate the emerging technologies the multimedia researchers are working so hard on today. On the other hand, more competent interaction designers and HCI practitioners should start working directly with the multimedia technology researchers, picking up those multimedia tools and algorithms with huge potential to design novel scenarios and applications that will forever change the way people work and play.

Acknowledgments. This work is supported by Science Foundation Ireland under grant 07/CE/I1147 and by Dublin City University Research Fellowship Scheme.

References

1. Ali, N.M., Smeaton, A.F., Lee, H., Brereton, P.: Developing, deploying and assessing the usage of a movie archive system. In: HCI Intl. 2009 - 13th International Conference on Human-Computer Interaction (2009)
2. Blighe, M.: Mo msaem foril: A web-based search and information service for museum visitors. In: Campilho, A., Kamel, M.S. (eds.) ICIAR 2008. LNCS, vol. 5112, pp. 485–496. Springer, Heidelberg (2008)

3. Browne, P., Czirjek, C., Gurrin, C., Jarina, R., Lee, H., Marlow, S., Donald, K.M., Murphy, N., O'Connor, N., Smeaton, A.F., Ye, J.: Dublin City University Video Track Experiments for TREC 2002. In: TREC 2002 - Text REtrieval Conference, MD, USA. National Institute of Standards and Technology (2002)
4. Cross, N.: Creative cognition in design: processes of exceptional designers. In: C&C 2002: Proceedings of the 4th Conference on Creativity & Cognition, pp. 14–19. ACM Press, New York (2002)
5. Cross, N.: Designerly Ways of Knowing. Birkhäuser, Basel (2006)
6. Cross, N.: Creative thinking in design: an introduction. In: SoD 2007: Proceedings of the 2007 Symposium on Science of Design, pp. 2–3. ACM Press, New York (2007)
7. Gaver, B., Dunne, T., Pacenti, E.: Design: Cultural probes. Interactions 6(1), 21–29 (1999)
8. Gurrin, C., Smeaton, A.F., Lee, H., McDonald, K., Murphy, N., O'Connor, N., Marlow, S.: Mobile access to the Físchlár-News Archive. In: Crestani, F., Dunlop, M.D., Mizzaro, S. (eds.) Mobile HCI International Workshop 2003. LNCS, vol. 2954, pp. 124–142. Springer, Heidelberg (2004)
9. Holtzblatt, K., Jones, S.: Contextual Inquiry: A Participative Technique for System Design, pp. 180–193. Lawrence Erlbaum, Hillsdale (1993)
10. Jaimes, A., Sebe, N., Gatica-Perez, D.: Human-centered computing: a multimedia perspective. In: MULTIMEDIA 2006: Proceedings of the 14th Annual ACM International Conference on Multimedia, pp. 855–864. ACM, New York (2006)
11. Lawson, B.: How designers think: the design process demystified, 4th edn. Architectural Press (2006)
12. Lee, H., Ferguson, P., Gurrin, C., Smeaton, A.F., O'Connor, N.E., Park, H.: Balancing the power of multimedia information retrieval and usability in designing interactive TV. In: UXTV 2008: Proc. Intl. Conf. Designing Interactive User Experiences for TV and Video, pp. 105–114. ACM, New York (2008)
13. Lee, H., Smeaton, A.F.: Interaction platform-orientated perspective in designing novel applications. In: Create 2009 - Creative Inventions and Innovations for Everyday HCI (2009)
14. Lee, H., Smeaton, A.F., O'Connor, N., Murphy, N.: User-Interface to a CCTV Video Search System. In: ICDP 2005 - IEE International Symposium on Imaging for Crime Detection and Prevention, pp. 39–43 (2005)
15. Lee, H., Smeaton, A.F., O'Connor, N.E., Jones, G.J., Blighe, M., Byrne, D., Doherty, A., Gurrin, C.: Constructing a SenseCam visual diary as a media process. Multimedia Sys. J. 14(6), 341–349 (2008)
16. Lee, H., Smeaton, A.F., O'Connor, N.E., Smyth, B.: User evaluation of Físchlár-News: An automatic broadcast news delivery system. ACM Transactions on Information Systems 24(2), 145–189 (2006)
17. Ljungblad, S., Holmquist, L.E.: Transfer scenarios: grounding innovation with marginal practices. In: CHI 2007, pp. 737–746. ACM, New York (2007)
18. Norman, D.: Technology first, needs last: The research-product gulf. Interactions: Exploring Aspects of Design Thinking XVII(2) (2010)
19. O'Connor, N., Duffy, T., Ferguson, P., Gurrin, C., Lee, H., Sadlier, D., Smeaton, A.F., Zhang, K.: A content-based retrieval system for UAV-like video and associated metadata. In: SPIE Defence and Security Conference 2008 (2008)
20. O'Connor, N., Lee, H., Smeaton, A.F., Jones, G., Cooke, E., le Borgne, H., Gurrin, C.: Físchlár-TRECVid2004: Combined text- and image-based searching of video archives. In: ISCAS 2006 - IEEE International Symposium on Circuits and Systems (2006)

21. O'Hare, N., Smeaton, A.F.: Context-aware person identification in personal photo collections. IEEE Transactions on Multimedia, Special Issue on Integration of Context and Content for Multimedia Management (2009)

22. Rogers, Y., Bellotti, V.: Grounding blue-sky research: how can ethnography help? Interactions 4(3), 58–63 (1997)

23. Sadlier, D., Lee, H., Gurrin, C., Smeaton, A.F., O'Connor, N.: User-feedback on a feature-rich photo organiser. In: WIAMIS 2008 - 9th Intl. Workshop. Image Analysis for Multimedia Interactive Services (2008)

24. Sadlier, D., O'Connor, N.: Event detection in field sports video using audio-visual features and a support vector machine. IEEE Transactions on Circuits and Systems for Video Technolog 15(10), 1225–1233 (2005); (Pereira, F., van Beek, P., Kot, A.C., Ostermann, J. (eds.))

25. Sav, S., Jones, G., Lee, H., O'Connor, N., Smeaton, A.F.: Interactive experiments in object-based retrieval. In: Sundaram, H., Naphade, M., Smith, J.R., Rui, Y. (eds.) CIVR 2006. LNCS, vol. 4071, pp. 1–10. Springer, Heidelberg (2006)

26. Sengers, P., Gaver, B.: Staying open to interpretation: engaging multiple meanings in design and evaluation. In: DIS 2006, pp. 99–108. ACM, New York (2006)

27. Shneiderman, B., Plaisant, C., Cohen, M., Jacob, S.: Designing the user interface: strategies for effective Human-Computer Interaction, cf. 3.4 Development methodologies; 3.5 Ethnographic observation, and 3.7 Scenario development, 5th edn. Addison-Wesley, Reading (2009)

28. Smeaton, A.F., Lee, H., Foley, C., McGivney, S.: Collaborative video searching on a tabletop. Multimedia Systems Journal 12(4), 375–391 (2006)

29. Smeaton, A.F., Over, P., Doherty, A.: Video shot boundary detection: Seven years of trecvid activity. Computer Vision and Image Understanding (2009)

30. Wolf, T.V., Rode, J.A., Sussman, J., Kellogg, W.A.: Dispelling "design" as the black art of CHI. In: CHI 2006, pp. 521–530. ACM, New York (2006)

31. Zimmerman, J., Forlizzi, J., Evenson, S.: Research through design as a method for interaction design research in HCI. In: CHI 2007: Proceedings of the SIGCHI Conference on Human Factors in Computing Systems, pp. 493–502. ACM, New York (2007)

Metadata Aggregation for Personalized Music Playlists

A Multi-layered Architecture for an In-Car Prototype

Clemens Hahn[1,2], Stéphane Turlier[1,3], Thorsten Liebig[2],
Sascha Gebhardt[1,4], and Christopher Roelle[1]

[1] BMW Group Research and Technology, Munich, Germany
[2] Ulm University, Faculty of Computer Science, Ulm, Germany
[3] Eurécom, Multimedia Communications Department, Sophia-Antipolis, France
[4] University of Munich, Department of Informatics, Munich, Germany

Abstract. The growing amount of digital music content and the increasing connectivity of vehicles raise new challenges in terms of media access for vehicle drivers. Creating easily a personalized playlist in vehicles involves a unified representation of various metadata, combined with a mobile architecture addressing media resolution and aggregation issues. This paper analyzes the technical aspects of mobile access to music metadata and its use in a personalized playlist generation scenario. A prototype illustrates this study and gives first results.

Keywords: Metadata, content aggregation, mobile architecture, playlist creation.

1 Introduction

Music is one of the most consumed media assets in vehicles. The increasing vehicle internet connectivity is bringing more multimedia content to the mobile use every day. Digital music assets are nowadays distributed on-demand by internet services for their consumption.

A typical use case in a modern vehicle is: The driver wants to quickly select specific online digital music tracks, in order to create a playlist corresponding to his tastes of the moment. Since his primary task is to drive a vehicle, this selection process has to provide first class user guidance in terms of minimal interaction, presentation and explanation. While driving, he wants to be able to influence the composition of the playlist by choosing alternative tracks or music styles, without having to reformulate the whole selection query.

The vehicle integration and adaptation of such services is raising a lot of technical challenges in terms of software architecture, network infrastructure and usability. We will address the following aspects in this paper:

G. Leitner, M. Hitz, and A. Holzinger (Eds.): USAB 2010, LNCS 6389, pp. 427–442, 2010.

- provide the user with playlist generation techniques that require few interactions but still allow granularity.
- define an efficient architecture, adapted to the mobile use and the vehicle
  requirements.
- make use of internet cloud metadata from external providers while containing
  the software complexity overhead.

We will first present the problem of playlist creation for vehicles in section 2 and
describe the state of the art in section 3. After a technical discussion about the
different sources of music metaknowledge according to their integrability into
a mobile architecture in section 4 and we will propose a prototype of playlist
generation, that takes into account architecture constraints for the aggregation
of content, as well as techniques that allow the user to take advantage of it and
consume easily music in a vehicle.

2   Using Metaknowledge to Create Music Playlists

From a user's point of view, the creation of a playlist is an optimization problem
between the time necessary to create the playlist and the quantity of music assets
which are available. Important parameters are the quantity and the quality of
available information that helps the user to make his decisions. We will discuss
in this section the different kinds of criteria that can be used to create a playlist
and explain how a mobile device like a vehicle can access them.

2.1   Techniques for the Creation of Music Playlists

Digitalized music is a media asset that can be sorted and selected through different techniques [2].

Creating Playlists Based on Music Similarity

- **acoustic similarity:** different low-level features (MFCCs or MPEG-7) can
  be extracted from the audio signal and using data mining techniques to
  compute similarity, [10], [9].
- **expert opinion:** the music genome project [24] has identified more than
  400 musical attributes that are analyzed by experts and saved in a database.
- **social information:** Social services allow users to share free-text tags,
  tracks, artists or genre favorites, playlists and to write comments. They often
  implement implicit relevance feedback mechanisms based on the monitoring
  of the user behavior (like the scrobbling protocol [13] from Last.FM[1]). Based
  on this information, it is possible to compute playlist co-occurrence [3], or
  to analyze common tags between playlists.

---

[1] http://www.last.fm/

Creating Playlists Based on Filtering Criteria

- **artistic performance:** The semantic description of music performances [19] can help to define playlist creation criteria: author information, performer, instrument, year of release, etc.
- **high-level acoustic features:** Based on the accoustic features mentioned previously, MPEG-7 defines high-level descriptors such as *Timbre*, *Melody* and *Tempo*. They can be considered as understandable for all users, even those with minimal music expertise.
- **genre:** Genres are defined on cultural and historical backgrounds [14]. They define commonly accepted cultural properties of music composition and performance.
- **mood:** A mood is a long lasting personal affect. The energy-stress [22], or valence-arousal [21] models have been developed by psychology research to semantically describe it. Regarding music the Moodswing [11] proposes a technique to select music according to the mood.
- **web crawled information:** The world wide web is an important source of comments on musical performances. Analyzing it allows to identify the popularity of an artist (how often the artist has been quoted in musical reviews) and his hotness (how he he has been quoted the last week).

2.2 Accessing Media Information Knowledge

Accessing the information we have defined in 2.1 is a crucial step to its aggregation and its use in playlist generation. This section describes the different types of multimedia metaknowledge sources that can be used to filter music tracks. In our context, metaknowledge means every kind of knowledge about the content that can help in selecting it among others through one or several criteria. We draw a distinction between metadata that is extracted from the content, metacontent that is delivered together with the content and metainformation that can be linked to the content.

Agent Self Extracted Metadata. A first option to access knowledge is to extract it directly from the content (see table 1). Low-level features as well as some high-level features can be accessed this way.

In spite of their advantages, we believe that the metadata extraction has currently too many shortcomings to be integrated as such in a vehicle. This is the reason why we decided not to use this technique in our prototype. However, we will consider in section 4.3 other external services that propose to deliver metacontent extracted from the content itself.

Co-delivered Metacontent. Metacontent like the performing artist, or a cover art illustration is delivered together with the audio content (see table 2). This knowledge is tightly linked to the value chain (see 4.1) of the music distribution;

Table 1. Self extracted metadata

Playlist creation	Integration in a mobile device
Advantages	
The quality of the metadata is entirely based on the quality of the extraction. The more features can be extracted, the more criteria can be used. A lot of algorithms based on similarity are available.	Extracting information directly in the client limits the need of internet connectivity.
Disadvantages	
Low-level descriptors are useful for the computation of music similarity but cannot be used as such as filtering criteria by a user with no music expertise. Pure acoustic based music selection has shown some limits and underperforms, methods based on high-level data[5].	The extraction of metadata in a multi-layered architecture does not scale to the aggregation role. Considering the chain value, the dynamic computation of such features in a client or in an aggregator does not scale to the increasing amount of available content.

from the producer to the publisher and to the online provider. It mainly consists in expert information: track name, artist name, album name, year of release. The ID3 tags were one of the first attempts to propose a standard way to deliver track, artist, album and genre information, within the MP3 mediacontainer. Afterwards then other formats have been proposed based on structured binary information of the mediacontainer, or XML formats.

Separately Delivered Metainformation. In the past years, an increasing amount of internet services aimed at federating new sources of metainformation without providing music data themselves. We can distinguish:

- textual information based on web crawling.
- music similarity: it can be based on automated music analysis (Gracenote), expert annotations (Music Genome Project), or social information (playlist-co-occurrence).
- social tagging and classification, like Last.fm or Finetune who allow their user to give free-text tags to the tracks or the artists, and compare user profiles based on the listening behavior.

Since they do not propose the content themselves (see table 3), they all need to implement some kind of identification in order to deliver the metacontent for a specific music track. This identification can be based:

- either on extracted metadata: computation of a unique fingerprint of the track [4],[1];

Table 2. Co-delivered metacontent

Playlist creation	Integration in a mobile device
Advantages	
Correctness: Co-delivered metacontent has usually a very good quality in terms of reliability.	This type of metacontent does not need any extra processing neither on client side nor on aggregation side.
Disadvantages	
Consistency: spelling differences between different providers may lead an aggregating recommender system to propose twice the same artists or oppositely to underestimate his importance. Completeness: for taxonomic values like genre or mood, the inner structure (number of genre, hierarchy, dependency between semantic concepts) can vary a lot between providers.	The whole content need to be requested even if only the metadata is necessary.

- or on the co-delivered textual metacontent: the metadata is available through a search engine using the name of the track, or the name of the artist performing it.

3   Related Work

The music information and retrieval (MIR) research has already presented recommender systems to help users to create playlists. The *Simple Playlist Generator* [15] proposes to create a playlist based on a seed song. Using the user's skipping behavior [16], it is possible to infer implicit relevance feedback and improve the playlists.

In the field of data visualization, the development of user interfaces for the display of music libraries such as in [12] or [8], has also lead indirectly to propose clients capable of creating music playlist by selecting regions on a map.

A third important aspect in the literature are the recommender systems based on user input filters. Satisfly [17] proposes to select the variance around a genre, an interpret, or an album, as well as a desired tempo or a specific time period (*i.e.* 60', 70', etc.). Musiclens [7] uses other original metadata like the intention of the music, importance of the voice or number of instruments.

Most of this research effort has focused on finding innovative ways to use metaknowledge for the creation of playlists. However, they gave rather little focus to the analysis of the quality of the metaknowledge for an online scenario

Table 3. Separately delivered metainformation

Playlist creation	Integration in a mobile device
Advantages	
Those data are independent from the content provider, so they are not influenced by commercial orientations and it allows addressing simultaneously different content providers. Some kind of information like popularity, can only be gathered through transverse crawling methods (web information, radio charts, etc.), that content providers do not provide.	Most of those services can be abstracted and aggregated in a multi-layered architecture.
Disadvantages	
Correctness: folksonomy and other user generated content need often extraprocessing of normalization [18]. The lack of consistency in the co-delivered metacontent may cause problem to retrieve linked metainformation.	The architecture of such system is less efficient than former systems, since the query of new metadata requires bidirectional exchange of information.

where the content changes every day, and the way to integrate it efficiently in a mobile infrastructure. Moreover, most of them did not address the topic of vehicle clients which have limited user interaction possibilities.

4   Prototype

Before giving the details of our prototype we think it is important to analyze what are the different sources of content and metacontent that we need in order to perform playlist generation in a vehicle using daily changing on-demand media.

4.1   Role Definition

The music industry is a complex ecosystem that has been dramatically changed by the digitizing of music assets [20]. The generation of playlists and more generally the selection and display of media content can be schematically positioned at the end the value chain, after the production and publication of content (see figure 1).

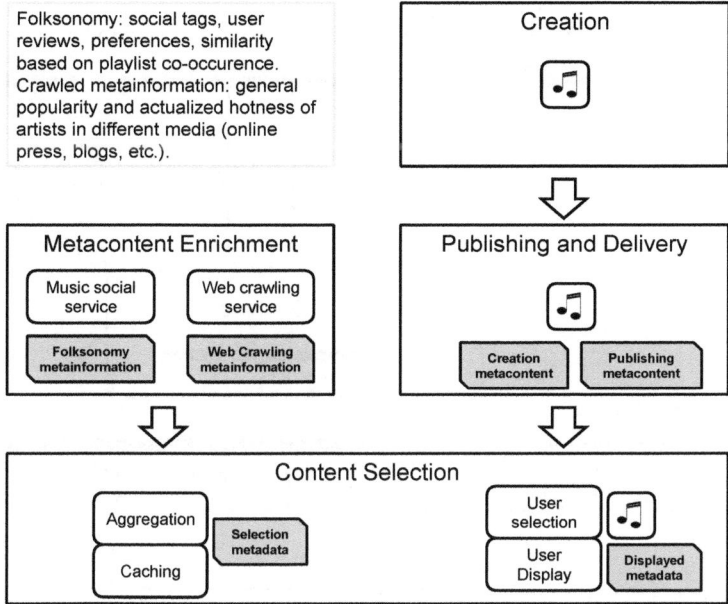

Fig. 1. Extension of the value chain, with internet services

With the development of internet as a media distribution channel, new services have emerged which do not propose content but rather metadata. We identify mainly two categories of them.

– Web crawlers and cloud services: They provide metadata based on information gathered from the web.
– Social services: They provide information based on social services.

On the one hand, the increasing amount of information available through this services simplifies some processing tasks for the clients as we announced in 2.1 but on the other hand they involve a multiplication of interfaces which would lead to a serious overhead in the software complexity of vehicle clients, and increase the latency needed to access those services. New functional roles need to be developed in order to achieve:

– The aggregation of multiple providers, like music providers and metacontent providers while maintaining a low software complexity.
– The caching of metacontent to interconnect structured information and provide reactive user interfaces.

4.2 Functional Architecture

Our prototype focuses on the implementation of a multilayered architecture.

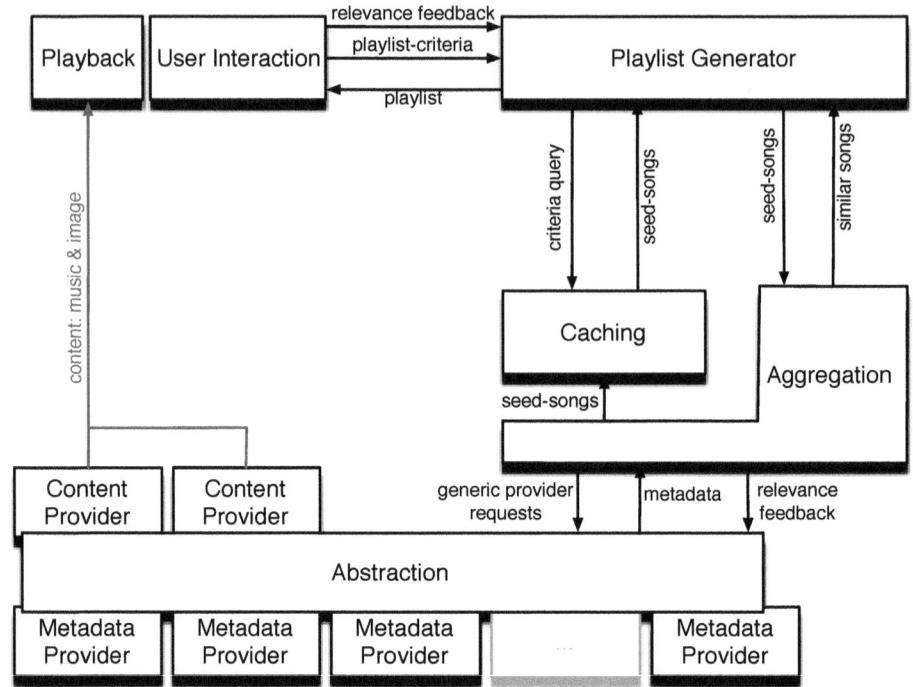

Fig. 2. The functional components of the architecture for generating playlists in a mobile environment

Abstraction. Since the prototype uses different kinds of metadata- and content-provider to have access to a comprehensive set of knowledge, it needs to access them all in a common way. This component abstracts their functionalities by providing common functions like *search for track* or *similar tracks for* a specific song to other software components. Thereby the precise implementation of the several providers is hidden to the frontend and the playlist generator.

Aggregation. The data is collected and merged from different providers through the abstraction component. This component builds up information entities which hold all required metadata. The set of required metadata is defined by the caching component.

During the aggregation of data different metadata sources have to be assembled. Our prototype uses metadata provided by experts as well as metadata provided by the so called folksonomies. To assemble them the system has to consider factors like spelling differences in track or artist names and the various kinds of identifiers.

Caching. This component caches a representative sample of the digital available music of our content providers. In order to best support the user in his playlist generation process, the system must react to the user interactions very fast. Short reaction times reduce the risk of distraction from the primary task of the vehicle-driver. Thereby, it reduces the cognitive disorder.

These cached information permits a multi-criteria playlist generation. The cached tracks have to support the following attributes:

- name of track, artist and album;
- year of release;
- genre and mood information;
- ratings of the popularity;
- user specific ratings;
- album cover;
- download URL of the audio data.

The Aggregation component provides this component with metadata, collected from different providers. This data collections and caching process is scheduled as a background process, independently from the playlist generation process.

Playlist Generator. This component receives from the vehicle, resp. from the driver, a set of criteria which are the constraints for the desired playlist. By matching these criteria with cached songs it receives some seed-songs. These seed-songs provide the starting-point of the generated playlist. Combined with similar tracks to these seed-songs (over the Aggregation and Abstraction component), a playlist is automatically built up (for details see section 4.2 - the interlacing strategy).

User Interaction & Playback. By interacting with this component the user can control the whole system. As described he can select different criteria for his playlist. He can combine the following criteria in order to tell the system his current music tastes:

- **Genre:** A hierarchicaly structured tree with 8 top level genres like *Rock, Pop, Jazz, Classical* and so on;
- **Mood:** A set of 25 moods, ordered in a valence-arousal grid;
- **Popularity:** A three stepped scale from *underground* over *mainstream* to *hot*;
- **Year:** A period of time or the exact year of publication;
- **Origin:** A personalized option like music from the own repository or loved songs.

For each selected criteria a preview of the playlist is presented. The songs of the preview derive from the caching component. Therefore they can be displayed very fast.

After the user has selected all his playlist constraints, the Playlist Generator builds up a list of tracks which fit these criteria. Thereupon the Generator returns

Table 4. Similar tracks for two seed song, collected from Last.fm's web service

seed song 1: Mando Diao - Gloria		seed song 2: Kasabian - Fast Fuse	
T1,1 Mando Diao	High Heels	T1,2 Kasabian	Take Aim
T2,1 The Libertines	Can't Stand Me Now	T2,2 Arctic Monkeys	Fire and the Thud
T3,1 Johnossi	Man Must Dance	C4 **Editors**	**Munich**
C1 **The Kooks**	**Do You Wanna**	T3,2 White Lies	Death
T4,1 Sugarplum Fairy	She	T4,2 Franz Ferdinand	Turn It On
T5,1 The Hives	Walk Idiot Walk	T5,2 Arctic Monkeys	Potion Approaching
C2 **The Hives**	**Tick Tick Boom**	C1 **The Kooks**	**Do You Wanna**
T6,1 Johnossi	18 Karat Gold	T6,2 The Libertines	Can't Stand Me Now
T7,1 Razorlight	Wire To Wire	C3 **Razorlight**	**America**
C3 **Razorlight**	**America**	C2 **The Hives**	**Tick Tick Boom**
C4 **Editors**	**Munich**	T7,2 Kaiser Chiefs	The Angry Mob

the playlist to the user. Each track of the list has a download URL attribute. So the vehicle can request the songs directly from the content providers and playback them.

Query Adaption via Preference Relaxation. In the case that a filter combination will not produce any results due to conflicting criteria the search query is gradually relaxed along the path of the category taxonomy. In particular, the most specific categories are replaced with their respective more general super categories until there are matching results which can be combined to a playlist of reasonable size. This approach is easily extensible to more sophisticated relaxation mechanism which incorporates additional domain knowledge into account such as those described in [23] for instance.

Fast Filter Criteria Preview through Pre-Cached Content. In order to support the driver in his playlist generation process a preview of the desired playlist will be offered. Each time the filter criteria changes a new preview demonstrates its influence on the final result.

The user can add as many filters as he wants, while filters from different categories are linked by a logical AND and filters from the same category are linked by a logical OR. We expect the user to naturally assume that kind of linkage.

Track Interlacing Strategy and Parallel Metadata Aggregation. Once a preview has been requested, the backend starts automatically a playlist generation process in background and saves the results. If the user is pleased with the preview, the playlist is transferred from the backend to the frontend, otherwise, it is deleted.

Since we are using different metadata providers to generate the playlist we had to develop an algorithm to combine the results. The playlist generation

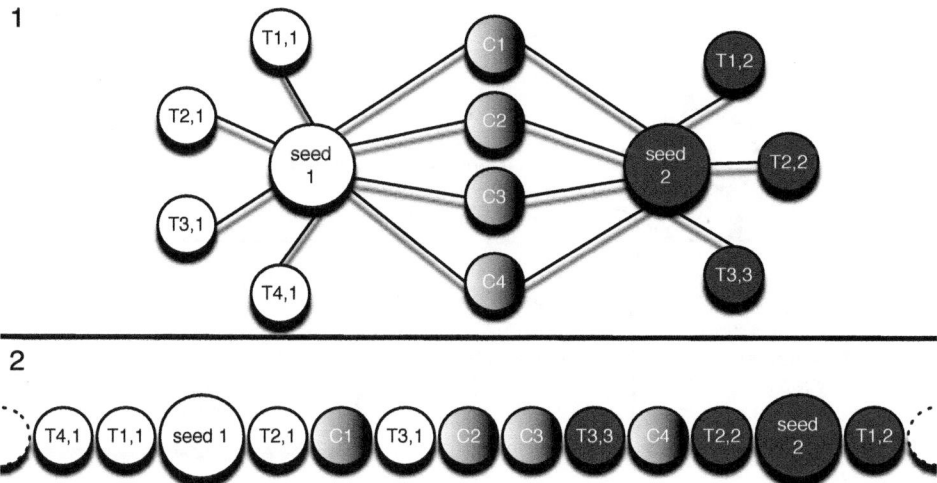

Fig. 3. The interlacing method to generate playlists with smooth track-to-track inter-sections. At the top two seed-songs with similar tracks (T) and common similar tracks (C). At the bottom the generated playlist with interlaced tracks for two seed-songs.

process is based on the preview tracks which consist in a list of n seed songs; $S[0] = \{s_1, s_2, ..., s_n\}$. For every s_k there is set of m_k recommendations $\mathcal{R}_{s_k} = \{t_{1,k}, t_{2,k}, ..., t_{m_k,k}\}$ which is retrieved from metadata providers. Our algorithm process incrementally and takes the first seed song s_1 and searches in $s_2, ..., s_n$ a song s_k such that the cardinal of $\mathcal{C}_{s_1,s_k} = \mathcal{R}_{s_1} \cap \mathcal{R}_{s_k}$ is maximum, that is to say that the recommendations of s_1 and s_k have the maximum of tracks in common (see figure 3-1). The algorithm then carries on with the set $S[1] = \{s_k, s_2, ..., s_{k-1}, s_{k+1}, ..., s_n\}$ where s_1 has been removed, until $S[n-1]$ when the set of seed songs is exhausted. This way, we create an ordered listed chain of seed-songs $S' = \{s_1, s'_2..., s'_n\}$ where s'_k are a permutation of s_k and sets of common songs which can have different cardinality $\mathcal{C}_{s_i,s_j}$. A playlist can be created by placing the common songs between the seed songs as following: s'_i, $\mathcal{C}_{s'_{i+1},s'_i} \setminus \mathcal{C}_{s'_i,s'_{i-1}}$, s'_{i+1}, $\mathcal{C}_{s'_{i+2},s'_{i+1}} \setminus \mathcal{C}_{s'_{i+1},s'_i}$, where $\mathcal{C}_x \setminus \mathcal{C}_y$ is the difference between the sets C_x and C_y.

The figure 3-2 and the table 4 illustrate how the remaining tracks that are not common to the seed songs (*i.e.* they belong to the complementary of $\mathcal{C}_{s'_i,s'_{i+1}}$ in $\mathcal{R}_{s'_i} \cup \mathcal{R}_{s'_{i+1}}$) are interlaced between the common tracks completing the result, in order to create a playlist smoothly going from a seed song to another.

In order to deliver a playlist to the user as fast as possible, the collections of similar songs are (a) parallel retrieved and (b) the playlist generation is split in multiple parts. The parallel request for similar tracks accelerates the generation

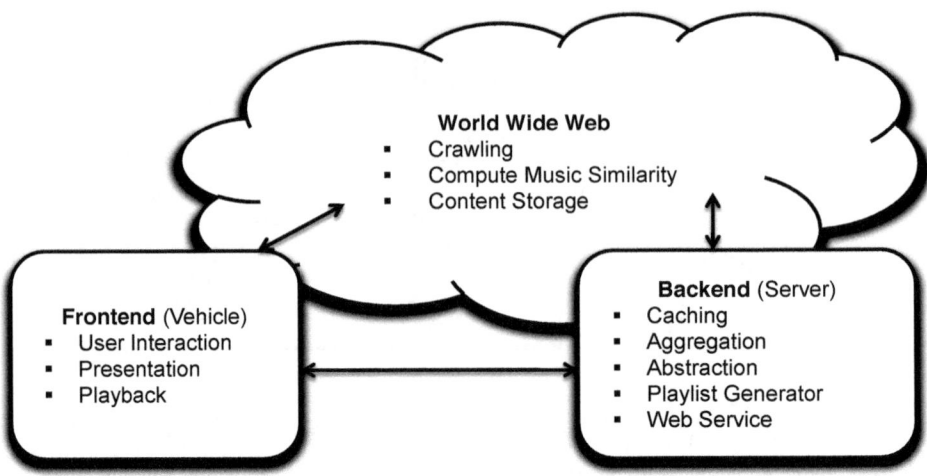

Fig. 4. The hardware architecture of the prototype

process. Depending on the latency of the service providers, waiting for the response takes a significant amount of time in generating the playlist. By splitting up the playlist a first part of it can be delivered in an acceptable delay to the user. Thereupon, while listening to the first tracks of the playlist, the other parts can be built up in background.

4.3   Deployment Architecture for a Mobile Use

The presented functional components have to be deployed on an adequate hardware architecture. The prototype is split into two main applications: firstly the graphical user interface (the so called frontend), with whom the user can interact in the car and secondly a server (backend). A conceptual model of this architecture is presented in figure 1. The discussed functional components are mapped to the corresponding hardware components.

Frontend. The UI-Prototype we implemented for the frontend is written in Flash. The input/output-devices used in the prototype are the controller knob (a push-shift-rotate controller) for input and the central information display (CID) for visual output. The music playback performs over the car audio system. The flash application runs in a Web-Browser based on Webkit and specifically developed to read commands from the controller. Commands are forwarded to the flash run-time using JavaScript. The browser is capable of handling gzip compression over HTTP, which helps reducing the latency of exchanging requests.

We use a 7 Series BMW for our experimental vehicle. It is equipped with an UMTS router and the described visual and haptic interface. A picture of the user interface in the vehicle is presented in figure 5.

Backend. We installed on a server a servlet container (Glassfish) and a relational database (MySQL). The functional component *Caching* is mapped to the relational database. The components *Abstraction*, *Aggregation* and *Playlist Generator* are deployed in the servlet container . The *Abstraction* handles the access to the several providers by implementing the web service API over WSDL or REST. The *Aggregation* and *Playlist Generator* implement the business logic.

World Wide Web. The several providers for metadata and audio/image-content reside in the world wide web. These providers aggregate dynamically metadata by crawling the web for music related content. They also support services to identify tracks and deliver similar music to given seed-songs. We use the music-catalog from Rhapsody[2] with over 9 Mio. songs as content-provider as well as metadata-provider. Additionally Gracenote[3] supplies the prototype with mood-information. The social network Last.fm and the web crawler The Echo Nest complete the list of the metadata providers that we have used.

The backend offers a web service that can be accessed by the frontend. This service is designed in a RESTful style [6]. The data is transferred between front- and backend in XML format over HTTP.

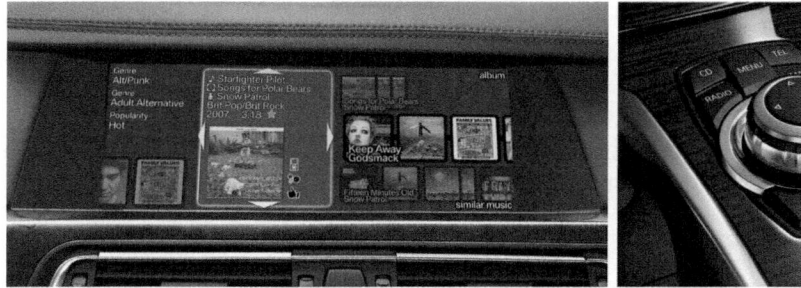

Fig. 5. The experimental vehicle. left: graphical user interface, right: controller knob.

First Results. We monitored the response time of the server to the client based on the simulation of 1000 user preview queries that generated around 1600 queries from the frontend to the backend, with a number of playlist criteria from 1 to 6. As depicted in figure 6, the response time does not depend of the number of criteria (still it is only database selects on the different rows of the track table) and remains reasonable from user experience since the user does not have to wait longer than 3 seconds. The variability in the results can be explained by the jitter of mobile communications, the very changing latency of internet web services. In order to permit an almost immediate start of the final playlist, its first three tracks are always composed of cached tracks, while

---

[2] http://www.rhapsody.com

[3] http://www.gracenote.com

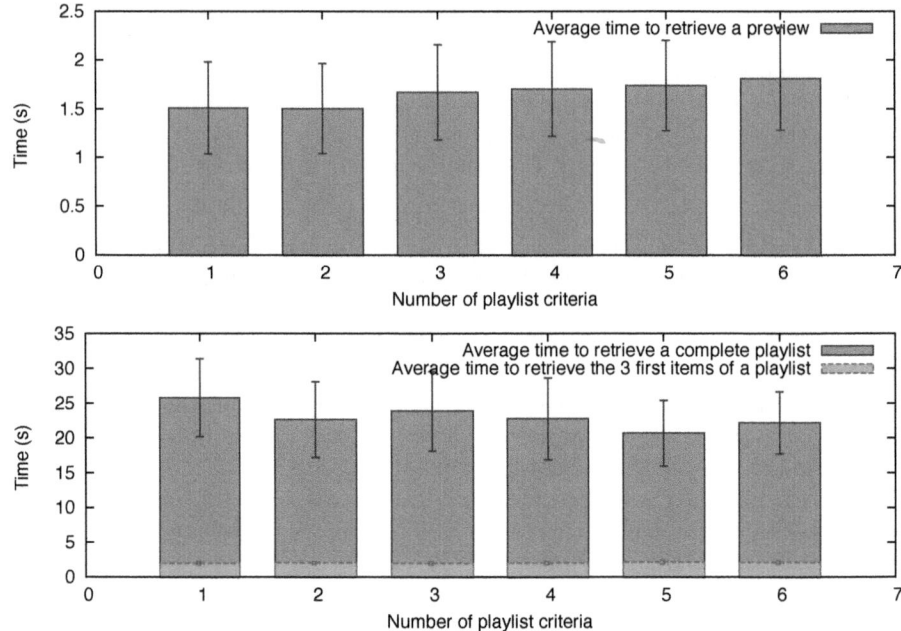

Fig. 6. Response time for the preview and the playlist over 1000 user queries

our system retrieves additional metadata in the background with the algorithm described formerly. As a result, the rendering of the playlist can start right after the preview.

5   Conclusion and Future Works

We have analyzed the issues encountered when tackling the topic of personalized playlist creation in a vehicle. Our vehicle scenario involves usability aspects like selecting different metadata filters to create a playlist, overcoming the latency of some internet services and proposing the user alternative choices to modify the final result.

We have presented a prototype to illustrate how the main functional components, user display, caching, aggregation and abstraction can be deployed in a mobile architecture. We have noticed that even if this deployment gives satisfying results it could be improved to provide a more reactive interface for the preview of user queries.

We believe that new web technologies that will be implemented in mobile devices like HTML 5 browsers or Adobe Air, allow the development of efficient caching methods on the client side. Combined with a synchronization mechanism with our backend, a future version of our client will be able to give immediate previews of user queries avoiding the latency of backend requests.

References

1. Allamanche, E.: Content-based identification of audio material using mpeg-7 low level description. In: ISMIR (2001)
2. Berenzweig, A., Logan, B., Ellis, D.P.W., Whitman, B.P.W.: A large-scale evaluation of acoustic and subjective music-similarity measures. Computer Music Journal 28(2), 63–76 (2004)
3. Bernhardsson, E.: Implementing a Scalable Music Recommender System. Master's thesis (2009)
4. Cano, P., Batlle, E., Kalker, T., Haitsma, J.: A review of algorithms for audio fingerprinting. VLSI Signal Processing 41(3), 271–284 (2005)
5. Celma, O.: Music Recommendation and Discovery in the Long Tail. Ph.D. thesis, Universitat Pompeu Fabra, Barcelona, Spain (2008), http://mtg.upf.edu/~ocelma/PhD/doc/ocelma-thesis.pdf
6. Fielding, R.: Architectural styles and the design of network-based software architectures. Ph.D. thesis, Citeseer (2000)
7. Finetunes: musiclens - in tune with you (2010), http://finetunes.musiclens.de/ (accessed June 9, 2010)
8. van Gulik, R., Vignoli, F.: Visual playlist generation on the artist map. In: Proceedings of the International Conference on Music Information Retrieval ISMIR, Citeseer (2005)
9. Haitsma, J., Kalker, T.: A highly robust audio fingerprinting system. In: ISMIR (2002)
10. Kastner, T., Allamanche, E., Herre, J., Hellmuth, O., Cremer, M., Grossmann, H.: Mpeg-7 scalable robust audio fingerprinting (May 2002)
11. Kim, Y., Schmidt, E., Emelle, L.: Moodswings: A collaborative game for music mood label collection. In: Proc. Intl. Symp. Music Information Retrieval (2008)
12. Lillie, A.S.: MusicBox: Navigating the space of your music. Master's thesis, School of Architecture and Planning, Massachusetts Institute of Technology (September 2008)
13. Audioscrobbler Ltd. Audioscrobbler. The social music technology playground (2010), http://www.audioscrobbler.net/ (accessed June 9, 2010)
14. Pachet, F., Cazaly, D.: A Taxonomy of Musical Genres. In: Proceedings of the 1st Conference of Content-Based Multimedia Information Access (RIAO), Paris, France (April 2000)
15. Pampalk, E., Gasser, M.: An implementation of a simple playlist generator based on audio similarity measures and user feedback (2006)
16. Pampalk, E., Pohle, T., Widmer, G.: Dynamic playlist generation based on skipping behavior. In: Proc. of Int. Symposium on Music Information Retrieval (2005)
17. Pauws, S., van de Wijdeven, S.: User evaluation of a new interactive playlist generation concept. In: Proc. Sixth International Conference on Music Information Retrieval (ISMIR 2005), Citeseer, vol. 11, p. 15 (2005)
18. Peters, I., Weller, K.: Tag gardening for folksonomy enrichment and maintenance. Webology 5(3) (2008)
19. Raimond, Y.: A Distributed Music Information System. Ph.D. thesis, Queen Mary, University of London (November 2008)
20. Rayport, J., Sviokla, J.: Exploiting the Virtual Value Chain. The McKinsey Quarterly (1), 21–22 (1996)

21. Russell, J.: A circumplex model of affect. Journal of personality and social psychology 39(6), 1161–1178 (1980)
22. Thayer, R.: The biopsychology of mood and arousal. Oxford University Press, USA (1989)
23. Wagner, M., Liebig, T., Noppens, O., Balzer, S., Kellerer, W.: Towards Semantic-based Service Discovery on Tiny Mobile Devices
24. Westergren, T.: The music genome project (2010),
    `http://www.pandora.com/mgp.shtml` (accessed June 9, 2010)

Instant Video Browsing: A Tool for Fast Non-sequential Hierarchical Video Browsing

Manfred del Fabro, Klaus Schoeffmann, and Laszlo Böszörmenyi

Institute of Information Technology, Klagenfurt University, Austria
{manfred,ks,laszlo}@itec.uni-klu.ac.at

Abstract. We introduce an easy-to-use video browsing tool which assists users in getting a quick overview of videos as well as in finding segments of interest. It provides a parallel and a tree-based view for browsing the content of videos – or even video collections – in a hierarchical, non-sequential manner. The tool has a plug-in architecture and can be extended both by further presentation methods and by video analysis algorithms.

1 Introduction

Video browsing is an appealing approach to find out whether a video or some parts of it are of interest and where the most interesting segments are located within a video. Usually, video browsing solutions are based on content analysis of the underlying video. Almost all proposed solutions use shot segmentation as a first step and provide browsing mechanisms based on the shot structure. Content analysis – of a newly stored video file – takes quite an amount of time. In some scenarios, e.g. when only a quick overview of the content of a video is required, it is an overkill to perform a deep content analysis. If single shot videos are browsed, shot detection does not help at all. Examples for single shot videos can be typically found in surveillance applications. For such scenarios it is much better to provide quick, yet powerful, interactive navigation means.

Several video browsing tools have been proposed in the recent years. While some of them try to improve navigation with extended timeline sliders (e.g. [1][2], others show content abstractions that can help users to more quickly locate desired segments [3][4]). Some other tools facilitate browsing by an index of extracted keyframes, typically at different levels of granularity (e.g. [5]), or by providing smart fast-forwarding features (e.g. [6]). A comprehensive review on video browsing applications can be found in [7].

We propose a novel approach for instant video browsing that requires no content analysis at all. Our application can immediately and efficiently be used for scenarios where a quick inspection of a newly recorded video is required. While video retrieval tools typically perform much better and provide better content-based search functions, they first need to perform a deep content analysis step requiring a lot of processing time (often in dimensions of several hours). Users, who just quickly want to get an overview of a new video or to find some specific

G. Leitner, M. Hitz, and A. Holzinger (Eds.): USAB 2010, LNCS 6389, pp. 443–446, 2010.

segments in it do usually not accept long delays before they can use the tool. From a preliminary user study [8] we know that users in such situations rather employ common video players for interactive browsing although they provide only poor navigation features. The tool proposed in this paper has been designed to provide a real alternative to common video players for such situations.

2   Instant Video Browsing

Our tool divides every video into as many parts of equal length, as there are video windows opened on the screen. The number of windows (n) can be increased or reduced by the user with a single click. Two different views are available for browsing the content: a *parallel* and a *tree based view*. With both of them it is possible to traverse the content in a hierarchical way down, until the frame level is reached, and up again.

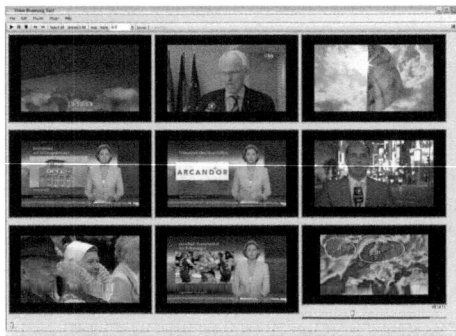

Fig. 1. Parallel View

An example of the parallel view is given in Figure 1, where a news video is divided into nine parts of equal length. If one of the parts is selected by clicking the right mouse button, the user gets down into a deeper level with more details. That means that the selected part is divided into n parts of equal length again. To get a coarser view again, it is possible to go back to a higher level. The parallel view only shows one level of the browsing hierarchy at a glance. In contrast the tree based view shows all levels simultaneously in a treelike structure, thus the context of the video windows is better preserved. Figure 2 shows an example[1] of the tree based view with a highlight video of a soccer match. Each row represents one level of the browsing hierarchy. The browsing history from the top to the bottom level is preserved by coloring the selected video parts on each layer with a green border. This should help the user to quickly find an alternative browsing path. If a part is selected, a new row that shows only that part is added to the

---

[1] The red lines between the horizontal window rows have been added to the screen shot for a better visualization of the tree-based browsing concept.

tree. Browsing through the content of a video this way can be compared with navigating through a tree structure. Having found the required scene the user may select the starting point of it as the new root. This enables the user to quickly locate a number of interesting scenes in a video.

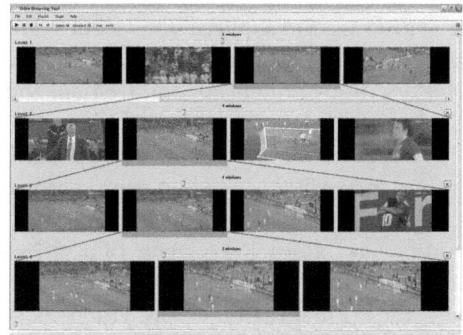

Fig. 2. Tree Based View

Beyond hierarchical browsing, the tool also offers parallel playback. All shown parts or only selected ones can be watched in parallel and the playback speed can be adjusted. The slider at the bottom of the container window can be used to scroll through selected videos in parallel. The users can get an impression of the whole video in a fraction of the overall duration. The audio playback is only enabled for one single selected video window (where the mouse points at). The ability to play the audio stream only of parts regarded to be interesting, helps the users in getting a better browsing experience.

The introduced views are not limited to single video files. They can be applied to small video collections as well. Opening a video archive adds an additional level to the browsing hierarchy, which means that on the first level all videos of the selected collection are shown, serving as starting point for hierarchical browsing of the whole video archive.

Another feature of our video browser is that segments of interest can be selected and stored in a playlist for later use. Moreover, selected segments can also be exported as a single file, which can be opened with a common video player. Thus, our browser is also a "poor men's" video cut tool.

Our video browsing tool offers a simple plug-in architecture. With new plug-ins it can be extended by further presentation views and also by video analysis and video processing algorithms. By combining different plug-ins it can be easily adjusted to the needs of the users and the peculiarities of different video domains.

Regarding the performance of the tool we can state that at least nine videos can be decoded and played in parallel with normal playback speed on a standard desktop computer (Pentium 4 2GHz, 1GB RAM).

3   Conclusion

The presented tool focuses on easy to use video browsing concepts for instant usage. The parallel view can be used to get an overview of the content of a video by using parallel playback or parallel scrolling. The tree view provides mechanisms for quickly exploring different search paths within a video and thus it is better suited for searching for a particular scene. Both approaches refrain from content analysis and work for single-shot videos as well. They provide a flexible user interface for non-sequential hierarchical video browsing and are suggested particularly for situations, in which video analysis is not adequate (e.g. due to lack of rich semantics) or would take too much time.

In future we are going to perform another user study to compare our video browser with other video players to measure the retrieval performance for situations where a user wants to get a quick overview of a video or a video collection. Furthermore, we plan to integrate several lightweight video analysis plug-ins to be able to perform a better segmentation of the videos. Users will be able to decide whether they use the instant approach or a more sophisticated one, based on fast video analysis steps.

References

1. Hürst, W.: Interactive audio-visual video browsing. In: Proceedings of the 14th annual ACM International Conference on Multimedia, pp. 675–678. ACM, New York (2006)
2. Dragicevic, P., Ramos, G., Bibliowitcz, J., Nowrouzezahrai, D., Balakrishnan, R., Singh, K.: Video browsing by direct manipulation. In: CHI 2008: Proceeding of the Twenty-Sixth Annual SIGCHI Conference on Human Factors in Computing Systems, pp. 237–246. ACM, New York (2008)
3. Barbieri, M., Mekenkamp, G., Ceccarelli, M., Nesvadba, J.: The color browser: a content driven linear video browsing tool. In: IEEE International Conference on Multimedia and Expo., ICME 2001, pp. 627–630 (2001)
4. Schoeffmann, K., Taschwer, M., Boeszoermenyi, L.: The video explorer: a tool for navigation and searching within a single video based on fast content analysis. In: Proceedings of the First Annual ACM SIGMM Conference on Multimedia Systems, pp. 247–258. ACM, New York (2010)
5. Chang, L., Yang, Y., Hua, X.S.: Smart video player. In: 2008 IEEE International Conference on Multimedia and Expo., pp. 1605–1606 (April 23-26, 2008)
6. Cheng, K.Y., Luo, S.J., Chen, B.Y., Chu, H.H.: Smartplayer: user-centric video fast-forwarding. In: CHI 2009: Proceedings of the 27th International Conference on Human Factors in Computing Systems, pp. 789–798. ACM, New York (2009)
7. Schoeffmann, K., Hopfgartner, F., Marques, O., Boeszoermenyi, L., Jose, J.M.: Video browsing interfaces and applications: a review. SPIE Reviews 1(1) (2010)
8. Schoeffmann, K., Boeszoermenyi, L.: Interactive Video Browsing of H.264 Content Based on Just-in-Time Analysis. In: Angelides, M.C., Mylonas, P., Wallace, M. (eds.) Advances in Semantic Media Adaptation and Personalization, vol. 2, pp. 159–180. CRC Press, Boca Raton (February 2009)

An Experimental Investigation of the Akamai Adaptive Video Streaming

Luca De Cicco and Saverio Mascolo

Dipatimento di Elettrotecnica ed Elettronica, Politecnico di Bari,
Via Orabona n.4, Bari, Italy
ldecicco@gmail.com, mascolo@poliba.it

Abstract. Akamai offers the largest Content Delivery Network (CDN) service in the world. Building upon its CDN, it recently started to offer High Definition (HD) video distribution using HTTP-based adaptive video streaming. In this paper we experimentally investigate the performance of this new Akamai service aiming at measuring how fast the video quality tracks the Internet available bandwidth and to what extent the service is able to ensure continuous video distribution in the presence of abrupt changes of available bandwidth. Moreover, we provide details on the client-server protocol employed by Akamai to implement the quality adaptation algorithm. Main results are: 1) any video is encoded at five different bit rates and each level is stored at the server; 2) the video client computes the available bandwidth and sends a feedback signal to the server that selects the video at the bitrate that matches the available bandwidth; 3) the video bitrate matches the available bandwidth in roughly 150 seconds; 4) a feedback control law is employed to ensure that the player buffer length tracks a desired buffer length; 5) when an abrupt variation of the available bandwidth occurs, the suitable video level is selected after roughly 14 seconds and the video reproduction is affected by short interruptions.

1 Introduction and Related Works

Nowadays the Internet, that was originally designed to transport delay-insensitive data traffic, is becoming the most important platform to deliver audio/video delay-sensitive traffic. Important applications that feed this trend are YouTube, which delivers user-generated video content, and Skype audio/video conference over IP. In this paper we focus on adaptive (live) streaming that represents an advancement *wrt* classic progressive download streaming such as the one employed by YouTube. With download streaming, the video is a static file that is delivered as any data file using greedy TCP connections. The receiver employs a player buffer that allows the file to be stored in advance *wrt* the playing time in order to mitigate video interruptions. With adaptive streaming, the video source is adapted on-the-fly to the network available bandwidth. This represents a key advancement *wrt* classic download streaming for the following reasons: 1) live video content can be delivered in real-time; 2) the video quality can be continuously adapted to the

G. Leitner, M. Hitz, and A. Holzinger (Eds.): USAB 2010, LNCS 6389, pp. 447–464, 2010.
© Springer-Verlag Berlin Heidelberg 2010

network available bandwidth so that users can watch videos at the maximum bit rate that is allowed by the time-varying available bandwidth.

In [8] the authors develop analytic performance models to assess the performance of TCP when used to transport video streaming. The results suggest that in order to achieve good performance, TCP requires a network bandwidth that is two times the video bit rate. This bandwidth over provisioning would systematically waste half of the available bandwidth.

In a recent paper [6] the authors provide an evaluation of TCP streaming using an adaptive encoding based on H.264/SVC. In particular, the authors propose to throttle the GOP length in order to adapt the bitrate of the encoder to the network available bandwidth. Three different rate-control algorithms for adaptive video encoding are investigated. The results indicate that the considered algorithms perform well in terms of video quality and timely delivery both in the case of under-provisioned links and in the case of competing TCP flows.

In this paper we investigate the adaptive streaming service provided by Akamai, which is the worldwide leading Content Delivery Network (CDN). The service is called High Definition Video Streaming and aims at delivering HD videos over Internet connections using the Akamai CDN. The Akamai system is based on the *stream-switching* technique: the server encodes the video content at different bit rates and it switches from one video version to another based on client feedbacks such as the measured available bandwidth. It can be said that the Akamai approach is the leading commercial one since, as we will see shortly, it is employed by the Apple HTTP-based streaming, the Microsoft IIS server, the Adobe Dynamic Streaming, and Move Networks. By encoding the same video at different bitrates it is possible to overcome the scalability issues due to the processing resources required to perform multiple on-the-fly encoding at the price of increasing storage resources. HTTP-based streaming is cheaper to deploy since it employs standard HTTP servers and does not require specialized servers at each node.

In the following we summarize the main features of the leading adaptive streaming commercial products available in the market.

IIS Smooth Streaming [9] is a live adaptive streaming service provided by Microsoft. The streaming technology is offered as a web-based solution requiring the installation of a plug-in that is available for Windows and iPhone OS 3.0. The streaming technology is codec agnostic. IIS Smooth Streaming employs stream-switching approach with different versions encoded with configurable bitrates and video resolutions up to 1080p. In the default configuration IIS Smooth Streaming encodes the video stream in seven layers that range from 300 kbps up to 2.4 Mbps.

Adobe Dynamic Streaming [4] is a web-based adaptive streaming service developed by Adobe that is available to all devices running a browser with Adobe Flash plug-in. The server stores different streams of varying quality and size and switches among them during the playback, adapting to user bandwidth and CPU. The service is provided using the RTMP streaming protocol [5]. The supported video codecs are H.264 and VP6 which are included in the Adobe Flash plug-in. The advantage of Adobe's solution is represented by the wide availability of Adobe Flash plug-in at the client side.

Apple has recently released a client-side *HTTP Adaptive Live Streaming* solution [7]. The server segments the video content into several pieces with configurable duration and video quality. The server exposes a playlist (.m3u8) containing all the available video segments. The client downloads consecutive video segments and it dynamically chooses the video quality employing an undisclosed proprietary algorithm. Apple HTTP Live Streaming employs H.264 codec using a MPEG-2 TS container and it is available on any device running iPhone OS 3.0 or later (including iPad), or any computer with QuickTime X or later installed.

Move Networks provides live adaptive streaming service [2] to several TV networks such as ABC, FOX, Televisa, ESPN and others. A plug-in, available for the most used web browsers for Windows and Mac OS X, has to be installed to access the service. Move Networks employs VP7, a video codec developed by On2, a company that has been recently acquired by Google. Adaptivity to available bandwidth is provided using the stream-switching approach. Five different versions of the same video are available at the server with bitrates ranging from 100 kbps up to 2200 kbps.

The rest of the paper is organized as follows: Section 2 describes the testbed employed in the experimental evaluation; in Section 3 we show the main features of the client-server protocol used by Akamai in order to implement the quality adaptation algorithm; Section 4 provides a discussion of the obtained results along with an investigation of the dynamics of the quality adaptation algorithm; finally, Section 5 draws the conclusions of the paper.

2   Testbed and Experimental Scenarios

The experimental evaluation of Akamai HD video server has been carried out by employing the testbed shown in Figure 1. Akamai HD Video Server provides a number of videos made available through a demo website [1]. In the experiments we have employed the video sequence *"Elephant's Dream"* since its duration is long enough for a careful experimental evaluation. The receiving host is an Ubuntu Linux machine running 2.6.32 kernel equipped with NetEm, a kernel module that, along with the traffic control tools available on Linux kernels, allows downlink channel bandwidth and delays to be set. In order to perform traffic shaping on the downlink we used the Intermediate Functional Block pseudo-device IFB[1].

The receiving host was connected to the Internet through our campus wired connection. It is worth to notice that before each experiment we carefully checked that the available bandwidth was well above 5 Mbps that is the maximum value of the bandwidth we set in the traffic shaper. The measured RTT between our client and the Akamai server is of the order of 10 ms. All the measurements we report in the paper have been performed after the traffic shaper (as shown in Figure 1) and collected by dumping the traffic on the receiving host employing

---

[1] http://www.linuxfoundation.org/collaborate/workgroups/networking/ifb

`tcpdump`. The dump files have been post-processed and parsed using a Python script in order to obtain the figures shown in Section 4.

The receiving host runs an `iperf` server (TCP Receiver) in order to receive TCP greedy flows sent by an `iperf` client (TCP Sender).

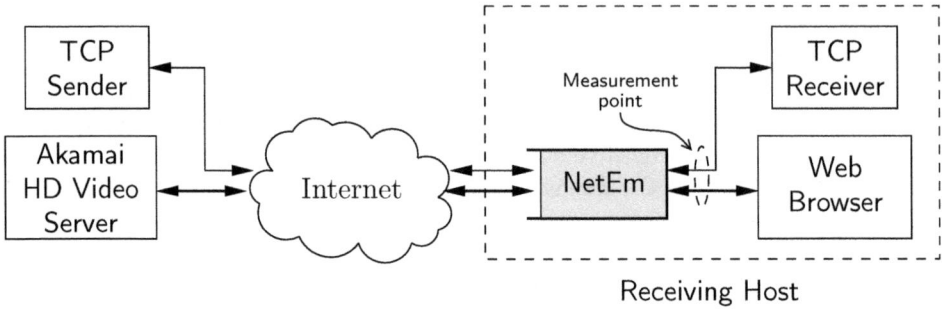

Fig. 1. Testbed employed in the experimental evaluation

Three different scenarios have been considered in order to investigate the dynamic behaviour of Akamai quality adaptation algorithm:

1. Akamai video flow over a bottleneck link whose bandwidth capacity changes following a step function with minimum value 400 kbps and maximum value 4000 kbps;
2. Akamai video flow over a bottleneck link whose bandwidth capacity varies as a square wave with a period of 200 s, a minimum value of 400 kbps and a maximum value of 4000 kbps;
3. Akamai video flow sharing a bottleneck, whose capacity is fixed to 4000 kbps, with one concurrent TCP flow.

In scenarios 1 and 2 abrupt variations of the available bandwidth occur: even though we acknowledge that such abrupt variations are not frequent in real-world scenarios, we stress that step-like variations of the input signal are often employed in control theory to evaluate the key features of a dynamic system response to an external input [3]. The third scenario is a common use-case designed to evaluate the dynamic behaviour of an Akamai video flow when it shares the bottleneck with a greedy TCP flow, such as in the case of a file download. In particular, we are interested in assessing if Akamai is able to grab the fair share in such scenarios.

3   Client-Server Quality Adaptation Protocol

Before discussing the dynamic behaviour of the quality adaptation algorithm employed by Akamai, we focus on the client-server protocol used in order to implement this algorithm.

To this purpose, we analyzed the dump file captured with `tcpdump` and we observed two main facts: 1) The Akamai server employs TCP in order to transport the video flows and 2) a number of HTTP requests are sent from the client to the server throughout all the duration of the video streaming. Figure 2 shows the time sequence graph of the HTTP requests sent from the client to the Akamai server reconstructed from the dump file.

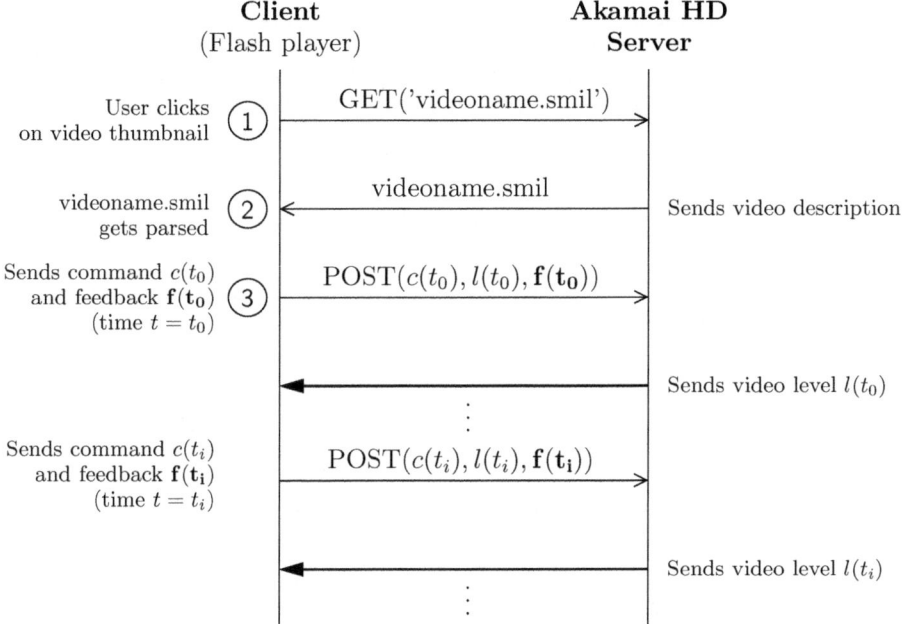

Fig. 2. Client-server time sequence graph: thick lines represent video data transfer, thin lines represent HTTP requests sent from client to server

At first, the client connects to the server [1], then a Flash application is loaded and a number of videos are made available. When the user clicks on the thumbnail (1) of the video he is willing to play, a GET HTTP request is sent to the server pointing to a Synchronized Multimedia Integration Language 2.0 (SMIL) compliant file[2]. The SMIL file provides the base URL of the video (`httpBase`), the available levels, and the corresponding encoding bit-rates. An excerpt of this file is shown in Figure 3.

Then, the client parses the SMIL file (2) so that it can easily reconstruct the complete URLs of the available video levels and it can select the corresponding video level based on the quality adaptation algorithm. All the videos available on the demo website are encoded at five different bitrates (see Figure 3). In particular, the video level bitrate $l(t)$ can assume values in the *set of available*

---

[2] `http://www.w3.org/TR/2005/REC-SMIL2-20050107/`

```
<head>
 <meta name="title" content="Elephants Dream" />
 <meta name="httpBase"
       content="http://efvod-hdnetwork.akamai.com.edgesuite.net/"/>
 <meta name="rtmpAuthBase" content="" />
</head>
<body>
 <switch id="Elephants Dream">
  <video src="ElephantsDream2_h264_3500@14411" system-bitrate="3500000"/>
  <video src="ElephantsDream2_h264_2500@14411" system-bitrate="2500000"/>
  <video src="ElephantsDream2_h264_1500@14411" system-bitrate="1500000"/>
  <video src="ElephantsDream2_h264_700@14411" system-bitrate="700000"/>
  <video src="ElephantsDream2_h264_300@14411" system-bitrate="300000"/>
 </switch>
</body>
```

Fig. 3. Excerpt of the SMIL file

video levels $L = \{l_0, \ldots, l_4\}$ at any given time instant t. Video levels are encoded at 30 frames per second (fps) using H.264 codec with a group of picture (GOP) of length 12. The audio is encoded with Advanced Audio Coding (AAC) at 128 kbps bitrate.

Table 1. Video levels details

Video level	Bitrate (kbps)	Resolution (width×height)
l_0	300	320x180
l_1	700	640x360
l_2	1500	640x360
l_3	2500	1280x720
l_4	3500	1280x720

Table 1 shows the video resolution for each of the five video levels l_i, that ranges from 320×180 up to high definition 1280×720.

It is worth to notice that each video level can be downloaded individually issuing a HTTP GET request using the information available in the SMIL file. This suggests that the server does not segment the video as in the case of the Apple HTTP adaptive streaming, but it encodes the original raw video source into N different files, one for each available level.

After the SMIL file gets parsed, at time $t = t_0$ (3), the client issues the first POST request specifying five parameters, two of which will be discussed in detail here[3]. The first POST parameter is cmd and, as its name suggests, it specifies a

---

[3] The remaining three parameters are not of particular importance. The parameter v reports the HDCore Library of the client, the parameter g is fixed throughout all the connection, whereas the parameter r is a variable 5 letters string that seems to be encrypted.

command the client issues on the server. The second parameter is `lvl1` and it specifies a number of feedback variables that we will discuss later.

At time $t = t_0$, the quality adaptation algorithm starts. For a generic time instant $t_i > t_0$ the client issues commands via HTTP POST requests to the server in order to select the suitable video level. It is worth to notice that the commands are issued on a separate TCP connection that is established at time $t = t_0$. We will focus on the dynamics of the quality adaptation algorithm employed by Akamai in the next section.

3.1 The `cmd` Parameter

Let us now focus on the commands the client issues to the server via the `cmd` parameter.

Table 2. Commands issued by the client to the streaming server via `cmd` parameter

Command	Number of arguments	Occurrence (%)
c_1 throttle	1	˜80%
c_2 rtt-test	0	˜15%
c_3 SWITCH_UP	5	˜2%
c_4 BUFFER_FAILURE	7	˜2%
c_5 log	2	˜1%

Table 2 reports the values that the `cmd` parameter can assume along with the number of command arguments and the occurrence percentage.

We describe now the basic tasks of each command, and leave a more detailed discussion to Section 4.

The first two commands, i.e. `throttle` and `rtt-test`, are issued periodically, whereas the other three commands are issued when a particular event occurs. The periodicity of throttle and `rtt-test` commands can be inferred by looking at Figure 4 that shows the cumulative distribution functions of the interdeparture times of two consecutive `throttle` or `rtt-test` commands. The Figure shows that `throttle` commands are issued with a median interdeparture time of about 2 seconds, whereas `rtt-test` commands are issued with a median interdeparture time of about 11 seconds.

`throttle` is the most frequently issued command and it specifies a single argument, i.e. the *throttle percentage* $T(t)$. In the next Section we will show that:

$$T(t) = \frac{\bar{r}(t)}{l(t)} 100 \qquad (1)$$

where $\bar{r}(t)$ is the maximum sending rate at which the server can send the video level $l(t)$. Thus, when $T(t) > 100\%$ the server is sending the video at a rate that is greater than the video level encoding rate $l(t)$. It is important to stress that in

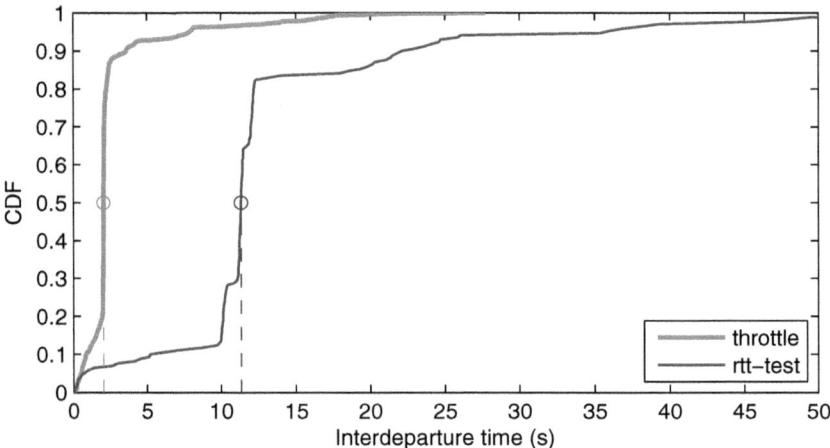

Fig. 4. Cumulative distribution functions of interdeparture time between two consecutive **throttle** or **rtt-test** commands

the case of live streaming it is not possible for the server to supply a video at a rate that is above the encoding bitrate since the video source is not pre-encoded. A traffic shaping algorithm can be employed to bound the sending rate to $\bar{r}(t)$. We will see in detail in Section 4 that this command plays a fundamental role in controlling the receiver buffer length.

The **rtt-test** command is issued to ask the server to send data in greedy mode. We conjecture that this command is periodically issued in order to actively estimate the end-to-end available bandwidth.

The **SWITCH_UP** command is issued to ask the server to switch from the current video level l_j to a video level l_k characterized with an higher encoding bitrate, i.e. $k > j$. We were able to identify four out of the five parameters supplied to the server: 1) the estimated bandwidth $b(t)$; 2) the bitrate l_k of the video level the client wants to switch up; 3) the video level identifier k the client wants to switch up; 4) the filename of the video level l_j that is currently playing.

The **BUFFER_FAIL** command is issued to ask the server to switch from the current video level l_j to a video level l_k with a lower encoding bitrate, i.e. $k < j$. We identified four out of the seven parameters supplied with this command: 1) the video level identifier k the client wants to switch down; 2) the bitrate l_k of the video level the client wants to switch down; 3) the estimated bandwidth $b(t)$; 4) the filename of the video level l_j that is currently playing.

The last command is **log** and it takes two arguments. Since this command is rarely issued, we are not able to explain its function.

3.2   The lvl1 Parameter

The **lvl1** parameter is a string made of 12 feedback variables separated by commas. We have identified 8 out of the 12 variables as follows:

1. **Receiver Buffer size** $q(t)$: it represents the number of seconds stored in the client buffer. A key goal of the quality adaptation algorithm is to ensure that this buffer never gets empty.
2. **Receiver buffer target** $q_T(t)$: it represents the desired size of the receiver buffer size measured in seconds. As we will see in the next Section the value of this parameter is in the range $[7, 20]$s.
3. unidentified parameter
4. **Received video frame rate** $f(t)$: it is the frame rate, measured in frames per second, at which the receiver decodes the video stream.
5. unidentified parameter
6. unidentified parameter
7. **Estimated bandwidth** $b(t)$: it is measured in kilobits per second.
8. **Received goodput** $r(t)$: it is the received rate measured at the client, in kilobits per second.
9. **Current video level identifier:** it represents the identifier of the video level that is currently received by the client. This variable assumes values in the set $\{0, 1, 2, 3, 4\}$.
10. **Current video level bitrate** $l(t)$: it is the video level bitrate measured in kilobits per second that is currently received by the client. This variable assumes values in the set $L = \{l_0, l_1, l_2, l_3, l_4\}$ (see Table 1).
11. unidentified parameter
12. **Timestamp** t_i: it represents the Unix timestamp of the client.

4 The Quality Adaptation Algorithm

In this Section we discuss the results obtained in each of the considered scenarios. Goodput measured at the receiver and several feedback variables specified in the lvl1 parameters will be reported. It is worth to notice that we do not employ any particular video quality metric (such as PSNR or other QoE indices). The evaluation of the QoE can be directly inferred by the instantaneous video level received by the client. In particular, the higher the received video level $l(t)$ the higher the quality perceived by the user. For this reason we employ the received video level $l(t)$ as the key performance index of the system.

In order to assess the efficiency η of the quality adaptation algorithm we propose to use the following metric:

$$\eta = \frac{\hat{l}}{l_{max}} \qquad (2)$$

where $\hat{l}$ is the average value of the received video level and $l_{max} \in L$ is the maximum video level that is below the bottleneck capacity. The index is 1 when the average value of the received video level is equal to l_{max}, i.e. when the video quality is the best possible with the given bottleneck capacity.

An important index to assess the Quality of Control (QoC) of the adaptation algorithm is the transient time required for the video level $l(t)$ to match the available bandwidth $b(t)$.

In the following we will investigate the quality adaptation control law employed by Akamai HD network in order to adapt the video level to the available bandwidth variations.

4.1   The Case of a Step-Like Change of the Bottleneck Capacity

We start by investigating the dynamic behaviour of the quality adaptation algorithm when the bottleneck bandwidth capacity increases at time $t = 50$ s from a value of $A_m = 500$ kbps to a value of $A_M = 4000$ kbps. It is worth to notice that $A_m > l_0$ and that $A_M > l_4$ so that we should be able to test the complete dynamics of the $l(t)$ signal. Since for $t > 50$s the available bandwidth is well above the encoding bitrate of the maximum video level l_4 we expect the steady state video level $l(t)$ to be equal to l_4. The aim of this experiment is to investigate the features of the quality adaptation control. In particular we are interested in the dynamics of the received video level $l(t)$ and of the receiver buffer length $q(t)$. Moreover, we are interested to validate the command features described in the previous Section.

Figure 5 shows the results of this experiment. Let us focus on Figure 5 (a) that shows the dynamics of the video level $l(t)$ and the estimated bandwidth $b(t)$ reported by the lvl1 parameter. In order to show their effect on the dynamics of $l(t)$, Figure 5 (a) reports also the time instants at which BUFFER_FAIL and SWITCH_UP commands are issued.

The video level is initialized at l_0 that is the lowest available version of the video. Nevertheless, at time $t = 0$ the estimated bandwidth is erroneously overestimated to a value above 3000 kbps. Thus, a SWITCH_UP command is sent to the server. The effect of this command occurs after a delay of 7.16 s when the channel level is increased to $l_3 = 2500$ kbps that is video level closest to the estimated bandwidth initialized at $t = 0$. By setting the video level to l_3, which is above the channel bandwidth $A_m = 500$ kbps, the received buffer length $q(t)$ starts to decrease and it eventually goes to zero at $t = 17.5$ s. Figure 5 (e) shows that the playback frame rate is zero, meaning that the video is paused, in the time interval $[17.5, 20.8]$ s. At time $t = 18.32$ s, a BUFFER_FAIL command is finally sent to the server. After a delay of about 16 s the server switches the video level to $l_0 = 300$ kbps that is below the available bandwidth A_m. We carefully examined each BUFFER_FAIL and SWITCH_UP command and we have found that to each BUFFER_FAIL command corresponds a decrease in the video level $l(t)$. On the other hand, when a SWITCH_UP command is issued the video level is increased. Moreover, we evaluated the delays incurring each time such commands are issued. We found that the average value of the delay for SWITCH_UP is $\tau_{su} \simeq 14$ s, whereas for what concerns the BUFFER_FAIL command the average value is $\tau_{sd} \simeq 7$ s. These delays pose a remarkable limitation to the responsiveness of the quality adaptation algorithm.

By considering the dynamics of the received frame rate, shown in Figure 5 (e), we can infer that the quality adaptation algorithm does not throttle the frame rate to shrink the video sending rate. We can conclude that the video level $l(t)$

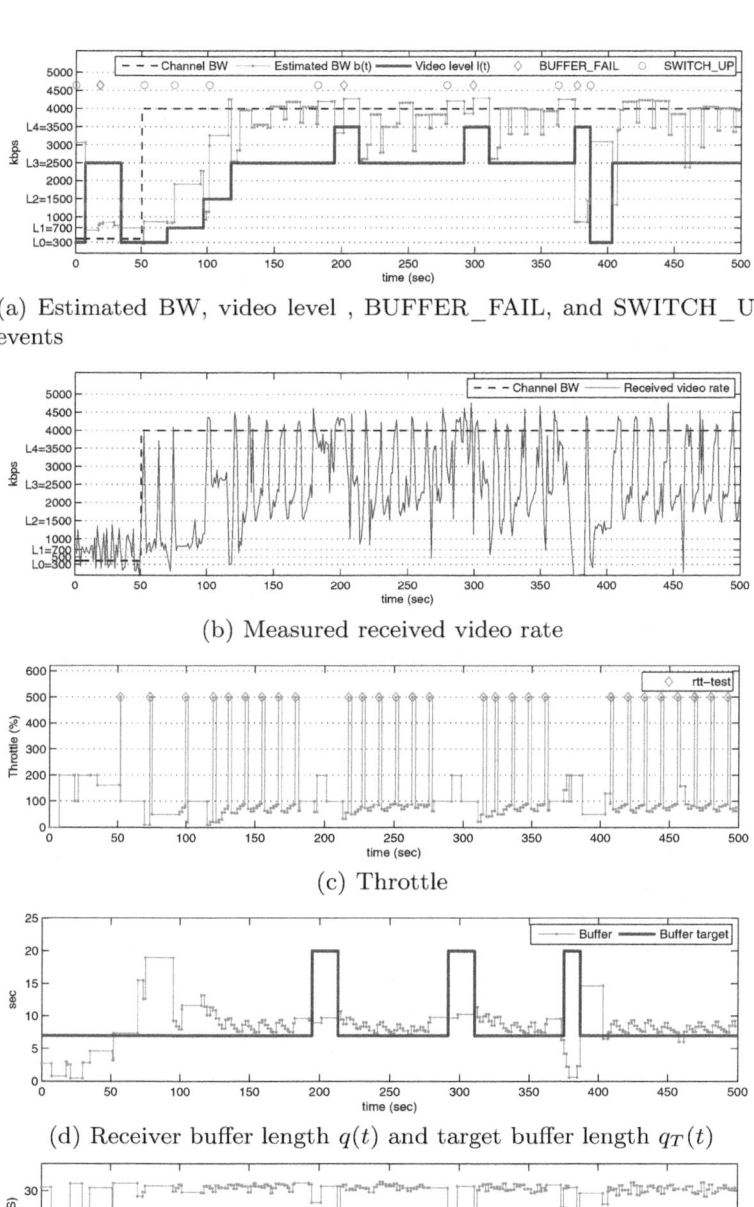

(a) Estimated BW, video level , BUFFER_FAIL, and SWITCH_UP events

(b) Measured received video rate

(c) Throttle

(d) Receiver buffer length $q(t)$ and target buffer length $q_T(t)$

(e) Frame rate $f(t)$

Fig. 5. Akamai adaptive video streaming response to a step change of available bandwidth at $t = 50s$

is the only variable used to adapt the video content to the network available bandwidth.

Let us now focus on the dynamics of the estimated bandwidth $b(t)$. When the bottleneck capacity increases to $A_M = 4000$ kbps, $b(t)$ slowly increases and, after a transient time of 75 s, it correctly estimates the bottleneck capacity A_M. Figure 5 (a) shows that SWITCH_UP commands are sent to select level l_i when the estimated bandwidth $b(t)$ becomes sufficiently greater than l_i. Due to the large transient time of $b(t)$, and to the delay τ_{su}, the transient time required for $l(t)$ to reach the maximum video level l_4 is around 150 s. Even though we are not able to identify the algorithm that Akamai employs to adapt $l(t)$, it is clear that, as we expected, the dynamics of the estimated bandwidth plays a key role in controlling $l(t)$. Finally, to assess the performance of the quality adaptation algorithm, we evaluated the efficiency η by using equation (2), finding a value of 0.676 and the average absolute error $|q_T(t) - q(t)|$ that is equal to 3.4 s.

Another important feature of Akamai streaming server can be inferred by looking at Figure 5 (c) that shows the throttle signal $T(t)$ and time instants at which rtt-test commands are issued. The figure clearly shows that each time a rtt-test command is sent, the throttle signal is set to 500%. By comparing Figure 5 (b) and Figure 5 (c) we can infer that when a rtt-test command is sent the received video rate shows a peak which is close to the channel capacity, in agreement with (1). Thus, we can state that when the throttle signal is 500% the video flow acts as a greedy TCP flow. For this reason, we conjecture that the purpose of such commands is to actively probe for the available bandwidth.

In order to validate equation (1), Figure 6 compares the measured received video rate with the maximum sending rate that can be evaluated as $\bar{r}(t) = \frac{T(t)}{100}l(t)$. The figure shows that equation (1) is able to model quite accurately the maximum rate at which the server can send the video. Nevertheless, it is important to stress that the measured received rate is bounded by the available bandwidth and its dynamics depends on the TCP congestion control algorithm.

The last feature we investigate in this scenario is the way the throttle signal $T(t)$ is controlled. In first instance, we conjecture that $T(t)$ is the output of a feedback control law whose goal is to make the difference between the target buffer length $q_T(t)$ and the buffer length $q(t)$ as small as possible. Based on the experiments we run, we conjecture the following control law:

$$T(t) = \max\left((1 + \frac{q_T(t) - q(t)}{q_T(t)})100, 10\right) \tag{3}$$

The throttle signal is 100%, meaning that $\bar{r}(t) = l(t)$, when the buffer length matches the buffer length target, i.e. when $q_T(t) = q(t)$. When the error $q_T(t) - q(t)$ increases, $T(t)$ increases accordingly in order to allow the maximum sending rate $\bar{r}(t)$ to increase so that the buffer can be filled.

Figure 7 compares the measured throttle signal with the dynamics obtained by using the conjectured control law (3). Apart from the behaviour of the throttle signal in correspondence of the rtt-test commands that we have already commented above, equation (3) recovers with a small error the measured throttle signal.

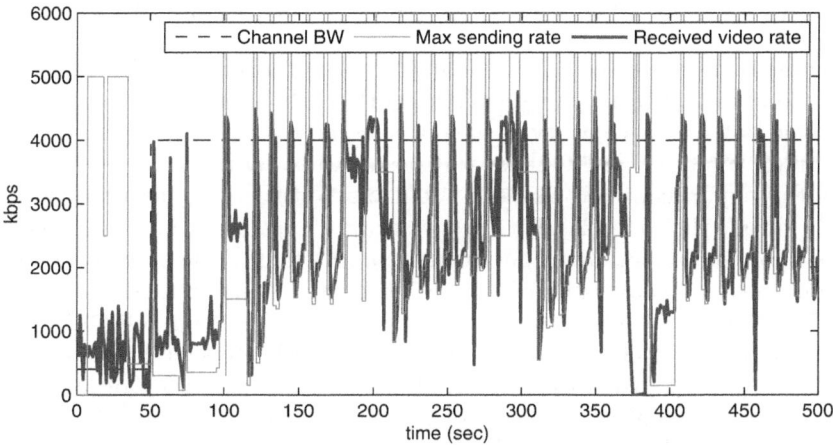

Fig. 6. Maximum sending rate $\bar{r}(t)$ and received video rate dynamics when the available bandwidth varies as a step function

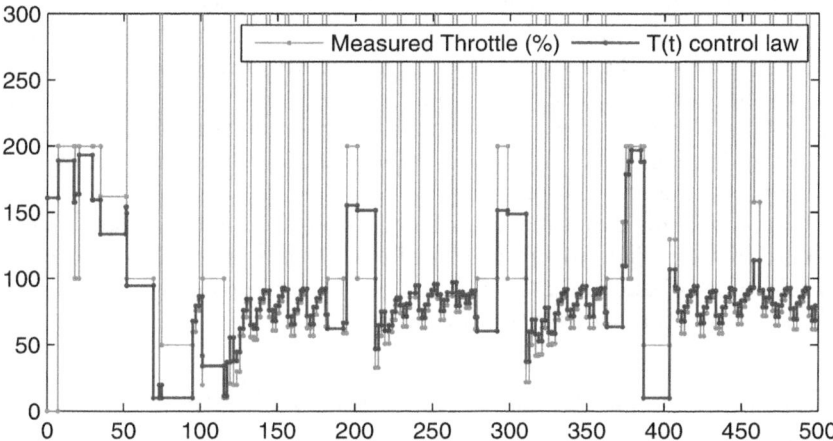

Fig. 7. Measured throttle signal $T(t)$ compared to the conjectured control law, eq. (3)

To summarize, the main results of this experiment are the following: 1) the only variable used to adapt the video source to the available bandwidth is the video level $l(t)$; 2) the video level $l(t)$ takes around 150 s to match the available bandwidth; 3) when a BUFFER_FAIL command is sent to switch the video level down, the server takes $\tau_{sd} \simeq 7$ s to actuate this command; 4) when a SWITCH_UP command is sent to switch the video level up, the server takes $\tau_{su} \simeq 14$ s to actuate the command; 5) when a rtt-test command is issued the throttle signal is set to 500% allowing the video flow to act as a greedy TCP flow to actively probe for the available bandwidth; 6) a feedback control law is employed to ensure that the player buffer length $q(t)$ tracks the desired buffer length $q_T(t)$.

4.2   The Case of a Square-Wave Varying Bottleneck Capacity

In this experiment we show how the quality adaptation algorithm reacts in response to abrupt drops/increases of the bottleneck capacity. Towards this end, we let the bottleneck capacity to vary as a square-wave with a period of 200 s, a minimum value $A_m = 400$ kbps and a maximum value $A_M = 4000$ kbps. The aim of this experiment is to assess if Akamai adaptive video streaming is able to quickly shrink the video level when an abrupt drop of the bottleneck capacity occurs in order to guarantee continuous reproduction of the video content.

Figure 8 shows the results of this experiment. Let us first focus on Figure 8 (a): when the first bandwidth drop occurs at time $t \simeq 208$ s, a BUFFER_FAIL is sent to the server after a delay of roughly 7 s in order to switch down the video level from l_3 to l_0. After that, a switch-down delay τ_{sd} of 7 s occurs and the video level $l(t)$ is finally switched to l_0. Thus, the total delay spent to correctly set the video level $l(t)$ to match the new value of the available bandwidth is 14 s. Because of this large delay an interruption in the video reproduction occurs 13 s after the bandwidth drop as it can be inferred by looking at Figure 8 (d) and Figure 8 (e). The same situation occurs when the second bandwidth drop occurs. In this case, the total delay spent to correctly set the video level is 16 s. Again, 13 s after the second bandwidth drop, an interruption in the video reproduction occurs. We found an efficiency $\eta = 1$ when the bandwidth is $A_m = 400$ kbps, i.e. the quality adaptation algorithm delivers the best possible quality to the client. On the contrary, during the time intervals with bandwidth $A_M = 4000$ kbps, the efficiency is roughly 0.5. Finally, in this scenario the average absolute error $|q_T(t) - q(t)|$ is equal to 3.87 s.

To summarize, this experiment has shown that short interruptions affect the video reproduction when abrupt changes in the available bandwidth occur. The main cause of this issue is that the video level is switched down with a delay of roughly 14 s after the bandwidth drop occurs.

4.3   The Case of One Concurrent Greedy TCP Flow

This experiment investigates the quality adaptation algorithm dynamics when one Akamai video streaming flow shares the bottleneck capacity with one greedy TCP flow. The bottleneck capacity has been set to 4000 kbps, a video streaming session has been started at $t = 0$ and a greedy TCP flow has been injected at time $t = 150$ s and stopped at time $t = 360$ s.

Figure 9 (a) shows the video level dynamics $l(t)$ and the estimated bandwidth $b(t)$. Vertical dashed lines divide the experiment in three parts.

During the first part of the experiment, i.e. for $t < 150$ s, apart from a short time interval $[6.18, 21.93]$ s during which $l(t)$ is equal to $l_4 = 3500$ kbps, the video level is set to $l_3 = 2500$ kbps. The efficiency η in this part of the experiment is 0.74.

When the second part of the experiment begins ($t = 150$ s), the TCP flow joins the bottleneck grabbing the fair bandwidth share of 2000 kbps. Nevertheless, the estimated bandwidth $b(t)$ decreases to the correct value after 9 s. After an

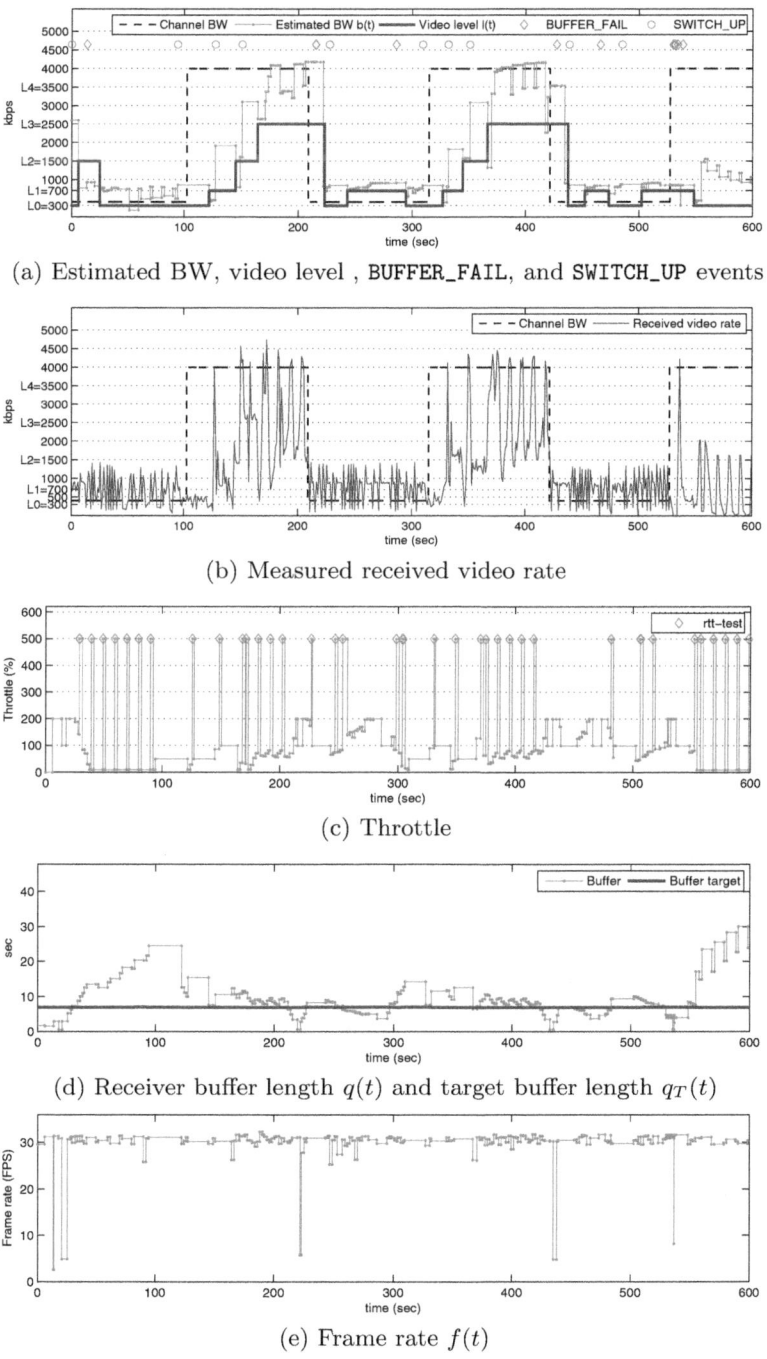

(a) Estimated BW, video level , BUFFER_FAIL, and SWITCH_UP events

(b) Measured received video rate

(c) Throttle

(d) Receiver buffer length $q(t)$ and target buffer length $q_T(t)$

(e) Frame rate $f(t)$

Fig. 8. Akamai adaptive video streaming response to a square-wave available bandwidth with period 200 s

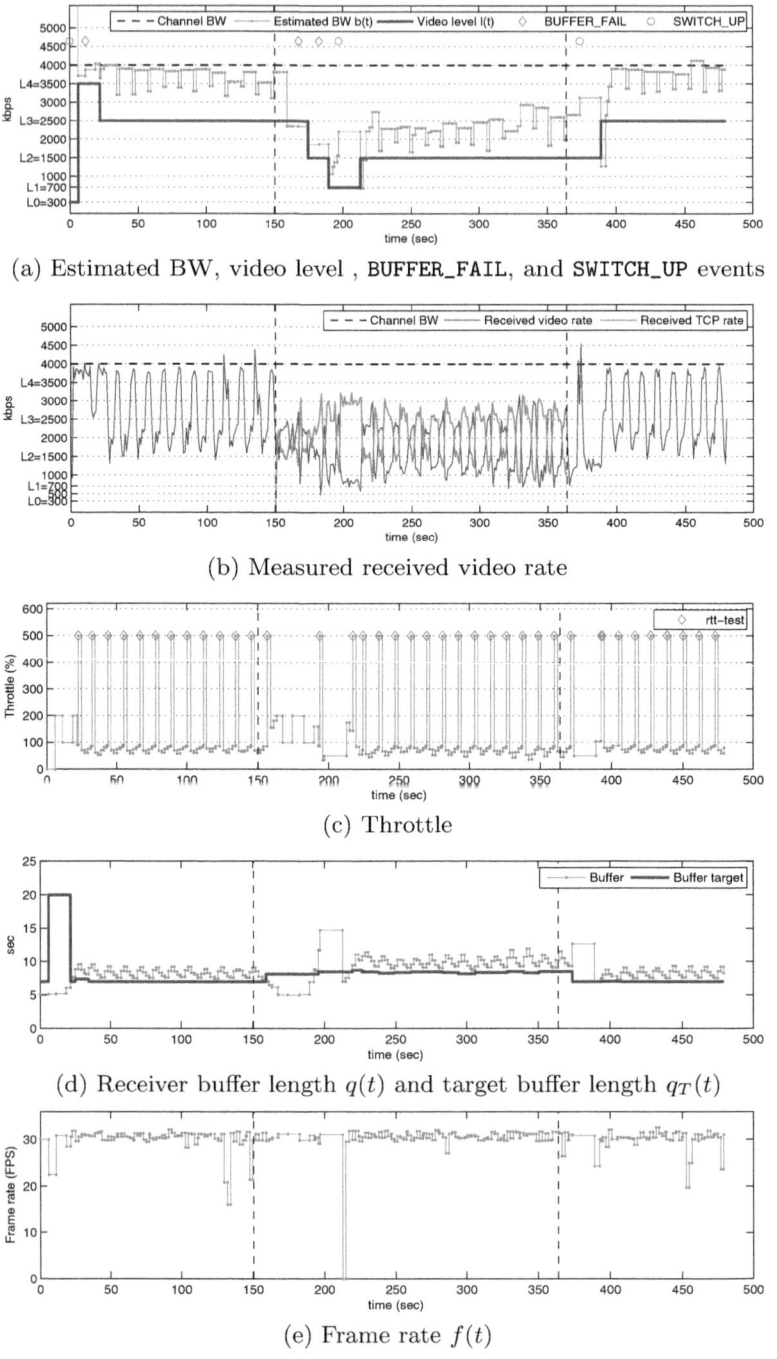

(a) Estimated BW, video level , BUFFER_FAIL, and SWITCH_UP events

(b) Measured received video rate

(c) Throttle

(d) Receiver buffer length $q(t)$ and target buffer length $q_T(t)$

(e) Frame rate $f(t)$

Fig. 9. Akamai adaptive video streaming when sharing the bottleneck with a greedy TCP flow

additional delay of 8 s, at $t = 167$ s, a `BUFFER_FAIL` command is sent (see Figure 9 (a)). The video level is shrunk to the suitable value $l_2 = 1500$ kbps after a total delay of 24 s. In this case, this actuation delay does not affect the video reproduction as we can see by looking at the frame rate dynamics shown in Figure 9 (e). At time $t = 182$ s a second `BUFFER_FAIL` command is set and the video level is shrunk after the usual delay $\tau_{sd} \simeq 7$ s at time $t = 189$ s. At time $t = 193$ s an `rtt-test` command is issued so that for a short amount of time the video flow becomes greedy (see Subsection 4.1). At time $t = 196$ s the bandwidth is estimated to 2200 kbps so that a `SWITCH_UP` command is sent and at $t = 212$ s the video level is switched up to the suitable value of $l_2 = 1500$ kbps. The efficiency η in this part of the experiment is 1, i.e. the best video quality has been provided.

Finally, when the TCP flow leaves the bottleneck at time $t = 360$ s, the level is switched up to $l_3 = 2500$ kbps with a delay of 26 s. In this part of the experiment the efficiency is 0.69.

To summarize, this experiment has shown that the Akamai video streaming flow correctly adapt the video level when sharing the bottleneck with a greedy TCP flow.

5   Conclusions

In this paper we have shown the results of an experimental evaluation of Akamai adaptive streaming. The contribution of this paper is twofold: firstly, we have analyzed the client-server protocol employed in order to actuate the quality adaptation algorithm; secondly, we have evaluated the dynamics of the quality adaptation algorithm in three different scenarios.

For what concerns the first issue, we have identified the POST messages that the client sends to the server to manage the quality adaptation. We have shown that each video is encoded in five versions at different bitrates and stored in separate files. Moreover, we identified the feedback variables sent from the client to the server by parsing the parameters of the POST messages. We have found that the client sends commands to the server with an average interdeparture time of about 2 s, i.e. the control algorithm is executed on average each 2 seconds.

Regarding the second issue, the experiments carried out in the three considered scenarios let us conclude that Akamai uses only the video level to adapt the video source to the available bandwidth, whereas the frame rate of the video is kept constant. Moreover, we have shown that when a sudden increase of the available bandwidth occurs, the transient time to match the new bandwidth is roughly 150 seconds. Furthermore, when a sudden drop in the available bandwidth occurs, short interruptions of the video playback can occur due to the a large actuation delay. Finally, when sharing the bottleneck with a TCP flow, no particular issues have been found and the video level is correctly set to match the fair bandwidth share.

References

1. Akamai hd network demo,
   http://wwwns.akamai.com/hdnetwork/demo/flash/default.html
2. Move networks hd adaptive video streaming, http://www.movenetworkshd.com
3. De Cicco, L., Mascolo, S.: A Mathematical Model of the Skype VoIP Congestion
   Control Algorithm. IEEE Trans. on Automatic Control 55(3), 790–795 (2010)
4. Hassoun, D.: Dynamic streaming in flash media server 3.5. (2009),
   http://www.adobe.com/devnet/flashmediaserver/articles/
   dynstream_advanced_pt1.html
5. Adobe Systems Inc. Real-Time Messaging Protocol (RTMP) Specification (2009)
6. Kuschnig, R., Kofler, I., Hellwagner, H.: An evaluation of TCP-based rate-control
   algorithms for adaptive internet streaming of H. 264/SVC. In: Proceedings of the
   First Annual ACM SIGMM Conference on Multimedia Systems, pp. 157–168. ACM,
   New York (2010)
7. Pantos, R., May, W.: HTTP Live Streaming. IETF Draft (June 2010)
8. Wang, B., Kurose, J., Shenoy, P., Towsley, D.: Multimedia streaming via TCP: An
   analytic performance study. ACM Transactions on Multimedia Computing, Communications, and Applications (TOMCCAP) 4(2), 1–22 (2008)
9. Zambelli, A.: IIS smooth streaming technical overview. Microsoft Corporation
   (2009)

A Social Approach to Image Re-targeting Based on an Interactive Game

Mathias Lux, Laszlo Böszörmenyi, and Alexander Müller

Klagenfurt University, Universitätsstr. 65-67, 9020 Klagenfurt, Austria
{mlux,laszlo}@itec.uni-klu.ac.at, lexe1@edu.uni-klu.ac.at

Abstract. Resolution of digital images is on the rise, but screens of mobile devices are still small. Therefore, image adaptation and especially image re-targeting for browsing images is still a challenging research topic. In this short paper we report work in progress on a social interactive game that can be used to identify meaningful portions of images. Based on preliminary evaluation we propose that these areas, found by our game, should be retained in an image re-targeting process.

Keywords: Games with a purpose, digital images, image re-targeting.

1 Introduction

The availability of cheap imaging devices supports the enormous growth of digital photos. With the internet and mobile devices like smart phones or portable multimedia players people can upload and access images virtually anywhere. Still, one problem is yet unsolved: how to present a big image on a small screen, e.g. a 10 megapixel image on a 0.5 megapixel screen. Approaches include scaling (just making the image much smaller), moveable viewports (scrolling the image with the small screen; just a small part of the image is shown), cropping, image re-targeting (selecting the most important section of the image), and hybrid approaches combining two or all of the aforementioned. Especially image re-targeting is a challenging task. It is typically based on visual attention models, which try to find spots and areas in images people look at in a first glance, or spots that carry the *most information*. These areas are retained, while others are scaled and cropped.

In this short work-in-progress paper we present an interactive game with a purpose [1]. It tries to tackle the problem of semantic image re-targeting by uncovering the same picture to two players at the same time. The image is slowly uncovered and the players can guess the image contents using game controllers. Based on multiple runs with different players the statistics of the regions that have been uncovered, when people could guess the correct answer we can infer the semantically most important region of the image. Supported by a preliminary evaluation we state that this region is a good candidate for being retained in an image re-targeting process. Our short paper first gives a brief overview on related work, then presents the actual game, discusses the results of a preliminary evaluation and concludes our findings at last.

G. Leitner, M. Hitz, and A. Holzinger (Eds.): USAB 2010, LNCS 6389, pp. 465–470, 2010.

2   Related Work

This work falls in the broad category of *human computation* [7]. Prominent examples for human computation are reCaptchta [11] and Peekaboom [10], whereas the latter is a so called *game with a purpose*. The term *game with a purpose* or short *GWAP* has been coined by Louis von Ahn in 2006 in a widely recognized publication [1]. The author also describes in a subsequent publication the main design patterns and critical issues in GWAPs [9].

As there are so many different GWAPs in many different domains available, we focus on the most widely recognized ones solving computational problems in multimedia. One of the earliest approaches is the ESP game [8], which generates descriptive tags for images. Two distant players look at the same image and guess tags. If both guess the same tags the overall score of both players improves. The game was later adopted by Google and offered as the Google Image Labeler[1]. Another one of the most prominent is Peekaboom [10], a multiplayer game for creating metadata on objects in pixel images.

Our game presented in this article focuses on the problem of finding regions in an image to be retained in the process of image re-targeting. Re-targeting selects the most important sections of an image and is often based on a visual attention model like for instance [3] or [6]. Seam carving for instance is a promising and fast method to re-target an image [2]. It is based on an energy map, where each and every pixel has an "energy value". Based on backtracking "seams" of pixels with minimum energy are found and "carved" from the image. Other approaches include for instance automatic pan and scrolling like in [4] or [5].

3   The Game

Our game features very simple game mechanics. Two players play on one screen in a competitive image guessing game. Each of the players has a game controller. A set of five images is sequentially slowly uncovered and the players guess the right answer out of four different given answers (see also Fig. 1) using colored buttons of the game controller. For each correct answer a score point is awarded to the player. In case of wrong answers players lose score points. Winner is the player with the highest score after all five images have been shown. Players can then choose to play another game with five new pictures.

The way images are uncovered alternates with different images. Possible uncovering options are (i) from one of the four corners, (ii) from one of the sides, and (iii) from the center (see also Fig. 2). Note that the mode of uncovering the image is selected automatically. We employ the bottom up visual attention model of [6] to determine the portions of the image with the highest visual attention. The uncovering mode then tries to show these portions at earliest possible time. So if most of the visual attention can be found in the bottom right area, the image is uncovered starting from there.

---

[1] URL: http://images.google.com/imagelabeler/

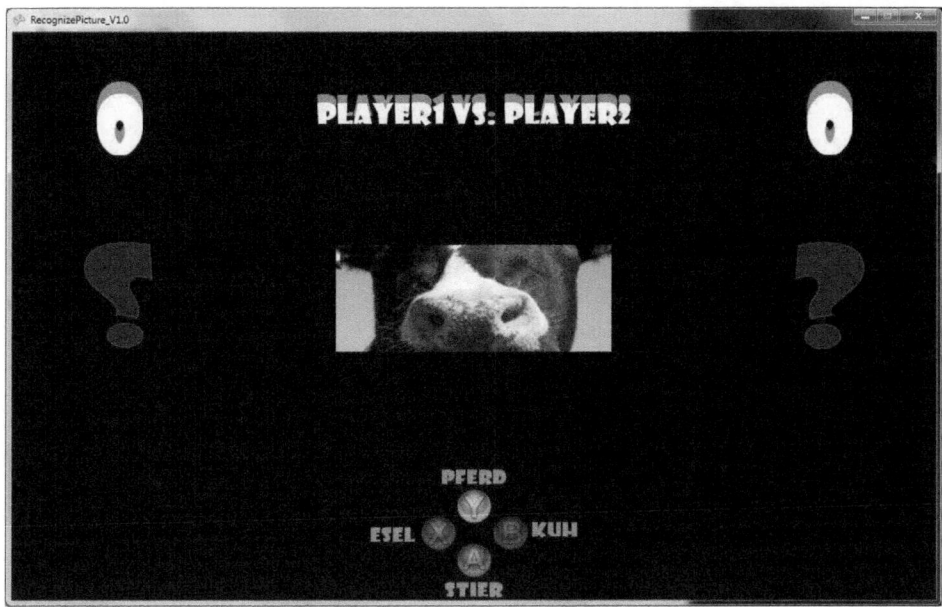

Fig. 1. Screenshot of the game showing the main screen. In this case the image gets uncovered from the center. On the top the names of the players are given along with their already achieved scores. The icons for the answers resemble the according buttons on the game controller. The labels translated from german to english in clockwise order starting from the topmost are *horse*, *cow*, *bull*, and *donkey*.

In addition to the actual game a server application allows for data management and gathering as well as basic statistical analysis of the games played. The analysis offers a simple visualization of the intersection and union of pixel sets that have been uncovered when a correct answer has been given. An example can be seen in Fig. 3: the red rectangle indicates the intersection, which can be interpreted as the minimum set of pixels to be uncovered to interpret the content correctly for given the right answer. The non-black pixels – including the pixels in the red rectangle – give union of pixel sets that have been uncovered at the time of a correct answer.

4   Discussion

The approach has only been tested in an exploratory way: in a heuristic evaluation with 4 participants. In groups of two they played the game two times (resulting in ten different images to be shown to the players) and gave feedback on the game mechanics. Resulting analysis of three different images can be seen in Fig. 3. For all three of the shown examples the approach worked well. The cow can be easily recognized by its nose, also for the joystick only a small part in the center is necessary for geeks, while others have to take a closer look at the

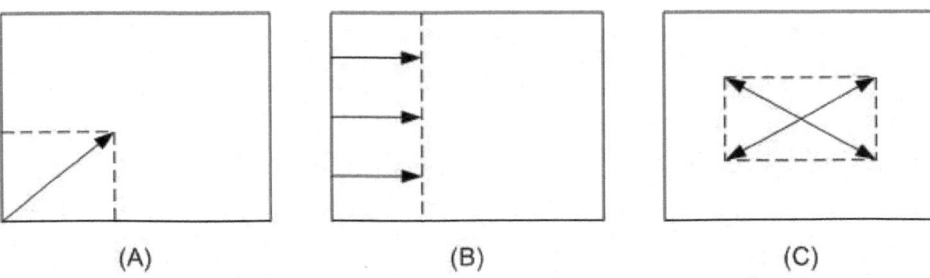

Fig. 2. Modes for uncovering the images depicted. Note that for mode (A) and mode (B) four different variations are possible (based on each corner and side of the image).

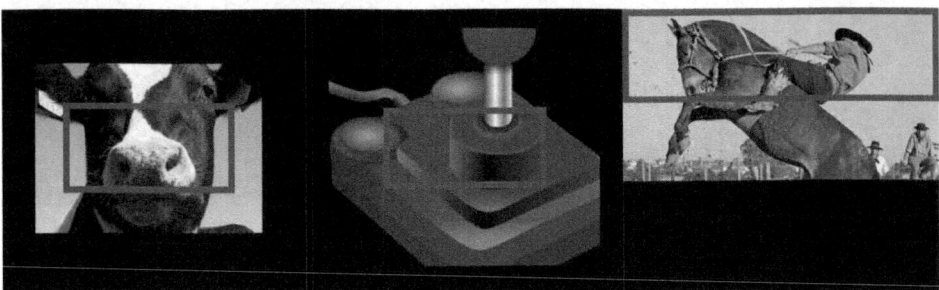

Fig. 3. Analysis of three sample pictures: The set of pixels within the red box are the intersection of pixels needed for the right answers. The pixels not being black are the union set of the pixels needed for the right answer.

picture. The rightmost image in Fig. 3 has been uncovered from the top and the intersection and union set show that less than a third of the image is needed to infer the answer *rodeo*.

What we found within our preliminary evaluation is rather encouraging. The game based approach shows some advantages to an automatic approach based on the visual attention model. As can be seen in Fig. 4 the visual attention is more or less distributed over the whole picture. Our software infers that uncovering from center is a valid option, however, people start to note that it is not a tiger only as they can see the eyes. The analysis Fig. 4 shows that the correct answers have only been given when players can see the eyes (cp. red rectangle in part (B) of Fig. 4). However, uncovering from the center leads to relatively big intersection and union sets. Therefore we assume that the uncovering process has to be varied over multiple games – especially for images with spatially distributed peaks of attention values.

A negative aspect is that the outcome is heavily depending on the set of possible answers presented. While cat and tiger can be easily mistaken in the example given in Fig. 4, the distinction between cat and elephant is rather easy based on few pixels in the center. This is quite a hard problem as it heavily

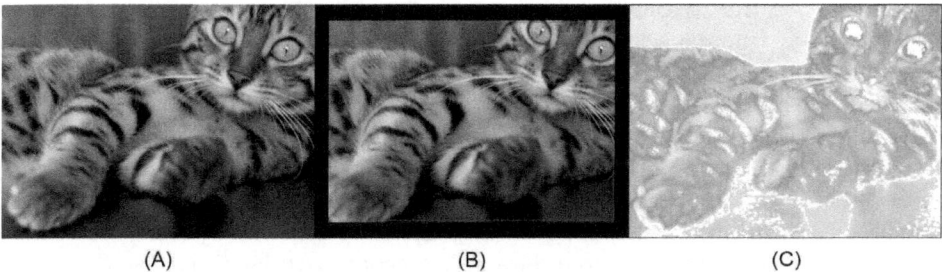

Fig. 4. Example of a kitten typically mistaken as a tiger. (A) shows the original picture, (B) shows the game results analysis and (C) shows the visual attention: dark pixels have higher attention values.

depends on the actual meaning an image has to convey. Image semantics can differ over many scenarios for one single image.

Our preliminary evaluation indicated that there is potential in the approach. While this is greenhouse work and no large scale evaluation has been undertaken we still can formulate hypotheses based on the preliminary results and plan for evaluation to support or reject the hypothesis. Our hypothesis is that *our game based approach allows for significantly better image re-targeting when the semantics of an image have to be retained compared to the classical approaches scaling, cropping and seam carving.* We plan to test the hypothesis based on a set of images in two stages. First we gather a set of test images and data on the images by letting people play the game with the test data set. Subsequently we employ for all images of the test data set (i) scaling, (ii) cropping, (iii) seam carving, and (iv) re-targeting based on the games results. In the second stage we do a quantitative study, where participants rate the semantic value of the re-targeted images compared to the original.

5   Summary

We have presented a GWAP, which can be used to find areas of images, that express more semantics than others. We propose this as a social approach to select meaningful portions of an image, which should be retained in a image re-targeting process. We hypothesize that this approach leads to semantically more meaningful miniature images than classical thumbnail approaches like cropping or scaling, or even seam carving. An exploratory discussion of the approach and first results has been presented.

In our opinion the approach has certain potential. Critical – as with all GWAPs – is that the game mechanics have to provide *enough fun* to encourage gaming, thus enough data can be gathered. A potential setting for such games are social platforms, where small and simple games are common. Also the selection of possible answers is critical. One can possibly cope with that based by alternating the "wrong" answers – even automatically, for instance based on Google Sets[2], where a set of words can be automatically created based on a few examples.

Future work includes work on the game itself, including the variation of uncovering methods and a more fine grained analysis of the regions, as well as the large scale evaluation outlined in Section 4. An interesting question for our proposed tool is the applicability of the approach to large scale image repositories. Future research might also focus on a possible transition a (semi-) automatic approach based on the gathered data able to cope with large data sets.

Acknowledgements

This work was supported by the Lakeside Labs GmbH, Klagenfurt, Austria and funding from the European Regional Development Fund and the Carinthian Economic Promotion Fund (KWF) under grant 20214/17097/24774.

References

1. von Ahn, L.: Games with a purpose. Computer 39(6), 92–94 (2006)
2. Avidan, S., Shamir, A.: Seam carving for content-aware image resizing. ACM Trans. Graph. 26(3), 10 (2007)
3. Itti, L., Koch, C., Niebur, E.: A model of saliency-based visual attention for rapid scene analysis. IEEE Trans. Pattern Anal. Mach. Intell. 20(11), 1254–1259 (1998)
4. Liu, F., Gleicher, M.: Video retargeting: automating pan and scan. In: MULTI-MEDIA 2006: Proceedings of the 14th Annual ACM International Conference on Multimedia, pp. 241–250. ACM, New York (2006)
5. Liu, H., Xie, X., Ma, W.-Y., Zhang, H.-J.: Automatic browsing of large pictures on mobile devices. In: MULTIMEDIA 2003: Proceedings of the Eleventh ACM International Conference on Multimedia, pp. 148–155. ACM, New York (2003)
6. Stentiford, F.: An estimator for visual attention through competitive novelty with application to image compression. In: Proc. Picture Coding Symposium, pp. 101–104 (April 2001)
7. von Ahn, L.: Human computation. In: K-CAP 2007: Proceedings of the 4th International Conference on Knowledge Capture, pp. 5–6. ACM, New York (2007)
8. von Ahn, L., Dabbish, L.: Labeling images with a computer game. In: CHI 2004: Proceedings of the SIGCHI Conference on Human Factors in Computing Systems, pp. 319–326. ACM, New York (2004)
9. von Ahn, L., Dabbish, L.: Designing games with a purpose. ACM Commun. 51(8), 58–67 (2008)
10. von Ahn, L., Liu, R., Blum, M.: Peekaboom: a game for locating objects in images. In: CHI 2006: Proceedings of the SIGCHI Conference on Human Factors in Computing Systems, pp. 55–64. ACM, New York (2006)
11. von Ahn, L., Maurer, B., McMillen, C., Abraham, D., Blum, M.: reCAPTCHA: Human-Based Character Recognition via Web Security Measures. Science 321(5895), 1465–1468 (2008)

---

[2] URL: http://labs.google.com/sets

Vicarious Learning with a Digital Educational Game: Eye-Tracking and Survey-Based Evaluation Approaches

Effie Lai-Chong Law[1], Elke E. Mattheiss[2],
Michael D. Kickmeier-Rust[3], and Dietrich Albert[3]

[1] University of Leicester, United Kingdom
[2] CURE, Austria
mattheiss@cure.at
[3] University of Graz, Austria
elaw@mcs.le.ac.uk,
{michael.kickmeier,dietrich.albert}@uni-graz.at

Abstract. The paper presents an empirical study with a digital educational game (DEG) called 80Days that aims at teaching geographical content. The goal of the study is twofold: (i) investigating the potential of the eye-tracking approach for evaluating DEG; (ii) studying the issue of vicarious learning in the context of DEG. Twenty-four university students were asked to view the videos of playing two micro-missions of 80Days, which varied with regard to the position of the non-player character (NPC) window (i.e. lower right vs. upper left) and the delivery of cognitive hints (i.e. with vs. without) in this text window. Eye movements of the participants were recorded with an eye-tracker. Learning effect and user experience were measured by questionnaires and interviews. Significant differences between the pre- and post-learning assessment tests suggest that observers can benefit from passive viewing of the recorded gameplay. However, the hypotheses that the game versions with cognitive hints and with the NPC window on the upper left corner can induce stronger visual attention and thus better learning effect are refuted.

Keywords: Eye-tracking, visual attention, game-based learning, vicarious learning, evaluation methodology, user experience, cognitive load.

1 Introduction

The inception of eye-tracking technique can be dated back almost a century ago when it was primarily deployed in the field of psychology. In the recent decade, the advance of computer technology has rendered this technique much less invasive, much more reliable and less costly than earlier on. Consequently, eye-tracking is increasingly adopted in various research fields for investigating people's visual attention in a range of contexts. The main assumption underpinning the use of eye-tracking in scientific research is the relationship between the gaze pattern (e.g., number of fixation, fixation duration, scanpath) and its underlying cognitive processes. In the field of human-computer interaction (HCI) the use of eye-tracking is deemed promising [1], for instance, in usability research [2] and website design [3, 4]. This coincides with the trend in HCI of tapping the potential of psycho-physiological measures for understanding

G. Leitner, M. Hitz, and A. Holzinger (Eds.): USAB 2010, LNCS 6389, pp. 471–488, 2010.
© Springer-Verlag Berlin Heidelberg 2010

user experience (e.g., [5, 6]) given the increasing emphasis on triangulating subjective experiential data with objective observational ones and the ongoing debates about correlations between these types of measures (e.g., [7, 8]) – an issue we look into in this study.

Eye-tracking enables researchers to study how users direct their focus or attention when acting upon an interactive system. It is considered especially challenging in the case of digital game because of dynamically changing user interfaces during gameplay [9], making the capture and analysis of eye-tracking data much more complicated and error-prone than otherwise. This practical hindrance may account for the relatively low number of eye-tracking studies on visual attention while playing videogames in general (e.g., [10]) and digital educational games in particular. We aim to provide and validate a methodological solution, namely, videotaping the game scenarios to provide a constant set of interfaces. This approach supports well the primary aim of our study to understand how people's visual attention varies with certain features of the game design, viz. the location of the main text window and the nature of the content delivered in it.

Another aim of our research study is to observe the effect of vicarious learning; whether people can gain conceptual knowledge by simply viewing instead of actively interacting with the scenarios of a digital educational game (DEG). According to [11], in vicarious multimedia environments, observers are not the addressees of the educational material. In other words, they can neither control the source of the material (i.e. the game) nor interact with it in any way [12]. However, they can cognitively engage in such an environment by actively processing the incoming information and integrating it into their existing knowledge schema [13]. We aim to investigate this specific phenomenon in our study by asking participants to view recorded gameplay of some DEG scenarios. Such an investigation is deemed relevant for the design of online multiplayer DEGs, which become increasingly popular thanks to the advent of social software like Facebook and YouTube. Similarly, it is intriguing to explore the question whether a viewer can empathize with a player's user experience (i.e. vicarious experience; e.g., [14]); this kind of empathy presumably enables software designers and other stakeholders to identify design issues and remedies [15]. Note that qualitative data on vicarious experience will be dealt with in another publication.

We address the aforementioned challenges in our empirical study with a DEG called 80Days (Section 3). Prior to presenting the details of our study, we review the related work (Section 2) and discuss their relevance to our results subsequently (Section 4). Implications for our future work are described in Section 5.

2   Related Work

2.1   Eye-Tracking

Visual attention has a long tradition in psychology. As a survival mechanism for living in complex environments, human vision comprises two basic processes – perception (i.e. bottom up) and cognition (i.e. top-down). El-Nasr and Yan [16] describe how these processes orchestrate in the context of 3D videogames. Accordingly, while saliency of objects can grab players' attention (bottom-up), the higher goal-orientation (top-down) in games is more effective for attracting attention. The big challenge for the authors was to develop a new methodology to analyse eye-tracking data in a complex 3D environment, which differed considerably from the stimuli used in eye-tracking experiments conducted until then. In eye-tracking studies, fixations (i.e. moments when eyes are relatively stationary and encoding of information takes place) and saccades (i.e. when quick eye movements occurring between fixations without any information intake) are two basic metrics [17]. A multitude of derivatives such as scanpath (i.e. sequence of fixations in a target area) are available [2]. While these eye-tracking measures are commonly used, their interpretations remain malleable [1].

Specifically, fixation measures include two attributes: duration and number (or frequency), which are inversely related. Mean fixation duration is normally used as an indicator of information complexity and task difficulty [18]. For a specific time slot (say one second), if a person fixates on a certain stimulus to process it, then less time is left for the other stimuli and the number of fixation thus becomes low. Longer fixation (i.e. lower number of fixation) implies higher task difficulty and thus higher cognitive workload [19, 20]. However, considering the complexity of computer games, relationships between these variables can be very different.

A common goal of eye-tracking studies is to understand how visual attention manifest as eye-tracking data is related to cognitive processes. Some evidence can be found in the work of Jennett and her colleagues [9], who investigated the immersion in a videogame with the aid of eye-tracking technology. They found that a decrease in eye movements measured with the number of fixation per second in the immersive condition as compared to an increase in a non-immersive control condition. The authors claim that in an immersive game the attention of the players becomes more focused on visual components relevant to the game (i.e. fixate on a selected set of objects within a specific timeslot), and in a non-immersive activity the individuals more likely get distracted by other items (i.e. fixate at various objects within a specific timeslot). In addition, they observe that their participants tended to change the nature of the game given (i.e. alter the game rule to make it more engaging), rendering it difficult to predict fixation behaviour. A similar observation was noted by Sundstedt and his colleagues [5] in their eye-tracking study with a maze videogame. They argue that such a *player-effect* (we coin it) of redefining a given game-task undermines the predictive power of saliency maps [21]. However, in a non-game situation, the validity threat posed by the player effect seems insignificant [3] or the non-game-based task can more effectively be controlled because of its lower complexity and dynamicity.

Furthermore, the eye-tracking study of Buscher et al. [3] on the user's browsing behaviour of web pages reveals some interesting observation. Specifically, with the research question about the distribution of visual attention, they divide a webpage into ten regions: a 3x3 grid plus the fold region (which can only be seen when scrolling down a page). They notice that the right third region (the lowest right corner) attracts almost no visual attention during the first second of each webpage view, suggesting participants' low expectations of information content on the right side of most web pages. This finding seems consistent with those of the previous studies that identify triangular or F-shaped scan patterns on web pages [22, 23].

2.2 Vicarious Learning

According to Gholson and Craig [24], vicarious learning is defined as "knowledge acquisition under conditions in which learners are not addressed and are physically passive" (p.120). Accordingly, learners do not physically interact with the source of the content they are attempting to master. However, they can cognitively engage in the content, albeit with different depths of processing, depending on a range of personal factors (e.g., pre-existing knowledge schema) and other situational variables (e.g., provision of reflective questions). Presumably, the relative knowledge gain is determined by how deep the incoming information is processed. In fact, the notion of vicarious learning is not new but was put forward in the field of educational psychology about half-a-century ago by the renowned psychologist Bandura [25]. Originally, it was applied to study how children acquired aggressive behaviour through social modeling. Later on, the notion was further refined and known as observational (or social) learning (e.g., [26, 27]). More recent work has focused on identifying effective approaches to support the constructive processes during vicarious learning in the domain of computer-based instruction (CBI) [11, 12, 28]. CBI generally involves multimedia presentations [13, 29] in which learners receive information being presented in different modalities including visual, auditory, and textual stimuli.

DEGs in particular draw heavily on the advantages of multimedia for educational purposes. Specifically, in the case of our study, provision of cognitive intervention (i.e. offering hints but not giving away answers) can serve as a kind of support for the constructive process in vicarious learning. Furthermore, some previous studies report the non-significant difference in spatial reasoning and visual attention between active gamers and their passive counterparts [5, 30, 31].

3   Method

3.1   Design

The experiment includes two independent variables. A 2x2 mixed factorial design was employed. Firstly, as a between-subject factor or independent variable (IV), the position of the NPC-window is varied (lower right corner versus upper left corner). Secondly, cognitive interventions are delivered or not (a within-subject factor). Table 1 illustrated the experimental design and the number of subjects.

Table 1. A 2x2 mixed factorial design with the variations of the two independent variables (IV) 'cognitive intervention' and 'NPC-window position'

| | | IV2: Cognitive Intervention (within-subject) ||
		With	Without
IV1: NPC-Window Position (between-subject)	Lower right	n = 12	
	Upper left	n = 12	

Dependent variables (DV) include a range of different measures, which are roughly categorized as two types: objective eye-tracking data and subjective survey-based self-reported data. Each of the related measures will be described subsequently.

3.2 Participants

Altogether 24 participants took part in the study (17 female and 7 male). Participants were between 18 and 27 years old ($M = 21.65$, $SD = 2.92$). Most of them were psychology students at a university in Europe. They were recruited through an announcement in a psychology lecture and got a course credit for taking part in the study. Participation was voluntary and participants were fully debriefed at the end of the experiment.

3.3 Material

The testing material was derived from a digital educational game prototype called 80Days, which was developed under the auspices of a R&D project. The game teaches geographical content (e.g., cities and countries) based on an alien story to school children of 10 to 14 years old. The player takes the role of a 14-year-old boy, who gets hijacked by a friendly alien named Feon (a non-player character, NPC). The boy was asked to help Feon write a travelogue about the Earth. Together they fly a UFO round the globe. The player has to perform four micro-missions (MM) to collect geographical information with some of which being provided by Feon or the boy's aunt (another NPC) in the form of verbal messages on the NPC-communication-text-window. Furthermore, Feon provides cognitive intervention (i.e. adaptive hint) to support the player to resolve impasses encountered in the game. Besides studying the effect of enabling or withdrawing cognitive intervention, we aim to evaluate the effect of the location of the NPC-communication-window on visual attention.

Recorded game session. The eye movements of the participants are recorded while they watch a video of a game session. Only parts of the game are used to ease the extraction and analysis of relevant data. They include the introduction (which is not analysed) and two micro-missions (called MM2 and MM3) of the game. The position of the NPC-window is the same for each participant in both missions (either lower right or upper left). The cognitive interventions are 'on' in one of the missions and 'off' in the other mission. The player's (the notional 12-year old boy is not visible at all in the game) learning performance in the recorded game session is identical for all the experimental groups. To eliminate noise data, the voice of Feon is turned off and the text is only displayed in the NPC-communication-window.

Essentially the game play switches between two situations: (1) In the flying situation (see Fig. 1) the player flies with the UFO over Europe with the aid of the cursor keys. A Head-up display (HUD) is shown on the screen, with a compass in the middle, a communication window with the NPCs on the lower right side, a section of the map on the upper right side, and a computer text window on the lower side of the display. (2) In the map desk situation (see Fig. 2) the player has to label points with city or country names on a map. The NPC and computer text window, which provides the player with information, are the same like in the flying situation. On the upper right side is a list with options for city names.

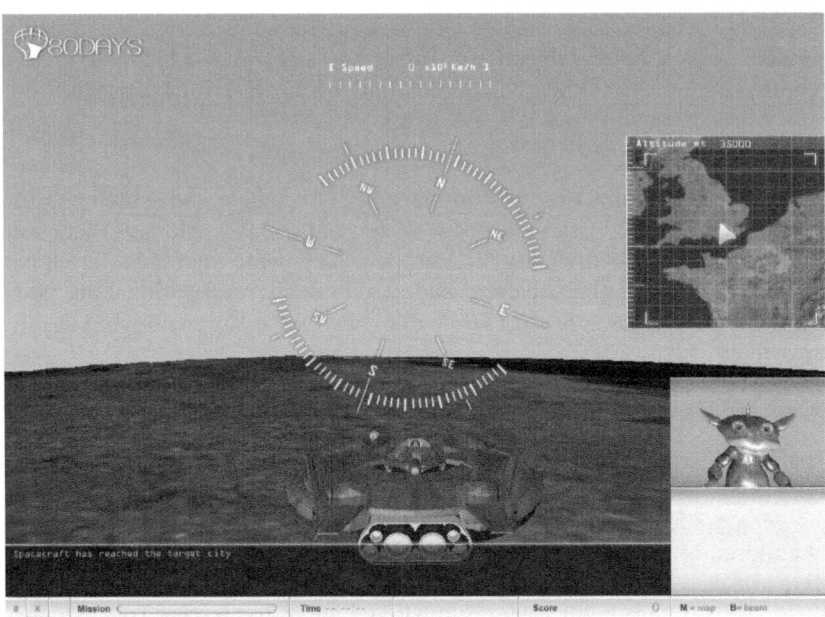

Fig. 1. Flying situation of the 80Days demonstrator game with the NPC-window in the lower right corner

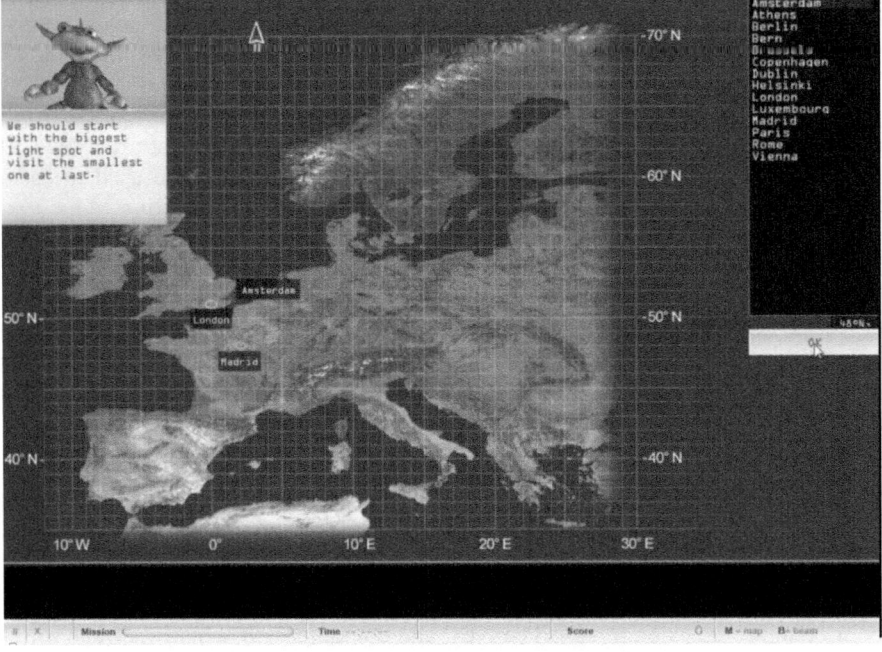

Fig. 2. Map desk situation of the 80Days demonstrator game with the NPC-window in the upper left corner

Eye Tracker. The participants' eye movements were recorded with a Tobii 1750 Eye Tracker with the Clearview software system. This eye tracker works with an infrared light source (in contrast to head mounted systems). To avoid a substantial loss of data a chin rest was used to restrain head movements.

Learning Assessment. To measure the effect of vicarious learning from watching the recorded game, a learning assessment test was administered before and after viewing the video. We developed the test with reference to the content of the game. It consisted of a map of Europe with nine countries being marked with dots. The task was to enter in a table the following information for each of these countries: its name, the name and location of its capital, its European Union (EU) membership, and some specific characteristics (e.g., the largest area in EU). The information of five of these countries is provided in the game whereas the remaining four serve as distractor and control.

Subjective Measures. To measure different aspects of the participants' attitudes towards and perceptions of the game, *after-mission questionnaires* (AMQ), *free recall exercises, NASA-TLX (Task Load Index)* and *semi-structured interviews* were conducted. Specifically, AMQ is divided into two parts: Part A consists of ten questions addressing how the participant interprets the notional player's performance in and perceptions of the game. Part B consists of five questions (Table 2) corresponding to their counterparts in Part A, albeit from the first instead of the third person perspective, including the micro-mission's ease-of-use, enjoyability, duration, understandability, and usability problems (qualitative, not to be reported here). Each question is rated with 5-point nominal scale. In the subsequent analysis, we focus on Part B; comparisons between Part A and Part B will be dealt with in another publication. As the qualitative data collected with AQM and the other instruments are not addressed in the current paper, the related measures are not elaborated here.

Table 2. Questions for evaluating four perceived qualities of the game

▪ How *easy* would you find this Mission?   (Answer options: Very difficult, Difficult, Medium, Easy, Very easy)
▪ How *enjoyable* would you find this Mission?   (Answer options: Not at all, A bit, Medium, Quite a lot, Very much)
▪ How *would* you find the duration of this Mission?   (Answer options: Too long, Somewhat longer than I prefer, Appropriate, Somewhat shorter   than I prefer, Too short)
▪ How easy would it be for you to *understand* the instructions in the Mission?   (Answer options: Very difficult, Difficult, Medium, Easy, Very easy)

Furthermore, the *perceived cognitive load* for watching the recorded game was assessed by the standardized questionnaire NASA-TLX (Task Load Index). NASA-TLX is a subjective workload assessment tool developed by Hart and Staveland [32] with established psychometric properties. It allows users to perform subjective workload assessments on users working with various human-machine systems. NASA-TLX is a multi-dimensional rating procedure that derives an overall workload score based on a weighted average of ratings on six subscales (i.e. Mental Demands, Physical Demands,

Temporal Demands, Own Performance, Effort and Frustration) and each is measured with a 21-point scale.

3.4 Procedure

The whole experimental procedure took about 90 minutes (see Table 3). After receiving some general instructions in the beginning of the session, the participants filled out the pre-learning assessment test. Then the eye-tracking measurement was started, first with calibration. After watching the introduction of the 80Days game prototype (which was not analysed), the participants were asked to view video recordings of 12-year-old children playing an educational computer game on geography. Additionally, the following instruction was given with the purpose of sustaining the participants' motivation for the viewing task:

> *"Please follow the recordings closely as if you were playing the game yourself. Please try to remember the content of the recordings as you will be asked to complete some recall exercises later on."*

After a mission had been played, free recall exercise, after-mission questionnaire (AMQ) and NASA-TLX questionnaire were administered. The eye-tracking measurement was then halted. The testing session was completed with the post-learning assessment test, a background questionnaire, and a semi-structured interview.

Table 3. Experimental procedure

Activity	Duration
Introduction, general instruction, questions	~ 5 minutes
Pre-learning assessment	~ 5 minutes
Calibration of the eye tracker	~ 2 minutes
Watching video of the intro	~ 5 minutes
Viewing video of micro-mission 2 (MM2)	~16 minutes
Free recall exercise	~4 minutes
After-mission questionnaire (AMQ)	~ 7 minutes
NASA-TLX questionnaire	~ 3 minutes
Viewing video of micro-mission 3 (MM3)	~ 7 minutes
Free recall exercise	~ 4 minutes
After-mission questionnaire	~ 7 minutes
NASA-TLX questionnaire	~3 minutes
Post-learning assessment	~ 5 minutes
Background demographic questionnaire	~ 4 minutes
Interview, debriefing and Thank You	~ 13 minutes
Total	~ 90 minutes

3.5 Hypotheses

With reference to the literature review (Section 2), we assume that the lower the number of fixations per second (i.e. the longer the fixation duration), the higher the visual attention is and the more information processing takes place. Furthermore, vicarious learning can occur when passively viewing the recorded gameplay. Besides, different combinations of NPC-window position and availability of cognitive intervention can lead to different perceptions of the game, including its ease of use, enjoyability, duration, and understandability.

With these assumptions, the following hypotheses are formulated:

H1:   The number of fixations per second will be significantly smaller when NPC-window is positioned at the upper left than when it is at the lower right.

H2:   The number of fixations per second will be significantly smaller when cognitive intervention is on than when it is off.

H3:   There will be significant differences in scores between the post- and pre-learning assessment tests (i.e. learning gain).

H4:   There will be significant differences between the four experimental conditions in terms of the participants' perceived qualities of the game: (a) enjoyability; (b) ease of use; (c) duration; (d) understandability.

H5:   Participants' perceived cognitive load will be significantly different between the four experimental conditions.

H6:   There will be significant correlation between the number of fixations per second and learning gain.

H7:   There will be significant correlations between the perceived game qualities and the number of fixations per second.

H8:   Participants' perceived cognitive load will be significantly correlated with the number of fixations per second.

H9:   Participants' perceived cognitive load will be significantly correlated with the learning gain.

To verify these nine hypotheses, a series of 2-way mixed design ANOVAs with the between-factor 'NPC-position' (lower right vs. upper left) and the within-factor 'cognitive intervention' (on vs. off) were conducted. In addition, Pearson correlations among these variables were computed to identify potential relationships between the objective and subjective measures.

4   Results and Discussions

4.1   Visual Attention: Number of Fixations

As mentioned earlier, the two measures of fixations – duration and frequency (per second) – are inversely related. We use the number of fixations per second to conduct statistical analyses. The number of fixations per second is computed by averaging the total number of fixations over the total viewing time for both micro-missions MM2 and MM3. Table 4 displays the results under the four conditions.

Table 4. Average viewing duration and number of fixations per sec in the four conditions

			IV2: Cognitive Intervention (within-subject)	
			With	Without
IV1: NPC-Window Position (between-subject)	Lower right	Total viewing time (sec)	703.5	642.5
		No. of fixation per sec.	2.32	2.15
	Upper left	Total viewing time (sec)	678.5	631.5
		No. of fixation (per sec)	2.44	2.57

Specifically, a non-parametric procedure was applied, because the condition of equal co-variances in the groups was not given (Box-test). However, the findings do not differ from those of ANOVA. Hence, the respective averages are reported (see Fig. 3). The Wilcoxon test shows no significant difference between the two cognitive intervention groups ($Z = -0.71$; $p > 0.05$). For the position of the NPC-window the Mann-Whitney-Test revealed a significantly higher number of fixations per second for the upper left position than for the lower right ($Z = -2.10$; $p < 0.05$). The higher the number of fixations per second the shorter the fixation duration is, and it can imply that the participants do not spend much time in processing the information presented. Put differently, it seems that the lower right corner is a relatively more favourable location for positioning the NPC-window in terms of enabling the uptake of the content. However, as pointed out in the foregoing literature review, interpretations of eye-tracking data are somewhat malleable. Due to the complexity of computer games, the result may imply the exact opposite. According to [9], a high immersion goes along with a decrease in the number of fixations per second; this would indicate a higher immersion in the lower right than in the upper left group. An alternative explanation is the arrangement of the objects in the game (see Fig. 1 and 2). In the upper left NPC-window position the distance to the other relevant objects (e.g., map) is higher than for the lower right condition, which would require a higher number of eye movements to follow the game.

H1:   The hypothesis was refuted. The opposite trend was observed with the number of fixations per second being significantly higher in the upper left than the lower right. Alternative explanations are plausible.

H2:   The hypothesis was refuted. No significant difference was detected. The presence/absence of cognitive interventions or hints seems not play a role in influencing visual attention.

4.2   Learning Effect, Perceived Game Qualities and Cognitive Load

The analysis of the learning assessment (see Fig. 4) shows a significant effect for the geographical skills taught by the micro-mission MM2 ($t = -5.73$; $df = 23$; $p < 0.001$) and MM3 ($t = -6.828$; $df = 23$; $p < 0.001$). As expected, participants did not improve skills which were not taught by the game ($t = 0.401$; $df = 23$; $p > 0.05$). The ANOVA shows no significant difference, irrespective of the variables 'cognitive intervention' ($F(1) = 0.983$; $p > 0.05$) or 'NPC-window position' ($F(1) = 0.242$; $p > 0.05$).

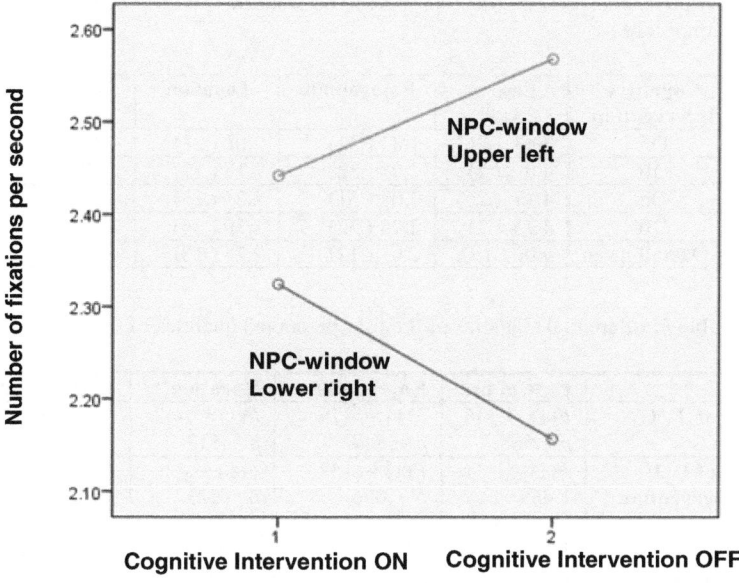

Fig. 3. The number of fixations per second in the four different experimental groups

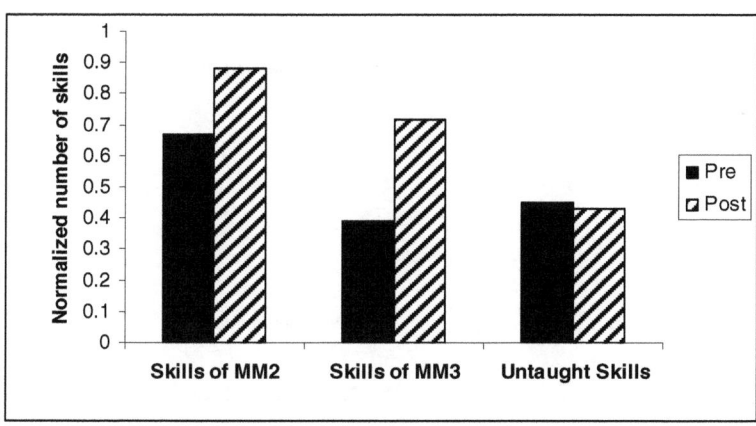

Fig. 4. Relative number of skills correct in the pre- and respectively post-learning assessment (MM = micro-mission)

Furthermore, results of 2-way mixed design ANOVA show no significant difference in the four perceived qualities of the game except for Understandability (After-Mission Questionnaires; Section 3.3); Table 5 and Table 6 display the related descriptive and inferential statistics, respectively. While the perceived ease-of-use and understandability of the instructions were high, the perceived enjoyability was relatively low and the duration of the game was somewhat too long.

Table 5. Descriptive statistics of the four perceived qualities of the game under different experimental conditions

NPC-Window	Cognitive Intervention	Ease of Use	Enjoyability	Duration	Understandability
Lower Right	On	3.83 (.26)	1.83 (.31)	2.08 (.28)	4.25 (.28)
	Off	4.0 (.2)	2.0 (.32)	2.17 (.17)	4.67 (.17)
Upper Left	On	4.17 (.26)	2.08 (.31)	2.25 (.28)	4.33 (.28)
	Off	4.25 (.2)	2.08 (.32)	2.50 (.36)	4.5 (.17)
	Overall mean	4.06 (.19)	2.0 (.12)	2.25 (.18)	4.44 (.19)

Table 6. Inferential statistics of the four perceived qualities of the game

	Ease of use	Enjoyability	Duration	Understandability
Main effect of IV1: NPC-window	$F(1) = .336$ $p = .568$	$F(1) = .379$ $p = .544$	$F(1) = .442$ $p = .513$	$F(1) = 3.08$ $p = .093$
Main effect of IV2: cognitive intervention	$F(1) = 1.469$ $p = .238$	$F(1) = .157$ $p = .696$	$F(1) = .42$ $p = .523$	$F(1) = .022$ $p = .885$
Interaction effect between the two IVs	$F(1) = .037$ $p = .849$	$F(1) = .379$ $p = .544$	$F(1) = .111$ $p = .743$	$F(1) = .566$ $p = .46$

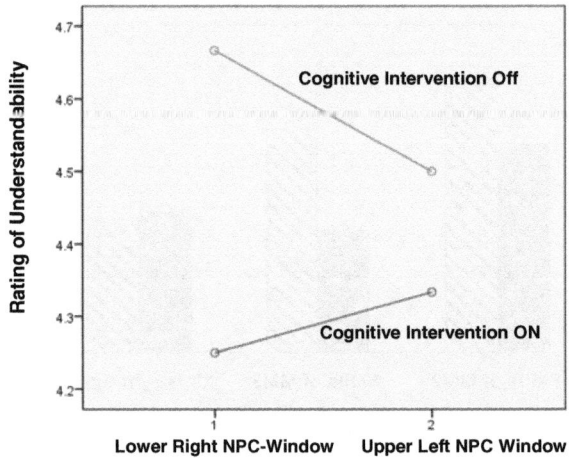

Fig. 5. Rating of Understandability in relation to the NPC-window position and availability of cognitive intervention

As illustrated in Figure 5, the quality Understandability is rated significantly higher when the cognitive intervention is off than when it is off; it is explicable because the amount of text to be viewed is apparently less when the cognitive intervention is off.

With regard to the perceived cognitive load – no significant effect could be found in all the six attributes (i.e. mental demand, physical demand, temporal demand, performance, effort, and frustration). Hence, the position of the NPC-window and the presence of cognitive interventions seem to have no influence on the learning effect and the perceived task load. Table 7 displays the perceived cognitive load for the task of viewing video recording. Note that the maximum rating is 21 with the leftmost and rightmost anchors being labelled as "very low" and "very high", respectively. Generally speaking, the task was perceived to be low in mental demand, causing low level of frustration, workable at quite a relaxing pace, and low in difficulty. However, the level of physical demand was about average (probably straining the eye muscles), but the participants' perceived level of success was above average.

H3:   The hypothesis was supported. The significant difference indicated that the vicarious learning by passively viewing the recorded gameplay was effective.

H4:   The hypothesis was mostly refuted. Among the four perceived qualities of the game, only Understandability had a moderately significant within-subject difference with the higher understandability being shown when the cognitive intervention was off. No interaction effect between the two IVs on the four perceived game qualities was detected.

H5:   The hypothesis was refuted. The perceived task load did not differ significantly among the four experimental conditions.

Table 7. Perceived task load (viewing video recording) for the two micro-missions (MM) with respect to the six dimensions of NASA-LTX

		Mental	Physical	Temporal	Performance	Effort	Frustration
MM2	Mean	8.2	10.7	5.4	13.8	7.9	7
	SD	4.8	6.1	4.6	5.3	4.9	6.3
MM3	Mean	6.4	7.6	5.6	15.2	6.4	6.1
	SD	4.1	6.1	4.4	3.8	3.8	5.2

4.3   Correlations between Measures

To find potential relationships between the different measures Pearson correlations were calculated. Three significant correlations have been found (see Table 8). The number of fixations per second was significantly correlated with the perceived performance and perceived effort expended. In other words, the higher the participants rated the question "How successful were you in accomplishing what you were asked to do?" (*performance*), the lower was their number of fixations when viewing the video (i.e. higher visual attention). Similarly, the same relationship was observed for the question "How hard did you have to work to accomplish your level of performance" (*effort*). This result seems consistent with Jennett et al.'s [9], since the successful and engaged learners tended to show a lower number of fixations per second, implying a higher degree of immersion. Furthermore, the lower the rating of mental demand ("How mentally demanding was the task?") the higher the learning effect of viewing the game was. This result seems intuitive, because a high mental demand may corrupt a potential learning effect. However, the subjectively perceived perform-ance and effort did not correlate significantly with the objectively measured learning gain. Participants might interpret the term "performance" to a wider scope than learn-ing the geographical content, which might entail limited effort.

In contrast to our expectation, no significant correlation could be detected between the number of fixations per second and the learning gain in terms of the differences in scores between pre- and post-learning assessment tests, irrespective of MM2 or MM3. Such insignificance may imply that the fixation frequency (or duration) does not re-flect the relative depth of information processing. Alternatively, it might be attributed to the ceiling effect, given that the participants had already possessed on average 52% of the skills covered by MM2 and MM3 prior to viewing the game.

Furthermore, correlations between the four perceived qualities of the game and the number of fixations per second were also computed. Loosely speaking, moderately significant negative correlation was detected for Understandability ($r = -0.269$, $p<.1$) but not for the other three qualities. In other words, the higher the understandability the lower the number of fixations per second was, implying that the participants had viewed the objects of interest for a longer period of time. The insignificant and weak correlations between these subjective game quality measures and the objective eye-tracking data suggest that the validity of the items gauging the former and the inter-pretation of the latter need to be further investigated. Specifically, as each of the four qualities was gauged by only single item, one may challenge the validity of such measurement (cf. Hassenzahl's [33] arguments about the holistic judgment of the highly subjective evaluative constructs such as *beauty* and *goodness* of which the fuzziness and dynamicity are comparable to *enjoyability* but stronger than *ease-of-use*). This issue will be explored in our future work.

H6: The hypothesis was rejected. The fixation frequency did not reflect the depth of information processing and the possible ceiling effect of the learning gain.

H7: The hypothesis was mostly refuted. Only one of the four perceived qualities of the game was moderately correlated with the number of fixations per second.

H8: The hypothesis was partially supported with two of the three relevant attributes (i.e. performance, effort) of cognitive load being significantly correlated with the strength of visual attention

H9: The hypothesis was partially supported with one of the three relevant attributes (i.e. mental demand) of cognitive load being significantly correlated with the learning effect.

Table 8. Pearson correlations between number of fixations, learning effect, and perceived task load (n.s. = no significant correlation)

	Number of fixations per second	Learning effect
Mental demand	n.s.	-0.40 ($p < 0.01$)
Performance	-0.30 ($p < 0.05$)	n.s.
Effort	-0.31 ($p < 0.05$)	n.s.

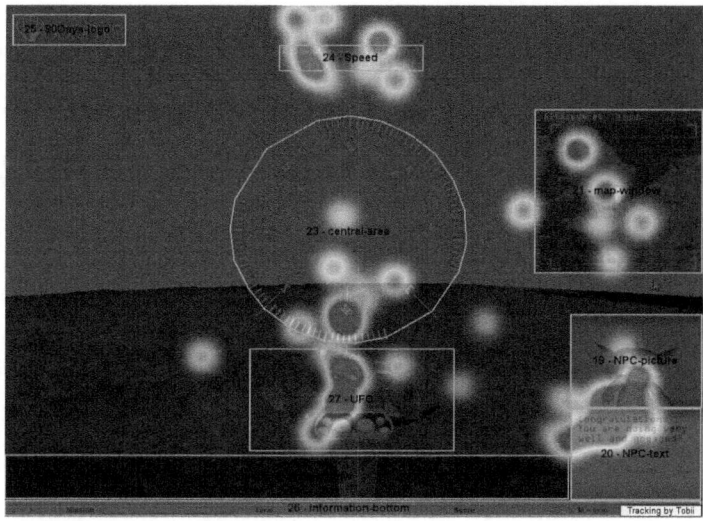

Fig. 6. Hot Spot analysis of the visual attention in the flying situation of the 80Days demonstrator game

5   Conclusion

Here we revisit the two major research goals of the current pilot study. First, with regard to the potential of eye-tracking for evaluating digital educational games, we primarily used the key eye-tracking metric – number of fixations per second – to understand how visual attention could be related to the learning effect and other usability and user experience attributes. No clear picture, however, has emerged that this eye-tracking metric could relate to the extent of learning effect in the existing context – vicarious learning by viewing the recorded gameplay. However, it does not exclude such a relationship, which might be masked by the ceiling effect (i.e. participants' relatively high pre-knowledge). Furthermore, while the position of NPC-window was shown to have some impact on visual attention, the availability of cognitive intervention (i.e. textual hints) did not make significant difference in it. It seems to suggest that layout is more effective than content for capturing user attention, even for adult learners. Furthermore, the mixed picture about the interrelations between the objective eye-tracking measure and supposedly related subjective survey-based measures is consistent with the current literature. In other words, there remains a lack of a working model to predict as well as explain relationships between quality attributes. Nevertheless, the malleability of interpreting eye-tracking data can be seen as a limitation, as shown by alternative explanations for the number of fixations per second with respect to participants' behavioural goals (i.e. actively taking in information or staring without seeing). Presumably, further calibration with a large volume of empirical data, given the increasing interest in eye-tracking, is called for. Second, concerning the issue of vicarious learning, our empirical findings demonstrate that it is feasible for passive viewers of a digital educational game to acquire knowledge. This finding corroborates with the past studies on computer-based instruction and game. However, the research design of the current study does not allow us to answer the question whether the effect of vicarious learning is comparable or even stronger than that of active learning. Comparative experimental studies in this direction are planned as our future work.

In this study, we report the quantitative findings. Data related to the most relevant areas of interest (AOIs) - like the NPC-window - will be analysed in the next step, in terms of a Hot Spot analysis (see Figure 6) and the number of fixations per second on the various AOIs. A limitation of the present research is the involvement of adult participants (owing to various organizational constraints) instead of children of representative age groups, who will be recruited for our further investigations. The aim of this upcoming study is also to compare different saliencies of instructional objects in terms of their efficiency and attention attraction. Furthermore, the issue of vicarious experience will be explored with the qualitative data collected in this and to be collected in the future work.

Acknowledgments

The research and development introduced in this work is funded by the European Commission under the seventh framework programme in the ICT research priority, contract number 215918 (80Days, www.eightydays.eu) and the Austrian Federal Ministry of Science and Research.

References

1. Jacob, R.J.K., Karn, K.S.: Eye Tracking in Human-Computer Interaction and Usability Research: Ready to Deliver the Promises. In: Hyona, R., Deubel (eds.) The Mind's Eye: Cognitive and Applied Aspects of Eye Movement Research, Elsevier, Oxford (2003)
2. Poole, A., Ball, L.J.: Eye tracking in HCI and Usability Research. In: Ghaoui, C. (ed.) Encyclopedia of Human-Computer Interaction. Idea Group Inc., Pennsylvania (2006)
3. Buscher, G., Cutrell, E., Morris, M.R.: What Do You See When You're Surfing? Using Eye Tracking to Predict Salient Regions of Web Pages. In: Proceedings of CHI 2009, pp. 21–30 (2009)
4. Cutrell, E., Guan, Z.: What Are You Looking for? An Eye-Tracking Study of Information Usage in Web Search. In: Proceedings of CHI 2007, pp. 407–416 (2007)
5. Sundstedt, V., Stavrakis, E., Wimmer, M., Reinhard, E.: A Psychophysical Study of Fixation Behavior in a Computer Game. In: Creem-Regehr, S., Myszkowski, K. (eds.) Proceedings of the 5th Symposium on Applied Perception in Graphics and Visualization, pp. 43–50 (2008)
6. Nacke, L.E., Grimshaw, M.N., Lindley, C.A.: More Than a Feeling: Measurement of Sonic User Experience and Psychophysiology in a First-Person Shooter Game. Interacting with Computers 22(5) (2010)
7. Hornbæk, K., Law, E.L.-C.: Meta-Analysis of Correlations among Usability Measures. In: Proceedings of CHI 2007, pp. 617–626 (2007)
8. Lin, T., Hu, W.: Do Physiological Data Relate to Traditional Usability Indexes? In: Proceedings of OZCHI 2005, Canberra, Australia (23-25, 2005)
9. Jennett, C., Cox, A.L., Cairns, P., Dhoparee, S., Epps, A., Tijs, T., Walton, A.: Measuring and Defining the Experience of Immersion in Games. International Journal of Human Computer Studies 66(9), 641–661 (2008)

10. Johansen, S.A., Noergaard, M., Janus, R.: Can Eye Tracking Boost Usability Evaluation of Computer Games? In: Proceedings of CHI 2008, Workshop on Evaluating User Experience in Game (2008)
11. Gholson, B., Witherspoon, A., Morgan, B., Brittingham, J.K., Coles, R., Graesser, A.C., Sullins, J., Craig, S.D.: Exploring the Deep-Level Reasoning Questions Effect during Vicarious Learning among Eighth to Eleventh Graders in the Domains of Computer Literacy and Newtonian Physics. Instructional Science 37, 487–493 (2009)
12. Craig, S.D., Sullins, J., Witherspoon, A., Gholson, B.: The Deep-Level Reasoning Effect: the Role of Dialogue and Deep-Level-Reasoning Questions during Vicarious Learning. Cognition and Instruction 24, 565–591 (2006)
13. Mayer, R.E.: Multimedia Learning. Cambridge University Press, New York (2001)
14. Marsh, T.: Vicarious Experience: Staying There Connected With and Through Our Own and Other Characters. In: Williams, S.H.P.J. (ed.) Gaming as Culture: Social Reality, Identity and Experience in Role-Playing, Collectible, and Computer Games, Jefferson, NC, McFarland, pp. 196–213 (2005)
15. Wright, P., McCarthy, J.: Empathy and Experience in HCI. In: Proceedings of CHI 2008, pp. 637–646 (2008)
16. El-Nasr, M.S., Yan, S.: Visual Attention in 3D Video Games. In: Proceedings of ACE 2006, Hollywood, California, USA (2006)
17. Land, M.F.: Eye Movements and the Control of Actions in Everyday Life. Progress in Retinal and Eye Research 25, 296–324 (2006)
18. Rayner, K.: Eye Movements and Information Processing: 20 Years of Research. Psychological Bulletin 124(3), 343–372 (1998)
19. Nakayama, M., Takahashi, K., Shimizu, Y.: The Act of Task Difficulty and Eye-Movement Frequency for the Oculo-Motor Indices. In: Eye Tracking Research & Applications (ETRA) Symposium, pp. 43–51. ACM, New York (2002)
20. Pan, B., Hembrooke, H.A., Gay, G.K., Granka, L.A., Fuesner, M.K., Newman, J.K.: The Determinants of Web Page Viewing Behavior: an Eye-Tracking Study. In: Proceedings of 2004 Symposium on Eye Tracking Research & Applications, pp. 147–154 (2004)
21. Peters, R.J., Itti, L.: Beyond Bottom-up: Incorporating Task-Dependent Influences into a Computational Model of Spatial Attention. In: Proceedings of IEEE Conference on Computer Vision and Pattern Recognition, pp. 1–8 (2007)
22. Hotchkiss, G., Alston, S., Edwards, G.: Eye Tracking Study (2006), http://www.enquiro.com/eyetrackingreport.asp (retrieved March 15, 2010)
23. Nielsen, J.: F-Shaped Pattern for Reading Web Content (2006), http://www.useit.com/alertbox/reading_pattern.html (retrieved March 15, 2010)
24. Gholson, B., Craig, S.D.: Promoting Constructive Activities that Support Vicarious Learning during Computer-Based Instruction. Educational Psychology Review 18, 119–138 (2006)
25. Bandura, A.: Social Learning through Imitation. In: Jones, M.R. (ed.) Nebraska Symposium of Motivation, pp. 211–269. University of Nebraska Press, Lincoln (1962)
26. Bandura, A.: Social Foundations of Thought and Action: A Social Cognitive theory. Prentice Hall, Englewood Cliffs (1986)
27. Rosenthal, R.L., Zimmerman, B.J.: Social Learning and Cognition. Academic Press, New York (1978)

28. McNamara, D.S., McDaniel, M.: Suppressing Irrelevant Information: Knowledge Activation or Inhibition? Journal of Experimental Psychology: Learning, Memory, & Cognition 30, 465–482 (2004)
29. Craig, S.D., Driscoll, D., Gholson, B.: Constructing Knowledge from Dialog in an Intelligent Tutoring System: Interactive Learning, Vicarious Learning, and Pedagogical Agents. Journal of Educational Multimedia and Hypermedia 13, 163–183 (2004)
30. Melanson, B., Kelso, J., Bowman, D.: Effects of Active Exploration and Passive Observation on Spatial Learning in a CAVE, Department of Computer Science, Virginia Tech., pp. 1–11 (2001), http://eprints.cs.vt.edu:8000/archive/00000602/ (retrieved March 15, 2010)
31. Keehner, M., Hegarty, M., Cohen, C., Khooshabeh, P., Montello, D.R.: Spatial Reasoning with External Visualizations: What Matters is What You See, not Whether You Interact. Cognitive Science 32(7), 1032–1099 (2009)
32. Hart, S.G., Staveland, L.E.: Development of a Multi-Dimensional Workload Rating Scale: Results of Empirical and Theoretical Research. In: Hancock, P.A., Meshkati, N. (eds.) Human Mental Workload, pp. 139–183. Elsevier, Amsterdam (1988)
33. Hassenzahl, M.: The interplay between beauty, goodness, and usability in interactive products. Human Computer Interaction 19, 319–349 (2004)

iPhone/iPad Human Interface Design

Martin Ebner, Christian Stickel, and Josef Kolbitsch

CIS / Dept. Social Learning
Graz University of Technology
Steyrergasse 30/I,
A-8010 Graz
martin.ebner@tugraz.at, stickel@tugraz.at,
josef.kolbitsch@tugraz.at

Abstract. In this tutorial, we will present the Human Interface Guidelines for both iPhone and iPad and offer hands-on experience in designing user interfaces for these devices. We will also discuss how to integrate the guidelines in higher education and give examples from our lecture on iPhone application development. The goal of the tutorial is to provide the participants with a basic understanding of the iPhone Human Interface Guidelines and enable them to review and design iPhone apps according to the standards.

Keywords: Usability, design, human computer interaction, mobile devices.

1 Introduction

Taking a closer look at the market of mobile devices, it can be seen that the largest growth rates can be found among mobile devices with mobile Internet connections. According to the latest AdMob Mobile Metrics report, *"the mobile Internet devices category experienced the strongest growth of the [smartphones, feature phones, mobile Internet devices], increasing to account for 17% of traffic in AdMob's network in February 2010."* [4]. Platforms for mobile phones such as Symbian, Android, and iPhone OS become increasingly popular [7]. With the special capabilities of these platforms on the one hand and the restrictions of mobile environments on the other hand, user design principles and mobile usability testing needs to be reconsidered [1], [2], [3].

New interaction and usage paradigms, for instance, on the iPhone have an impact on the way end users interact with ubiquitous devices according to [6]. Jakob Nielsen coined the current situation appropriately, *"Mobile Web 2009 = Desktop Web 1998"* [5].

2 Motivation

Considering the opportunities on, and distribution of, Apple's iPhone and iPod Touch, Graz University of Technology decided to give a lecture on iPhone development to provide students with a fundamental and comprehensive of mobile device development.

G. Leitner, M. Hitz, and A. Holzinger (Eds.): USAB 2010, LNCS 6389, pp. 489–492, 2010.

The lecturers aimed not only to teach the actual programming skills required, but also to put an emphasis on usability and user interface design principles. This was achieved by a dual approach: human computer interface guidelines were taught, and a cooperation with a secondary level design school was struck. The design school's experience was support students in user interface design.

Students implemented iPhone apps for real-world problems from two domains: business applications and educational applications. The lecturers attempted to find out if it is possible to create useful and valuable apps during a lecture series, and how innovative usability can be brought to the next generation of programmers. Based on the insights from this lecture, this tutorial will provide information on the outcome of the lecture, the teaching process, and the content taught.

3 Description of the Topic

iPhone, iPod Touch, and iPad are sophisticated mobile devices using "multi touch" technology, which enables advanced and intuitive user interactions based on gestures [10]. It is frequently said to be more intuitive than other mobile devices which results not only from the large touch screen or the flashy behavior of the elements. A key factor of this appraisal is the flat hierarchy with only one top level menu and one physical button. This single button provides an all time consistent way to the top menu. Since it's a small mobile device the interface aims to be as simple and consistent as possible. The balance between an exciting interface with intuitive interactions and practical functionality can be held account for adding an emotional appeal, which in the end might explain its success on the consumer market.

iPhone OS is the operating system running on these devices. In order to create applications for iPhone OS, developers have to use the iPhone SDK that is freely available at the Apple Developer Connection web-site. The SDK includes several tools for software development, whose most important parts are Xcode and Interface Builder. Interface Builder allows developers to design applications with an extensive library of interface objects. However, in order to create applications with the typical "look and feel" developers need to know about the recommended use of these UI elements. The iPhone Human Interface Guidelines therefore explain which kind of applications can be developed. Broken into four sections, it introduces developers to some of the concepts and paradigm shifts that they'll need to grasp before developing for the iPhone. The HIG help incorporating the key aspects of the iPhone's unique UI into development.

4 Tutorial Procedure

In this half-day tutorial, participants will be given an introduction to the fundamental human interface design principles for iPhone and iPad apps. This tutorial will help designing and reviewing iPhone and iPad apps, with a focus on the creation of an exceptional user experience. Participants are HCI practitioners, educators as well as PhD students in the field.

The tutorial will have three parts. In the first part, Apple's iPhone Human Interface Guidelines are presented and examples from the lecture on iPhone application development held at Graz University of Technology are given. In the second part, the tutorial participants will practically utilize the guidelines in a sample iPhone application, will evaluate the design of the sample interface, and come up with ideas to improve the app. The outcome of this analysis and improvement process will be discussed in the third part of the tutorial.

4.1 Guidelines

In the first part, an overview of the iPhone/iPad guidelines is given [8], and several essential parts are discussed in depth. Therefore we will share examples from the lecture "Advanced Topics of Media Technologies" in which iPhone application development is taught at Graz University of Technology. The topics in this first part will be: planning an iPhone app, user-centered design, elements of typical iPhone UIs, and design of the actual UI. Since Apple frequently applies user-centered design in software development, participants owning an iPhone, iPod Touch, or iPad are invited to think about the principles in their favorite apps and will be encouraged to demonstrate them to the fellow participants.

4.2 UI Design

The second part is a hands-on tutorial during which participants will be able to design the interface of a new iPhone app. The topic of this app will either be defined by the presenters or can cover a genuine idea raised by the participants. The sketching can be done with pen and paper on pre-printed templates or with an iPhone mockup tool (e.g., [9]). Material for the UI design phase will be provided.

The design phase will introduce the technologies particularly available on the iPhone—from multitouch to accelerometers. During this phase, also the limited resources available on mobile devices will be taken into account where appropriate—the relatively low CPU speed, a limited amount of memory, potentially slow network connections, limited screen size.

4.3 Discussion and Analysis

In the third part, the participants of the tutorial will present and discuss the results from the previous parts and evaluate the apps according to the guidelines. Furthermore a deeper insight in the teaching process is provided to give participants the possibility to plan a lecture or a workshop on their own. On request, an introduction to the administrative steps for iPhone development courses required by Apple can be given.

5 Conclusion

This tutorial will enable participants to get a detailed introduction on both the theoretical background and the practical aspects of UI design on the iPhone OS platform. With the information provided during this tutorial, participants will be able to teach UI design for iPhone and iPad, will be able to organise and administer a university-level course on this topic and will be capable of producing the required course materials.

References

[1] Kjeldskov, J., Stage, J.: New techniques for usability evaluation of mobile systems. International Journal of Human-Computer Studies 60(5-6), 599–620 (2004)

[2] Zhang, D.S., Adipat, B.: Challenges, methodologies, and issues in the usability testing of mobile applications. International Journal of Human-Computer Interaction 18(3), 293–308 (2005)

[3] Venkatesh, V., Ramesh, V., Massey, A.P.: Understanding usability in mobile commerce - Ramifications for wireless design: 'E' not equal 'M'. Communications of the ACM 46(12), 53–56 (2003)

[4] AdMob, AdMob Mobile Metrics Report (February 2010), http://metrics.admob.com/wp-content/uploads/2010/03/AdMob-Mobile-Metrics-Feb-10.pdf (last visited April 2010)

[5] Nielsen, J.: Mobile Web, = Desktop Web 1998, Alertbox, http://www.useit.com/alertbox/mobile-usability.html (last access: February 15, 2009)

[6] Weiser, M.: The computer for the twenty-first century. Scientific American 265(3), 94–104 (1991)

[7] Admob Mobile Metrics (January 2009), (report can be downloaded), http://metrics.admob.com/

[8] iPhone Human Interface Guidelines, http://developer.apple.com/iphone/library/documentation/UserExperience/Conceptual/MobileHIG/MobileHIG.pdf

[9] iPhone Mockup tool, http://iphonemockup.lkmc.ch/

[10] Apple's iPhone 3GS has 99 percent satisfaction rate, http://www.appleinsider.com/articles/09/08/14/apples_iphone_3gs_has_99_percent_satisfaction_rate.html (last visited March 2010)

On the Paradigm Shift of Search on Mobile Devices: Some Remarks on User Habits

Marcus Bloice, Markus Kreuzthaler, Klaus-Martin Simonic, and Andreas Holzinger

Institute for Medical Informatics, Medical University of Graz, Austria
{marcus.bloice,markus.kreuzthaler,
klaus.simonic,andreas.holzinger}@medunigraz.at

Abstract. This paper addresses a paradigm shift in the way the web is being searched. This shift is occurring due to the increasing percentage of search requests being made from mobile devices, changing the way users search the web. This change is occurring for two reasons: first, users of smart phones are no longer searching the web relying on generic, horizontal search engines as they do on the desktop, and second, smart phones are far more aware of the user's context than desktop machines. Smart phones typically include multiple sensors that can describe the user's current context in a very accurate way, something the standard desktop machine cannot normally do. This shift will mean changes for the information retrieval community, the developers of applications, the developers of online services, usability engineers, and the developers of search engines themselves.

1 Introduction

As device mobility, power and capability increases, and the amount of web-based information continues to rise, more and more searches are being performed by users on the move, especially in certain areas such as healthcare. This paper will discuss the implications that this usage shift will have on developers and users alike, and will investigate the ways in which search is changing from a text based, horizontal search paradigm, to a context aware, vertical search paradigm.

2 Mobile Information Retrieval

In the *Future of the Internet III* report [1] the authors claim that the mobile device will be the primary connection tool to the Internet for most people in the world by 2020. According to [2] there exists two major concepts that differentiate mobile IR from standard IR, and each comes with its typical research fields: *Context Awareness* and *Content Adaption*.

Context Awareness deals with the fact that smart embedded devices have features that can make them aware of the user's situation at any given moment. This means that time, location, social status (via a social network), and camera input, etc., can be

G. Leitner, M. Hitz, and A. Holzinger (Eds.): USAB 2010, LNCS 6389, pp. 493–496, 2010.
© Springer-Verlag Berlin Heidelberg 2010

used to shrink the search space or the space for an information need. Recent work completed by [3] involved making music recommendations based on the context from which the information retrieval process is started.

Content Adaption concerns how to visualize the results of an information need in a user friendly way, by optimizing content to suit the limited screen space on mobile devices. For example, in [4] the authors developed a block importance model to differentiate the segments of web pages in order to extract and present more condensed search results to mobile users.

Besides context awareness and adaption, mobile information retrieval systems must also make use of hardware components and device information: these include, but are not limited to, power awareness, multiple sensors and sensor fusion, computing power, and screen size.

3   Paradigm Shift and Its Impact

According to Nielsen[1], iPhone users have installed an average of 37 apps per device. For the most part these apps are games, but fewer still are apps that focus on what is known as horizontal search. Horizontal search is what is typically performed by most search engines, such as Google, Yahoo!, and Bing when a user makes a search request. Vertical search, on the other hand, is search performed on a much more focused information need. This is typically the case with mobile apps, as the context of the user's information need is already very well known, and the app itself can narrow the search space dramatically. In other words, users are focusing on apps to fulfill information needs, and are not relying on broader, more generic search engines to do this.

Other statistics show that search via traditional portals such as Google is in decline. According to comScore[2], there has been a 90% increase, in data measured over the same three month period in 2009 and 2010, in search usage through applications. It was also found that searches performed through the browser have increased by only 50%, with other areas such as social network access increasing by 90% in the same period. So while search usage is increasing rapidly on mobile devices, the usage of horizontal, web-based search engines is not increasing at the same rate. In fact, search is being accessing increasingly through apps, because apps are far better at knowing the user's context than a search field in a browser. To slow this trend, developers of search engines will need to be able to deliver more specific results depending on context, location, direction, time, and other contextual parameters.

Also of interest is the location of the search field itself within the interface design of some mobile devices. Search, while being a primary feature, may not necessarily have a primary position within interfaces, Apple's iOS being a notable example. The web search field on Apple's mobile OS occupies a secondary position within the interface, available through the browser. Google, on the other hand, and rather unsurprisingly, have not done this with their Android operating system. On Android, search has a central position on the device's "desktop". However, it remains to be seen

---

[1] http://blog.nielsen.com/nielsenwire/online_mobile/
the-state-of-mobile-apps/

[2] http://www.comscore.com/Press_Events/Press_Releases/2010/6/
Social_Networking_Ranks_as_Fastest-Growing_Mobile_Content_Category

whether users will embrace the search bar in the same way in which they have on the desktop, where almost all browsers make search a fundamental aspect of the entire user experience.

Of course, other ways of searching that do not make use of a standard text search field are being developed. Google, and others, are working hard to cater for users of mobile devices by offering products and services that are more at home on smart phones and tablets. A number of applications written by Google recently, including Google Goggles, Google Voice Search or Google Barcode Search, are typical examples of how search engine companies are making use of device components to transform information needs in new ways.

Considering the domain of medicine, Mobile IR also has the potential to alter the traditional interaction between the doctor and the hospital information system. As stated in [5] and [6] delivering content to mobile devices in an optimized way ensures increased legibility, but combining this knowledge with the enhanced context awareness of newer devices would ensure an even more tailored view of patient records for the medical professional. Health information systems developers must make their systems capable of much more than just text-based search: they must make their systems capable of taking many more parameters into account when a doctor performs a search, such as the doctor's whereabouts, to ensure more concise results are returned for a particular patient or situation.

4 Conclusion

The way in which search habits are changing on mobile devices will affect several areas of research. Information retrieval itself will be impacted greatly, as designers of such retrieval systems will have to cater for the increasing amounts of context information available to them from these new devices. This means that methods should be developed that will try to shrink the information space according to parameters supplied regarding the user's context. Developers of native applications for mobile devices must take into account the paradigm shift of search on mobile devices. They should understand that users expect applications to make full use of their context and that may not be as willing to perform horizontal searches to fulfill their information needs.

Content providers, who provide their services on the Web, must also be aware of how search is changing. They must ensure that they make available their content in such a way as to make it easy for application developers to a) have direct access to the information they provide (by providing RESTful services, for example), and b) make it easy for developers to supply the user context to the service. If content providers can allow context to be supplied along with the search term, it should be possible to return better results to the application. User interface designers must also be aware that users may not embrace the ubiquitous search field that is central to the user experience on all browsers in the same way on mobile devices. More innovative interfaces will have to be developed. Developers of applications for mobile devices will have two choices in this matter. An application could either search for content and filter the returned results according to the context of the user, or supply the user's context to the information provider along with the information need, in order to get more concise results back from the provider. In most cases it would be desirable to receive more concise results back, simply for bandwidth and speed reasons. Content providers must therefore carefully consider how they will make their information available, and consider how they will design their content APIs to allow the user context to be submitted along with the actual search request. Last, developers of search engines must make it possible for applications to be able to supply user context to the search engine as a list of parameters.

Another developing trend is the ability of web-based applications to make use of device information and user context. HTML5's *geolocation* specification allows for web-based applications to determine the location associated with device accessing the website. Future work will consider the amount of context information that web-based applications can determine in comparison to natively programmed applications. Furthermore, future work is also planned to perform usability testing, where test users will be asked to perform searches on an iPhone or similar smart phone. Their behavior will be monitored to determine whether users are more willing to use apps rather than a generic search engine when searching, if a suitable, more specific, app is also available to them. Perhaps users will only resort to searching the web directly when a suitable app is not available.

References

1. Anderson, J.Q., Rainie, L.: The Future of the Internet III,
   `http://www.pewinternet.org/Reports/2008/`
   `The-Future-of-the-Internet-III.aspx` (last access 2010-07-15)
2. Tsai, F.S., Etoh, M., Xie, X., Lee, W.C., Yang, Q.: Introduction to Mobile Information Retrieval. IEEE Intelligent Systems 25(1), 11–15 (2010)
3. Su, J.H., Yeh, H.H., Yu, P.S., Tseng, V.S.: Music Recommendations Using Content and Context Information Retrieval. IEEE Intelligent Systems 25(1), 16–26 (2010)
4. Xie, X., Miao, G., Song, R., Wen, J.R., Ma, W.Y.: Efficient Browsing of Web Search Results on Mobile Devices Based on Block Importance Model. In: Pervasive Computing and Communications, Third IEEE International Conference on Pervasive Computing and Communications, pp. 17–26 (2005)
5. Holzinger, A., Errath, M.: Mobile computer Web-application design in Medicine: some research based guidelines. Universal Access in the Information Society 6(1), 31–41 (2007)
6. Holzinger, A., Hoeller, M., Bloice, M., Urlesberger, B.: Typical Problems with developing mobile applications for health care: Some lessons learned from developing user-centered mobile applications in a hospital environment. In: Filipe, J., Marca, D.A., Shishkov, B., Sinderen, M.v. (eds.) International Conference on E-Business (ICE-B 2008), pp. 235–240. IEEE, Los Alamitos (2008)

Leveraging the Semantic Web for Intelligent and Adaptive Education

Vlado Glavinić[1], Marko Rosić[2], and Marija Zelić[2]

[1] Faculty of Electrical Engineering and Computing, University of Zagreb, Unska 3,
10000 Zagreb, Croatia
[2] Faculty of Science, University of Split, Teslina 12,
21000 Split, Croatia
vlado.glavinic@fer.hr,
{marko.rosic,marija.zelic}@pmfst.hr

Abstract. Knowledge is considered a foundation of all aspects of society and economy in general, and the need for fast, relevant and just-in-time learning is more important than ever. However, current educational systems face difficult challenges when it comes to interoperability, reusability, adaptivity, as well as knowledge sharing and management. This paper presents a novel approach to the development of educational systems based on the integration of Semantic Web technologies and the agent technology through an open e-learning architecture named SWEA. SWEA is to provide a distributed, dynamic and adaptive learning environment.

Keywords: Educational systems, Semantic Web, agent technology, adaptivity.

1 Introduction

In today's knowledge society, knowledge is considered a foundation of all aspects of society and economy in general, and the need for fast, relevant and just-in-time learning is more important than ever. In addition, the emergence of Internet and the World Wide Web has provided users with access to vast volumes of distributed data and information services. Furthermore, users with a wide variety of background, skills, interests and learning styles are using computers for quite diverse purposes. Consequently, there is a need for effective pedagogical methods and tools for finding, filtering, aggregating and presenting suitable information to users.

In order to improve the effectiveness of the learning process, educational systems have to become more intelligent and adaptive, enabling delivery of individualized, comprehensive and dynamic learning content and activities in real time. However, current systems face difficult challenges when it comes to interoperability, reusability, adaptivity, as well as knowledge sharing and management [1]. In order to address the aforementioned issues, present-day efforts attempt to combine AI techniques with the latest research and development initiatives, such as the Semantic Web [2]. Semantic Web-based educational systems are considered to be the next generation of educational systems that use Semantic Web technologies in order to provide personalized, intelligent and cost-effective learning environments [3].

G. Leitner, M. Hitz, and A. Holzinger (Eds.): USAB 2010, LNCS 6389, pp. 497–500, 2010.

This paper presents a novel approach to the development of educational systems based on the integration of Semantic Web technologies and the agent technology. We elaborate on the impact of this integration, and propose an open e-learning architecture named SWEA (Semantic Web-based E-learning Architecture). SWEA is to provide a distributed, dynamic and adaptive learning environment that can be configured on-the-fly, with intelligent agents searching, composing and invoking semantic Web services relevant for the current user and her/his learning context.

2 Semantic Web Technologies and Agent Technology

Present-day applications shift the focus from standalone computer systems to entire networks of open, distributed and dynamic systems. The agent technology is considered one of the most innovative approaches to modeling distributed software systems. Accordingly, the systems comprise autonomous and proactive components, i.e. agents, which support effective behavior in real-world, dynamic and open environments.

In addition to this highly dynamic environment, the Web keeps getting larger both in size as well as diversity. Consequently, there is a greater need to automate many tasks, such as finding, filtering and reasoning about Web resources. The Semantic Web is an initiative led by the W3C to extend the present-day Web by defining the meaning (i.e. semantics) of data and services on the Web in a way that software entities, e.g. agents, can understand and reason about them. The backbone technology of the Semantic Web are ontologies that formally specify semantic annotations.

The goal of semantic Web services is to ensure semantically rich descriptions of the services, hence enabling automation of service discovery, composition and execution. Unlike traditional Web services, semantic Web services are described by ontology-based expressions which describe the intended meaning of the service (e.g. "the service accepts an author name and returns the list of her/his books") and also enable reasoning of service capabilities. Given the fact that semantic Web services remain passive until invoked, it is safe to conclude that they depend on higher-level software entities, e.g. agents, to understand and use them.

As there is no comprehensive study on an overall e-learning architecture based on the integration of the agent technology and Semantic Web technologies, our objective is to use the aforementioned technologies so as to model a distributed, dynamic and highly adaptive learning environment. The imposed technological infrastructure inherently addresses the aforementioned issues in the development of (educational) systems. For instance, Web services offer benefits in terms of platform/vendor neutrality and ensure interoperable machine-to-machine interaction. The agent technology complements the Web service technology by providing a high-level degree of autonomy, cognitive abilities and proactive behavior. The Semantic Web acts as the underlying infrastructure, enabling agents to understand and use semantic annotations of data and services. Agents, semantic Web services and ontologies are separate components which can be deployed across the Web. Obviously, such an approach offers great possibilities in terms of system modularity, reusability and interoperability, consequently lowering the respective development costs.

3 SWEA E-Learning Architecture

The SWEA architecture can be viewed as a three-layer decomposition comprising (Fig. 1): (i) the presentation layer, (ii) the application layer, and (iii) the data layer.

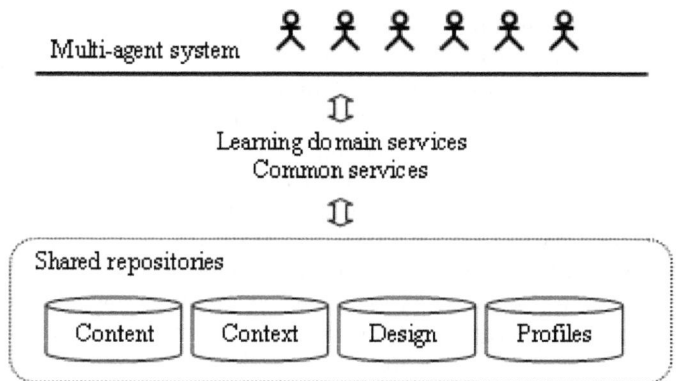

Fig. 1. SWEA e-learning architecture

The *data layer* in SWEA contains shared repositories of content, content structure, learner profiles and contextual information, along with related ontologies. Various adaptive systems are exploiting ontologies for the purpose of user modeling as well as context modeling, so as to enable adequate adaptations of the learning process. Some of the most quoted ontologies are the Dolog's learner ontology [4], CoOL (Context Ontology Language) [5], etc.

The *application layer* in SWEA consists of two sub-layers. The semantic Web services sub-layer encompasses services that retrieve and update content from the shared repositories. Our idea stems from the e-Framework for Education and research [6], an international effort to establish a service-oriented approach to the development of computer systems. SWEA puts the services defined by e-Framework (common services, learning domain services) in the Semantic Web context, hence enabling their automated discovery, composition and invocation. The agent-based sub-layer can be viewed as an application that efficiently and effectively utilizes resources from the underlying layers. Agents are to perform specialized tasks by interacting with other agents, configuring the services and managing the entire life cycle of the learning process. The agents base their operation on automated discovery and invocation of the services relevant for the current user and her/his learning context, thus providing a high-level functionality of the architecture. The basic agents in SWEA are: broker agent, course manager agent, semantic search agent, communication agent, collaboration agent, administration agent, authoring agent, profile agent, and system agents.

The *presentation layer* encompasses different agents deployed on user terminals, such as: personal agent, tracker agent, and monitoring agent. The agents provide personalized access to various functional models (e.g. learning, authoring or administration) as well as extensive local support. They are also engaged in communication, negotiation and information sharing with the agents from the application layer so as to support the user in accomplishing her/his tasks.

4   Conclusion and Future Work

Present-day educational systems face difficult issues in terms of their monolithic infra-structure, limited or no support for interoperability and reusability, as well as low level of adaptive and intelligent behavior. Recent initiatives in the development of educational systems are investigating the use of Semantic Web technologies for addressing the aforementioned issues. The Semantic Web ensures a comprehensive framework for representing data and services on the Web in such a way that computers are able to understand and reason about them. The deployment of software entities, e.g. intelligent agents, on the Semantic Web enables intelligent and adaptive system behavior that can accommodate a wide variety of users. This paper considers the latest initiatives and presents a novel approach to the development of e-learning systems through an open e-learning architecture named SWEA. SWEA is based on the integration of the agent technology and the Semantic Web. The agents, semantic Web services and data can be viewed as separate components distributed across the Web and offered in different parts of the world by different organizations and the academia. The components are configured and assembled dynamically for a specific objective, thus making SWEA highly modular. The learning experience is intelligent and adaptive because the agents base their actions on user profiles and contextual information. Our future work involves the definition of thorough specifications for each layer and the development of complex prototype systems. Each system component is to be tested in terms of performance, usability, effectiveness and user satisfaction.

Acknowledgements. This paper describes the results of research being carried out within the project 036-0361994-1995 *Universal Middleware Platform for e-Learning Systems*, as well as within the program 036-1994 *Intelligent Support for Ubiquity of e-Learning Systems*, both funded by the Ministry of Science, Education and Sports of the Republic of Croatia.

References

1. Rodrigues, M., Novais, P., Santos, M.F.: Future challenges in intelligent tutoring systems - a framework. In: Méndez-Vilas, A. (ed.) Recent Research Developments in Learning Technologies, Formatex, Badajoz, pp. 929–934 (2005)
2. The World Wide Web Consortium: W3C Semantic Web Activity (2010), http://www.w3.org/2001/sw
3. Devedžić, V.: Semantic Web and Education. Springer, Berlin (2006)
4. Dolog, P., Nejdl, W.: Challenges and Benefits of the Semantic Web for User Modelling. In: Proc. Workshop on Adaptive Hypermedia and Adaptive Web-Based Systems at the 12th International World Wide Web Conference, Budapest, pp. 1–12 (2003)
5. Strang, T., Linnhoff-Popien, C., Frank, K.: CoOL: A Context Ontology Language to enable Contextual Interoperability. In: Stefani, J.-B., Demeure, I., Hagimont, D. (eds.) DAIS 2003. LNCS, vol. 2893, pp. 236–247. Springer, Heidelberg (2003)
6. The e-Framework for Education and Research (2009), http://www.e-framework.org

Semantic Mash-Up Personal and Pervasive Learning Environments (SMupple)

Ahmet Soylu[1], Fridolin Wild[2], Felix Mödritscher[3], and Patrick De Causmaecker[1]

[1] K. U. Leuven, Department of Computer Science, CODeS, iTec, Kortrijk, Belgium
{Ahmet.Soylu,Patrick.DeCausmaecker}@kuleuven-kortrijk.be
[2] The Open University, Knowledge Media Institute, Milton Keynes, United Kingdom
f.wild@open.ac.uk
[3] Vienna University of Economics and Business, Department of Information Systems,
Vienna, Austria
felix.moedritscher@wu.ac.at

Abstract. Personal Learning Environments have emerged as a complementary, even challenging, paradigm to Adaptive Learning Systems. We consider the mash-up era as an appropriate approach for a successful realization of digital personal learning environments. However, mash-ups are also accompanied by critical technical and usability challenges. In this paper, we try to identify some of these challenges and present our solution approach which results in Semantic Mash-up Personal and Pervasive Learning Environments (SMupple).

Keywords: Personal Learning Environments, Mash-up, Ontologies, Embedded Semantics, Workflows, Pervasive Computing.

1 Introduction

Adaptive Learning Systems (ALSs), in general, focuses on automatically, often intrusively, changing the system behavior, according to the learner's needs and other characteristics and aiming at adapting the learning material and its presentation. However, it is already apparent that it is not possible to predefine adaptation rules for all different usage contexts. Furthermore, Wild and his colleagues [1] claim that adaptation technologies take away experiences from end-users (learners) thus prohibiting the development of important competences. In this respect, Personal Learning Environments (PLEs) emerge as a complementary, even challenging, paradigm to the ALSs. Wild et al [1] value learning environment as an important aspect of the learning process and consider it as an output of learning rather than a mere input. Digital learning environments can be composed of different applications, artifacts, and people etc. The individual at the centre modifies this environment through interacting with it, intending to positively influence her social, self, methodological, and professional competences and to change her potentials for future action. In other words, a learner actively or passively creates her own personal learning environment. In short, one can argue that PLEs aim at replacing the physical learning environment while ALSs focus on replacing the instructor.

G. Leitner, M. Hitz, and A. Holzinger (Eds.): USAB 2010, LNCS 6389, pp. 501–504, 2010.

Considering PLEs, learners acknowledge the abundance and variety of web applications, services and data sources to be used within their environments. Moreover, different technological devices, like mobile phones, digital media solutions, tablet PCs, intelligent household appliances, etc. are expected to be connected to the Web and serve their functionalities through embedded web servers or gateways coupled with the internal functions of available devices, possibly, with RESTful APIs [2]. This leads us to extend PLE paradigm to Personal and Pervasive Learning. Here, mash-up approaches enable users to design their ubiquitous and personal learning environments through combining functionalities and data available on the Web. However this leads to some challenges. In this paper, we identify these important challenges and present our solution approach, which builds on semantic technologies and, referring to [1], is called Semantic Mash-up Personal and Pervasive Learning Environments (SMupple).

2 Approach

We consider the mash-up paradigm to be crucial for realizing the PLE vision within the infinite space of the Web. However, before moving forward with our approach, we believe that a conceptual description of a personal learning environment and identification of basic requirements for a digital PLE shall be useful for situating important challenges. On a conceptual level, a user (learning) environment can be seen as space of entities, including people, artifacts, tools, learning objects etc., available to the learner. Each of these entities is attached with several possible activities; additionally composite activities and composite entities encompass several other entity-activity pairs and entities respectively. In that space learners derive their personal (sub-) environments, orchestrate member entities for their goals through maintaining data and interaction flows between these entities, and continuously refine the PLEs as a result of their activities and often through their own implicit formative assessment methods. A PLE can be further partitioned into disjoint or overlapping clusters with respect to varying goals of learners. Learners often shift their focus from one cluster to another according to their current goals. From this perspective, a mash-up personal and pervasive learning environment enables learners to construct their digital learning environments spanning various digital web resources and web-enabled devices encapsulated through widget like constructs.

Considering mash-ups, they can be created at client-side (i.e., at browser) or at web server-side. We identify two different types of mash-ups: (1) dashboard type (e.g., [1]), (2) box type (e.g., [3]). The former is usually created at the client-side where different applications are placed to the learner browser as widgets (all visible). Data and events can be moved from one widget to another one mainly through inter widget communication on the client, occasionally also through server-sided synchronization mechanisms. The latter mash-up type is usually created and provided by a server, combining the different applications into one single user experience (only the resulting application is visible). Data and events can be moved from one application to other application through server-sided synchronization mechanisms. The end product can also be used for developing other mash-ups of both types.

With respect to above descriptions and by considering the existing implementations [4], we identified several challenges. These challenges and our approach is described in three tiers which is partially depicted in Fig. 1.

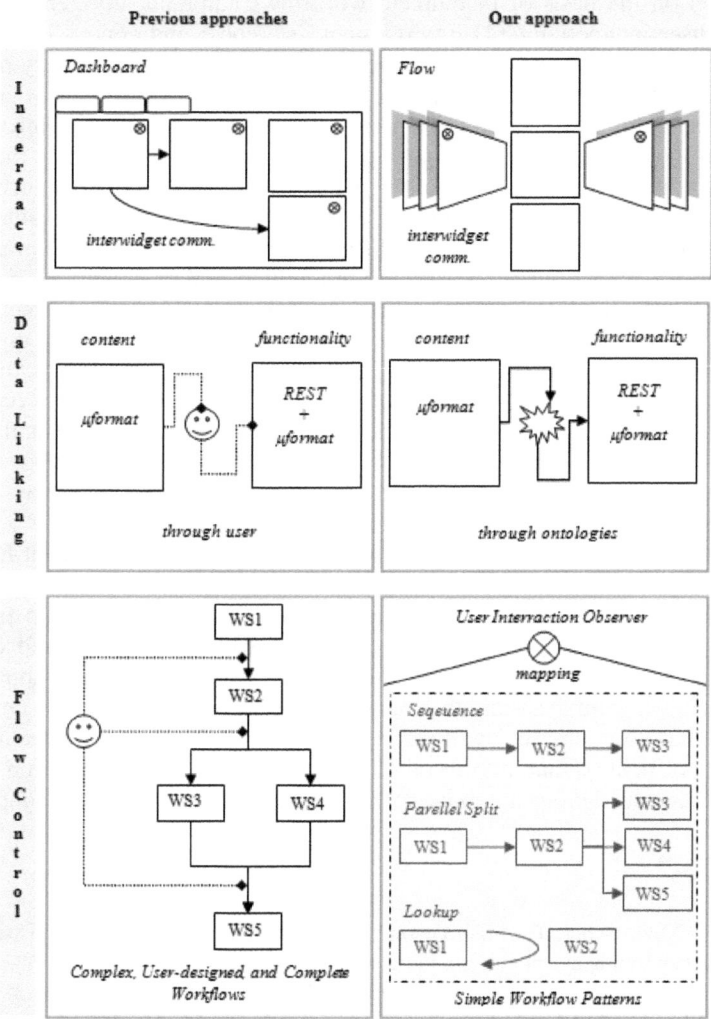

Fig. 1. Presentation and comparison of different approaches along the three tiers

Seven challenges have been identified each mapping to at least one tier: (1) composition/integration (services, applications and data), (2) inter widget communication. The first two challenges deal with data links between different applications, through server-sided synchronization or inter widget communication based on syntactic means, which is not sufficient for automated integration and composition of services leaving a huge burden to the end-user. Accordingly, injecting semantics through ontologies and embedded semantics technologies (e.g., microformats) may serve well for automated linking (e.g., [3, 5]). (3) Workflow management: this challenge is related to typical mash-up composition and requires users to define full workflows thus cognitively overloading the learner. Therefore, it is important to enable mash-up composition on the basis of incomplete workflows automatically generated through observing user interactions. (4) Environment awareness and control [6]: in physical environments users manage a limited number of entities with a relatively high awareness, however the Web offers an almost infinite amount of resources; therefore it is crucial to maintain awareness and control of one's space, so that the links between a learner and the environment stay tight. (5) Ease of orchestration: since the learner is confronted with more resources, learners should not experience a cognitive overload while managing the space. (6) Engaging learner experience: learners should feel comfortable through their experiences with PLEs. Hence identification and amalgamation of engaging and easy-to-use end-user design facilities and metaphors are required. (7) Adaptive guidance and support: this challenge is necessitated from the fact that learning process and end-user design of the environments requires adequate machine support, in terms of non-invasive adaptations, and recommendations. At this point, a formalized representation of the user's context through an ontology is promising with respect to "intelligent" guidance and end-user environment design. For the usability concerns, we approach a new type of mash-ups, a "flow" (see Fig. 1). Unlike dashboard type mash-ups, it tries to provide a reflection of the workflow among the widgets and the clustered nature of the learning environment.

We have elaborated on a scripting language and a design environment for realizing box like mash-ups addressing users ranging from experts to naïve. Our end-user tests, particularly on the interface mockup, have revealed that the mash-up paradigm is quite new, and hard to grasp for non-experts. Developing natural and easy-to-use design environments stands as a main challenge. However, apart from appropriates of design facilities, setting a smooth balance between machine and user control is required, so that users are not overloaded or not totally dominated by the machine. In that sense, we believe that automated data linking and workflow creation, as well as adaptive recommendations are more promising than strong, rule-based adaptation.

References

1. Wild, F., Mödritscher, F., Sigurdarson, S.E.: Designing for Change: Mash-Up Personal Learning Environments. eLearning Papers (9) (2008) ISSN: 1887-1542
2. Dillon, T., Talevski, A., Potdar, V., Chang, E.: Web of Things as a Framework for Ubiquitous Intelligence and Computing. In: Zhang, D., Portmann, M., Tan, A.-H., Indulska, J. (eds.) UIC 2009. LNCS, vol. 5585, pp. 1–10. Springer, Heidelberg (2009)
3. Sheth, A.P., Gomadam, K., Lathem, J.: SA-REST: Semantically Interoperable and Easier-to-Use Services and Mashups. IEEE Internet Computing 11, 91–94 (2007)
4. Taivalsaari, A.: Mashware: The future of web applications. Sun Microsystems (2009)
5. Kopecky, J., Gomadam, K., Vitvar, T.: hRESTS: An HTML Microformat for Describing RESTful Web Services. In: International Conference on Web Intelligence and Intelligent Agent Technology (WI-IAT 2008), pp. 619–625 (2008)
6. Spiekermann, S.: User Control in Ubiquitous Computing: Design Alternatives and User Acceptance. Shaker Verlag, Aachen (2008)

Model of a Touchscreen Interaction Benchmark Test Supporting Usability Awareness in Mobile Application Development Process

Vlado Glavinic[1], Sandi Ljubic[2], and Mihael Kukec[3]

[1] Faculty of Electrical Engineering and Computing, University of Zagreb,
Unska 3, HR-10000 Zagreb, Croatia
vlado.glavinic@fer.hr
[2] Faculty of Engineering, University of Rijeka,
Vukovarska 58, HR-51000 Rijeka, Croatia
sandi.ljubic@riteh.hr
[3] Polytechnic of Varazdin,
Jurja Krizanica 33, HR-42000 Varazdin, Croatia
mihael.kukec@velv.hr

Abstract. In order to create high quality and easy-to-use mobile software, the process of mobile device applications (MDAs) development must be accommodated to usability challenges. As present-day MDAs mostly target smartphones, with touchscreen ones increasingly gaining popularity, the primary focus in improving this process should include support for usability awareness at the earliest possible development phase for this class of mobile devices. In this paper we propose a model interaction benchmark test providing both quantitative and qualitative usability feedback at the elementary touchscreen action level.

Keywords: Mobile applications, mobile HCI, touchscreen interaction, usability.

1 Introduction

The nature of current mobile software development processes is intensely iterative, and within a framework environment like that, appropriate usability studies are either conducted following the deployment phase when it is usually too late, or intentionally pushed off and eventually ignored. As noted in [1], this results in usability to become only an add-on fix or upgrade, rather than the initial software product driver, thus forcing us to make usability issues an integral part of the development process.

Mobile applications are presently being developed using desktop computers and rich development tools coupled with mobile phone emulators. It is then plausible to ask oneself to what extent, by using emulators, does the experience of running and testing a mobile application correspond to its natural environment and true context of execution? In such a standard development process it is likely that certain usability issues will not come to the developer's attention. Hence, it can be claimed that some of usability problems mostly arise from the way mobile applications are being developed.

G. Leitner, M. Hitz, and A. Holzinger (Eds.): USAB 2010, LNCS 6389, pp. 505–508, 2010.

2 Mobile Applications and Usability Issues

As it is necessary to provide the ground for usability awareness early in the implementation phase, we have devised several test scenarios thus creating a suitable benchmark application. Test scenarios correspond to what we believe to be the basic factors of usability, common to all touchscreen applications: (i) optimal size of touchscreen objects, (ii) finding and selecting a particular target, (iii) feasibility of having screen objects located near the edge of the screen, (iv) touchscreen based drag-and-drop actions, and (v) activation of a sequence of closely placed GUI control commands.

2.1 Interactive Object Size and Occlusion

Interface designers and developers can ask themselves what is actually the acceptable size of an interactive object on a touchscreen device? Experimental results presented in [2] show that reducing the size of the interactive screen object from the nearly ideal 22 mm to 7.2 mm results in a negative performance impact of 25% along with a 6-7% increase in the need to correct erroneous actions thus carried out. Using experimental methods, Parham, Karlson and Bederson [3] determined the size of 9.6 mm as satisfactory for objects on a small touchscreen for discrete tasks. They state that "the error rates could not be discriminated statistically with target sizes $\geq$ 9.6 mm in discrete tasks and key sizes $\geq$ 7.7 mm in serial tasks".

A touchscreen device can be operated in two ways: either stylus or fingers. If fingers are involved, the problem arises with the occlusion of screen objects underneath the finger touching the screen [4]. Depending on screen size, users can cover a significant portion of the screen with their fingers. To understand whether an action was performed correctly, the user must consequently completely remove her/his finger from the screen surface, which hinders her/him to perform actions in a fast manner. It is certainly possible to reduce the impact of occlusion with an appropriate arrangement of interactive screen objects, but only if this issue is properly confronted with both in the design and in the development process as a whole.

2.2 Objects Near the Edge of the Screen and Drag-and-Drop Like Techniques

Interface objects that are located along the edge of the screen of the mobile device can be difficult to reach. This is especially true when the thumb of the hand holding the device is used to tap onto screen objects. It is very likely that because of the distance the user will experience difficulties reaching objects in the far corners of the device. Objects in the near corners of the screen will possibly be equally inaccessible because of the need to use some effort in bending the thumb to tap on the object.

Interaction techniques similar to drag-and-drop can be applied to a touchscreen to improve speed and accuracy of target selection [5]. Contemporary touchscreen interfaces for mobile phones combine *First contact* and *Take-off* strategies [6] in order to enable users to quickly activate the proper option. The technique is proven to be successful in case of rather big screen objects such as menu items and icons, but because of finger size it shows a poor performance when handling smaller objects. The method can be further improved by providing visual aids as a means of indirect target selection. Visual aid in form of some kind of a cursor drawn on screen is just another interactive object, and consequently all the aforementioned problems apply again: object size, occlusion and difficulties with target selection near the screen edge. Albinson and Zhai [7] have later suggested the use of *Cross-Keys* which is a form of visual aid for selecting small on-screen targets with a low error rate in object selection.

3 MDA Development Process and Usability Awareness

Testing and evaluation of MDA functionality is performed by porting the executables to a mobile device. The main disadvantages of this process is linking interface and interaction design to a smaller number of widgets since it is very unpractical to test an MDA on a variety of mobile devices, and it is literally impossible to predict or restrict the final set of devices on which it will be run. As opposed to real mobile device usage, the MDA development process can be based on the utilization of emulator platforms. When developing MDAs relying on touchscreen interaction on emulator platforms, it is obvious that the best possible way for both application testing and evaluation is to use a touch sensitive monitor. In such a working setup there is no need for porting executables on the physical device. Furthermore, various emulators can be installed within the available Interactive Development Environment (IDE), thus making possible to quickly verify both application performance and interaction characteristics on different mobile device platforms and models.

No matter which developing framework and emulator platform is being used, it is quite hard to quantitatively specify how well the user experience is supported by emulation in accordance with the respective physical mobile device. Evidently, while testing the application using emulators and touch sensitive screens, some of the eventual interaction design flaws can remain untraceable, and consequently overseen.

Problems derived from emulator-based development environments are becoming even more considerable with changing the application's context of use. To be exact, MDAs are generally designed and implemented in a nonflexible setting (similar to laboratory conditions); hence it is very demanding for developers to anticipate interaction performance of the application in all possible contexts of use, and as a result discrepancy of application usability can be expected while comparing the interaction effects in the developer's working environment and the target user's working context.

4 Conclusion and Future Work

Within our research we especially focus on touchscreen interaction based MDAs, while the central motivation factor is to enhance a touchscreen application development process by providing support for usability awareness. For this purpose, and specifically addressing the domain of touchscreen mobile devices, we are developing a benchmark test model for evaluating the respective interaction and obtaining both a quantitative and a qualitative feedback on the usability of elementary touchscreen actions.

Furthering the above work we are implementing the benchmark model, primarily focusing on improving the user interaction logging system. Additionally, we plan to apply the benchmark test prototype in real usability evaluation environments, where we are going to carry out appropriate testing within two framework setups: (i) using real touchscreen mobile devices, and (ii) interacting with device emulators on a touch sensitive monitor. With the results thus collected, we expect to get a better insight into the correlation between real devices and emulator-based touchscreen interaction effects. We will use special care in considering the correlation between usability issues and context-of-use, as evaluation within laboratory conditions may not give fully consistent results for more sophisticated context-aware mobile applications.

Acknowledgments. This paper describes the results of research being carried out within the project 036-0361994-1995 *Universal Middleware Platform for e-Learning Systems*, as well as within the program 036-1994 *Intelligent Support to Omnipresence of e-Learning Systems*, both funded by the Ministry of Science, Education and Sports of the Republic of Croatia.

References

1. Scott, K.M.: Is Usability Obsolete? ACM Interactions. XVI 3, 6–11 (2009)
2. Lee, S., Zhai, S.: The Performance of Touch Screen Soft Buttons. In: Proc. 27th Int'l Conf. Human Factors in Computing Systems (CHI 2009), pp. 309–318. ACM Press, New York (2009)
3. Parhi, P., Karlson, A.K., Bederson, B.B.: Target Size Study for One-Handed Thumb Use on Small Touchscreen Devices. In: Proc. 8th Conf. Human-computer interaction with mobile devices and services (MobileHCI 2006), pp. 203–210. ACM Press, New York (2006)
4. Roudaut, A., Hout, S., Lecolinet, E.: TapTap and MagStick: improving one-handed target acquisition on small touch-screens. In: Proc. Working Conf. Advanced Visual Interfaces (AVI 2008), pp. 146–153. ACM Press, New York (2008)
5. Roudaut, A., Lecolinet, E., Guiard, Y.: MicroRolls: expanding touch-screen input vocabulary by distinguishing rolls vs. slides of the thumb. In: Proc. 27th Int'l Conf. on Human Factors in Computing Systems (CHI 2009), pp. 927–936. ACM Press, New York (2009)
6. Potter, R.L., Weldon, L.J., Shneiderman, B.: Improving the Accuracy of Touch Screens: An Experimental Evaluation of Three Strategies. In: Proc. SIGCHI Conf. Human Factors in Computing Systems (CHI 1988), pp. 27–32. ACM Press, New York (1988)
7. Albinsson, P., Zhai, S.: High Precision Touch Screen Interaction. In: Proc. SIGCHI Conf. Human Factors in Computing Systems (CHI 2003), pp. 105–112. ACM Press, New York (2003)

Information System User Interface Complexity

Marko Rosic[1], Sasa Mladenovic[1], and Luka Borojevic[2]

[1] Faculty of Science, University of Split, Teslina 12,
21000 Split, Croatia
{Marko.Rosic,Sasa.Mladenovic}@pmfst.hr
[2] Ecsat d.o.o., Zrinsko-Frankopanska b.b.,
21000 Split, Croatia
Luka.Borojevic@ecsat.hr

Abstract. This paper examines problems and solutions related to the integration of the HCI perspective in software engineering and production. The goal is to bridge the gap between software engineers and HCI professionals by improving mutual understanding of their respective fields of interest. An information system is a complex system that can be modelled by means of the multilevel theory. The user interface design is a design problem without a single proper solution. There is no standard user interface look and feel, so that a multilevel user interface model is proposed. The user interface design is approached through hierarchical levels making it possible to choose between multiple developments methodologies. Case study: A highway automatic toll collection system user interface design proves that the multilevel approach can bridge the gap between developers and designers making team members use their respective strong points.

Keywords: HCI, software engineering, requirement elicitation, complexity, multilevel model, user interface, highway toll collection system.

1 Introduction

A system is made of any combination of interacting elements, which are themselves systems. Interacting elements can be people (a person, a group of people, organizations of people), intangible elements (methods, approaches, theories, software, processes, concepts, ideas), and tangible elements (computers, network devices, mechanical devices, sensors, vehicles) [1]. There are many definitions of complex systems [2], [3], but all agree that complex systems achieve missions, goals or functions through intricate interactions between elements. Individual elements cannot achieve the same properties therefore the whole is greater than the sum of the parts, with system properties emerging. Emergent phenomena are conceptualized as occurring on the macro level, in contrast to the micro-level components and processes out of which they arise [4]. In this paper the complexity theory is used to improve the overall software user interface in specific system integrator production environments. System integrators choose between already existing and newly developed components that are integrated into the final system at the end. Such a final system is heterogeneous, resulting in heterogeneous user interfaces.

G. Leitner, M. Hitz, and A. Holzinger (Eds.): USAB 2010, LNCS 6389, pp. 509–512, 2010.
© Springer-Verlag Berlin Heidelberg 2010

2 Information System Complexity and User Interface

Development of complex systems requires the collaboration between team members arriving from different communities. Although the team is heterogeneous, from the domain knowledge point of view, satisfying the user is the goal shared by all team members. The correctness of the user interface is essential since the interface is the point at which the system is perceived by the user [5]. Regardless of the programmer expertise, if the user interface is poorly done, the user is confused and frustrated with the system [6]. User interface implementation elements are limited by people (team members), intangible (software) and tangible (hardware) elements. In heterogeneous team engineers are focused on functionality, scalability and efficiency of the design proposed (since the programmer is responsible for the realization), while HCI professionals are more oriented toward usability and suitability of the solution proposed, looking at the functionality as a black box not knowing or caring how the system works. To team members inexperienced in the HCI field, good design can seem subjective, just a matter of personal taste[7]. Given the purpose of the product, its target market, and its desired performance specifications, the design team attempts to create a product form that will be successful [8]. Taking all mentioned above into account, design can be defined as service craft, not self-expression, in contrast to art [9]. At this point all team members have a clear understanding of both strong and weak points, which makes it possible to create a multilevel user interface model. When implementing the user interface in the real world it has to be noted that software systems that solve problems or implement computer applications in the real world are known as E-Type systems following the eight laws of software evolution [10]. User interface development is usually organized by a life cycle model describing and guiding activities from the initial idea to the final implementation and performance testing, as for example the waterfall model [11]. The problem with this approach is that the model requires correct and complete understanding of the complete user interface design project from the beginning, as correcting a mistake made in a previous phase is a difficult and expensive task. To overcome these restrictions, many new models, especially in software development, have been suggested [12], [13].

3 Case Study: Highway Automatic Toll Collection System User Interface

A highway electronic toll collection information system (ETC-IS) is defined as the technology that allows electronic tracing of toll payments regardless of payment method and user type. The task was to design the automatic toll collection payment system user interface for the customer Autocesta Rijeka-Zagreb (ARZ), to be used on the Demerje plaza. After several meetings and discussions, the common vocabulary has been defined to avoid ambiguities during meetings and brainstorming. The existing procedure for dealing with cashless payment failures has been identified and decomposed into toll collector steps. Following the information system multilevel modeling, the existing ETC-IS is represented as a hierarchical cone. The multilevel approach to user interface creation takes into account different limitations imposed by the technology and users. The low fidelity user prototype resulted in customers' request for changes in functionality, proving that the user's perception of the system is mainly related to the user interface. Instead of using a specific high fidelity user interface prototyping tool [14], like in other projects [15], the rapid application development environment has been used [16]. The breakthrough was achieved by accepting the idea of a virtual terminal proposed by the programmers' team. User interface evaluation has been conducted on the high fidelity user prototype and after reviewing all suggestions and objections, the accepted changes have been implemented in the final product user interface of the virtual toll collector terminal. Even if satisfied at the beginning, most users will be able to objectively and subjectively evaluate system user interface only after they have used the system in practice for some period so we have concluded our research by providing toll collectors with questionnaires. Questionnaire related to perceived usualness and ease of use, [17] has been provided to toll collectors using the new virtual toll collector terminal. The computer system usability questionnaire, [18], [19] gave the team a more general feedback needed for the generalization of the user interface and the concept of virtual toll collection terminal and implementation of ideas presented in other systems. Results have shown that users perceived virtual toll collection terminal as useful, easy to learn and use. They are satisfied with the system and they would recommend it to others.

4   Conclusion

In this paper, the information system user interface is recognized as a complex system. Bridging the gap between HCI experts and software engineers will result in enhancement of the overall information system perceived usefulness and ease of use which is crucial for acceptance of the new solution. By implementing the multilevel theory to both the information system and the user interface modeling, a common methodology and language is defined for these experts. The multilevel approach integrates that which is seen as purely academic and purely industrial and practical parts into a whole that is greater than the sum of its parts. The information system chosen as the study case is representative of heterogeneous systems that are used continuously throughout the year. The specific highway environment limited the user interface design choices, adding additional pressure to the team. The highway automatic toll collection system user interface has proved that the multilevel approach supports easy communication and interaction between team participants resulting in an added-value product, recognizable on the market. The virtual toll collector terminal as a product emerged from the interaction between users, user interface experts and software engineers using multilevel modeling. This proves that teams working in software production have to embrace a multidisciplinary approach to be successful in the ever demanding market. HCI is the field that has to be integrated into standard software development methodologies to allow moving up to the next level of information system products, just like what we are witnessing now in the field of the telecommunication industry.

References

1. Couture, M., Valcartier, D.: Complexity and chaos-State-of-the-art; Overview of theoretical concepts. Minister of National Defence, Canada (2007)
2. Simon, H.A.: The Sciences of the Artificial 1969. The MIT Press, Cambridge (1981)

3. Johnson, J.: Can Complexity Help Us Better Understand Risk? Risk Management-Leicester- 8, 227 (2006)
4. Goldstein, J.: Emergence as a construct: History and issues. Emergence 1, 49–72 (1999)
5. MacColl, I., Carrington, D.: User interface correctness. Crossroads 3, 9–13 (1997)
6. Bessiere, K., Ceaparu, I., Lazar, J., Robinson, J., Shneiderman, B.: Understanding Computer user frustration: Measuring and Modeling the disruption from poor designs (2003)
7. Lawson, B.: How designers think: the design process demystified. Elsevier, Amsterdam (2006)
8. Bloch, P.H.: Seeking the ideal form: Product design and consumer response. The Journal of Marketing 59, 16–29 (1995)
9. Long, J., Dowell, J.: Conceptions of the Discipline of HCI: Craft, Applied Science, and Engineering. In: People and Computers V: Proceedings of the Fifth Conference of the British Computer Society Human-Computer Interaction Specialist Group, University of Nottingham, September 5-8, p. 9. Cambridge University Press, Cambridge (1989)
10. Lehman, M.M., Ramil, J.F.: Rules and tools for software evolution planning and management. Annals of Software Engineering 11, 15–44 (2001)
11. Boehm, B.W.: Software Engineering Economics. Prentice-Hall, Englewood Cliffs (1981)
12. Gomaa, H.: The impact of rapid prototyping on specifying user requirements. ACM Sigsoft Software Engineering Notes 8, 17–27 (1983)
13. Floyd, C.: A systematic look at prototyping. Approaches to Prototyping, 1–18 (1984)
14. GUI Design and Software Prototyping Tools - Caretta Software, Caretta software (2010)
15. Mlačić, G., Mladenović, S., Mladenović, M.: Toll collection system integrator world wide expirience. In: Proceedings 29th Conference on Transportation Systems with International Participation Automation in Transportation, Zagreb-Ploče, Croatia, Sarajevo, pp. 48–51. KoREMA, Bosnia and Herzegovina (2009)
16. Ousterhout, J.K.: Scripting: Higher-level programming for the 21st century. IEEE Computer 31, 23–30 (1998)
17. Davis, F.D.: Perceived usefulness, perceived ease of use, and user acceptance of information technology. MIS Quarterly 13, 319–340 (1989)
18. Lewis, J.R.: IBM computer usability satisfaction questionnaires: psychometric evaluation and instructions for use. International Journal of Human-Computer Interaction 7, 57–78 (1995)
19. Lund, A.M.: Measuring usability with the USE questionnaire. Usability and User Experience 8 (2001)

Technical Expertise and Its Influence on the Acceptance of Future Medical Technologies: What Is Influencing What to Which Extent?

Martina Ziefle and Anne Kathrin Schaar

Human Technology Centre (Humtec)
RWTH Aachen University, Aachen
Theaterplatz 14, 52062 Aachen
{Ziefle,Schaar}@humtec.rwth-aachen.de

Abstract. In this research we examine the influence of technical expertise on future medical technology. Technical expertise is assumed to positively influence the acceptance of modern technologies, and there is evidence within the information and communication technology (ICT) sector for this. While no one would seriously dispute this basic impact of technical expertise on technology acceptance, it is far from clear what the main drivers of technical expertise are. In order to understand the complex nature of expertise on the one hand and its impact on the acceptance of other technology domains on the other, an empirical approach was undertaken. 100 participants (19–75 years) participated in a survey, in which the acceptance of a medical mobile device was explored. Outcomes show (1) that technical expertise is a highly complex construct entailing different facets (knowledge, motivational, emotional and pragmatic components), which are influenced by age and gender of respondents (2) technical expertise in the ICT domain decisively modulates acceptance of medical technology. Interestingly, a low technical expertise does not only reduce the acceptance of the pro-using arguments, but is specifically related to a high confirmation of contra-using arguments.

Keywords: Technical expertise, technical literacy, perceived technical competence, distrust in technology, technology acceptance, medical technology, ICT.

1 Introduction

One of the most important social and societal challenges already in these days, but also in the near future is the contemporaneous occurrence of three major developments: the aging of societies, the ubiquity of mobile wireless technologies and a considerable broadening of technical using contexts (context diversity) and user groups (user diversity). Old and increasingly older users will have to use technologies in many contexts, ranging from information and communication technology (ICT), over mobility services to medical technologies [1], [2]. The usage of these technologies is to a considerably lesser extent voluntary than it had been in former times; increasingly ICT usage represents a necessity for older people in order to have access to social life

G. Leitner, M. Hitz, and A. Holzinger (Eds.): USAB 2010, LNCS 6389, pp. 513–529, 2010.

and to maintain an independent living at home. Especially in Western Europe, the imbalance of generations is noticeable and we have to expect a prominent arising of this phenomenon, in combination with personal and structural societal consequences. In this context a lack of caregivers is anticipated and in the opposite a huge number of old and frail persons that are reliant on help [3], [4]. This future scenario makes it essential to think about possible solutions, which entail a complex bunch of measurements on different societal levels.

Future medical technologies in combination with mobile ICT usage might be one promising solution in this supply shortfall [5], [6]. Due to their overall availability, mobile (medical) technologies are assumed to be especially suited to maintain or even enhance older and chronically ill people's mobility, independence and safety. Also, the increasing shortage in the available caring staff- relatives, nurses, caregivers, or physicians could be relieved by mobile electronic assistance, as patients could be remotely cared. Mobile digital medical assistants could also help to minimize hospital stays, and, in so doing enable not only patients an independent life in a domestic environment, but also a relief of the threatening overcharging of sickness funds [5]. Currently, different kinds of mature and sophisticated medical assistive technologies are available to enhance older and ill peoples.

However, recent experience shows that it is not predominately the technical barrier, which hampers a successful rollout and a broad responsiveness of users. Rather, far-reaching acceptance barriers are prevalent which represent serious obstacles to technical solutions [7], [8], [9]. One major reason for this reluctant acceptance and a still negative evaluation might be due to the fact that current developments in this sector are predominately focusing on technical feasibility, inspired by technical disciplines, in combination with medical and computer science knowledge, while the "human factor" and the consideration of users' needs in these systems are fairly underdeveloped [10], [11], [12].

Still, a barrier free and broadly accepted utilization of mobile devices is supposed to happen "along the way". This attitude ignores the enormous difficulties of older users to handle technical devices properly and their hesitant technology acceptance, but also the considerable knowledge gap about the genesis of technical experience.

1.1 Acceptance of Medical Technology

Talking about the acceptance of technology in general is practiced meanwhile for about 25 years [14]. Especially the 1980ies and 1990ies, with the diffusion of computers and the Internet, pushed the subject as a prominent issue in research of different scientific disciplines (e.g. psychology, sociology, economics, anthropology, linguistics, and cultural studies). As technology cycles are increasingly faster, technology acceptance continued to be a key research issue. Technical products are only successful on the long run if users perceive them as useful and easy to use, e.g. [15], [16], [17], [18].

Though research has made significant efforts in explaining and predicting technology acceptance of ICT, the knowledge about factors, determinants and situational aspects impacting acceptance is still limited. With the increasing diversity of users (age, gender, technical generation, culture), the diversity of technical systems (visible vs. invisible, local vs. distributed) and using contexts (fun and entertainment, medical, office, mobility), more aspects are relevant for understanding users' acceptance – beyond the ease of using a system and the perceived usefulness. In addition, studies dealing with technology acceptance had been mostly considered ICT within the working context, and it is highly disputable if outcomes might be transferable to other technology and using contexts.

Furthermore, most studies are limited to technology acceptance of young, experienced and technology-prone persons - a user group whose technology acceptance patterns seem not to apply to the broad variety of users nowadays confronted with technology. Technology is no longer an issue for a small number of interested people. Nowadays the usage of technology concerns everyone, men as well as women, and not only young people but also the older ones. Also, the using conditions are different compared to former times, especially in the medical sector: here, (mobile) technology covers vital and essential parts of life, and the usage is not voluntary any more, but highly correlated with involuntariness and dependency.

Recently, research started to include the using context in combination with different technology types in their impact on technology acceptance. Increasingly it is understood that technology acceptance is neither static, nor independently from the specific using context in which a technology is applied [12], [10]. Also, the impact of user diversity and the different abilities and restrictions that influence acceptance receive attention [11]. Among the user characteristics, age and gender effects had been identified to considerably impact the technology acceptance, and, as a strong moderator, users' expertise of technology, which decisively determines the way users handle and evaluate technical devices [17], [18], [19], [20].

1.2 Technical Expertise

Computer expertise is definitively one of the most important user characteristics that influence the quality of human-computer interaction. Studies revealed that users with a high level of technical expertise show considerably higher performance when using technical devices [21], [22], [23], [24], [25], independently of the type of technology: performance advantaging expertise effects had been found for the interaction with personal computers, the Internet, as well as mobile devices (mobile and smart phones). Also, it had been found that users with higher technical expertise revealed a higher technology acceptance in terms of perceived ease of using a device and usefulness [26], [27], [28], [29], [30].

Focusing on the nature of the expertise effect it is assumed that experts in a specific domain are able to reach higher performance levels, because they possess highly organized knowledge structures, more sophisticated procedural knowledge structures, more elaborated mental models and problem solving strategies, which enable them to analyze problems thoroughly and to develop flexible solutions and alternatives [21], [24], [25], [28], [29]. Bransford et al. [31] outlined six main characteristics of expertise: First of all an expert is able to recognize attributes and important patterns of information, which cannot be seen by a novice (especially meta key patterns). Second an expert has acquired a vast proportion of content knowledge [28], [29], [32]. And this knowledge is organized in ways that make a reflected understanding of subject matter possible. Third the knowledge an expert has cannot be divided into single isolated facts. Further it is instead possible to reflect contexts of applicability. The fourth point of an expert's characteristic says, that an expert is able to demand its knowledge with little costs. But although an expert is absolutely in his topic it doesn't mean in the other way that he/she is able to teach others his/her knowledge. The last aspect of an experts characteristics is that an expert has varying levels of flexibility in his/hers approach to new situations.

Although computer expertise and its effect on performance had been studied thoroughly [21], [22], [23], [24], [25], the underlying concept of expertise and its measurement are not exactly defined yet. In most studies computer experience is determined by subjective reports of length and frequency of computer use [33], [34], [35], [36], [37]. This kind of assessment is based on the simplified assumption that expertise can be understood as a function of the time spent operating a device.

Furthermore, this conceptualization of expertise leaves open what knowledge structures are acquired while interacting with the technology and how these knowledge components constitute the nature of expertise. However, it is highly questionable that the time spent at a computer automatically leads to an acquisition of computer-relevant knowledge. Therefore, instead of defining experience by the assessment of quantitative aspects (duration and frequency) of computer usage, possibly qualitative aspects like domain-specific knowledge concepts should be assessed [33], [38].

In addition, there are more questions in the context of operationalisation of computer expertise as a main predictor of performance and acceptance of technology. Studies showed that motivational and emotional factors of human computer interaction are also involved in technical expertise [13], [16], [17]: People with a high self-confidence when using technical devices show higher levels of technical interest in general, and a lower computer anxiety. While both factors are not directly related to computer expertise, there is though an indirect relation: users with high levels of technical self-confidence and low computer anxiety levels show a considerably better performance when interacting with technical devices and the better performance is also correlated to a higher level of computer expertise.

Furthermore, across studies the measuring of "computer"- expertise referred to very different types of technical devices, different using contexts of technology as well as different generations of technology (covering a time frame from 1980 until today). It is more than questionable if technical expertise with former devices may be transferred to current devices. The expertise, which had been acquired in former times, may have a considerable short half-life. In this context the factor users' age becomes an important part. The relationship between age and technology is always to be dealt with the view on general changes in (technical-) history. It is not fully known in how far technical expertise formed by a specific former technology may be transferred to more recent technical devices. Yet, a basic transferability had been identified: It was found that computer expertise was also impacting the performance when handling mobile phones [36], [37], [38]. Beyond a basic positive effect on performance, computer expertise had also a positive effect on technology acceptance, especially on the perceived ease of using technical devices [10], [13].

However can we assume that the expertise effect, which refers to information and communication technologies, is transferable to other domains (e.g. medical technology), which might have completely different using characteristics?

Taken together: On a first sight, technical expertise is a concise construct, which is assumed to positively influence the acceptance of modern technologies. However, there is a lot of vagueness with this assumption. While no one would seriously dispute a basic impact of technical expertise on technology acceptance, it is far from clear what is the main driver of expertise: is it the increased technical literacy (declarative knowledge) of persons, which advantages the interaction with technology? It is an increased proficiency in how to handle technical devices (procedural knowledge, [28])? Or is it the perceived trust into own abilities, or the self-reported competence or even the interest in technical developments, which is mainly responsible for the advantaging effect of expertise? Furthermore, is the expertise effect limited to one technology context (e.g. ICT) or can we expect that expertise in one domain may be transferred to other domains (e.g. medical technology)?

1.3   Questions Addressed in the Present Study and Working Model

The current paper aimed for an explorative study of the different facets of technical expertise, their relation among each other and their impact on medical technology. The research model is visualized in Figure 1.

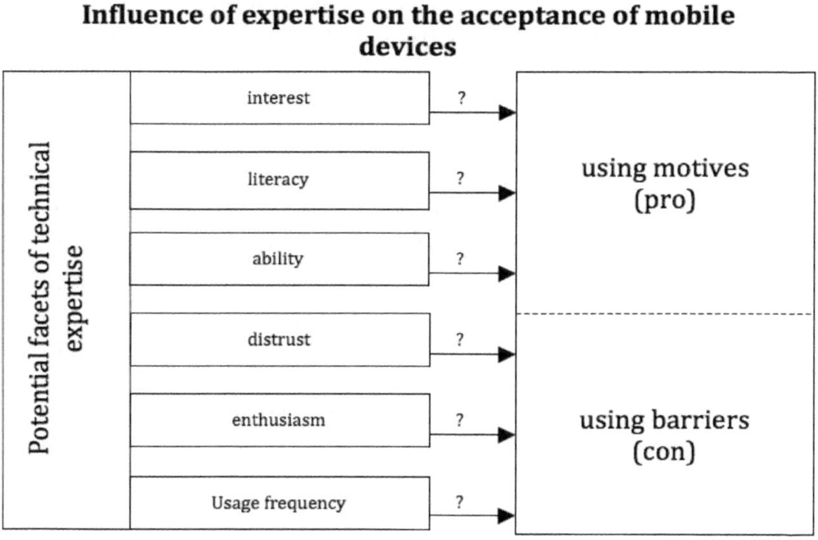

Fig. 1. Research model

Relying on the literature and the different aspects of computer expertise, which were found to be influential across studies, we measured motivational aspects (interest in technology), emotional aspects (enthusiasm when using technology, trust in technology) as well as cognitive aspects of technical expertise (self-reported technical literacy and ability when handling technical devices). Additionally, we assessed participants' reported frequency of using technical devices.

In a second step, we looked at the impact of the different expertise facets on technology acceptance of mobile medical devices. It is quite reasonable to assume that the acceptance of medical technology distinctly differs from acceptance-patterns of ICT for several reasons: First, medical devices are used not just for fun, but also because of (critical) health states [9], [10], [11]. Also, beyond its importance for patients' safety and the feeling of being safe, medical technology refers to "taboo-related" areas, which are associated with disease and illness [9]. Medical monitoring is often perceived as breaking into persons' intimacy and privacy spheres and often leads to a feeling of being permanently controlled [9], [10].

Recent studies [11], [13] showed that medical technology acceptance is a complex product out of positive and negative attitudes, which persist at the same time. Hence, both the positively connoted using motives as well as the negatively connoted using barriers should be assessed to get a complete picture. The following questions were guiding our research and data analysis:

-    Which aspects form expertise in the domain of ICT to which extent?
-    Are there inter-correlations between motivational, emotional and cognitive aspects of ICT-expertise?
-    Is ICT expertise (and if so, which facets) predictive to the acceptance of medical technology?
-    Which aspects of the acceptance of medial technology are formed by ICT expertise: The pros (using motives) or the cons (usage barriers)?

2   Method

In order to examine a large number of participants and to consider the diversity within the sample we have chosen the questionnaire method in combination with a scenario technique. Our participants were instructed into a medical scenario:

> "Imagine you came down on with diabetes mellitus and from now on forced to check your blood sugar meter several times a day. Imagine further that your medical device has the option to select the collected data via WLAN. This technical solution offers you the opportunity to collect and analyze your data easily. In addition to that you could also use the option you could send your body health parameters to your doctors, without being forced to bring them personally".

2.1   Variables

As independent variables different aspects of technical expertise were selected.

-   *Interest in technology* and *technology enthusiasm* as motivational components
-   *Technical literacy* and *perceived ability when handling technical devices* as cognitive components and
-   *Distrust in technology* as an emotional component.

Dependent variable was the acceptance for medical technology, operationalized by five pro and con statements, each. The statements reflected arguments collected in focus groups (prior to the questionnaire study), and covered different aspects of the usage of medical technology, including safety, reliability, ease of use issues as well social and financial aspects (items are described in detail in section 2.2.).

2.2 Questionnaire-Instrument

The questionnaire was arranged in four main sections: The first part included demographic data concerning gender, age, and educational level. The second section of the questionnaire inquires information about the technical expertise of the participants and attitude towards technology. First we asked for the frequency of using technology in a private or in a job related context. On a five-point scale the participants had to evaluate their frequency (1 = very little to 5 = very often). In this context we also asked for information about the possession of different devices (ICT and medical technology), the frequency of usage and the ease of use. Additionally participants rated the general attitudes toward technology (Table 1).

Table 1. Components of technical expertise (1 = very low to 6 =very high)

Interest for Technology...
My technical interest is…
My enthusiasm for technology is…
My technical literacy is…
My ability in dealing with technology is…
My distrust against technology is…

The third section of the questionnaire was concerned with the technology acceptance for a medical device, including both, "pro" using motives (Table 2) as well as "cons", i.e. usage barriers (Table 3).

Table 2. Pro Items for medical device(1 = complete confirmation to 6 complete rejection)

The following arguments might supporting the usage of the device...
I feel save, when a medical devices controls my body functions constantly.
I am sure that the most innovative devices are solid.
I want an easy instruction manual.
I expect a positive feedback of my social surrounding.
I would use the device, if the sickness funds pay for them.

Table 3. Con items (1 = complete confirmation to 6 = complete rejection)

The following arguments might hinder the usage of the device...
I feel observed, when a medical devices permanently documents my body functions.
I fear that a new medical device is not matured.
I am afraid, that the new devices are not easy to use.
I fear that my surrounding doesn't support my technical device
I fear that the devices would be expensive.

2.3 Participants

The intention in the recruitment procedure was to survey users of a wide age range and health status in order to explore and to compare their motives and barriers about future healthcare solutions.

A total of 100 participants between 19 and 75 years volunteered to take part in the study. The purpose in the recruitment procedure was to survey users of a wide age range in order to compare their motives and barriers about future healthcare solutions. For younger participants (N = 49), ranging between 19 and 30 years of age, 65.3% were females, 34.7% male. Regarding the middle-aged group (31 to 55 years of age, N = 35), 62.9% were female and, 37.1% male. Finally, for the older participants (N = 29), between 56 to 75 years of age, 57.5% was female and 42.5% was male. Participants were reached through the authors' social network and corresponded to notices posted on campus and in public places of the city. The educational level of our participants was rather high. 59% (N = 59) declared to have an academic degree. 24% (N = 24) have at least the A-school level. Regarding the health condition, 45% of our sample reported to be healthy. 33% had one or two chronic illnesses and 22% were affected by comorbidity[1].

3   Results

Outcomes were analyzed by ANOVA procedures and Spearman rank correlations. First, we analyzed the independent variables regarding their influence on technical expertise. Then, we examine whether there is a direct influence of technical expertise on the evaluation of the smart devices - blood sugar meter.

3.1   Aspects of Technical Expertise

Before we look at the inter-correlations of the different aspects of expertise, we descriptively analyzed the different aspects of expertise, in order to learn the degree of each of the aspects as well as the distribution within the sample. Outcomes are visualized in Figure 2 and 3.

As can be seen from Figure 2, the motivational aspects of expertise, interest in and enthusiasm for technology showed similar patterns. Only few persons reported to have very low and low interest/enthusiasms for technical issues. The majority (about 70%) ranked themselves with 3, 4 or 5 points out of 6 points possible.

Regarding the distrust, we see a "perfect" distribution (normal distribution): more than 40% reported to have a medium degree of distrust in technology in general.

Regarding the cognitive components of technical expertise (Figure 3) - the reported literacy and the handling competence – we also found quite similar patterns. While only few participants stated to have a "very low" declarative (technical literacy) and procedural knowledge (handling competence), about 80 % of participants ranked their literacy and handling competence with 3, 4 and 5 ("high") points out of 6 ("very high") points possible.

---

[1] Presence of one or more diseases in addition to a primary disease.

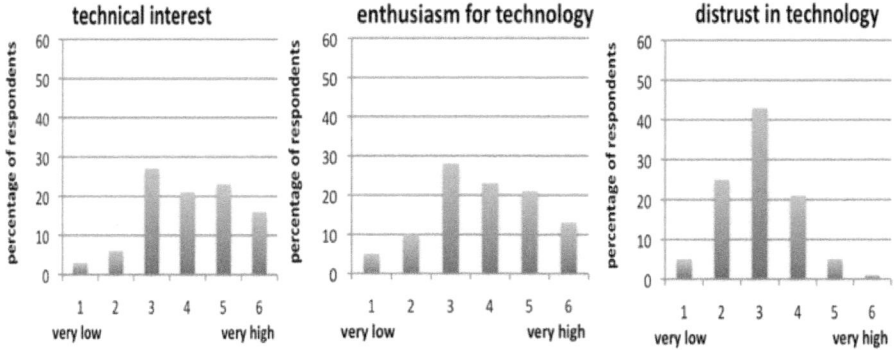

Fig. 2. Descriptive outcomes in different expertise facets: left: interest in technology; center: enthusiasm for technology; right: distrust in technology (N = 100)

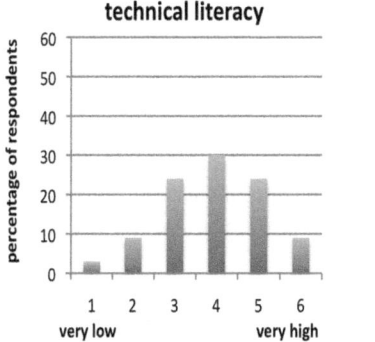 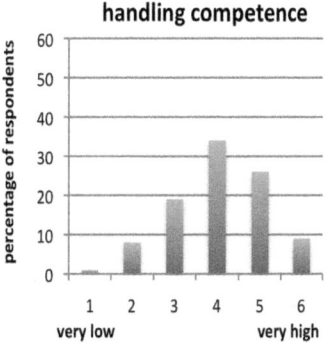

Fig. 3. Descriptive outcomes in different expertise facets: left: technical literacy; right: reported competence when handling technical devices; (N = 100)

In a second step, we looked at the relations between and across the single components. According to correlation outcomes, all expertise facets revealed high intercorrelations. Figure 4 illustrates the statistic connections between the relevant items, revealing that cognitive, emotional and motivation aspects do significantly contribute to the concept of technical expertise.

In order to reduce the number of factors for further analysing of the relation between expertise and acceptance of medical technology, we selected one motivational, two cognitive aspects and one emotional aspect of expertise: Interest in technology, technical literacy, ability (handling competence) and the perceived distrust in technology.

As in many studies technical expertise had been determined by reports of length and frequency of computer/device use, we now analyze whether the simplified assumption that expertise can be understood as a function of the time spent operating the device, can be validated. We asked for the possession and the usage frequency of

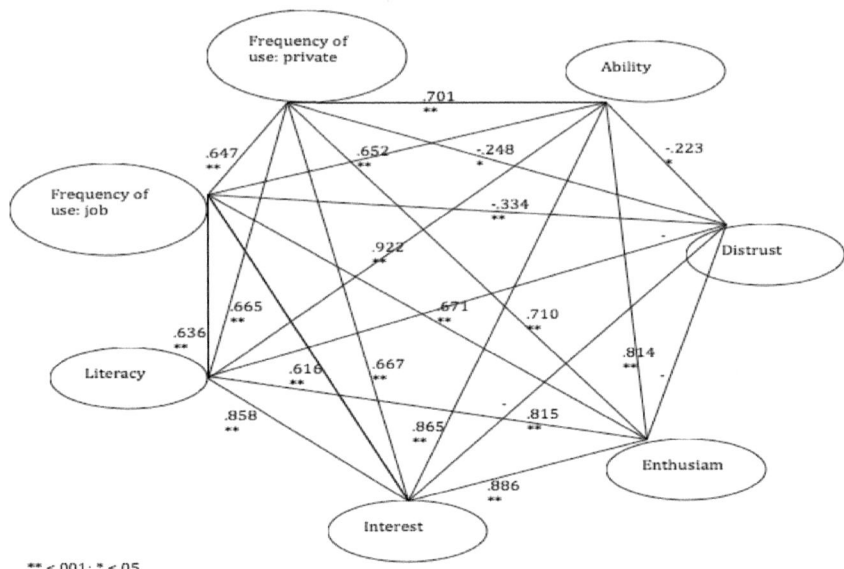

Fig. 4. Inter-correlations between expertise aspects. Device usage refers to a mobile phone.

ICT (PC, mobile phone, fax, digital camera) and medical devices (blood pressure / sugar meter, hearing aid, pulse watch), as well as the reported ease of use (Table 4).

Table 4. Correlations (Ease of use, frequency of device usage and technical expertise)

Expertise Items	Ownership	Evaluation: Ease of use		Frequency of using	
			Correlation coefficient significance		Correlation coefficient significance
		computer	-.711	.000	.211	.04
Reported Interest	ns	mobile phone	-.468	.000	.267	.009
		camera	-.409	.000	.324	.002
		computer	-.692	.000	.175	.084
Reported Literacy	ns	mobile phone	-.494	.000	.292	.004
		camera	-.364	.000	.284	.006
		computer	-.748	.000	.248	.015
Reported Ability	ns	Mobile phone	-.520	.000	.262	.010
		camera	-.394	.000	.331	.002
		computer	.278	.005	-.278	.005
Reported Distrust	ns	mobile phone	.259	.010	-.224	.027
		camera	.217	.037	-	-

For the ownership, no significant relations to neither of the expertise aspects were found. Also, the usage frequency of medical devices did not reveal statistically significant relations to the extent of technical expertise.

Though, regarding some ICT devices (PC, mobile phone, and digital camera), significant correlations between expertise and ease of use ratings and well as frequency of usage were found. Thus, we can conclude that for common ICT devices, frequency of usage and ease of use ratings show a basic interrelation to the technical expertise, operationalized as interest in technology, literacy in technology, handling competence when using technical devices, and distrust in technology

Another meaningful finding in this context is that expertise components are highly correlated to gender, and less pronounced to age. Regarding age, we only found one relation: with increasing age, the distrust in technology raises ($r = .23$; $p < .05$). In contrast, gender showed to be highly connected to expertise components. Women report to have a lower interest in technology ($r = .43$; $p < .05$; a lower self-reported handling competence ($r = .58$; $p < .05$) and also a lower self-reported technical literacy ($r = .52$; $p < .05$) in contrast to male respondents. Interestingly, the level of distrust is not different between both gender groups.

In the following, we now focus on the influence the technical expertise aspects on the acceptance of medical technology, taking a blood sugar meter as an example, thus an external mobile device, which may have similar attributes than the mobile phone.

3.2 Technical Expertise and Its' Influence on the Acceptance of Medical Technology

In order to learn something about the influence of the technological expertise and its influence on the acceptance of future medical technology we picked the following items to prove whether they have an influence on the evaluation of the pro or con arguments: reported interest (motivational component), reported literacy (cognitive component), reported ability/handling competence (cognitive component), and distrust (emotional component). Each of the expertise components was dichotomized by the median in a "high" and a "low group" (e.g. high interest, low interest).

In a first step, we looked at the main effects (ANOVA procedures) of expertise aspects on the acceptance of medical technology, separated for the pros and the con items Secondly we analyzed the influence of the expertise components on the single items of the pro using arguments and the using barriers (using Spearman rank correlations).

Main effects of expertise facets on the medical device blood sugar meter

First of all, the pro-using arguments are focussed at. While the ANVOA revealed no significant effect for the interest in technology, the technical literacy and the handling competence, the distrust in technology ($F (5,92) = 3$; $p < .05$) revealed to be a main driver for the pro-using motivation of medical technology. When looking at the usage barriers, the interest in technology was significantly impacting the using barriers of medical technology ($F (5,88) = 2.4$; $p = .05$), the technical handling competence ($F (5,98) = 4.9$; $p < .05$) as well as the distrust ($F (5,92) = 5.1$; $p < 0.05$) significantly influenced the negative connoted acceptance of medical technology. Comprising statistical analyses, the more distrust in technology persons report, the lower is their pro-using motivation and the higher their reluctance if not refusal to use medical technology if necessary. Beyond the distrust in technology, which was found to impact both, the pros and the cons, the reported competence in handling technical devices and the interest in technology was influencing exclusively the using barriers, thus the reluctance of using medical technology. The lower the interest in technology and the lower the self-reported handling competence with ICT technology, the higher is the unwillingness to accept medical technology.

Influence of expertise facets on the pro and con items in detail

So far, we considered all pro-using items and all con-using items as a total score. As it might be insightful to get a deeper insight into the relative extent of (dis-) agreement for the specific pros and cons, we used correlation analyses to find out the relative relation between expertise components and the single items with the expertise components. As can be seen from Figure 5, for the pro items there are only two statistically significant relations between the expertise component *distrust in technology* on the one hand and the pro-using argument *"I feel save if a device checks my vital values constantly"* and the pro-using argument *"I would use the device if the sickness fund pays for it"* on the other hand. Apparently, for persons having high distrust levels, there are two arguments which militate in favour of using the medical device: the public sickness funds pay for it, which could be interpreted by high distrust persons that the reliability in the devices is high and that they are constantly informed about their own health status and vital parameters, respectively.

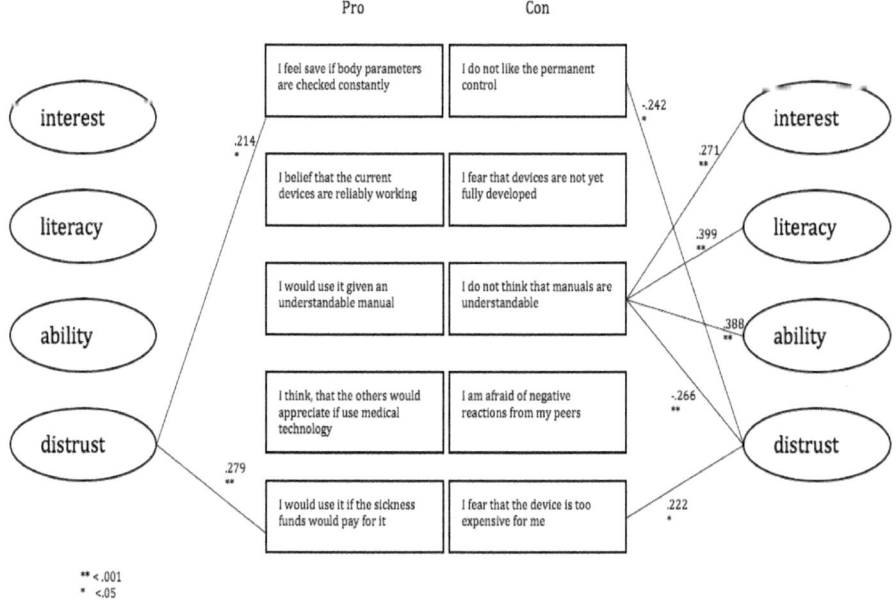

Fig. 5. Intercorrelations between pros (left) and cons (right) and expertise components

When looking at the usage barriers (right side in Figure 5), all facets of expertise showed significant correlations. Thus it can be concluded that participants with high levels of distrust, low levels of technical interest, technical literacy, and a low self-reported handling competence when using ICT technologies tend to refuse the usage of medical technology and to overestimate the negative aspects in contrast to the positive using argumentations.

4 Discussion and Suggestions for Future Research

The aim of the present study was to analyze the impact of expertise on the acceptance of medical technology, taking a mobile blood sugar device as an example. The following questions were guiding our research: (1) Is ICT expertise (and if so, which facets) predictive to the acceptance of medical technology? (2) Are there inter-correlations between motivational, emotional and cognitive aspects of ICT-expertise? (3) Which aspects of the acceptance of medial technology are formed by ICT expertise: The pros (using motives) or the cons (usage barriers)?

Before findings of the research are discussed within implications for research, application and future research demands, it should be noted that the topic "acceptability of medical technology" is highly sensitive. People asked to participate in this research showed a high interest for the topic and a high willingness to participate, independently of generation and gender. Apparently, a high public awareness for the societal needs of medical technology is present as well as a high motivation to express own opinions and fears connected to its usage. On the basis of the results we now can answer the research questions:

(1) On the one hand we now can clearly say that technical expertise, operationalized by four components - interest in technology, technical literacy, handling competence and distrust in technology in general- is in fact impacting the acceptance of medical technology. The higher the technical expertise the higher is the acceptance of medical technology and the higher the intention to use the medical device. Apparently, there is a basic transferability of the positive expertise effect from one domain (information and communication technology to another quite different domain: medical technology.

(2) When asking which of the facets of expertise, the cognitive, the emotional and the motivational part, we now can say that the emotional part (distrust in technology) is the strongest player for both, the pro-usage and the contra-usage motivation of medical technology. Beyond the emotional component, also cognitive and motivational factors) play also a role, especially in the unwillingness to accept medical technology. This findings lead to the final point, which is the most important one in our perspective.

(3) Expertise, especially the missing or low technical expertise, is nearly exclusively related to the high confirmation of using barriers and the not-acceptance of medical technology. Conversely, the pro-using arguments and the positive expectations when using medical technology nearly play no role for persons with a low extent of technical expertise. From this it can be derived that it is not specifically the acceptance of medical technology, which is problematic. Rather, the low technical expertise with ICT technology and the low self-confidence of persons when

interacting with common ICT devices acts as a general brake which is then transferred to the medical technology application context.

Even though this study revealed detailed insights into differential components and effects of technical expertise on the acceptance of a medical mobile device, still there are many duties for future research:

Other technology contexts: This study mainly concentrated on one medical technology, a mobile external device (blood sugar meter). This was selected because many people - though not chronically ill - know diabetes as a quite popular disease as well as the disease's handling by means of a blood sugar device and therefore should have sufficient shared knowledge and experience. However, future studies will have to concentrate on other forms of mobile technology, which are not that prominent yet. Currently, mature medical technical solutions cover smart artifacts, a promising context for medical technology, as all-day objects equipped with special functions like sensors, memory and communications skills and are assumed to be appropriate in disease handling (e.g., Smart Sofa [39], Smart Pillow [40] and Smart Dishes [41]). Another technological context regards 'wearable computing', that makes the computer to an integral part of everyday clothing [42]. Future studies will have to study technology acceptance for this new forms of medical technology.

User diversity: Another research duty regards user diversity, beyond technical expertise. In this study we did not differentiate in a detailed way whether other user characteristics may affect acceptance outcomes. This, however, is of prominent interest considering the complexity of personal and individual factors, which might impact acceptance of technology. As opposed to the past, when mostly sophisticated and technology prone professionals were the typical end-users of technical products, now broader user groups have access to technology. Still, the development of technology in general seems to be limited to dominantly young, technology experienced, Western, middle- and upper class males [43], [44]. Although the vital importance of ensuring that a technology produced is both usable and acceptable for a diverse user group is known in the meanwhile, the recognition of the importance of users' diversity is only slowly influencing mainstream usability studies and not yet considered within the development of technical products. Design approaches thus have to undergo a radical change taking current societal trends into account, which have considerable impact for the inclusion of a diverse user group.

Thus, it is a central claim that mobile displays are designed to be in line with older users' specificity and diversity [45]. Design approaches should therefore take the user-perspective seriously. The duty of further research efforts is to fill the knowledge gap, and to systematically integrate user diversity—age, gender, social and cultural factors—into usability approaches.

Self-reported technical expertise vs. factual expertise: It should be kept in mind that the expertise-aspects, which were assessed in this research, are exclusively subjective and represented users' judgments about own abilities and attitudes. Users taking part in this study evaluated their own technical interest, literacy, their competencies when handling technical devices as well as their distrust in technology. However, so far, we do not have an external validation of the respective high or lower expertise levels. In addition, the real expertise level of participants should be determined by a psychometric testing procedure [33].

Acknowledgements

Authors would like to thank all respondents having taken the time to patiently fill in the questionnaire, to vividly discuss the sensitive topic with us and openly share their perspectives. In addition we thank Christina Vedar for her research support.

This research had been funded by the Excellence Initiative of the German federal and state governments.

References

1. Leonhardt, S.: Personal Healthcare Devices. In: Mukherjee, S., et al. (eds.) Malware: Hardware Technology Drivers of Ambient Intelligence, pp. 349–370. Springer, Dordrecht (2006)
2. Ziefle, M., Röcker, C.: Acceptance of Pervasive Healthcare Systems: A comparison of different implementation concepts. In: Workshop User-Centred-Design of Pervasive Health Applications (UCD-PH 2010). 4th ICST Conference on Pervasive Computing Technologies for Healthcare 2010 (2010)
3. Wittenberg, R., Malley, J., Comas-Herrera, A., Fernandez, J.L., King, D., Snell, T., Pickard, L.: Future Demand for Social Care, 2005 to 2041: Projections of Demand for Social Care and Disability Benefits for Younger Adults in England, Report to the Strategy Unit (Cabinet Office) and the Department of Health, PSSRU Discussion paper 2512, Personal Social Services Research Unit, London (2008)
4. Wittenberg, R., Comas-Herrera, A., Pickard, L., Hancock, R.: Future Demand for Long-Term Care in England. PSSRU Research Summary (2006)
5. Weiner, M., Callahan, C.M., Tierney, W.M., Overhage, M., Mamlin, B., Dexter, A.: Using Information Technology To Improve the Health Care of Older Adults. Ann. Intern. Med. 139, 430–436 (2003)
6. Schmitt, J.M.: Innovative medical technologies help ensure improved patient care and cost-effectiveness. International Journal of Medical Marketing 2(2), 174–178 (2002)
7. Bohn, J., Coroama, V., Langheinrich, M., Mattern, F., Rohs, M.: Social, Economic, and Ethical Implications of Ambient Intelligence and Ubiquitous Computing. In: Weber, W., Rabaey, J., Aarts, E. (eds.) Ambient Intelligence, pp. 5–29. Springer, Heidelberg (2005)
8. Ziefle, M., Röcker, C., Wilkowska, W., Kasugai, K., Klack, L., Möllering, C., Beul, S.: A Multi-Disciplinary Approach to Ambient Assisted Living. In: Röcker, C., Ziefle, M. (eds.) E-Health, Assistive Technologies and Applications for Assisted Living: Challenges and Solutions. IGI Global, Hershey (2010)
9. Ziefle, M., Schaar, A.K.: Gender differences in attitudes towards invasive medical technology. Electronic Journal of Health Informatics (2010, in press)
10. Ziefle, M., Wilkowska, W.: Technology acceptability for medical assistance. Full Paper at the 4th ICST Conference on Pervasive Computing Technologies for Healthcare 2010 (2010)
11. Gaul, S., Ziefle, M.: Smart Home Technologies: Insights into Generation-Specific Acceptance Motives. In: Holzinger, A., Miesenberger, K. (eds.) USAB 2009. LNCS, vol. 5889, pp. 312–332. Springer, Heidelberg (2009)
12. Arning, K., Ziefle, M.: Comparing apples and oranges? Exploring users' acceptance of ICT- and eHealth-applications. In: Proceedings of the International Conference on Healthcare Systems, Ergonomics and Patient Safety, Straßbourg, France [CD-ROM] (2008)

13. Wilkowska, W., Ziefle, M.: Which factors form older adults' acceptance of mobile information and communication technologies? In: Holzinger, A., Miesenberger, K. (eds.) USAB 2009. LNCS, vol. 5889, pp. 81–101. Springer, Heidelberg (2009)
14. Davis, F.D.: Perceived usefulness, perceived ease of use, and user acceptance of informarion technology. MIS Quaterly 13, 319–334 (1998)
15. Brosnan, M.J.: The impact of computer anxiety and self-efficacy upon performance. Journal of Computer Assisted Learning 14, 223–234 (1998)
16. Busch, T.: Gender differences in self-efficacy and attitudes toward computers. Journal of Educational Computing Research 12, 147–158 (1995)
17. Ziefle, M., Bay, S.: Transgenerational Designs in Mobile Technology. In: Lumsden, J. (ed.) Handbook of Research on User Interface Design and Evaluation for Mobile Technology, pp. 122–140. IGI Global, Hershey (2008)
18. Arning, K., Ziefle, M.: Different Perspectives on Technology Acceptance: The Role of Technology Type and Age. In: Holzinger, A., Miesenberger, K. (eds.) USAB 2009. LNCS, vol. 5889, pp. 20–41. Springer, Heidelberg (2009)
19. Vicente, K.J., Hayes, B.C., Williges, R.C.: Assaying and isolating individual difference in searching a hierarchical file system. Human Factors 29, 349–359 (1987)
20. Westerman, S.J.: Individual differences in the use of command line and menu computer interfaces. International Journal for Human Computer Interaction 9, 183–198 (1995)
21. Chi, R., Glaser, R., Farr, M.J.: The Nature of Expertise. Lawrence Erlbaum, Hillsdale (1988)
22. Downing, R.W., Moore, J.L., Brown, S.W.: The effects and interaction of spatial visualization and domain expertise on information seeking. Computers in Human Behaviour 21, 195–209 (2005)
23. Mayer, R.E.: From novice to expert. In: Helander, M.G., Landauer, T.K., Prabhu, P. (eds.) Handbook of Human Computer Interaction, pp. 781–795. Elsevier, Amsterdam (1997)
24. Ye, N., Salvendy, G.: Quantitative and qualitative differences between experts and ices in chunking computer software knowledge. International Journal of Human Computer Interaction 6, 105–118 (1994)
25. Chi, M.T.H., Feltovich, P.J., Glaser, R.: Categorization and representation of physics problems by experts and novices. Cognitive Science 5, 121–152 (1981)
26. Arning, K., Ziefle, M.: Understanding differences in PDA acceptance and performance. Computers in Human Behaviour 23(6), 2904–2927 (2007)
27. Arning, K., Ziefle, M.: Ask and you will receive: Training older adults to use a PDA in an active learning environment. International Journal of Mobile Human-Computer Interaction 2(1), 21–47 (2010)
28. Harvey, L., Anderson, J.: Transfer of declarative knowledge in complex information processing domains. Human Computer Interaction 11(1), 69–96 (1996)
29. Kent, P., Vaubel, R., Gettys, C.F.: Inferring User Expertise for Adaptive Interfaces. Journal Human-Computer Interaction 5(1), 95–117 (1990)
30. Hanisch, K., Kramer, A., Hulin, C.: Cognitive representations, control, and understanding of complex systems: a field study focusing on components of users' mental models and expert/novice differences. Ergonomics 34(8), 1129–1145 (1991)
31. Bransford, J.D., Brow, A.L., Cocking, R.R.: How People Learn: Brain, Mind Experience and School. National Academy Press, Washington (1999)
32. Dunphy, B.C., Williamson, S.L.: Pursuit of expertise. Towards an Educational Model for Expertise Development. Advances in Health Sciences Education 9, 107–127 (2004)

33. Arning, K., Ziefle, M.: Assessing computer experience in older adults: Development and validation of a computer expertise questionnaire for older adults. Behaviour and Information Technology 27(1), 89–93 (2008)
34. Potosky, D., Bobko, P.: The Computer Understanding and Experience Scale: a self-report measure of computer experience. Computers in Human Behavior 14(2), 337–348 (1998)
35. Vu, K.-P., Hanley, G., Strybel, T., Proctor, R.W.: Metacognitive Processes in Human-Computer Interaction: Self-Assessments of Knowledge as Predictors of Computer Expertise. International Journal of Human-Computer Interaction 12(1), 43–71 (2000)
36. Arning, K., Ziefle, M.: Effects of cognitive and personal factors on PDA menu navigation performance. Behaviour and Information Technology 28(3), 251–268 (2009)
37. Ziefle, M.: The influence of user expertise and phone complexity on performance, ease of use and learnability of different mobile phones. Behaviour and Information Technology 21(5), 303–311 (2002)
38. Ziefle, M., Schroeder, U., Strenk, J., Michel, T.: How young and older users master the use of hyperlinks in small screen devices. In: Proceedings of the SIGCHI Conference on Human Factors in Computing Systems 2007, pp. 307–316. ACM, New York (2007)
39. Legon, J.: 'Smart Sofa' Aimed at Couch Potatoes (2003), http://www.cnn.com/2003/TECH/ptech/09/22/smart.Sofa/index.html2003
40. Ferguson, G.T.: Have your objects Call My Objects. Havard Business Review 80(6), 138–143 (2003)
41. Cook, D.J., Das, S.K.: How Smart are our Environments? An UpdateLook at the State of the Art. Journal of Pervasive and Mobile Computing 3(2), 53–73 (2007)
42. Horter, H., Linti, C., Loy, S., Planck, H., Kotterba, B., Günther, U.: Health Wear – Sensorische Textilien zur Erfassung von Vitalparametern. In: Proceedings of the Second German Congress on Ambient Assisted Living (AAL 2009), January 27-28. VDE, Berlin (2009) (CD ROM)
43. Asada, H.H., Shaltis, P., Reisner, A., Rhee, S., Hutchinson, R.C.: Mobile Monitoring with Wearable Photoplethysmographic Sensors. IEEE Engineering in Medical and Biology Magazine 22(3), 28–40 (2003)
44. Choong, Y.Y., Salvendy, G.: Implications for Design of Computer Interfaces for Chinese Users in Mainland China. International Journal of Human-Computer Interaction 11(1), 29–46 (1999)
45. Ziefle, M., Jakobs, E.-M.: New challenges in Human Computer Interaction: Strategic Directions and Interdisciplinary Trends. In: 4th International Conference on Competitive Manufacturing Technologies, South Africa, University of Stellenbosch, pp. 389–398 (2010)

Author Index